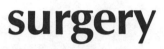

# surgery

The National Medical Series for Independent Study

# surgery

EDITORS

**Bruce E. Jarrell, M.D.**

*Associate Professor of Surgery*
*Jefferson Medical College*
*Thomas Jefferson University*
*Attending Surgeon*
*Thomas Jefferson University Hospital*
*Philadelphia, Pennsylvania*

**R. Anthony Carabasi, III, M.D.**

*Associate Professor of Surgery*
*Jefferson Medical College*
*Thomas Jefferson University*
*Attending Surgeon*
*Thomas Jefferson University Hospital*
*Philadelphia, Pennsylvania*

A WILEY MEDICAL PUBLICATION
**JOHN WILEY & SONS**
New York • Chichester • Brisbane • Toronto • Singapore

*Harwal Publishing Company, Media, Pennsylvania*

**Library of Congress Cataloging in Publication Data**
Main entry under title:

Surgery.

(The National medical series for independent study)
(A Wiley medical publication)
    Includes index.
    1. Surgery—Examinations, questions, etc.
2. Surgery—Outlines, syllabi, etc.   I. Jarrell, Bruce E.
II. Carabasi, R. Anthony.   III. Series.   IV. Series:
Wiley medical publication.   [DNLM: 1. Surgery—
examination questions.   2. Surgery—outlines.
WO 18 S9583]
RD37.2.S96   1986      617′.0076        85-26501
ISBN 0-471-82342-2

©1986 by Harwal Publishing Company, Media, Pennsylvania

10 9 8 7 6 5 4 3

# Dedication

We would like to dedicate this book to our wives, Leslie S. Robinson, M.D., and Jane Marko Carabasi, B.S.N., M.S., R.N. The many hours that we devoted were hours that obviously came from their time. Without their support and understanding, this effort would surely have failed.

# Contents

# Contributors

**Demetrius H. Bagley, M.D.**
Associate Professor of Urology and
    Radiology
Jefferson Medical College
Thomas Jefferson University
Attending Urologic Surgeon
Thomas Jefferson University Hospital
Philadelphia, Pennsylvania

**Bikash Bose, M.D.**
Instructor in Neurosurgery
Jefferson Medical College
Thomas Jefferson University
Philadelphia, Pennsylvania
Attending Neurosurgeon
Medical Center of Delaware
Newark, Delaware

**R. Anthony Carabasi, III, M.D.**
Associate Professor of Surgery
Jefferson Medical College
Thomas Jefferson University
Attending Surgeon
Thomas Jefferson University Hospital
Philadelphia, Pennsylvania

**Maryalice Cheney, M.D.**
Resident in General Surgery
Thomas Jefferson University Hospital
Philadelphia, Pennsylvania

**Herbert E. Cohn, M.D.**
Professor of Surgery
Jefferson Medical College
Thomas Jefferson University
Vice-Chairman, Department of Surgery
Thomas Jefferson University Hospital
Philadelphia, Pennsylvania

**Anthony V. Coletta, M.D.**
Instructor in Surgery
Jefferson Medical College
Thomas Jefferson University
Philadelphia, Pennsylvania
Assistant Attending Surgeon
Bryn Mawr Hospital
Bryn Mawr, Pennsylvania

**Scott M. Goldman, M.D.**
Instructor in Surgery
Jefferson Medical College
Thomas Jefferson University
Attending Surgeon
Thomas Jefferson University Hospital
Philadelphia, Pennsylvania

**Eric L. Hume, M.D.**
Assistant Professor of Orthopedic Surgery
Jefferson Medical College
Thomas Jefferson University
Attending Orthopedic Surgeon
Thomas Jefferson University Hospital
Philadelphia, Pennsylvania

**Bruce E. Jarrell, M.D.**
Associate Professor of Surgery
Jefferson Medical College
Thomas Jefferson University
Attending Surgeon
Thomas Jefferson University Hospital
Philadelphia, Pennsylvania

**Charles J. Lamb, M.D.**
Resident in Cardiothoracic Surgery
University Hospital of Cleveland
Cleveland, Ohio

**Martha Shenot Matthews, M.D.**
Chief Resident in General Surgery
Thomas Jefferson University Hospital
Philadelphia, Pennsylvania

**John H. Moore, Jr., M.D.**
Resident in Plastic Surgery
Eastern Virginia Graduate School of
  Medicine
Norfolk, Virginia

**Michael J. Moritz, M.D.**
Research Fellow and Instructor in Surgery
Jefferson Medical College
Thomas Jefferson University
Philadelphia, Pennsylvania

**John S. Radomski, M.D.**
Resident in General Surgery
Thomas Jefferson University Hospital
Philadelphia, Pennsylvania

**Francis E. Rosato, M.D.**
Professor and Chairman,
  Department of Surgery
Jefferson Medical College
Thomas Jefferson University
Attending Surgeon
Thomas Jefferson University Hospital
Philadelphia, Pennsylvania

**Robert T. Sataloff, M.D.**
Associate Professor of Otolaryngology
Jefferson Medical College
Thomas Jefferson University
Attending Surgeon
Thomas Jefferson University Hospital
The Graduate Hospital
Albert Einstein Medical Center,
  Mount Sinai-Daroff Division
Philadelphia, Pennsylvania

**Joseph R. Spiegel, M.D.**
Instructor in Otolaryngology
Jefferson Medical College
Thomas Jefferson University
Attending Surgeon
Thomas Jefferson University Hospital
The Graduate Hospital
Albert Einstein Medical Center,
  Mount Sinai-Daroff Division
Philadelphia, Pennsylvania

**Jerome J. Vernick, M.D.**
Clinical Professor of Surgery
Jefferson Medical College
Thomas Jefferson University
Attending Surgeon
Thomas Jefferson University Hospital
Philadelphia, Pennsylvania

**Charles W. Wagner, M.D.**
Head, Renal Transplantation Program
St. Christopher's Hospital for Children
Philadelphia, Pennsylvania

**Stephen M. Weiss, M.D.**
Associate Professor of Surgery
Jefferson Medical College
Thomas Jefferson University
Attending Surgeon
Thomas Jefferson University Hospital
Philadelphia, Pennsylvania

**David A. Zwillenberg, M.D.**
Assistant Professor of Otolaryngology
Jefferson Medical College
Thomas Jefferson University
Attending Surgeon
Thomas Jefferson University Hospital
Consultant in Otolaryngology
Wills Eye Hospital
Acting Director, Division of Otolaryngology
Albert Einstein Medical Center,
  Mount Sinai-Daroff Division
Philadelphia, Pennsylvania

# Preface

In keeping with the purpose of *The National Medical Series for Independent Study*, this book presents the core material of the specialty of surgery. The text is not meant to be all-inclusive and does not contain minutiae that we felt would be of little use to the reader. The authors have included not only didactic material but also facts that they find useful in clinical practice. Where controversy exists, we have attempted to present all sides fairly and to indicate factors that are essential in the decision-making process. We have also tried to stress situations in which surgeons and all others involved in patient care must work closely to make the most appropriate decisions regarding treatment.

*Surgery* was written primarily for students and residents in general surgery, but we anticipate that practicing surgeons as well as physicians in other specialties will find it a useful reference.

Bruce E. Jarrell
R. Anthony Carabasi, III

# Acknowledgments

The editors would first like to acknowledge Joseph S. Gonnella, M.D., Dean of Jefferson Medical College. Dr. Gonnella is nationally and internationally recognized as an expert in medical education, and his dedication to progress and excellence in this field has been our inspiration during the preparation of this book.

We would also like to express the admiration, appreciation, and affection that we feel for Francis E. Rosato, M.D., Samuel D. Gross Professor and Chairman of the Department of Surgery at Thomas Jefferson University. In our opinion, he is the ideal academic surgeon.

This work would not have been possible without the dedicated help of Mrs. Joanne Crouch, Mrs. Grace Hershman, and Ms. Rosina Froio. We gratefully acknowledge their assistance.

# Publisher's Note

The objective of the *National Medical Series* is to present an extraordinarily large amount of information in an easily retrievable form. The outline format was selected for this purpose of reducing to the essentials the medical information needed by today's student and practitioner.

While the concept of an outline format was well received by the authors and publisher, the difficulties inherent in working with this style were not initially apparent. That the series has been published and received enthusiastically is a tribute to the authors who worked long and diligently to produce books that are stylistically consistent and comprehensive in content.

The task of producing the *National Medical Series* required more than the efforts of the authors, however, and the missing elements have been supplied by highly competent and dedicated developmental editors and support staff. Editors, compositors, proofreaders, and layout and design staff have all polished the outline to a fine form. It is with deep appreciation that I thank all who have participated, in particular, the staff at Harwal—Debra L. Dreger, Jane Edwards, Gloria Hamilton, Jeanine Kosteski, Wieslawa B. Langenfeld, Keith LaSala, June A. Sangiorgio, Mary Ann C. Sheldon, and Jane Velker.

The Publisher

# Introduction

*Surgery* is one of six clinical science review books in a series entitled *The National Medical Series for Independent Study*. This series has been designed to provide students and house officers, as well as physicians, with a concise but comprehensive instrument for self-evaluation and review within the clinical sciences. Although *Surgery* would be most useful for students preparing for the National Board of Medical Examiners examinations (Part II, Part III, FLEX, and FMGEMS), it should also be useful for students studying for course examinations. These books are not intended to replace the standard clinical science texts but, rather, to complement them.

The books in this series present the core content of each clinical science area, using an outline format and featuring a total of 300 study questions. The questions are distributed throughout the book at the end of each chapter and in a pretest and post-test. In addition, each question is accompanied by the correct answer, a paragraph-length explanation of the correct answer, and specific reference to the outline points under which the information necessary to answer the question can be found.

We have chosen an outline format to allow maximal ease in retrieving information, assuming that the time available to the reader is limited. Considerable editorial time has been spent to ensure that the information required by all medical school curricula has been included and that each question parallels the format of the questions on the National Board examinations. We feel that the combination of the outline format and board-type study questions provides a unique teaching device.

We hope you will find this series interesting, relevant, and challenging. The authors, as well as the John Wiley and Harwal staffs, welcome your comments and suggestions.

# Pretest

## QUESTIONS

**Directions:** Each question below contains five suggested answers. Choose the **one best** response to each question.

1. What characteristic radiographic finding would be seen in a patient with a gallstone that has eroded into the duodenum?

(A) A widened duodenal C-loop
(B) Gallbladder calcification
(C) Evidence of gas-forming organisms in the retroperitoneum
(D) Air in the biliary tree
(E) A filling defect in the rectosigmoid colon

2. What is the most reliable method for precisely locating an upper gastrointestinal lesion that is responsible for a bleed?

(A) Upper GI series
(B) Exploratory laparotomy
(C) Upper gastrointestinal endoscopy
(D) Arteriography
(E) Radionuclide scanning

3. Arterial claudication is associated with all of the following conditions EXCEPT

(A) abnormal lipoprotein concentrations
(B) smoking
(C) hypertension
(D) pain in the toes and metatarsal heads
(E) absent extremity pulses

4. Ligation of the superior thyroid artery above the superior pole of the thyroid gland carries with it the risk of

(A) injury to the recurrent nerve
(B) injury to the vagus nerve
(C) devascularization of the inferior parathyroid gland
(D) injury to the hypoglossal nerve
(E) injury to the external branch of the superior laryngeal nerve

5. All of the following are indications for open fracture reduction and internal fixation EXCEPT

(A) open fracture
(B) functional requirements
(C) unsatisfactory closed reduction
(D) multiple trauma
(E) intra-articular fracture

6. All of the following statements regarding oral cholecystography are true EXCEPT

(A) it reliably demonstrates the presence of gallstones
(B) it demonstrates the common bile duct in many cases
(C) a normal gallbladder may fail to visualize if diarrhea or malabsorption is present
(D) failure to visualize the gallbladder indicates a nonfunctional gallbladder
(E) ultrasonography may be as reliable as oral cholecystography

7. An elderly man is brought to the emergency room because of massive bleeding from the rectum. The bleeding is most likely due to

(A) carcinoma of the colon
(B) diverticulosis
(C) diverticulitis
(D) ulcerative colitis
(E) colonic polyps

8. Treatment of an incarcerated congenital hernia involves

(A) immediate operation to prevent the reduction of necrotic intestine
(B) evaluation of the child's state of hydration, after reduction of the hernia
(C) observation after reduction of the hernia until the child is old enough to undergo surgery
(D) observation after reduction until the processus vaginalis has clearly fused
(E) surgery of the small intestine in both male and female patients

9. One of the most common causes of missed diagnosis in patients with an aldosterone-producing adenoma of the adrenal gland (Conn's syndrome) is

(A) failure to measure the postural response of serum aldosterone
(B) measurement of serum aldosterone before potassium repletion
(C) measurement of serum potassium after sodium loading
(D) failure to visualize a tumor on computed tomography (CT)
(E) failure to visualize a tumor on iodocholesterol scanning

10. An elderly woman is admitted with weakness, anemia, weight loss, and a palpable abdominal mass. She has a colon carcinoma. The most likely anatomic site is the

(A) rectum
(B) sigmoid colon
(C) left colon
(D) transverse colon
(E) cecum

11. Which vessel is most commonly associated with a posterior duodenal ulcer?

(A) Right gastroepiploic artery
(B) Common hepatic artery
(C) Gastroduodenal artery
(D) Superior mesenteric artery
(E) Middle colic artery

12. The best method to determine the effectiveness of pulmonary ventilation preoperatively is by

(A) arterial blood gas analysis
(B) serial spirometry
(C) pH determination
(D) expired lung $P_{CO_2}$
(E) pulmonary dead space

13. Likely causes of anuria following renal transplantation include all of the following EXCEPT

(A) acute tubular necrosis
(B) acute rejection
(C) ureteral obstruction
(D) azathioprine toxicity
(E) renal artery thrombosis

14. Which of the following situations requires true emergency care?

(A) Closed tendon rupture
(B) Comminuted fracture of the femur
(C) "Boxer's" fracture of the hand
(D) Open fracture of the ankle
(E) Subperiosteal hematoma of the tibia

15. The most effective way to prevent infection in a dirty traumatic wound is to

(A) administer tetanus toxoid
(B) administer intravenous antibiotics
(C) apply a skin graft
(D) repeat surgical debridement
(E) administer topical antibiotics

16. Achalasia of the esophagus is suspected on the basis of an x-ray film showing

(A) multiple strictures of the esophagus
(B) diffuse dilatation of the esophagus
(C) "corkscrew" appearance of the esophagus
(D) a diverticulum in the cricopharyngeal muscle
(E) reflux of barium into the esophagus

17. All of the following measures are likely to be helpful in the management of cerebral edema EXCEPT

(A) restricting fluids to two-thirds of maintenance
(B) administering osmotic agents (e.g., mannitol and glycerol)
(C) monitoring intracranial pressure (ICP)
(D) maintaining $P_{CO_2}$ in the 40 mm Hg to 45 mm Hg range
(E) administering barbiturates

18. All of the following components or qualities of stored whole blood tend to decrease over time EXCEPT

(A) red blood cell survival time
(B) potassium concentration
(C) pH
(D) platelet activity
(E) oxygen-carrying capacity

19. The most common indication for surgery in Crohn's disease is

(A) bowel obstruction
(B) enterovesical fistula
(C) intra-abdominal abscess
(D) enterocutaneous fistula
(E) gastrointestinal bleeding

20. What organism most frequently causes a urinary tract infection?

(A) *Staphylococcus aureus*
(B) *Staphylococcus epidermidis*
(C) *Escherichia coli*
(D) *Proteus mirabilis*
(E) *Pseudomonas aeruginosa*

21. Familial polyposis of the colon is most often associated with which of the following conditions?

(A) Carcinoma of the pancreas
(B) Carcinoma of the colon
(C) Granulomatous disease of the colon
(D) Pneumatosis cystoides intestinalis
(E) Sigmoid volvulus

22. A 5-year-old patient has a midline neck mass, which moves with swallowing and is located just below the hyoid. The mass is most likely to be a

(A) branchial cleft cyst
(B) cystic hygroma
(C) teratoma
(D) thyroglossal duct cyst
(E) laryngeal papilloma

23. The most common cause of death in patients with alcoholic cirrhosis following portal-systemic shunting is

(A) bleeding esophageal varices
(B) hepatic failure with encephalopathy
(C) malnutrition
(D) hepatocellular carcinoma
(E) cardiac failure with peripheral edema and ascites

24. Which treatment method is most appropriate for a patient with acute perirectal pain and with a tender, fluctuant perirectal area?

(A) Abdominoperineal resection
(B) Abdominal transsacral rectal resection
(C) Removal of an anal fissure
(D) Drainage of an abscess
(E) Antibiotic therapy alone

25. A 15-year-old girl is admitted with acute generalized abdominal pain. She gives a history of intermittent abdominal pain and anorexia with vomiting. Examination of her abdomen reveals a fullness in the right lower quadrant with localized tenderness. She has a temperature of 102° F, a white blood count of 18,000, and a hematocrit of 45%. What is the most likely diagnosis?

(A) Simple appendicitis
(B) Perforated appendicitis with abscess formation
(C) Ovarian tumor
(D) Ruptured ectopic pregnancy
(E) Intussusception

26. Which of the following presenting symptoms of breast cancer is the most common?

(A) Isolated axillary enlargement
(B) Nipple discharge
(C) Breast mass
(D) Mammographic findings of microcalcifications
(E) Nipple changes and desquamation

**Directions:** Each question below contains four suggested answers of which **one or more** is correct. Choose the answer

A   if **1, 2, and 3** are correct
B   if **1 and 3** are correct
C   if **2 and 4** are correct
D   if **4** is correct
E   if **1, 2, 3, and 4** are correct

27. True statements concerning cystic hygromas include which of the following?

(1) They are derived from embryonic lymph sacs
(2) They occur in the neck, groin, axilla, and mediastinum
(3) They may enlarge enough to cause respiratory distress
(4) Removal should include cranial nerve resection, since recurrence rates are high

28. The rate of wound healing may be influenced by multiple factors, including

(1) malnutrition
(2) previous radiation treatment
(3) poor vascularity
(4) anti-inflammatory drugs

29. Trauma is the leading cause of death among people under 35 years of age. Of trauma victims it can be said that

(1) over one-half of deaths result from motor vehicle accidents
(2) some 10% to 15% have serious multisystem injuries
(3) patient management requires adherence to an established order of priority
(4) prophylactic antibiotics and tetanus prophylaxis should be administered routinely

30. Common warts (verrucae vulgaris) exhibit which of the following characteristics?

(1) They occur most frequently in the third decade of life
(2) They are caused by papovaviruses
(3) Most will not resolve spontaneously and require treatment such as desiccation
(4) The fingers are the most common location

31. True statements concerning the anatomy of the parotid gland include which of the following?

(1) It is the largest of the salivary glands
(2) The fascia of the gland is quite tight
(3) The facial nerve and its branches run through the gland
(4) The gland has two true anatomic lobes separated by the facial nerve

32. Factors that improve the results of renal transplantation include

(1) an HLA-$D_R$–locus match
(2) donor-specific pretransplantation transfusions
(3) cyclosporine administration
(4) azathioprine administration

33. A transient ischemic attack is associated with

(1) cerebral embolus
(2) amaurosis fugax
(3) cerebrovascular accident
(4) residual neurologic deficits

34. True statements concerning hypersplenism include

(1) primary hypersplenism is more common in men than in women
(2) primary hypersplenism does not respond to splenectomy
(3) portal hypertension usually causes severe secondary hypersplenism
(4) splenic vein thrombosis can cause secondary hypersplenism and bleeding from esophageal varices

35. The surgical treatment of abdominal injuries involves

(1) a generous midline incision
(2) obtaining hemostasis as a first priority
(3) immobilization and palpation of the pancreas and duodenum if an upper abdominal retroperitoneal hematoma is present
(4) exploration of lower abdominal and pelvic retroperitoneal hematomas

36. The incidence of postoperative complications can be lowered by

(1) complete bed rest
(2) removal of all surgical tubes as soon as possible
(3) avoidance of pain medication
(4) careful hemostasis in the operating room

37. Indications for the surgical removal of urinary calculi include

(1) infection
(2) obstruction
(3) severe pain
(4) growth of a silent calculus

38. In the normal term infant, the ductus arteriosus closes within the first few days of life. If the ductus remains patent, the clinical features likely to result include

(1) a classic "machinery-like" murmur
(2) right-to-left shunt
(3) congestive heart failure
(4) coarctation of the aorta

39. A patient with acute pancreatitis is admitted to the hospital. Which of the following conditions might be likely to show up in the patient's history?

(1) Biliary tract stones
(2) Hyperlipidemia
(3) Alcohol ingestion
(4) Hypertension

40. The treatment of a stage $T_1$ laryngeal carcinoma might consist of

(1) cordectomy
(2) total laryngectomy
(3) radiotherapy
(4) chemotherapy

41. A 50-year-old man who ate a huge meal at a company banquet ended up in the emergency room with excruciating left upper abdominal pain radiating through to his back. The history reveals that his pain followed an episode of severe retching and vomiting. Which of the following studies would be ordered to provide the diagnosis?

(1) Chest roentgenogram
(2) Splenic radionuclide scan
(3) A Gastrografin swallow
(4) Celiac arteriogram

42. True statements about hepatic abscesses include

(1) the most common hepatic abscess in the United States is of bacterial origin
(2) amebic abscess is the most common hepatic abscess in third-world countries
(3) endocarditis can cause a hepatic abscess
(4) standard treatment for a solitary bacterial hepatic abscess is broad-spectrum antibiotic treatment alone

43. Clinical manifestations of gas gangrene include

(1) confusion or deliruim
(2) mildly increased leukocyte count
(3) characteristic foul odor of the wound
(4) onset 48 hours after injury

44. True statements concerning lipomas include which of the following?

(1) They can be found in any location of the body where fat is usually found
(2) Malignant transformation is common
(3) Simple excision is curative
(4) They can be caused by trauma to areas of fatty tissue

45. Factors that increase the risk of pulmonary embolism in patients undergoing surgery include

(1) deep venous thrombosis
(2) pregnancy
(3) obesity
(4) estrogen therapy

46. Conditions that are commonly seen in patients with chronic renal failure include

(1) anemia
(2) hypernatremia
(3) metabolic acidosis
(4) hypophosphatemia

47. Gastrointestinal fistulas may develop as a result of

(1) penetrating abdominal trauma
(2) congenital anomaly
(3) inflammation
(4) malignancy

SUMMARY OF DIRECTIONS

| A | B | C | D | E |
|---|---|---|---|---|
| 1, 2, 3 only | 1, 3 only | 2, 4 only | 4 only | All are correct |

48. Recommended nutrients for long-term parenteral nutrition include which of the following?

(1) Fat solution
(2) Amino acids
(3) Magnesium
(4) Plasma proteins

49. Functions of the spleen include

(1) removal of abnormal red blood cells
(2) storage of over one-half of the body's platelets
(3) production of opsonins and immunoglobulin M (IgM)
(4) production of new red blood cells

50. Chronic pancreatitis is often diagnosed by

(1) chronically elevated amylase levels
(2) chronic abdominal pain following episodes of acute pancreatitis
(3) the presence of gallstones
(4) the presence of pancreatic calcification

**Directions:** The groups of questions below consist of lettered choices followed by several numbered items. For each numbered item select the **one** lettered choice with which it is **most** closely associated. Each lettered choice may be used once, more than once, or not at all.

**Questions 51–55**

For each multiple endocrine adenomatosis (MEA) syndrome or pancreatic tumor, select the clinical feature that is most characteristic of it.

(A) Elevated serum calcium level
(B) Elevated serum thyrocalcitonin level
(C) Severe watery diarrhea
(D) Abdominal pain secondary to peptic ulceration
(E) Distorted body habitus

51. MEA type I (Wermer's syndrome)

52. MEA type II (Sipple's syndrome)

53. MEA type III (mucosal neuroma syndrome)

54. Pancreatic gastrinoma (Zollinger-Ellison syndrome)

55. Pancreatic cholera

**Questions 56–60**

The most common manifestations of ulcer disease are gastric ulcers and duodenal ulcers. These share certain characteristics but are dissimilar in other ways. For each phrase describing a characteristic of ulcer disease, select the most appropriate response.

(A) Gastric ulcer
(B) Duodenal ulcer
(C) Both
(D) Neither

56. The major cause is hypersecretion of gastric acid

57. Degeneration into cancer may occur

58. Complications include bleeding and perforation

59. Smoking and aspirin use are associated with an increased incidence

60. Surgery is the treatment of choice

# ANSWERS AND EXPLANATIONS

**1. The answer is D.** (*Chapter 9 II I 5 b*) Any abnormal communication between the biliary tree and the intestinal tract will produce air in the biliary tract. When a gallstone erodes into the intestinal tract, it is usually a large gallstone that slowly erodes into the duodenum, forming a scarred, well-established tract without gas-forming organisms. If a filling defect is present, it is usually in the terminal ileum, secondary to the large gallstone's obstruction of the lumen.

**2. The answer is C.** (*Chapter 4 III E 1*) Upper gastrointestinal endoscopy is the most versatile, reliable, and rapidly performed examination for precisely locating the site of upper gastrointestinal bleeding. Endoscopy can be used in most situations except when bleeding is massive, and it is useful when more than one type of pathology is present, which is often the case. An upper GI series, arteriography and radionuclide scanning are helpful but only in more selected cases. Exploratory laparotomy is most useful as a diagnostic procedure only when the bleeding is so rapid that exsanguination is imminent.

**3. The answer is D.** (*Chapter 13 I B 1 a, b, 2 a, b*) One of the most characteristic symptoms of peripheral vascular disease is claudication—that is, pain which commonly occurs in the calf muscles and less commonly in the buttocks and thigh muscles. Frequently, extremity pulses are diminished or absent. Risk factors related to claudication include smoking, hypertension, abnormal lipoprotein levels, and diabetes mellitus. Pain involving the toes or metatarsal heads is most commonly ischemic rest pain, a symptom of very severe peripheral vascular disease. It is usually a constant ache that frequently awakens the patient at night. It is not associated with calf or thigh pain.

**4. The answer is E.** (*Chapter 18 II E*) The external branch of the superior laryngeal nerve is intimately intertwined with the branches of the superior thyroid artery, necessitating ligation of the branches of the artery where they join the superior pole of the gland. Ligation at a more proximal level carries with it the risk of injury to the superior laryngeal nerve. The recurrent laryngeal and vagus nerves are well removed from injury during dissection in this area. Although 10% of superior parathyroid glands derive their blood supply from the superior thyroid artery and may be devascularized during mobilization of the superior pole of the gland, the inferior parathyroids are always supplied by the inferior thyroid artery and are not at risk of injury during dissection in this area. The hypoglossal nerve crosses the internal carotid artery at a much higher level and is not at risk at all during thyroid operations.

**5. The answer is A.** (*Chapter 32 III A 3 a, B 1*) An open fracture is a surgical emergency because of the risks of infection. Surgical management includes thorough debridement, use of appropriate prophylactic antibiotics, and, if needed, tetanus inoculation. Functional requirements—e.g., the need for an absolutely smooth contour within a joint—may call for open reduction and surgical fixation of a fracture, as may unsatisfactory results after closed reduction of a less complicated type of fracture. Internal fixation is valuable when early mobilization is especially important, as in patients with multiple injuries and in elderly patients.

**6. The answer is B.** (*Chapter 9 II D*) The oral cholecystogram will not demonstrate the common duct but it is very reliable for detecting either gallstones or other pathologic processes in the gallbladder. The dye must be absorbed to be concentrated in the gallbladder; thus, a normal gallbladder may fail to visualize in a patient with diarrhea or malabsorption. An ultrasonic examination is virtually as reliable as oral cholecystography for detecting pathologic conditions.

**7. The answer is B.** (*Chapter 7 XVII E 1*) Diverticulosis is one of the most common causes of massive lower gastrointestinal bleeding. Arteriovenous malformations of the right colon are another common cause. Carcinoma of the colon rarely causes massive bleeding, nor does ulcerative colitis or polyps. Diverticulitis is not associated with massive bleeding.

**8. The answer is B.** (*Chapter 33 II A 5*) A congenital inguinal hernia is due to nonfusion of the processus vaginalis, which is highly unlikely to fuse after birth. The treatment of an incarcerated hernia is reduction, hydration of the patient, and herniorrhaphy. Essentially all incarcerated hernias can be reduced without the fear of reducing a necrotic intestine. The hernia in a female contains ovary, not intestine, and therefore after reduction it can be treated in a less urgent fashion.

**9. The answer is B.** (*Chapter 19 VIII D 3 a*) One of the most common causes of missed diagnosis of Conn's syndrome is the measurement of plasma aldosterone levels before potassium repletion. Plasma aldosterone levels may not be elevated in the potassium-depleted patient but will usually become significantly elevated after potassium and sodium loading. Measuring the serum aldosterone levels after 4 hours of upright posture helps to differentiate primary hyperaldosteronism due to bilateral adrenal cortical hyperplasia from that due to adenoma. Computed tomography (CT) and iodocholesterol scanning are localization studies. Failure to visualize a tumor on either study would not preclude the diagnosis of primary hyperaldosteronism, since the diagnosis is primarily a biochemical one. Selective adrenal venous sampling could then be used for localization.

**10. The answer is E.** (*Chapter 7 XII E 1*) Cecal lesions are likely to be silent until they become very large. They cause heme-positive stools from a slow, chronic blood loss. The resultant anemia is so insidious in its onset that it often does not cause symptoms until late in the course.

**11. The answer is C.** (*Chapter 4 III F 4 d*) Duodenal ulcers that penetrate posteriorly usually have the gastroduodenal artery or one of its branches at the base of the ulcer. Although ulcers have the potential to erode into the right gastroepiploic, common hepatic, superior mesenteric, or middle colic artery, this is less common. Giant gastric ulcers also can penetrate into nearby arteries, especially the middle colic artery and the left gastric artery.

**12. The answer is A.** (*Chapter 3 II C*) Arterial blood gas analysis is the best and simplest method to determine effective ventilation. If the $PO_2$ is low, inadequate alveolar ventilation is taking place. If the $PCO_2$ is high in the absence of primary metabolic alkalosis, then $CO_2$ retention and inadequate gaseous exchange is taking place. In the presence of a low $PCO_2$ without a primary metabolic acidosis, hyperventilation is taking place.

**13. The answer is D.** (*Chapter 16 III B 1, 3; IV A 1; VI A 2 a, b*) Azathioprine toxicity is not associated with anuria; rather, it usually causes leukopenia. Acute tubular necrosis generally resolves in 7 to 14 days, resulting in normal renal function. However, the anuria associated with acute rejection is often irreversible and there is loss of the kidney. When anuria is present, a high index of suspicion is necessary to diagnose ureteral obstruction or renal artery thrombosis early enough to salvage the kidney.

**14. The answer is D.** (*Chapter 32 III B*) Open fractures constitute surgical emergencies not only because bone is relatively susceptible to infections, but more importantly because the devitalized soft tissue which inevitably accompanies open fractures is a likely target for a life-threatening anaerobic infection. Other orthopedic emergencies include vascular compromise, spinal cord injuries, and peripheral nerve injuries.

**15. The answer is D.** [*Chapter 1 IV C 4, D 6 c (1) (b), (2); VII A 4 b (1) (c), M 1*] The most effective way to prevent infection in a dirty traumatic wound is debridement with irrigation. Any person with a penetrating injury must receive tetanus prophylaxis if previous immunization cannot be documented; however, adequate debridement of devitalized tissue is also essential. Although prophylactic antibiotics can reduce the incidence of wound infections, they are probably of little benefit for grossly contaminated wounds. Topical antibiotics are used most appropriately for burns of the skin. Skin grafts are used to cover large open wounds that are covered by healthy granulation tissue.

**16. The answer is B.** (*Chapter 28 II B 3*) In achalasia, the normal peristalsis in the body of the esophagus is absent, resulting in diffuse esophageal dilatation that can be seen on x-ray films. A corkscrew appearance is characteristic of esophageal spasm; reflux of barium indicates inadequate functioning of the lower esophageal sphincter. A diverticulum visible in the area of the cricopharyngeal muscle is a Zenker's or pharyngoesophageal diverticulum, caused by dysfunction in the upper esophageal sphincter.

**17. The answer is D.** (*Chapter 31 VI D*) In patients who develop severe brain edema, fluids must be restricted and osmotic agents may be necessary to keep the serum osmolality in the 300 mOsm to 320 mOsm range. The use of intracranial pressure (ICP) monitoring helps in following the course of the edema and in determining the time for therapeutic intervention. The cerebral microvasculature is most responsive to changes in the arterial $PCO_2$. Hyperventilation (hypocapnia) reduces the cerebral blood volume and thus decreases the ICP almost instantaneously. In severe cases, $PCO_2$ has to be kept in the 20 mm Hg to 25 mm Hg range in order to control intracranial hypertension. Barbiturates can rapidly reduce the ICP, although their role in improving the eventual outcome is debatable.

**18. The answer is B.** (*Chapter 1 VI A 1–2*) There is a progressive increase in the potassium concentration of stored blood, which may reach 30 mEq/L after 3 to 4 weeks. This is an important consideration when massive transfusions are required and in patients with renal disease. Red blood cells gradually lose their ability to survive. For example, if blood is transfused after storage for 28 days, only 25% of the red cells will be viable 60 days after the transfusion. Oxygen transport is also reduced because of a decrease in cellular 2,3-diphosphoglycerate. The pH of stored blood gradually decreases, reaching about 6.7 after 4 weeks of storage. Platelets become inactive after only 24 hours.

**19. The answer is A.** (*Chapter 6 IV E 1–4*) Crohn's disease, a chronic inflammatory disease, can involve any area of the gastrointestinal tract. Its cause is unknown. Medical treatment is preferred, but surgical treatment, which is reserved for complications of the disease, ultimately becomes necessary in most cases. Small bowel obstruction is the most common complication necessitating surgery; however, surgery may also be required for fistulas or abscesses. Only rarely is Crohn's disease associated with significant bleeding.

**20. The answer is C.** (*Chapter 29 III B 2, D 2, E 1*) *Escherichia coli* is responsible for over 90% of all renal infections, both initial and recurrent. The presence of other organisms should raise the suspicion of prior antibiotic therapy or complicating factors such as anatomic abnormalities.

**21. The answer is B.** (*Chapter 7 XI E 1*) Total colectomy is recommended for patients with familial polyposis of the colon because all untreated patients will develop cancer. The resection should be done as early as the patient will accept it because cancer is inevitable.

**22. The answer is D.** (*Chapter 24 III B 3*) A midline neck mass that is mobile with swallowing is indicative of a thyroglossal duct cyst. These are infrahyoid in 65% of the cases, suprahyoid in about 20%, and at the hyoid in 15%. In one-half of the cases, they present by age 10. Branchial cleft cysts can occur anywhere between the external auditory canal and the clavicle. Cystic hygromas are found in the neck, most commonly in the posterior triangle, and are usually noted soon after birth. Teratomas are generally unilateral and cause tracheal compression or deviation. They are most commonly noted at birth. Laryngeal papillomas in children are usually multiple and may involve the airway from the epiglottis to the bronchi.

**23. The answer is B.** (*Chapter 9 I E 10 d, e*) Hepatic failure is the most common cause of death following a nonselective portal-systemic shunting procedure. It is related to a deprivation of portal blood in the liver. Portal blood appears to be necessary in the maintenance of hepatocellular function, and nonselective shunting always results in hepatofugal flow. A repeat of variceal hemorrhage following shunting is unusual if the shunt remains patent. Another common cause of death in cirrhotics is infection such as pneumonia or primary peritonitis. Malnutrition, hepatic carcinoma, and cardiac failure are less common causes of death in cirrhotics undergoing shunting procedures.

**24. The answer is D.** (*Chapter 7 XVIII E*) The patient has a perirectal abscess, which should be drained. Antibiotic therapy alone will not cure an abscess; adequate drainage is essential. Whether to drain a perirectal abscess in an outpatient setting or in the operating room is a matter of clinical judgment. Factors that must be considered are the severity of the patient's pain and the need for proper visualization of the involved region.

**25. The answer is B.** [*Chapter 4 I A 1 a (4), B 2 b (5)*] The most likely diagnosis is a perforated appendicitis with a periappendiceal abscess. The usual method of diagnosis is exploratory laparotomy with drainage of the abscess and removal of the appendix if it is identifiable. Simple appendicitis, ovarian tumor, ruptured ectopic pregnancy, and intussusception are much less likely in the setting described.

**26. The answer is C.** (*Chapter 23 III B 2*) Although axillary node enlargement, nipple discharge as well as nipple changes and desquamation, and microcalcifications may be signs of breast cancer, an isolated breast mass is the most common mode of presentation, occurring in 85% to 90% of patients. For this reason, routine physical examination as a means of surveillance in high-risk patients and the teaching of breast self-examination are the most important aspects of the management of this condition.

**27. The answer is A (1, 2, 3).** (*Chapter 12 II A*) Cystic hygromas are the most common benign tumors of the lymphatics. Derived from embryonic lymph sacs, they are seen during the first year of life. They occur most often in the neck, where they can become large enough to cause respiratory distress. Other, less common, sites are the groin, axilla, and mediastinum. Cranial nerves should not be sacrificed since these tumors are benign.

**28. The answer is E (all).** (*Chapter 1 IV D 1–4*) Wound healing may be influenced by a variety of factors. Young patients heal more rapidly than old patients, and malnutrition can impede wound healing even though the biologic needs of wounds take priority over those of the organ systems. Highly vascular regions, such as the face, heal more rapidly than regions of poor vascularity, such as the pretibial area. Anti-inflammatory drugs, such as steroids, delay wound healing if they are given the first few day after the injury; however, their effect is minimal if given after that time.

**29. The answer is E (all).** (*Chapter 2 I A*) Trauma is the leading cause of death among people under 35 years of age. More than one-half of deaths in this group result from motor vehicle accidents. Multisystem injuries occur in 10% to 15% of trauma victims. Mortality can be reduced by efficient handling of the injured patients; this begins with skilled emergency medical technicians, rapid transport of patients to trauma centers, and trauma centers that are staffed by professional personnel trained in delivering rapid care to seriously injured patients. Prophylactic antibiotics and tetanus prophylaxis should be administered to all patients suffering severe traumatic injuries.

**30. The answer is C (2, 4).** (*Chapter 30 II B 1*) Common warts occur most frequently in the second decade of life and may be transmitted by direct or indirect contact. They are caused by a member of the papovavirus family. The fingers are the most common location, and the lesions have a characteristic rough, elevated surface and can become tender. Many of these warts will resolve spontaneously, and only problematic lesions should be treated. This is usually accomplished by electrodesiccation or with caustic topical agents.

**31. The answer is A (1, 2, 3).** (*Chapter 26 I A, D, G*) The parotid is the largest salivary gland. The tight fascia is the reason for the severe pain that occurs if the gland swells acutely. The gland probably does not have two true lobes, although this concept is useful in planning resections of the parotid gland. The facial nerve runs through the gland, and preservation of the nerve is essential in surgery for benign conditions of the parotid gland.

**32. The answer is E (all).** (*Chapter 16 I D 3 d, 4 b; IV A 1, 5*) The successful outcome of any type of tissue transplantation is determined by the immunologic compatibility of the recipient and donor. The survival rate of an HLA-$D_R$–locus perfect match is 80% at 2 years. At 2 years post-transplantation, the success rate is over 90% for individuals who received preoperative transfusions from a donor-specific source. Long-term prophylactic immunosuppression has included the use of azathioprine; prednisone also may be used to suppress both cell-mediated and humoral immunity. However, the use of cyclosporine, which is associated with excellent graft survival, may surpass that of both of these traditional drugs.

**33. The answer is A (1, 2, 3).** (*Chapter 13 VIII C 1 a–c*) A transient ischemic attack (TIA) is an episode of focal neurologic symptoms. It is characterized by an abrupt onset (i.e., maximal symptoms occur in less than 5 minutes), a rapid recovery (i.e., within 24 hours), and no residual neurologic deficits. TIA is associated with generalized atherosclerosis, usually occurring secondary to a cerebral embolus. Motor and sensory deficits include aphasia, hemianopia, and amaurosis fugax (i.e., transient monocular blindness). The risk of a stroke following a TIA is 23% in 1 year and 45% in 5 years.

**34. The answer is D (4).** (*Chapter 11 III A 2, 3, B 1, 2*) Primary hypersplenism is a diagnosis of exclusion and is more common in women than in men. It can be cured by splenectomy. Portal hypertension is a common cause of hypersplenism, but it is usually mild and not clinically significant. Splenic vein thrombosis usually is a result of pancreatitis. It can lead to splenic congestion and resultant secondary hypersplenism. Varices in the distal esophagus develop from pressure transmitted via the short gastric veins between the spleen and the stomach. Bleeding may be severe. Splenectomy is curative and will stop both the bleeding and the hematologic complications.

**35. The answer is A (1, 2, 3).** [*Chapter 2 I C 6 c (8)*] A midline incision should be made for all abdominal explorations. Hemostasis should be controlled by clamping obvious bleeders and packing areas where the bleeding site is not immediately obvious. At this time, the anesthesiologist can catch up with volume loss and the patient can be stabilized before a systematic exploration is undertaken. Retroperitoneal hematomas in the pelvis should not be explored unless they show evidence of arterial pulsation or rapid expansion. In the upper abdomen, these retroperitoneal hematomas must be explored since they are frequently associated with injuries of the duodenum, pancreas, and bile ducts.

**36. The answer is C (2, 4).** (*Chapter 1 VIII B, C 1–6*) Early mobilization rather than complete bed rest will lower the risk of thrombophlebitis and pulmonary complications. All surgical tubes should be removed as soon as possible. Adequate but not excessive pain medication should be prescribed so that the patient remains alert enough to breathe deeply, cough, and move around. Adequate hydration is necessary; withholding fluids will not prevent pulmonary complications.

**37. The answer is E (all).** (*Chapter 29 Table 29-1*) The indications for the surgical removal of urinary calculi include infection, obstruction, severe pain, and growth of a silent calculus. When infection is present proximal to a calculus, antibiotic therapy should be instituted to control the infection and the urine should be drained. Removal of the calculus should be delayed until this time. A calculus should be removed if it is causing severe obstruction with potential renal damage. Temporary relief may be obtained by catheter drainage of urine. Mild pain from a urinary calculus can be controlled with analgesics. More severe pain that cannot be controlled satisfactorily is a major indication for removal of the calculus. Calculi can be monitored without specific treatment if they remain asymptomatic. Growth of a silent calculus during observation is also an indication for removal.

**38. The answer is B (1, 3).** (*Chapter 17 II B 2*) Hypoxia and certain prostaglandins may act to keep the ductus arteriosus patent in a newborn infant; it normally closes within the first few days of life. The history of patent ductus arteriosus is variable. Common presenting symptoms include dyspnea, fatigue, and palpitations, signifying congestive heart failure; however, many patients remain asymptomatic. On physical examination, a "machinery-like" murmur is usually heard; other signs include a widened pulse pressure and pounding peripheral pulses. Patent ductus may be seen in combination with other defects, such as ventricular septal defect and coarctation of the aorta, but it does not cause these defects.

**39. The answer is A (1, 2, 3).** (*Chapter 10 II B*) In addition to stones, alcohol ingestion, and hyperlipidemia, acute pancreatitis can be caused by trauma, oral diuretics such as the thiazides, and other drug therapies. Hypertension of itself does not show an association with pancreatitis.

**40. The answer is B (1, 3).** (*Chapter 25 VIII F 3*) Equal cure rates are provided with either cordectomy or radiation therapy. Cordectomy by laser is recommended by some authorities, but the procedure is still controversial. Hemilaryngectomy may be performed for some glottic lesions that involve the anterior commissure, but neither total laryngectomy nor chemotherapy is indicated.

**41. The answer is B (1, 3).** (*Chapter 4 I F 2, 3*) The patient has a classic history of Boerhaave's syndrome. In this disease, severe retching and vomiting of large amounts of food cause perforation of the intrathoracic esophagus, resulting in a left pleural effusion. Meglumine diatrizoate (Gastrografin) swallow will confirm the diagnosis of pleural effusion.

**42. The answer is A (1, 2, 3).** (*Chapter 9 I D 2, 3*) In the Western world, most hepatic abscesses are bacterial in origin. The primary source may be abdominal, but seeding from a distant focus of infection, such as a subacute bacterial endocarditis, can also be the cause. Amebic abscesses, caused by *Entamoeba histolytica*, are more common than bacterial abscesses in third-world countries. The standard treatment for a bacterial hepatic abscess is primarily surgical drainage. Besides removing infectious and necrotic matter, drainage allows identification of the infecting organism and, thus, more appropriate antibiotic therapy. Ultrasonically guided catheter drainage may also be effective if minimal necrotic debris is present.

**43. The answer is E (all).** (*Chapter 1 VII E 1–3*) Gas gangrene in most commonly caused by *Clostridium perfringens* in wounds where extensive destruction of tissue has occurred, where there is marked impairment of blood supply, if there is a delay in treatment or the wound is grossly contaminated, or if surgical debridement was inadequate. The average time of onset of symptoms is 48 hours after injury. The most common complaint is severe pain at the site of injury. The skin may appear normal, but the wound usually drains a serous fluid with a brownish color and a foul odor. The white blood cell count may be mildly elevated, and there may be mental changes, such as confusion or delirium.

**44. The answer is B (1, 3).** (*Chapter 30 II B 4*) Lipomas, which are tumors composed of fat cells, can be found in any area of the body where fat is usually found. They are most commonly found on the neck, shoulders, back, and thighs. Malignant transformation is extremely uncommon, and simple excision is curative.

**45. The answer is E (all).** (*Chapter 14 II A, C*) Pulmonary embolism is one of the most common causes of sudden death in hospitalized patients. Patients who are at increased risk of pulmonary embolism include the following: patients with deep venous thrombosis or varicose veins, pregnant women and women in the postpartum period, women undergoing estrogen therapy, obese patients, cancer patients, trauma patients, and patients who have had previous pulmonary embolism.

**46. The answer is B (1, 3).** (*Chapter 3 III A 1 a*) In patients with chronic renal failure, fluid and electrolyte homeostasis is altered. These patients usually retain fluids and thus have dilutional hyponatremia except in cases of chronic pyelonephritis where salt wasting and subsequent dehydration may be present. Metabolic acidosis as a result of the failure of the kidney to excrete phosphates can result in hyperphosphatemia.

**47. The answer is E (all).** (*Chapter 8 II A–E*) The causes of gastrointestinal fistulas are many. Fistula-forming abdominal trauma may be accidental or an inadvertent surgical injury; a gastrocutaneous fistula after splenectomy is an example. The most important fistulous congenital anomaly is a distal tracheoesophageal fistula with esophageal atresia. Crohn's disease is an inflammatory bowel disease that usually affects the ileum; a fistula connecting the ileum to another enteric site is a common late complication. Fistulas can develop because of the destruction of organs by tumors; for example, a colovesical fistula may occur in a patient with a large sigmoid colon cancer.

**48. The answer is A (1, 2, 3).** (*Chapter 1 II E 3 a, b; Table 1-6*) Parenteral nutrition can be used to provide all or part of a patient's nutrients for an indefinite period of time. Because it completely bypasses the gastrointestinal tract, parenteral nutrition is useful for patients who lack intestinal function. A hypertonic nutrient solution should include a fat solution as a source of calories and to prevent essential fatty acid deficiency; amino acids as a protein source, although short-chain peptides may also be used; and a variety of minerals, including magnesium. Plasma proteins, on the other hand, are not considered to be nutrients. Although albumin is sometimes included, it is often given to increase plasma oncotic pressure temporarily rather than as a nutrient source.

**49. The answer is B (1, 3).** (*Chapter 11 II A 2, B 1, 2*) Primarily the spleen functions as a blood filter that removes senescent or abnormal red blood cells and cellular debris and as a producer of opsonins and antibodies, particularly immunoglobulin M (IgM). Approximately one-third of the body's platelets are stored in the spleen. Under normal circumstances red blood cells are not produced by the spleen.

**50. The answer is C (2, 4).** (*Chapter 10 II A 2 d, C 4 a, E*) An elevated serum amylase level is diagnostic of acute, not chronic, pancreatitis; the serum amylase level is increased in 95% of pancreatitis patients during acute attacks. The presence of gallstones also does not help in making the diagnosis of chronic pancreatitis but may point to biliary tract disease. Chronic pancreatitis shows symptoms that are due to inflammation, fibrosis, and calcification. A history of unrelenting abdominal pain is usual in advanced cases of chronic pancreatitis. The damage to the pancreas may cause exocrine pancreatic insufficiency, leading to malabsorption and weight loss.

**51–55. The answers are: 51-A, 52-B, 53-E, 54-D, 55-C.** [*Chapter 22 I B 3 b, C 1 a, 2 a (2), 3 b; II C 2 a, D 1 a*] Multiple endocrine adenomatosis (MEA) syndromes are characteristic patterns of endocrine hyperfunction, which are inherited as autosomal dominant traits. In all MEA syndromes, the affected endocrine glands develop either hyperplasia, adenoma, or carcinoma.

MEA type I, or Wermer's syndrome, chiefly involves the parathyroid glands, pancreatic islet cells, and the pituitary gland. Hyperparathyroidism is present in 90% of patients, pancreatic tumors occur in 80%, and pituitary tumors occur in 65%. Most patients present with symptoms of peptic ulceration related to the pancreatic gastrinoma (Zollinger-Ellison syndrome) or with symptoms related to the pituitary tumor (e.g., acromegaly, galactorrhea, and Cushing's syndrome). The hyperparathyroidism usually is asymptomatic, evidenced only by an increased serum calcium level.

MEA type II, or Sipple's syndrome, involves medullary thyroid carcinoma (in all patients), pheochromocytoma (in 40% of patients), and parathyroid hyperplasia (in 60% of patients). Medullary thyroid carcinoma often is preceded by nonmalignant hyperplasia of the parafollicular C cells. An elevated serum thyrocalcitonin level is diagnostic. In the premalignant state, infusion of calcium and pentagastrin may be needed to demonstrate the abnormal thyrocalcitonemia.

MEA type III, or mucosal neuroma syndrome, is considered a variant of MEA type II, sharing with it the development of medullary thyroid carcinoma and pheochromocytoma. Patients with MEA type III are distinguished, however, by their characteristically distorted body habitus.

Pancreatic gastrinoma, or Zollinger-Ellison syndrome, is characterized by oversecretion of gastrin, most commonly due to a non-beta islet cell tumor. The excess gastrin stimulates hypersecretion of gastric acid, which ultimately results in peptic ulceration. Abdominal pain secondary to peptic ulceration occurs in 90% of patients. Diarrhea also is common.

Pancreatic cholera is believed to be caused by hypersecretion of vasoactive intestinal peptide (VIP) due to a pancreatic non-beta islet cell tumor. The syndrome sometimes is referred to as WDHA syndrome for its severe **w**atery **d**iarrhea, **h**ypokalemia, and **a**chlorhydria.

**56–60. The answers are: 56-B, 57-D, 58-C, 59-C, 60-D.** (*Chapter 5 III A 1–8, B 1–6*) The etiology of gastric ulcers is multifactorial, but damage to the gastric mucosal barrier appears to be the key. Reflux of bile into the stomach is thought to change the mucosal barrier, allowing gastric acid to enter the mucosa and injure it. Drugs such as ethanol, indomethacin, and salicylates can alter the mucosal barrier, and the combination of smoking and salicylate ingestion is strongly implicated in the development of gastric ulcers. Patients with gastric ulcers seem to have lower than normal rates of acid secretion. Although evidence suggests that gastric ulcer does not degenerate into carcinoma, gastric cancer will ulcerate in 25% of cases; thus, it is mandatory that nonhealing ulcers be examined histologically for signs of malignancy. Initial medical therapy is indicated for gastric ulcers; however, surgery is recommended if malignancy cannot be ruled out, if perforation or hemorrage occurs, or if medical therapy fails.

The major cause of duodenal ulcers is increased acid production. Smoking, caffeine ingestion, and aspirin use are all associated with an increased incidence of duodenal ulcer, but they have not proven to be causative. In the absence of complications, such as perforation, hemorrhage, or obstruction, medical management of duodenal ulcer is usually successful. Although stomach cancers can ulcerate and mimic ulcers, there is no evidence to suggest that benign ulcers can degenerate into cancer.

# Part I
# Introduction

# 1
# Surgical Principles

R. Anthony Carabasi, III
Herbert E. Cohn
Bruce E. Jarrell

John S. Radomski
Jerome J. Vernick
Stephen M. Weiss

## I. FLUID, ELECTROLYTE, AND ACID-BASE DISTURBANCES*

### A. General aspects

1. Fluid and electrolyte homeostasis is determined by the individual's intake and output, and is carefully and precisely regulated by the body during health.

2. The fluid and electrolyte losses and requirements of the normal healthy adult are shown in Table 1-1, and the normal distribution, volume, and electrolyte composition of body fluids are shown in Tables 1-2, 1-3, and 1-4.

3. In disease states, regulatory mechanisms often become impaired and imbalances occur. The surgeon frequently encounters these problems in patients because of the additional stress of surgery, the use of tubes that drain fluids which are not usually excreted, and a patient's inability to tolerate oral intake of fluids and nutrients.

### B. Fluid and electrolyte imbalance in surgical patients

1. Several **types of imbalance** can occur.
   a. **Isotonic hypohydration (dehydration)**, a proportionate loss of water and salt, is the most common type of deficit.
      (1) This imbalance can occur when patients have gastrointestinal losses without renal compensation, or when sweating is not compensated by adequate hypotonic fluid replacement.
      (2) Usual causes in surgical patients include vomiting and the presence of a Levin tube.
   b. **Hypertonic hypohydration** is the loss of water in excess of salt.
      (1) It can result from diarrhea, tube feeding, excess sweating, inadequate water intake, or corticosteroid therapy.
      (2) This imbalance is common in comatose patients who are not receiving fluid.
      (3) It can also occur in patients with diabetes insipidus (cerebral or renal), hyperosmolar coma, or protein or blood in the gastrointestinal tract.
   c. **Hypotonic hypohydration** is the loss of salt in excess of water. It can result from:
      (1) Gastrointestinal losses
      (2) Adrenal cortical insufficiency (as in Addison's disease)
      (3) Renal salt loss (as in excessive diuretic therapy)
      (4) Extravasation of fluid (as in pancreatitis, burns, or rapidly forming ascites)
      (5) Acute blood loss
      (6) Hypoalbuminemia
   d. **Hypervolemia**, an excess of circulating fluid (plasma), interstitial fluid, or intracellular fluid can result from the administration of intravenous fluid in excess of the body's needs and ability to excrete it.
   e. **Third-space loss** involves an obligatory loss of water, crystalloid, and colloid into an area of operative or pathologic injury. Examples are the edemas of cellulitis, peritonitis, operative injury, or burns. Recovery from capillary injury is marked by a spontaneous diuresis.

2. **Physiologic response to volume abnormalities**
   a. **Hypovolemia**, an abnormally low volume of body fluids, stimulates volume receptors in the juxtaglomerular apparatus, with the release of renin and thus of angiotensin.
      (1) This stimulates the adrenal cortex to secrete aldosterone. Aldosterone causes the kidney to retain sodium, raising the sodium concentration and osmolality of blood. This

---

*Author: Herbert E. Cohn

**Table 1-1.** Normal Daily Fluid and Electrolyte Losses and Requirements

| Substance | Losses/24 hr | | | | | Requirements/24 hr | |
| | | Insensible | | | | | |
| | Urine | Skin | Lungs | Feces | Total | Per kg of body weight | Total |
| --- | --- | --- | --- | --- | --- | --- | --- |
| Water | 1200–1500 ml* | 200–400 ml† | 500–700 ml† | 100–200 ml | 2300–2600 ml | 35 ml | ... |
| Sodium | 100 mEq‡ | 40 mEq/L of sweat | ... | ... | 80–100 mEq | 1 mEq | 60–80 mEq |
| Potassium | 100 mEq§ | ... | ... | ... | 80–100 mEq | 1 mEq | 60–80 mEq |
| Chloride | 150 mEq‡ | 40 mEq/L of sweat | ... | ... | 100–150 mEq | 1.5 mEq | ... |
| Bicarbonate | ... | ... | ... | ... | ... | 0.5 mEq | ... |

Note.—Calorie requirements include at least 100 g carbohydrates per 24 hours.
*25 ml/kg of body weight.
†10 ml/kg of body weight.
‡Varies with intake and with volume of urine and sweat. Autoregulated via renin–angiotensin–aldosterone system.
§Aldosterone increases excretion.

**Table 1-2.** Distribution of Body Water and Blood

| Compartment | Body Weight (%) |
|---|---|
| Total body water | 60–70* |
| Extracellular fluid | 20–25 |
|   Blood volume | 5–8† |
|     Red cell mass | 2–4 |
|     Plasma | 3–5 |
|   Interstitial fluid | 15–18 |
| Intracellular fluid | variable‡ |

*Percentage decreases as body fat increases.
†Percentage is greater in males than in females.
‡This figure cannot be measured easily.

**Table 1-3.** Volume of Various Body Fluids

| Substance | Volume (ml) |
|---|---|
| Saliva | 1500 |
| Gastric secretions | 2500 |
| Bile | 500–1500 |
| Pancreatic juice | 700 |
| Small bowel secretions | 3000 |
| Total | 8200–9200 |

stimulates the secretion of antidiuretic hormone (ADH) and results in water retention. This in turn will produce **hyponatremia** (abnormally low serum sodium concentration) if the patient continues to drink fluids.

(2) **Diuretics** can cause hypotonic dehydration by interfering with renal free-water clearance.

(3) If a patient with hyponatremia does not show signs of dehydration, it is likely that he or she is overhydrated and has dilutional hyponatremia, not a true sodium deficit.

  **b. Hypervolemia** suppresses aldosterone secretion, resulting in reduced tubular reabsorption of sodium, with a reduction in ADH secretion and consequently an increase in water excretion.

**3. Physiologic response to blood osmolality abnormalities**

  **a.** If plasma and glomerular filtrate are **hypertonic**, this stimulates osmoreceptors in the supraoptic nucleus to release ADH. The effect is to increase water resorption in the distal and collecting tubules, leading to the dilution of plasma and reduction of plasma osmolality.

  **b. Hypotonicity** leads to a decrease in ADH secretion, a decrease in tubular resorption of water, and an increase in urine volume with a loss of water in excess of electrolyte losses.

**C. Acid-base imbalance in surgical patients**

  **1.** In **metabolic acidosis**, bicarbonate ($HCO_3^-$) is used up or lost.

    **a.** Serum bicarbonate concentration is decreased and carbonic acid ($H_2CO_3$) is unchanged.

    **b.** The usual causes are vomiting, dehydration, starvation, diabetes, or renal failure.

**Table 1-4.** Electrolyte Composition of Body Fluids

| Substance | Electrolyte Content (mEq/L) | | | | | | | |
|---|---|---|---|---|---|---|---|---|
| | $Na^+$ | $K^+$ | $H^+$ | $Cl^-$ | $HCO_3^-$ | Protein* | $PO_4^-$ | $SO_4^-$ |
| Plasma | 142 | 4.5 | . . . | 100 | 25 | 16 | 2 | 1 |
| Gastric juice | | | | | | | | |
|   High-acid | 45 | 30 | 70 | 120 | 25 | . . . | . . . | . . . |
|   Low-acid | 100 | 45 | 0.015 | 115 | 30 | . . . | . . . | . . . |
| Intestinal juice | 120 | 20 | . . . | 110 | 30 | . . . | . . . | . . . |
|   Bile | 140 | 5 | . . . | . . . | 40 | . . . | . . . | . . . |
|   Pancreatic juice | 130 | 15 | . . . | . . . | 80 | . . . | . . . | . . . |
| Intracellular fluid | 10 | 150 | . . . | 5 | 10 | 60 | 100 | 20 |

*Subject to wide variation in gastric and intestinal fluids.

2. In **metabolic alkalosis**, there is an excess of bicarbonate.
   **a.** Serum bicarbonate concentration is increased and carbonic acid is unchanged.
   **b.** The usual causes are pyloric obstruction, potassium loss, or alkali excess.

3. In **respiratory acidosis**, carbon dioxide is retained in the body.
   **a.** Serum bicarbonate concentration is unchanged and carbonic acid is increased.
   **b.** The usual causes are chronic pulmonary disease, respiratory depression, or the effects of anesthesia.

4. In **respiratory alkalosis**, carbon dioxide excretion is increased.
   **a.** Serum bicarbonate concentration is unchanged and carbonic acid is decreased.
   **b.** The usual cause is hyperventilation.

**D. Determining the presence of fluid and electrolyte imbalance**

1. A **history** of vomiting (with or without bile) or diarrhea, especially if severe or prolonged, should alert one to the possibility of imbalance.

2. The **physical examination** should give attention to:
   **a.** The patient's present weight versus his or her normal weight
   **b.** Skin turgor
   **c.** Moistness of mucous membranes
   **d.** Venous filling
   **e.** Blood pressure and pulse
   **f.** Ocular tension

3. **Laboratory tests** of importance include:
   **a.** Hematocrit
   **b.** Urine specific gravity
   **c.** Sodium levels in urine and serum
   **d.** Central venous pressure
   **e.** Pulmonary wedge pressure

**E. Determining the amount of the deficit or imbalance**

1. A **volume (water) deficit** can be estimated clinically from the patient's body weight and appearance or can be calculated from the serum sodium level. The hematocrit also gives useful information.
   **a. Clinical estimates**
      **(1)** In **mild dehydration**, the patient loses 3% of the body weight and expresses thirst.
      **(2)** In **moderate dehydration**, 6% of the body weight is lost and clinical signs of dehydration are evident:
         **(a)** Marked thirst and dry mouth
         **(b)** No groin or axillary sweat
         **(c)** Loss of skin turgor
      **(3)** In **severe dehydration**, 10% of the body weight is lost, clinical signs of dehydration are marked, hypotension may be present, and the patient may be confused or delirious.
   **b. Body water calculation.** The formula is as follows:

$$\text{Body water} = \frac{\text{normal serum Na}^+}{\text{measured serum Na}^+} \times \text{normal body water,}$$

where normal body water = $0.6 \times$ body weight, and normal serum $Na^+$ = 140 mEq/L.

2. **Electrolyte deficits** are calculated after laboratory tests have provided the serum levels of the following ions: sodium, potassium, chloride, and bicarbonate.
   **a. Sodium, chloride**, and **bicarbonate deficits** are calculated using the following equation:

$$\text{Deficit} = \frac{\text{normal value (mEq/L) } -}{\text{observed value (mEq/L)}} \times \frac{\text{electrolyte distribution in body}}{\text{compartment (\%)} \times \text{body weight (kg),}}$$

where the sodium distribution = 60%, the chloride distribution = 20%, and the bicarbonate distribution = 50%. (Despite the fact that sodium is primarily an extracellular ion, the sodium space is considered to equal total body water because sodium controls total body osmolality. Therefore, 60% is used in the calculation.)
   **b.** The **potassium deficit** is figured differently. **With a normal blood pH:**
      **(1)** For every 1.0 mEq/L decrease in the potassium concentration at or above 3.0 mEq/L, consider the total body deficit as 100 to 200 mEq.

**(2)** For every 1.0 mEq/L decrease in the potassium concentration below 3.0 mEq/L, consider the total body deficit as **another** 300 to 400 mEq/l.

3. The type of **acid-base imbalance** is determined on the basis of the following formula for normal acid-base status:

$$\frac{Serum\ HCO_3^-}{Serum\ H_2CO_3} = \frac{20}{1} .$$

   **a.** A decrease in the "numerator" of this ratio (e.g., from 20/1 to 10/1) signifies **metabolic acidosis**.
   **b.** An increase in the "numerator" of this ratio (e.g., from 20/1 to 30/1) signifies **metabolic alkalosis**.
   **c.** An increase in the "denominator" of this ratio (e.g., from 20/1 to 20/2) signifies **respiratory acidosis**.
   **d.** A decrease in the "denominator" of this ratio (e.g., from 20/1 to 20/0.5) signifies **respiratory alkalosis**.

**F. Principles of managing fluid, electrolyte, and acid-base imbalances**

   **1. Priorities**
      **a.** Correct shock and restore blood volume to normal.
      **b.** Restore colloid osmotic pressure.
      **c.** Correct acid-base imbalance.
      **d.** Restore blood osmolality.
      **e.** Correct potassium deficits.
      **f.** Correct total body electrolyte disturbances (static debt) and establish daily maintenance.
      **g.** Establish daily caloric maintenance.

   **2. Deficit correction** is defined as the fluid and electrolyte therapy necessary to correct existing deficits.
      **a. Examples of existing deficits** include:
         **(1)** Blood volume deficit in acute or chronic blood loss
         **(2)** Extracellular or intracellular deficit in dehydration
      **b.** Fluid and electrolytes to replace existing deficits must be administered in addition to maintenance and replacement therapy in order to restore water, salt, and acid-base balance.
      **c.** Deficit correction has **top priority** in fluid and electrolyte therapy.

   **3. Replacement therapy** is defined as the fluid and electrolyte therapy necessary to replace abnormal (continuing) losses from or within the body (e.g., via drainage tubes).
      **a. Examples of continuing losses**
         **(1) Gastrointestinal losses**
            **(a)** If these are purely gastric (succus gastricus), a solution providing 0.45% sodium chloride plus 40 mEq potassium chloride per L is used for replacement.
            **(b)** If the fluid lost also contains intestinal juice (succus entericus), lactated Ringer's solution plus 10 mEq potassium chloride per L is used for replacement.
         **(2) Third-space loss**
            **(a)** The amount of loss varies with the magnitude of the injury.
            **(b)** Lactated Ringer's solution plus albumin is used for replacement.
      **b.** Continuing losses require **volume-for-volume replacement** and must be added to maintenance requirements.
      **c.** Replacement therapy has **second priority** in fluid and electrolyte therapy.

   **4. Maintenance therapy** is defined as the fluid and electrolyte therapy necessary to maintain fluid and electrolyte balance in an individual.
      **a.** If inadequate calories are provided, maintenance therapy should be associated with a weight loss of approximately 1/4 to 1/2 lb/day.
      **b.** Weight gain in the absence of adequate caloric intake connotes excessive fluid intake.

   **5.** Table 1-1 lists the daily maintenance requirements for fluid and electrolytes after existing deficits have been corrected. Table 1-5 lists commonly used electrolyte solutions and their principal uses.

**G. Clinical examples**

   **1. Maintenance therapy**
      **a.** This provides the fluid and electrolytes necessary to satisfy the normal requirements in the absence of abnormal losses.

**Table 1-5.** Commonly Used Parenteral Solutions

| Solutions | Na⁺ | K⁺ | Cl⁻ | HCO⁻₃ | Ca²⁺ | Principal Uses |
|---|---|---|---|---|---|---|
| | Electrolyte Content | | | | | |

| Solutions | Na$^+$ | K$^+$ | Cl$^-$ | HCO$^-_3$ | Ca$^{2+}$ | Principal Uses |
|---|---|---|---|---|---|---|
| | (mEq/L) | | | | | |
| 0.9% (isotonic) sodium chloride (saline)* | 154 | . . . | 154 | . . . | . . . | Correction of hyponatremia; ECF replacement |
| 0.45% (1/2 normal) sodium chloride* | 77 | . . . | 77 | . . . | . . . | Na$^+$ maintenance; gastric fluid replacement |
| Lactated Ringer's solution* | 130 | 4 | 109 | 28 | 3 | Best ECF replacement; correction of isosmolar deficit |
| 5% dextrose in water | . . . | . . . | . . . | . . . | . . . | Correction of insensible water loss; maintenance; correction of hyperosmolar dehydration |
| | (mEq/dl) | | | | | |
| 3% sodium chloride injection | 51 | . . . | 51 | . . . | . . . | Correction of symptomatic Na$^+$ deficit |
| 5% sodium chloride injection | 85 | . . . | 85 | . . . | . . . | Correction of symptomatic Na$^+$ deficit |
| | (mEq/ampul) | | | | | |
| 14.9% potassium chloride (20-ml ampul) | . . . | 40 | 40 | . . . | . . . | Additive for K$^+$ maintenance; correction of K$^+$ and acid-base imbalance |
| 7.5% sodium bicarbonate | 44.6 | . . . | . . . | 44.6 | . . . | Additive for GI losses; correction of metabolic acidosis |

Abbreviations.—ECF = extracellular fluid; GI = gastrointestinal.
*With or without 5% dextrose.

    **b. Example.** An average-sized (60-kg) woman has had an elective cholecystectomy. No nasogastric tube is placed and there is no T tube.
      **(1)** The patient's **normal daily requirements** would be calculated as follows:
        **(a)** Water: 35 ml/kg × 60 kg = 2100 ml
        **(b)** Sodium: 1 mEq/kg × 60 kg = 60 mEq
        **(c)** Potassium: 1 mEq/kg × 60 kg = 60 mEq
        **(d)** Chloride: 1.5 mEq/kg × 60 kg = 90 mEq
        **(e)** Bicarbonate: 0.5 mEq/kg × 60 kg = 30 mEq. (In a healthy individual, the bicarbonate buffer system is so efficient that one can ignore small bicarbonate requirements.)
      **(2)** The **intravenous (IV) fluid orders** would be as follows:
        **(a)** 1000 ml 5% dextrose in H$_2$O + 40 mEq KCl. (One should try not to exceed a concentration of 40 mEq K$^+$/L for maintenance.)
        **(b)** 650 ml 5% dextrose in H$_2$O + 20 mEq KCl
        **(c)** 450 ml 5% dextrose in lactated Ringer's solution
      **(3)** This will provide:
        **(a)** 2100 ml of H$_2$O
        **(b)** 58.5 mEq of Na$^+$ (4.5 × 13 mEq/dl)
        **(c)** 61.8 mEq of K$^+$ (40 mEq/L + 20 mEq/L + 1.8 mEq from lactated Ringer's solution)
        **(d)** 109 mEq of Cl$^-$ (49 mEq from lactated Ringer's solution + 60 mEq from KCl)
        **(e)** 12.6 mEq of HCO$_3^-$ (4.5 × 2.8 mEq/dl from lactated Ringer's solution)
      **(4)** In addition to the **type and quantity** of fluid ordered, the **rate of administration** should be stated (e.g., 100 ml/hr, 250 ml/hr, and so forth), depending on the volume of fluid required for a 24-hour period in a given patient.
      **(5)** Maintenance fluids can normally be delivered over an 8- to 10-hour period, and the IV line can then be removed, or can be capped if required for additional therapy.

  **2. Replacement therapy**
    **a.** This provides the fluid and electrolytes necessary to replace abnormal losses from the body or within the body.

**b. Example.** The same patient as in section G 1 b develops an ileus after her cholecystectomy, requiring insertion of a nasogastric tube. Over the next 24 hours, there is a recorded 1600 ml of nasogastric drainage, which is bile-stained. Serum electrolytes are normal.

(1) The patient's **requirements** would now be as follows:

(a) For **replacement**, she would require 1600 ml as 5% dextrose in lactated Ringer's solution + 10 mEq KCl/L.

(b) Her **maintenance** requirements would remain the same as in section G 1 b (1).

(2) Therefore, the **IV fluid orders** would become:

(a) 1000 ml 5% dextrose in $H_2O$ + 30 mEq KCl

(b) 1000 ml 5% dextrose in $H_2O$ + 30 mEq KCl

(c) 1000 ml 5% dextrose in lactated Ringer's solution + 10 mEq KCl

(d) 1000 ml 5% dextrose in lactated Ringer's solution + 10 mEq KCl to run at a rate of 170 ml/hr (600 ml is for replacement requirements and 400 ml is part of the maintenance requirements).

**3. Hypertonic dehydration**

**a.** In hypertonic dehydration, the serum sodium concentration is elevated.

**b. Example 1.** A moderately lean woman with an esophageal stricture has a serum sodium level of 160 mEq/L (normal: 140 mEq/L). Her present weight is 70 kg. Her requirements would be calculated as follows:

(1) Present body water:

$$\frac{140\ mEq/L}{160\ mEq/L} = 7/8 = 87.5\%\ of\ normal$$

(2) Water loss: 100% − 87.5% = 12.5%

(3) Patient's normal total body water: 70 kg × 60% = 42 L

(a) The formula used here is body weight × body water space.

(b) Although the patient's present weight was used instead of calculating her weight prior to dehydration, the error is minimal.

(4) Water deficit: 42 L × 12.5% = 5.3 L

(5) Fluid requirement: 2.7 L + 2.4 L = 5.1 L of fluid in next 24 hours, containing 70 mEq of sodium.

(a) The formula used here is 1/2 the water deficit (5.3 L/2) + normal daily fluid requirement (2.4 L).

(b) To this is added the normal daily sodium requirement (70 mEq).

**c. Example 2.** If this patient had diarrhea as well as an esophageal stricture and had presented with weakness, confusion, and hypotension, her requirements would be calculated as follows:

(1) Present body water:

$$\frac{140\ mEq/L}{160\ mEq/L} = 7/8 = 87.5\%\ of\ normal$$

(2) Water loss: 100% − 87.5% = 12.5%

(3) Patient's normal total body water: 70 kg × 60% = 42 L

(4) Water deficit: 42 L × 12.5% = 5.3 L

(5) However, the patient's clinical findings indicate that she now has a dehydration of at least 10% of her body weight. Therefore, the calculations are changed as follows (as before, using the patient's present weight instead of her normal weight gives a negligible error):

(a) Fluid loss: 10% of 70 kg = 7 L

(b) Isotonic fluid loss: 7 L − 5.3 L = 1.7 L

(c) Sodium loss (in isotonic fluid): 1.7 L × 140 mEq/L = 238 mEq

(d) 24-hour fluid requirement: 7 L/2 + 2.4 L = 5.9 L

(e) 24-hour sodium requirement: 238 mEq/2 + 70 mEq = 189 mEq

(6) This can be given as 4 L of 5% dextrose in water plus 1200 ml of normal saline.

**4. Isotonic dehydration**

**a.** In isotonic dehydration, the serum sodium concentration is normal.

**b. Example.** A short, obese alcoholic patient presents with vomiting due to gastritis and with a fever of 102.6° F due to pneumonitis. He is complaining of thirst and a dry mouth, and has no groin or axillary sweat. He is alert and normotensive. His weight is 100 kg; his serum sodium level is 140 mEq/L and his serum potassium level is 3.0 mEq/L. His requirements would be calculated as follows:

(1) Fluid loss: 6% (based on clinical findings)

(2) Isotonic fluid loss: 100 kg × 6% = 6 L

    **(3)** Sodium loss (in isotonic fluid): 140 mEq/L × 6 L = 840 mEq

    **(4)** 24-hour sodium requirement: 840 mEq/2 + 100 mEq = 520 mEq

    **(5)** 24-hour fluid requirement: 6 L/2 + 4.9 L = 7.9 L

        **(a)** The daily fluid requirement is 4.9 L instead of 3.5 L because of the patient's fever: Each 1-degree rise in temperature increases the daily fluid requirement by at least 10%.

        **(b)** The fluid and sodium replacement can be given as 3 L of 5% glucose in normal saline, 2 L of 5% dextrose in water, and 200 ml of normal saline.

            **(i)** Potassium chloride should be added as indicated, at 1/2 of the deficit plus the daily requirement (100 mEq), provided that urine flow is adequate.

            **(ii)** Thus, since the patient has a potassium deficit of 200 mEq (see section I E 2 b), (1/2 × 200) + 100 mEq of KCl would be divided among all the solutions.

**5. Hypotonic dehydration**

  **a.** In hypotonic dehydration, the serum sodium concentration is decreased.

  **b. Example.** A muscular 50-year-old man with polycystic kidney disease presents with hypotension, weakness, confusion, oliguria, and no axillary sweat.

    **(1)** His past medical record shows that he has polyuria, he has been eating a low-salt diet because of mild hypertension, his blood urea nitrogen has been stable at 40 mg/dl, and his blood carbon dioxide content has been 20 mmol/L.

    **(2)** He now has a metabolic acidosis with a blood carbon dioxide content of 15 mmol/L and a serum sodium level of 120 mEq/L. His body weight is 90 kg, and his urine output is 170 ml/day.

    **(3)** His requirements would be calculated as follows:

        **(a)** Hypotonic sodium deficit: 54 L × 20 mEq/L = 1080 mEq

            **(i)** The formula used here is $Na^+$ deficit × total body water [i.e., (ideal $Na^+$ − actual $Na^+$) × body weight × $Na^+$ space].

            **(ii)** For our patient, the figures used are:
$Na^+$ deficit: 140 mEq/L − 120 mEq/L = 20 mEq/L
Total body water: 90 kg × 60% = 54 L

        **(b)** Isotonic sodium deficit: 9 L × 140 mEq/L = 1260 mEq

            **(i)** Fluid loss: 10% (based on clinical findings)

            **(ii)** Isotonic fluid loss: 90 kg × 10% = 9 L

        **(c)** 24-hour sodium requirement:

$$\frac{(1080 \text{ mEq} + 1260 \text{ mEq})}{2} + 75 \text{ mEq} = 1245 \text{ mEq}$$

        **(d)** 24-hour water requirement: 9 L/2 + 600 ml = 5.1 L

            **(i)** The daily water requirement in an oliguric patient is reduced.

            **(ii)** The formula is 0.2 ml/kg body weight + preceding 24-hour output + 10% for each 1-degree rise in body temperature.

            **(iii)** For our patient, this would be (0.2 × 90 × 24) + 170 = 602, or 600 ml/day.

        **(e)** Bicarbonate requirement:

            **(i)** The ideal replacement solution should contain a sodium-to-chloride ratio of 1.4 to 1, particularly if the patient has acidosis.

            **(ii)** Therefore, since the patient's sodium requirement is 1245 mEq, the chloride requirement is:

$$\frac{1.4}{1} = \frac{1245 \text{ (mEq sodium)}}{x \text{ (mEq chloride)}}$$

$$x = \frac{1245}{1.4} = 890 \text{ mEq as sodium chloride.}$$

            **(iii)** The bicarbonate requirement is thus 1245 − 890 = 355 mEq as sodium bicarbonate.

    **(4)** The patient's requirements can be given as 8 vials of sodium bicarbonate (44 mEq/50 ml) added to 4.8 L of 5% dextrose in **0.9%** sodium chloride plus 200 ml of **5%** sodium chloride injection.

## II. NUTRITIONAL CONSIDERATIONS IN THE SURGICAL PATIENT*

  **A. Nutrient stores and body composition**

    **1. Fat** is the chief form of energy storage in the human body.

---

*Author: Stephen M. Weiss

    **a.** The standard 70-kg man has about 15 kg of fat, equivalent to about 135,000 kcal.

    **b.** Fat is necessary as a source of essential fatty acids—linoleic, linolenic, and arachidonic.

    **c.** During fasting, stored fat is metabolized to free fatty acids and ketone bodies, which are used for energy by most body tissues.

    **d.** Glycerol from fat is used for gluconeogenesis, providing energy for nerve cells and blood cells during fasting.

  **2. Carbohydrate** is present in several forms in the body, but in small amounts.

    **a.** Circulating glucose supplies about 80 kcal.

    **b.** Liver glycogen provides about 300 kcal of carbohydrate, which can be released into the circulation as glucose.

    **c.** Muscle glycogen contains 600 kcal of carbohydrate, which is expended during muscle contraction.

  **3. Protein** comprises about 6 kg of a 70-kg man, for a caloric value of 24,000 kcal. Body protein is present in several forms:

    **a.** Muscle (skeletal, smooth, and cardiac)

    **b.** Circulating proteins, such as albumin and antibodies

    **c.** Other molecules, such as enzymes

**B. Nutrient requirements**

  **1. Energy needs**

    **a.** Most hospitalized patients require between 35 and 45 kcal/kg of body weight/day [1 **kilocalorie (kcal)** = 1 Calorie (1 Cal) = 1000 calories].

    **b.** Basal caloric needs (e.g., for nonstressed persons at bed rest) are 25 to 35 kcal/kg/day.

    **c.** Patients with heightened metabolism, such as those with multiple injuries, sepsis, or extensive burns, may require 50 to 70 kcal/kg/day.

    **d. Sources of energy** include:

      **(1) Fat**, providing 9 kcal/g

      **(2) Carbohydrate**, providing approximately 4 kcal/g

        **(a)** Dextrose in intravenous solutions provides 3.4 kcal/g

        **(b)** One L of 5% dextrose in water contains 50 g of monohydrated dextrose and provides about 170 kcal.

    **e. Protein** provides 4 kcal/g, although it is not usually considered as a source of energy.

  **2. Protein requirements**

    **a.** The average 70-kg adult man loses about 70 g of protein per day.

      **(1)** This protein must be replaced in order to maintain protein equilibrium (or nitrogen equilibrium).

      **(2)** 6.25 g of protein are equivalent to 1 g of body nitrogen.

    **b.** A daily intake of 1 to 1.5 g of protein per kg of body weight will satisfy the requirements of most adult surgical patients.

    **c.** A restricted protein intake may be necessary in diseases that impair nitrogen excretion or metabolism, such as renal failure or hepatic cirrhosis.

    **d.** An increased protein intake is required in patients with conditions that cause excessive catabolism, such as sepsis, multiple fractures, or burns.

  **3.** A **calorie-to-nitrogen ratio** of 150 to 200 kcal per g of nitrogen is appropriate for surgical patients.

**C. Malnutrition**

  **1.** The **causes** of malnutrition in surgical patients are varied:

    **a. Increased catabolism**, in excess of nutrient intake (e.g., a patient with sepsis may be unable to increase his oral intake to provide sufficient calories and protein)

    **b. Nutrient losses** (e.g., a patient with cirrhosis can lose albumin in ascites fluid and become protein-depleted)

    **c. Decreased intake**, the most common reason for malnutrition (e.g., impaired taste perception, a common occurrence in cancer patients, results in diminished oral intake)

    **d. Decreased absorption** (e.g., patients with malabsorption syndrome, intestinal fistulas, or short bowel syndrome may not absorb ingested nutrients)

  **2.** Most commonly, patients are malnourished for a combination of reasons. For example:

    **a.** A patient with pancreatic cancer may be malnourished because of a decreased appetite, steatorrhea from pancreatic exocrine insufficiency, and increased nutritional requirements because of surgery.

    **b.** A trauma patient has a high expenditure of calories because of multiple injuries complicated by sepsis, yet is unable to eat because of prolonged ileus.

3. **Protein–calorie malnutrition**, the most common type of malnutrition in surgical patients, is characterized by diminished body stores of fat and protein. A marasmus-like state is characterized by depletion of body fat but relative sparing of visceral protein.

4. **Protein malnutrition**, sometimes considered a kwashiorkor-like state, is characterized by depletion of body protein with relative sparing of body fat, as may occur in an acutely ill, starved patient. Such patients may look well nourished or even obese, but can be profoundly malnourished.

D. **Evaluation of nutritional status** is an important aspect in the care of surgical patients.

1. The **history** and **physical examination** provide the most efficient means of assessing the patient's nutritional status.
   a. A history of weight loss, change in appetite, or gastrointestinal symptoms can be important.
   b. In the physical examination, malnutrition is suggested by muscle wasting, edema, or the loss of normal smooth skin contours over bony prominences. **Anthropometric measurements**, such as the triceps skinfold thickness to estimate body fat and midarm muscle circumference to estimate skeletal muscle mass, are useful but imprecise.
   c. **Indirect calorimetry** is useful to measure the caloric requirements of acutely ill patients: oxygen consumption and carbon dioxide production are measured and are used to calculate caloric expenditure.

2. **Laboratory tests** are also helpful.
   a. Serum albumin levels give an inexpensive measurement of visceral protein status. Total iron-binding capacity and levels of serum transferrin, prealbumin, and retinol-binding protein can also be used.
   b. The total lymphocyte count may be decreased in malnutrition, and a count below 1500/mm³ is associated with a poor prognosis.
   c. Delayed hypersensitivity to skin test antigens is correlated with nutritional status and with results of treatment, but the absence of delayed hypersensitivity is not specific for malnutrition.

3. The patient's current nutrient intake is an important aspect of nutritional assessment that can be ascertained relatively easily, whether the intake is oral or parenteral.

E. **Nutritional therapy**

1. **Oral feeding** of nutrients is the most efficient, most pleasant, least expensive, and most widely used form of therapy, both for hospital inpatients and for outpatients.
   a. The patient's actual caloric and protein intake should be determined and compared to estimated requirements.
   b. For patients whose oral intake is insufficient for their estimated needs, a variety of reasonably palatable oral supplements are available.

2. **Enteric feedings** are useful for patients whose digestive systems are functional but who are unable to take adequate nutrients by mouth.
   a. Several **routes** are available for administration:
      (1) **Feeding tubes** are soft, small-diameter tubes passed via the nose into the stomach or duodenum.
      (2) **Enterostomies** are surgically created openings into the stomach (**gastrostomy**), small bowel (**jejunostomy**), or esophagus (**esophagostomy**). Enterostomies are appropriate for long-term enteric feedings.
   b. **Nutrient solutions** are available in a variety of formulas that provide all the necessary nutrients in appropriate proportions. Most are nonhyperosmolar, reduced in residue, and lactose-free, and most are inexpensive.
   c. There are several potential **complications** of enteric feedings:
      (1) **Aspiration** can be avoided by eliminating large-volume, intermittent (bolus) feedings, and by feeding directly into the jejunum when patients are not alert.
      (2) **Diarrhea** is minimized by avoiding hyperosmolar or bolus feedings, and by taking care to prevent bacterial overgrowth in the nutrient solutions.

3. **Parenteral nutrition** (also called **intravenous hyperalimentation**) can be used to provide all or part of a patient's nutrients for an indefinite period of time.
   a. Because it completely avoids the gastrointestinal tract, parenteral nutrition is useful for patients who lack intestinal function and thus are likely to become malnourished.
   b. In this procedure, a central venous catheter inserted into the superior vena cava is used to administer a hypertonic nutrient solution whose components include:
      (1) A source of calories, usually a combination of carbohydrate (25% dextrose) and fat

(2) A protein source, typically a mixture of synthesized amino acids (protein hydrolysates were used in the past)

(3) Water in adequate amounts to satisfy maintenance requirements

(4) Vitamins, both water- and fat-soluble

(5) Trace metals, needed primarily as enzyme cofactors—zinc, copper, manganese, selenium, chromium

(6) Minerals and other nutrients—sodium, potassium, chloride, calcium, sulfate, phosphate, and magnesium

c. A typical prescription for parenteral nutrition is given in Table 1-6.

d. **Complications**, once considered common, can be minimized by experience and by careful metabolic monitoring.

(1) **Catheter-related complications**

(a) Pneumothorax, arterial puncture, or malpositioning the catheter can occur during attempts to insert the catheter. Complications are infrequent when the physician is experienced and the patient is cooperative, is well hydrated, and has normal blood coagulation.

(b) Great vein thrombosis can develop from a catheter's irritating the intima of the vena cava and subclavian vein. Thrombosis can be minimized by the use of soft catheters; some clinicians advocate adding small amounts of heparin to the infusion in order to minimize thrombosis.

(c) Sepsis increases in incidence with faulty catheter maintenance techniques. The most frequent pathogens (coagulase-positive and -negative staphylococci, candida) are normal skin flora.

(2) **Metabolic complications** can develop if either too much or too little of any nutrient is given, and can be minimized by supplying the patient's nutritional requirements and by judicious blood chemistry monitoring. The following complications are most common:

(a) **Water overload** occurs when a patient receives excessive fluid (usually via a peripheral vein) in addition to parenteral feeding. Weight gain in excess of 3 lb/week is usually from overhydration.

(b) **Hyperglycemia**, most likely to develop in a diabetic patient or a stressed patient, occurs when glucose is administered more rapidly than the patient's pancreas can tolerate.

**Table 1-6.** Prescription for Daily Total Parenteral Nutrition

| Infusion solution: | | |
| --- | --- | --- |
| Water | 2000 | ml |
| Dextrose | 500 | g |
| Carbohydrate calories | 1700 | kcal |
| Amino acids | 85 | g |
| Sodium | 70 | mEq |
| Potassium | 60 | mEq |
| Magnesium | 10 | mEq |
| Calcium | 10 | mEq |
| Acetate | 135 | mEq |
| Chloride | 70 | mEq |
| Phosphate | 30 | mEq |
| Copper | 1 | mg |
| Chromium | 0.01 | mg |
| Manganese | 0.5 | mg |
| Zinc | 10 | mg |
| IV fat solution 10%* | 500 | ml |
| Water- and fat-soluble vitamins | | |

**Schedule:**

Infuse solution over 12 hours

8:00 P.M.—Begin TPN infusion at 50 ml/hr for 30 minutes
8:30 P.M.—Increase rate to 170 ml/hr for 11 hours
7:30 A.M.—Decrease rate to 50 ml/hr for 30 minutes
8:00 A.M.—Stop TPN infusion
          Irrigate Hickman catheter with heparin 250 units/2.5 ml

*Provides 550 kcal/day.

(c) **Hypoglycemia** may occur in a glucose-intolerant patient if an infusion of hypertonic dextrose is suddenly stopped. Reactive hypoglycemia is not likely to occur in a patient who is not diabetic, even if the infusion is rapidly stopped.

(d) **Hepatic cholestasis** may develop in patients receiving high-caloric long-term total parenteral nutrition.

**e. Special parenteral solutions**

(1) Patients with oliguric renal failure may require:

(a) A higher dextrose concentration in a smaller daily volume

(b) Essential amino acids instead of mixed essential and nonessential amino acids

(2) Patients with liver failure may be given a high percentage of branched-chain amino acids (leucine, isoleucine, valine) to reduce the risk of encephalopathy.

(3) Formula modifications are also used in patients with sepsis, trauma, and congestive heart failure.

# III. SURGICAL TUBES*

**A. Postoperative drainage tubes.** Various types of tubes are used in surgery to permit drainage of material that is either abnormal, such as pus, or is a normal body fluid that cannot be handled normally by the body. Sometimes use of a tube is mandatory, such as a chest tube for a tension pneumothorax; in some situations, use is controversial.

**1. Types of drains**

**a. Closed drains** are tubes connecting a body cavity to a sealed reservoir.

(1) **Gravity drainage** allows whatever material that collects to drain out through the tube into a reservoir at a lower level. If the tube is allowed to remain filled, it will act as a siphon, suctioning material into the lower reservoir.

(2) An **underwater-seal drainage system** prevents air and fluid from reentering the body.

(a) It is used whenever the pleural space admits air, such as for a thoracotomy or pneumothorax.

(b) The end of the drainage tube is under water, in a sealed drainage bottle at floor level. The water prevents air from reentering the tube; the low level prevents fluid from siphoning back.

(3) **Suction drainage** applies a low level of suction at the distal end of the drainage tube. This will adequately drain a large production of fluid, such as develops in the gastrointestinal tract. It also promotes closure of "dead space," allowing better approximation of tissue surfaces.

**b. Open drains** are not sealed at either end. They allow bacteria and other materials access to the drained area, and as a result carry a higher risk of deep wound infection. Open drains have been used for many years, however, and are frequently part of the surgical routine in some centers.

**c. Sump drains** are dual-lumen catheters that allow air or irrigation fluid to enter through one lumen while suction is applied to the other lumen.

(1) When air is allowed to enter, a filter should be used to prevent the entrance of microorganisms.

(2) The entrance of air into the drain produces a sump effect; that is, free fluid is suctioned into the tube.

(3) Sump drains can be used as continuous irrigation catheters for closed spaces that are not accessible otherwise, such as deep abdominal abscesses.

**2. Conditions requiring drainage**

**a.** Drainage is clearly indicated in certain conditions. These include:

(1) Pneumothorax or any operative procedure that involves entering the pleural space. Chest tube drainage is absolutely indicated for a tension pneumothorax and for any patient on a ventilator following thoracotomy.

(2) A gastrointestinal tract that has been nonfunctioning for a prolonged period (more than 1 or 2 days). Nasogastric drainage, usually with a sump tube, is required.

(a) The decompression lessens abdominal distention, intestinal dilation, nausea, and vomiting.

(b) Drainage also allows a determination of the amount and type of fluid loss so that appropriate replacement can be made.

(3) Areas where extensive dissection has been performed in a closed space

(a) This applies to surgical procedures performed on solid organs such as the liver or a kidney where hemostasis is sometimes difficult and a postoperative hematoma is likely (see section III A 3 c).

---

*Authors: Bruce E. Jarrell and Jerome J. Vernick

          **(b)** It also applies to procedures such as mastectomies or skin flaps where there is a large raw area and little surrounding tissue to tamponade the bleeding.
     **(4)** Abscesses that do not communicate with the skin and thus do not provide direct access for local wound management
          **(a)** This usually involves a deep but well-walled-off abscess cavity, such as a subphrenic, subhepatic, or periappendiceal abscess.
          **(b)** Drains should not be relied upon to control a generalized infection such as cellulitis or suppurative peritonitis.
  **b.** Drains are often used after certain surgical procedures, although they are of unproven value:
     **(1)** In the gallbladder bed after cholecystectomy
     **(2)** In the pancreatic region after pancreatic surgery
     **(3)** In the duodenal stump after gastrectomy with Billroth II reconstruction [see section III A 4 c (3)]
     **(4)** In the pelvis after low anterior resection of the colon

**3. Caveats and complications**
  **a.** The presence of a drain does not guarantee the absence of an abscess or other collection. The foreign body reaction can isolate a drain from adjacent tissues, preventing blood, pus, or other fluid from having access to the lumen.
  **b.** Drains, and therefore the tissues that they traverse, can be colonized by microorganisms from exogenous sources. Drains increase the risk of infection in some settings, particularly where open drainage systems are used. Avoiding bacterial colonization requires careful wound care at the drain's exit site.
  **c.** A drain should not be regarded as a substitute for hemostasis. No drain will continue to function in the presence of active bleeding. Hematomas are likely to develop despite drainage if hemostasis is not adequate.
  **d.** A rigid drain may erode through the wall of a blood vessel or a hollow intestinal structure. This complication can be minimized by using soft drains and removing drains early.
  **e.** Excessive suction on a tube can also cause necrosis of nearby structures. Intermittent low-level suction is safer.
  **f.** A drain in direct contact with a fistula may perpetuate the fistula and prevent or delay its healing. The drain must be advanced beyond the fistula now and then if further healing is to occur.
  **g.** Drains may become detached from the skin and retract into the body, especially into the peritoneal cavity. Thus, they should always be firmly taped to the skin and should be marked with a radiopaque marker. A safety pin is also helpful to keep drains outside the body.

**4. Removal.** Drains should be removed when they have fulfilled their purpose.
  **a.** When the main risk of leakage has passed, following a surgical procedure, the drain is removed.
     **(1)** After a cholecystectomy, if a bile leak from a common duct injury is present, it should be evident in 1 or 2 days. Thus, drains are normally removed by the second day.
     **(2)** After urinary bladder procedures, a urinary leak will occur when the bladder catheter is removed. Thus, drains are removed a day after the catheter is removed.
  **b.** When a drain is used for postoperative fluid collections (blood, serum, lymph), it is removed when no further drainage occurs.
  **c.** When the drain is used as part of a reconstructive procedure, it is removed once the repair is safe.
     **(1)** Following common duct exploration, a T tube is used to drain the bile until spasm of the sphincter of Oddi has resolved. The T tube is removed when a cholangiogram documents free flow of bile into the duodenum.
     **(2)** Following total gastrectomy or esophagectomy, the esophageal anastomosis is drained internally with a nasogastric tube. If an anastomotic leak is going to occur, it usually does so within the first week. Therefore a "barium swallow" around the tube is performed to document that the anastomosis is intact and does not leak. The tube is removed if the repair is intact.
     **(3)** Following gastrectomy and Billroth II reconstruction, a major problem is disruption of the duodenal stump with subsequent formation of a duodenal–cutaneous fistula.
          **(a)** A tube is often placed within the duodenal lumen to prevent overdistention of the repaired duodenum, since this reduces the risk of disruption.
          **(b)** Once the patient has recovered from the surgical procedure, and if no signs of duodenal leakage have developed, the tube can be removed. This is usually not until 1 to 2 weeks after surgery.

**B. Other types of tubes**

1. A **rectal tube** is a large-caliber tube that is inserted into the rectum.
   a. The most common use is to relieve colonic distention from a colonic ileus or obstruction. It is the treatment of choice for sigmoid volvulus, where the tube is passed through the area of torsion under sigmoidoscopic visualization.
   b. Rectal tubes are best removed after several days because the thin-walled colon is very prone to pressure necrosis.

2. **Long intestinal tubes**, particularly the double-lumen **Miller-Abbott tube** and the single-lumen **Cantor tube**, are introduced through the nose and allowed to pass into the small intestine.
   a. Usually, a weight or bag is at the leading tip, allowing peristalsis to carry the tube distally. In the absence of bowel motility, such as with an ileus, the tube will generally not progress past the stomach.
   b. Long intestinal tubes are particularly useful for relieving small bowel obstruction.
      (1) Their use is for recurrent obstruction, particularly in the early postoperative period following laparotomy and the development of newly formed adhesions. The tubes are not used for a first episode of small bowel obstruction; laparotomy and lysis of adhesions should be performed in such cases.
      (2) Long intestinal tubes are less effective for late postoperative adhesions or for obstruction secondary to malignant disease.

3. Long intestinal tubes may also be inserted directly into the intestine at the time of laparotomy. The tube most commonly used is the **Baker jejunostomy tube**, which is passed through a hole in the jejunum and then distally through the bowel. It is used either to splint the bowel in situations where adhesions are likely to recur or to decompress a greatly distended bowel encountered at surgery.

4. **Cecostomy tubes** are large-caliber tubes that are surgically inserted into a distended cecum.
   a. Their most common use is in colonic ileus, where marked colonic distention produces a cecum that is greater than 11 cm in diameter, so that cecal rupture is imminent.
   b. Colonic obstruction secondary to a malignant process is better treated with a proximal diverting colostomy followed by colon resection.

5. **Gastrostomy tubes** are large tubes inserted into the stomach through the skin.
   a. Usually used for feeding purposes, they are also useful for prolonged gastric decompression, as in prolonged ileus.
   b. Once the tube is no longer necessary, it is removed. A tract forms between the skin and stomach but will close over in 6 to 24 hours if a tube is not reinserted.

6. **Cervical esophagostomy tubes** are placed into the esophagus distally and exit the skin in the neck region proximally. They function in much the same way as gastrostomy tubes.

7. **Jejunostomy tubes** are inserted into the jejunum as a surgical procedure or percutaneously. They exit on the abdominal wall and may be used for feeding purposes (see section II E 2).

8. **Gastroesophageal balloon tamponade tubes (Linton tube, Sengstaken-Blakemore tube)** are nasogastric tubes with inflatable balloons which are used to decompress bleeding esophageal varices (see Chapter 9, section I E 7 c).

9. **Tenckhoff peritoneal dialysis catheters** are permanent catheters inserted into the peritoneal cavity either for long-term dialysis therapy or for management of chronic ascites in patients with malignant disease. They may be inserted either percutaneously or surgically and can function for years if properly maintained with sterile technique.
   a. A Dacron cuff is glued to the Silastic catheter where it enters the peritoneum and also where it exits the skin.
   b. These cuffs become firmly incorporated into the surrounding tissue and function as a mechanical barrier to organisms entering at the exit site in the skin.

10. **Indwelling central venous catheters (Hickman catheters)** maintain access to the veins for prolonged periods.
    a. They are used for:
       (1) Long-term hyperalimentation in patients with nutritional problems
       (2) Chemotherapy and phlebotomy in patients with malignant diseases
    b. The Hickman catheter has a Dacron cuff like that of the Tenckhoff catheter and thus may function for many years. Both single- and double-lumen styles are available; they can be inserted percutaneously or surgically.

11. The **arteriovenous shunt (Scribner shunt)** is used for hemodialysis or plasmapheresis. It is a U-shaped cannula-and-tubing apparatus that is surgically inserted into an artery and a vein.

    **a.** The radial artery and a nearby vein are the usual vessels used.

    **b.** The patency of the ulnar artery should always be established before ligation and cannulation of the radial artery. This is done by means of the **Doppler test** or the **Allen test.**

        **(1)** The radial and ulnar arteries are occluded and the patient then exercises the hand.

        **(2)** The ulnar artery is released, and the patient is observed for blood flow into the hand.

        **(3)** If the hand blushes, then it has a dual blood supply.

## IV. WOUND HEALING.* 

Wound healing is the process in which incised or disrupted tissue undergoes repair, with restoration of intrinsic tissue strength and with resistance to infection and other external influences. It represents a process critical to the practice of surgery.

**A.** There are **three basic processes** involved in wound repair.

    **1.** Connective tissue in the form of **collagen is formed by fibroblasts** in a healing wound. Collagen is responsible for binding tissues together and, ultimately, is a major determinant of wound strength.

        **a.** Collagen is synthesized in the endoplasmic reticulum of fibroblasts. It is initially formed as protocollagen, a proline-rich collagen precursor, which is then hydroxylated to form collagen, a protein that contains glycine, proline, and hydroxyproline.

        **b.** Collagen is formed from three polypeptide chains found in a left-handed helix. The entire molecule is then twisted into a right-handed helix. Extensive cross-linking among molecules occurs and results in increased strength.

        **c.** Collagen synthesis requires ferrous iron, oxygen, ascorbic acid (vitamin C), and $\alpha$-ketoglutarate. Vitamin C deficiency leads to incompletely synthesized collagen.

    **2.** **Epithelial coverage of a wound occurs** as newly formed epithelial cells migrate onto the wound surface from the wound margin. Once covered, the wound becomes a barrier against infection from environmental organisms.

        **a.** **Fresh clean wounds have no resistance to infection** from surface contamination for the first 6 hours. By 5 days, the uncomplicated wound has the same resistance to infection as intact skin.

        **b.** Epithelium migrates slowly, and a **skin graft may be required** for complete wound healing to proceed at a more rapid rate.

    **3.** **Contraction occurs in the tissues of the wound**, helping the wound to close by decreasing its surface area. Contraction occurs in open wounds and generally is not important in healing by first intention (see section IV C 1). The **myofibroblast** exerts a contractile force within the wound and is responsible for wound contraction.

**B.** There are **three basic phases** that occur in healing which ultimately lead to the return of tissue strength.

    **1.** The **lag phase** occurs during the first several days.

        **a.** There is an **acute inflammatory response** with cellular migration into the wound. Neutrophils predominate for the first 24 to 48 hours, and macrophages become active by the third day. In addition to other functions, these cells are responsible for removing devitalized tissue in preparation for capillary ingrowth.

        **b.** There is no increase in wound strength during this time.

    **2.** The **proliferative phase** follows and is characterized by the migration of fibroblasts and capillaries into the wound. This phase lasts for 4 to 5 weeks.

        **a.** The fibroblasts begin to lay down collagen, which is usually detectable by the fourth day. Neutrophils and macrophages continue to be abundant in the wound.

        **b.** Capillary buds, originating in venules at the wound edges, grow across the wound to supply nutrients and oxygen to the cellular elements, particularly to the fibroblasts. Because of their rapid growth and immaturity, the capillaries remain highly permeable and susceptible to injury during this phase.

        **c.** **Wound strength** slowly increases during this phase and the next phase of healing.

            **(1)** After the first month, an uncomplicated wound has reached 50% of its final strength.

            **(2)** After the second month, the wound is at 75% of its final strength.

            **(3)** After the sixth month, the wound is at 95% of its final strength.

    **3.** The **maturation phase** of wound healing occurs when the cellular activity in the wound diminishes.

        **a.** Although the collagen content of the wound in this phase changes little, the wound continues to gain strength due to collagen cross-linking, remodeling, and contraction.

---

*Author: Bruce E. Jarrell

**b.** Wounds rarely attain the same breaking strength that was present in the tissue prior to the injury. Some wounds do reach 80% of the original strength, but this may require years.

**C.** Wounds are **managed clinically** by the following methods:

1. When possible, the edges of a wound are immediately approximated after injury. This procedure, known as **primary wound closure**, allows the wound to **heal by first intention**. Epithelialization occurs within 48 to 72 hours, and wound healing proceeds as described in section IV B.

2. **Second-intention wound healing** occurs when the wound edges are left unopposed and open. This procedure, known as **delayed** or **secondary closure**, allows necrotic and infected tissue to be readily accessible for surgical debridement. It is used primarily with grossly contaminated wounds.
   **a. Granulation tissue** forms on the wound surfaces when healing is by second intention. Granulation tissue is beefy, red, moist tissue that contains high numbers of inflammatory cells and capillaries.
   **b.** Granulation tissue is not sterile, but the large numbers of phagocytes act as a barrier to invasive infections. When the bacterial counts are as low as $10^4$ organisms per $mm^3$, usually either the wound can be closed, or a skin graft can be applied, or the tissue can support the ingrowth of epithelial cells.
   **c. Chronic granulation,** or **proud flesh,** is granulation tissue that is edematous, with an associated exudate. This tissue is less vascular than healthy granulation tissue and will not support epithelialization. It must be surgically removed and new granulation tissue allowed to form.

3. **Third-intention healing** occurs with **delayed primary closure**, used to close wounds with low-grade bacterial contamination. In this procedure, the wound is left open and observed for several days. If the wound edges are healthy by the third or fourth day, they are approximated, and wound healing progresses with very little delay.

4. **Skin grafts** (see also Chapter 30, section I D) may be used to cover open wounds that are large and covered by healthy granulation tissue.
   **a.** The graft is a segment of epidermis and dermis which has been surgically removed from another part of the body. When placed on a wound, the graft becomes vascularized from the underlying tissue. There are two thicknesses of grafts generally used.
      **(1)** A **split-thickness skin graft** is epidermis and a portion of the dermis and is usually 0.01 to 0.015 inches thick. A graft of this thickness allows the most rapid vascularization and is used on most wounds.
      **(2)** A **full-thickness skin graft** includes both epidermis and all of the dermis and is 0.02 to 0.025 inches thick. It is used more often in areas where cosmetic appearance is important.
   **b.** Movement between the graft and the wound disrupts the ingrowth of capillaries, making the graft fragile for weeks until firm adhesion occurs.

**D.** Wound healing may be **influenced by multiple factors**.

1. **Age**—younger patients heal more rapidly than older patients.

2. **Severe malnutrition** impedes wound healing. In general, however, wounds get priority for biologic needs over the organ systems.

3. **Vascularity**—highly vascular areas such as the face heal better than regions of poor vascularity such as the pretibial area.

4. **Anti-inflammatory drugs** such as steroids delay wound healing if they are given during the first several days of healing but have little effect on healing if given after that time.

5. **Adequate levels of oxygen** are necessary at the local wound area for unimpeded wound healing.
   **a.** Fibroblasts require oxygen to synthesize collagen, and phagocytes require oxygen to ingest and kill bacteria.
   **b.** Any process that interrupts the delivery of oxygen or other nutrients will impair healing; examples include hypoxemia, hypotension, vascular insufficiency, and local ischemia secondary to overtightened sutures.
   **c.** Radiation therapy causes obliteration of small vessels in the dermis, resulting in local ischemia and delayed wound healing.

6. **Local sepsis** is probably the most common and most important cause of delayed wound healing or wound breakdown.

    **a.** The **usual source of bacterial contamination** is the patient's own bacteria. Environmental sources account for only about 5% of wound infections.

    **b.** Wounds may be **classified** by the **degree of bacterial contamination**; the risk of infection in each type is given in section VII A 2.

        **(1)** A **clean wound** is one formed under relatively sterile conditions and in which the genitourinary, gastrointestinal, and tracheobronchial systems are not violated.

        **(2)** A **clean contaminated wound** occurs if one of these tracts is opened but minimal spillage has occurred. An example is a colectomy performed on the bowel that has been mechanically cleaned. These wounds may usually be closed with healing by first intention.

        **(3)** A **contaminated wound** is one in which gross contamination has occurred. Wounds in direct contact with purulent material have a 50% or greater incidence of infection and therefore are usually left open to heal by second or third intention. Examples include surgery for an intra-abdominal abscess or perforated appendicitis.

    **c.** **Prophylactic antibiotics** (see section VII A 3) may reduce the incidence of wound infections.

        **(1)** Antibiotics are probably of little benefit for clean wounds or for grossly contaminated wounds.

            **(a)** The only clean cases in which antibiotics are found to be beneficial are those in which an infection would be life-threatening, such as when using a vascular prosthesis.

            **(b)** For grossly contaminated wounds, antibiotics can be used to prevent soft tissue and systemic infections; however, debridement and irrigation are of prime importance in the management of this type of wound.

        **(2)** The **most appropriate use** is for clean contaminated wounds. The antibiotics should be given before or during the surgery. If they are given later than 3 hours after the wound is inoculated with bacteria, they have little effect.

        **(3)** The antibiotic used should be determined by the nature of the potential infecting organism. Bowel surgery patients should be treated with antibiotics effective against anaerobic and gram-negative organisms. Patients having upper torso surgery should be treated with antibiotics against gram-positive cocci.

**E.** **Wound dehiscence,** or **breakdown**, may occur in severely compromised wounds.

    **1.** It usually occurs early postoperatively when the wound strength is low and wound stresses are high due to such conditions as abdominal distention, ileus, or respiratory difficulties.

    **2.** Dehiscence may be the result of any of the factors discussed in section IV D. In addition, during normal healing, collagenases are released at wound edges as part of collagen deposition and remodeling. In the compromised patient, this may weaken the tissue in which sutures are placed, resulting in tissue failure. Patients with systemic diseases such as renal or hepatic failure also have a higher incidence of dehiscence.

**F.** **Scars** from wounds vary greatly.

    **1.** Most wounds continue to remodel for more than 1 year. A wound that is unsightly several weeks following surgery may be cosmetically acceptable months or years later.

    **2.** **Hypertrophic scars** are composed of dense fibrous tissue in the dermis of the wound skin. They result from wounds that heal with excessive collagen synthesis, causing an unsightly scar with a raised surface. The etiology is unknown.

    **a.** The scar is usually tense, reddish in color, and associated with itching, hyperesthesia, and tenderness.

    **b.** These scars occur most commonly in blacks, Orientals, and dark-skinned white patients, and are more common in younger patients.

    **c.** The scars are classified into two general categories.

        **(1)** An ordinary hypertrophic scar lies entirely within the confines of the wound. Histologically, it shows an increased amount of normal-appearing collagen and numerous mature fibroblasts. There is scant ground substance. The scar usually stabilizes after 3 months and even regresses slightly and softens.

        **(2)** A **keloid** is a scar that invades nearby normal tissue that was not previously involved in the wound. The scar continues to enlarge even after 6 months and does not usually regress or soften. Histologically, there are large swollen eosinophilic collagen bundles with abundant ground substance and scant fibroblasts.

    **d.** **Treatment** of these scars is very difficult. Excision of the scar may result in its recurrence. Steroid injections into the scar or following excision may prevent recurrence, as may radiation therapy.

## V. HEMOSTASIS*

**A.** Hemostasis is the physiologic process by which bleeding—that is, blood leakage from an injured vessel—is controlled. Hemostasis consists of four **components**: the vessel response, platelet (thrombocyte) activities, the coagulation mechanism, and the fibrinolytic system.

1. The **vessel response**, namely **vasoconstriction**, is the first hemostatic response to occur after an injury to a blood vessel. Vasoconstriction is due primarily to smooth muscle contraction.

2. **Platelet activity.** Following the onset of vasoconstriction, the platelets begin to **adhere** and **aggregate**, eventually forming a **platelet plug**.
   a. **Adherence**
      (1) The platelets adhere chiefly to exposed subendothelial collagen, a process requiring **von Willebrand factor**. This platelet factor is produced by the endothelial cells and is related to factor VIII of the coagulation cascade (see section V A 3).
      (2) At the same time, platelet granules release adenosine diphosphate (ADP), which promotes a loose platelet aggregation.
   b. **Aggregation**
      (1) Arachidonic acid is then released from platelet phospholipids, and is converted by cyclooxygenase to the unstable cyclic endoperoxides prostaglandin $G_2$ ($PGG_2$) and prostaglandin $H_2$ ($PGH_2$).
      (2) Thromboxane synthetase converts $PGH_2$ to thromboxane $A_2$, which in turn induces further ADP release and thus enhances platelet aggregation.
   c. **Platelet plug**. The aggregated platelets interact with thrombin, fusing together to form a plug.
   d. **Aspirin** inhibits the cyclooxygenase-mediated formation of $PGG_2$ and $PGH_2$, thus interfering with platelet aggregation and subsequent plug formation. This defect lasts for the life of the platelet (7 to 10 days).

3. The **coagulation system** converts prothrombin to thrombin and leads to the formation of the **fibrin clot**. Two systems of interacting factors are involved, the intrinsic and the extrinsic pathways (Fig. 1-1).
   a. The **intrinsic pathway** involves only normal blood components.
      (1) **Factor XII (Hageman factor)** becomes bound to a damaged vessel and is activated (factor XIIa).
      (2) In the presence of factor XIIa, prekallikrein, and high-molecular-weight kininogen, **factor XI,** is activated (XIa).
      (3) Factor XIa, together with calcium, activates **factor IX**, which joins with **factor VIII**, calcium, and platelet factor 3 to activate **factor X**.
      (4) Factor Xa and **factor V** together convert **prothrombin (factor II)** to **thrombin**.
      (5) Small peptides are then split from **fibrinogen (factor I)** by thrombin to produce **fibrin** monomers. These are cross-linked by **factor XIIIa** (activated by thrombin) to form a stable **clot**.
   b. The **extrinsic pathway** requires the presence of a tissue lipoprotein.
      (1) **Factor VII** forms a complex with calcium and **factor III** (thromboplastin, or tissue factor) to activate **factor X**.
      (2) The subsequent steps of the pathway are as described above. As Figure 1-1 shows, factors XII, XI, IX, and VIII are not involved.

4. There are **interactions** between the coagulation mechanisms and platelet activities. Platelet factor 3, released in the early stages of platelet adhesion, contributes to the factor IXa–VIIIa–calcium complex which activates factor X. Thrombin and subsequently fibrin lend strength to the final platelet plug.

5. The **fibrinolytic system.** The vasculature must have a mechanism to balance the clotting process in order to maintain the circulating blood in a fluid state.
   a. **Plasminogen**, an inactive protein, is converted to its active form, **plasmin**, by plasminogen activators.
   b. The vascular endothelium, whose disruption initiates both platelet adherence and the coagulation cascade, is probably the primary source of plasminogen activators.
   c. **Plasmin** digests fibrin, fibrinogen, and factors V and VIII.
   d. **Homeostatic function.** It appears likely that plasminogen becomes incorporated into a growing thrombus and eventually serves to eliminate the clot once its function is complete.

---

*Authors: R. Anthony Carabasi, III, and John S. Radomski

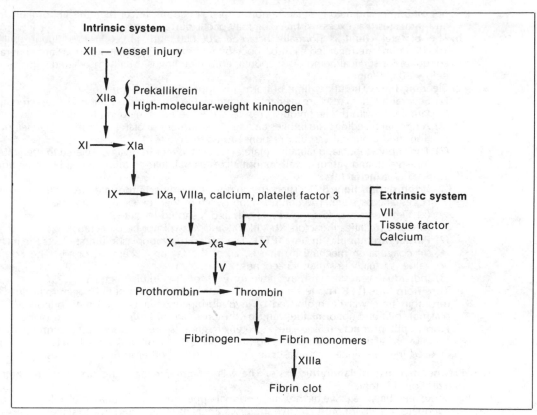

**Figure 1-1.** The coagulation cascade.

**B. Preoperative evaluation of hemostasis**

1. The **history.** Important for identifying potential bleeding problems are the personal medical history, the family history, and the drug ingestion history. Questions must be as direct as possible so that specific information is obtained.

   a. **Personal medical history.** The patient should be specifically asked about any bleeding problems that occurred after prior surgery, including circumcision, tonsillectomy, and dental extractions. Females should be asked about increased or excessive menstrual flow. Individuals with underlying hemostatic disorders are likely to have had problems in these areas.

   b. **Family history.** Because many coagulation disorders are inherited in an autosomal or sex-linked fashion, any history of spontaneous or postoperative bleeding in a relative warrants further investigation.

   c. **Drug history.** Aspirin, nonsteroidal anti-inflammatory drugs, quinidine, cimetidine, tranquilizers, and certain antibiotics can all affect platelet production or performance. Again, specific questions will yield important information. For instance, patients should be asked what over-the-counter preparations they are taking, since many patients do not realize that these often contain aspirin.

2. The **physical examination.** This should be thorough.

   a. Petechiae, ecchymoses, and purpura should be noted, as they are possible clues to platelet disorders.

   b. An enlarged spleen can sequester platelets and lead to excessive bleeding during surgery. Lymphadenopathy and hepatosplenomegaly may also be clues to a neoplasm of the reticuloendothelial system.

   c. Jaundice, ascites, spider angiomas, or hepatomegaly can indicate hepatic dysfunction. Because clotting factors are produced by the liver, hepatic disease can result in severe bleeding.

3. **Laboratory tests**

   a. The **peripheral blood smear**, besides giving information about red and white blood cell morphology, can also provide an estimate of the platelet count. Finding 15 to 20 platelets per oil immersion field indicates a normal platelet count; fewer than 5 is abnormally low and indicates that excessive bleeding may occur during surgery.

b. The **platelet count** is normally between 200,000 and 400,000/mm³. Counts below 100,000 mm³ are regarded as thrombocytopenic, but 70,000 platelets/mm³ are generally adequate for surgical hemostasis. Spontaneous bleeding is usually associated with counts below 20,000/mm³.

c. **Bleeding time.** The upper limit of normal is approximately 5 minutes.
  (1) Several standard tests are available, including the Duke and Ivy methods. Each requires familiarity with the technique if results are to be meaningful and reproducible.
  (2) A normal bleeding time implies an adequate number of platelets, normal platelet function, and a normal vascular response to an injury.
  (3) Thrombocytopenia, qualitative platelet defects (either intrinsic or related to drugs such as aspirin), and vascular wall abnormalities can all lead to a prolonged bleeding time.

d. **Tests of clotting factors**
  (1) **Prothrombin time (PT).** The prothrombin time reflects the integrity of the extrinsic coagulation system. The control value is determined by each laboratory.
    (a) Deficiencies of factors I, II, V, VII, and X should be detected.
    (b) Abnormalities in factors XI, VIII, IX, and XII will not be detected.
  (2) **Partial thromboplastin time (PTT).** The partial thromboplastin time reflects the intrinsic coagulation mechanism; that is, all of the factors except factor VII. The normal value is usually less than 45 seconds.
  (3) Individual assays are also available for each of the clotting factors.

e. **Thrombin time (TT).** This test measures the rate of conversion of fibrinogen to fibrin. The thrombin time will be prolonged by hypofibrinogenemia (< 100 mg fibrinogen/dl of plasma), by fibrin abnormalities, and by the presence of fibrin split products or heparin.

f. **Fibrin split products (FSP).** These protein fragments are released from fibrinogen and fibrin by the action of plasmin. The normal range is 0 to 10 mg/ml of plasma. FSP will be increased in disseminated intravascular coagulation and other fibrinolytic states.

4. **Preoperative use of laboratory tests.** There is disagreement among surgeons and hematologists on this topic.
  a. Some feel that a negative history and a normal-appearing blood smear or platelet count are adequate screens for most elective surgery. Others use the PT and PTT to screen preoperative patients further. In general, the PT and PTT will rarely be abnormal if the patient's bleeding history is negative and the peripheral smear is normal.
  b. Many hematologists feel that the bleeding time should be tested more frequently because the platelet count cannot detect qualitative platelet abnormalities.
  c. Ultimately, each physician must decide how much preoperative testing is warranted, based on the history and physical examination and the nature of the surgery that is planned.

C. **Disorders of hemostasis**

1. **Platelet disorders**
  a. **Thrombocytopenia** (platelet count below 100,000/mm³) is the most common cause of bleeding in the surgical patient. Spontaneous bleeding may occur with counts below 20,000/mm³; surgical hemostasis requires a level of at least 70,000/mm³. Thrombocytopenia can arise from a number of causes.
    (1) **Reduced production of platelets**, caused by bone marrow failure, can be congenital, as in Fanconi's syndrome, or can be due to the toxic effects of radiation or of drugs, especially chemotherapeutic agents. The marrow may also be replaced with leukemic or other neoplastic cells, or involved in a fibrotic process (myelofibrosis). **Treatment** is to eliminate the effects of the underlying drug or the disease if possible. If surgery is required, 8 units of platelets transfused just prior to the procedure should raise the count by 50,000 to 100,000/mm³. Postoperatively, the count should be maintained above 50,000/mm³.
    (2) **Faulty platelet maturation** can be secondary to megaloblastic anemia. **Treatment** is to replace the deficient vitamins—folate, B₁₂, or both.
    (3) **Abnormal platelet distribution** occurs with splenomegaly, in which the spleen contains more than the usual 30% of the circulating platelets (see Chapter 11).
    (4) **Increased platelet destruction or loss** can result from several causes:
      (a) **Autoimmune disorders** (idiopathic thrombocytopenic purpura, systemic lupus erythematosus)
      (b) **Drug hypersensitivity reactions**
        (i) Some drugs (quinidine, sulfonamides), acting as haptens, can form an anti-

gen–antibody complex that binds to the platelet membrane. Treatment is cessation of the drug.

    **(II)** Heparin is increasingly recognized as a cause of severe thrombocytopenia that appears to be antibody-related and can occur regardless of the duration, dose, route, or frequency of heparin administration. Platelet counts return to normal after the withdrawal of heparin. Patients receiving heparin should have platelet counts at least every other day.

  **(c) Disseminated intravascular coagulation** [see section V C 3 c (1)]

  **(d) Hemorrhage**, since platelets are lost, of course, along with all other blood components

**(5) Dilutional thrombocytopenia** can develop after large transfusions of banked blood, which contains few functional platelets.

**b. Abnormal platelet function** can produce hemostatic problems despite a normal platelet count.

  **(1) Causes** of functional platelet abnormalities include:

    **(a)** Uremia. Both acute and chronic renal failure often result in impaired platelet function, with prolonged bleeding time.

    **(b)** Cirrhosis of the liver

    **(c)** Idiopathic causes

    **(d)** Drug effects

      **(i)** Aspirin and other nonsteroidal anti-inflammatory drugs can adversely affect platelet aggregation by blocking the synthesis of the endoperoxides $PGG_2$ and $PGH_2$. If possible, patients should stop aspirin use at least 1 week prior to surgery.

      **(ii)** Penicillin G, carbenicillin, and ticarcillin can also impair platelet function.

  **(2)** Disorders of platelet function are **treated** by transfusion of normal platelets preoperatively, or by withdrawal of the offending drug if surgery can be delayed.

**2. Blood vessel wall abnormalities**, when serious, may prolong the bleeding time, although platelet count and function are usually normal.

  **a.** Scurvy and Cushing's syndrome each cause a defect in the blood vessel connective tissue, leading to weakened vessel walls. Henoch-Schönlein purpura, a hypersensitivity reaction, leads to inflammation of the capillaries, with increased permeability.

  **b.** Control of the disease process and awareness of the need for meticulous hemostasis in the operating room can minimize complications in these patients.

**3. Disorders of blood coagulation**

  **a. Congenital coagulation disorders.** Specific inherited deficiencies have been characterized for most of the clotting factors.

  **(1) Hemophilia A** is a deficiency of the procoagulant activity of factor VIII; its antigenic activity is usually normal. The PT is normal, but the PTT is usually prolonged. A sex-linked recessive disorder, hemophilia A has an incidence of about 1 per 10,000 population.

    **(a) Severity** depends on the degree of deficiency of factor VIII. Spontaneous bleeding can be avoided by plasma activity levels of at least 5%. Minor trauma may cause bleeding at levels between 5% and 25%, while surgical insult or major trauma is necessary to generate hemorrhage when levels are above 25% to 30%.

    **(b) Treatment** consists of providing appropriate levels of factor VIII for the situation. A synthetic analogue of antidiuretic hormone, desmopressin (1-deamino-8-D-arginine vasopressin, or dDAVP), can elevate factor VIII levels threefold in hemophiliacs who have at least 1% factor VIII activity. **Inhibitors of factor VIII** may develop in a hemophiliac and must be screened for prior to surgery.

  **(2) Von Willebrand's disease** (pseudohemophilia) can be transmitted as either an autosomal dominant or a recessive trait.

    **(a)** The endothelium releases decreased amounts of factor VIII. This results in a defect in platelet adherence to subendothelial structures and an abnormal bleeding time. The antigenic activity of factor VIII is reduced as well as its procoagulant activity.

    **(b)** Unlike hemophilia, in which the factor VIII level remains constant, the level may vary in von Willebrand's disease.

    **(c)** The purified factor VIII used in classic hemophilia does not contain the **von Willebrand factor (factor VIII R:WF)** and is therefore ineffective for treatment. Cryoprecipitate provides both portions of the factor VIII complex and corrects the bleeding disorder. It should be started the day before surgery to correct the bleeding time.

  **(3) Hemophilia B (Christmas disease)** is a sex-linked deficiency of factor IX. It occurs about one-tenth as often as hemophilia A. The manifestations, severity, and treatment are similar to those of hemophilia A. The PTT is usually prolonged. Prothrombin complexes used for treatment may contain activated factors which may precipitate thrombus formation; some manufacturers advocate adding small amounts of heparin.

    **(4) Factor XI deficiency (Rosenthal's syndrome)** is a rare autosomal dominant disorder. The PTT is abnormal; the PT is normal.

    **(5) Factor XII deficiency** is usually asymptomatic.

    **(6) Factor XIII deficiency** can be either autosomal dominant or sex-linked recessive. Fibrin monomers fail to cross-link, and the resulting weak clot will dissolve in 5 M urea. The PT and PTT are both normal.

    **(7) Factor V deficiency** is an autosomal recessive trait. Factor V is manufactured in the liver but, unlike most liver factors, factor V is not vitamin K–dependent. Both the PT and PTT are prolonged.

    **(8) Factor X deficiency** is an autosomal recessive disorder. The PT and PTT are prolonged.

    **(9) Factor VII deficiency** is also inherited as an autosomal recessive trait. The PT is abnormal; the PTT is normal.

  **(10) Hypoprothrombinemia (factor II deficiency)**, a rare autosomal recessive disorder, prolongs both the PT and PTT.

  **(11) Fibrinogen deficiency (afibrinogenemia)** is inherited in an autosomal recessive fashion; qualitatively **abnormal fibrinogen (dysfibrinogenemia)** is autosomal dominant. In both types, the PT, PTT, and TT are all prolonged. A fibrinogen level of 100 mg/dl is needed for hemostasis.

**b. Surgery in the patient with a congenital disorder of coagulation**

    **(1) Prerequisites.** Before elective surgery, support must be available from a hematology consultant and from a coagulation laboratory capable of performing rapid factor assays. An adequate replacement supply of the specific needed factor must be on hand.

      **(a)** Fresh frozen plasma, cryoprecipitate, and numerous factor concentrates are available in various strengths, so the strength must be known.

      **(b)** Levels of specific factors are expressed as a percent of normal activity. Levels above 30% are considered hemostatic and tests of coagulation are usually in the normal range. Factor concentrates are measured in units; one unit is the amount of factor present in 1 ml of plasma with 100% activity.

    **(2) Plan for surgery.** The plasma level of the deficient factor should be brought to 100% of activity at the time of surgery, after which the level should be kept above 60% for 4 days, and then above 40% for 4 more days or until all sutures, clips, tubes, and drains are removed. The factor levels are monitored by assays, and replacement therapy is based on the factor's half-life.

**c. Acquired disorders of the coagulation system**

    **(1) Disseminated intravascular coagulation (DIC)** results from the simultaneous activation of the coagulation and fibrinolytic systems. It occurs as a consequence of a severe underlying disorder such as sepsis, malignancy, trauma, shock, or serious obstetrical complications.

      **(a) Presentation.** As the coagulation and fibrinolytic systems are activated, platelets and clotting factors are consumed and fibrin split products are released. Clinically, there is usually widespread hemorrhage. The PT and PTT are usually prolonged. The presence of thrombocytopenia, hypoprothrombinemia, and elevated fibrin split products helps confirm the diagnosis.

      **(b) Treatment.** Most important is to control the underlying disease process. Beyond this, there is controversy.

        **(i)** Some advocate the use of heparin to halt coagulation, believing that additional platelets and clotting factors would "fuel the fire."

        **(ii)** However, in the face of diffuse hemorrhage it would appear more prudent to provide maximum support, including platelets, fresh frozen plasma, and cryoprecipitate, while aggressively attacking the underlying disease process.

    **(2) Vitamin K deficiency.** The liver requires vitamin K in order to synthesize factors II, VII, IX, and X.

      **(a)** A deficiency of vitamin K is common in surgical patients and results from poor nutrition, antibiotic therapy that alters the gut's normal flora, obstructive jaundice with blockage of bile salts, or parenteral nutrition without vitamin K supplementation.

      **(b)** Vitamin K in doses of 10 to 20 mg should begin to correct the defect in 8 to 12 hours. The dose is repeated, if possible, every 12 hours until the PT is corrected. For emergency surgery, the first dose is supplemented with fresh frozen plasma.

    **(3) Liver disease.** All factors except factor VIII are reduced. Vitamin K will not be helpful if there is severe hepatocyte dysfunction.

    **(4) Exogenous anticoagulants** (heparin, warfarin) will obviously cause clotting defects.

**D. Bleeding during surgery.** This can result from local factors or generalized disorders.

    **1. Local factors**

        **a.** If bleeding is from one site, such as the wound surface, it is most likely due to a **failure of local hemostasis** (e.g., an unligated vessel).

        **b.** The problem should be identified and corrected.

            **(1) Direct pressure** by finger or packs will usually control local bleeding until the source can be clearly identified. Once isolated, severed vessels can be clamped and then ligated, suture-ligated, or secured with metal clips, depending upon their size.

            **(2) Electrocautery**, although quicker than ligating, may cause more tissue necrosis if used improperly.

            **(3) Chemical aids**

                **(a) Epinephrine** produces local vasoconstriction, but its use is limited by its systemic effects.

                **(b) Thrombin**, applied topically, is effective because it induces the production of fibrin. Thrombin is frequently applied by means of gelatin foam (Gelfoam).

                **(c) Oxidized cellulose materials (Oxycel, Surgicel)** serve as a scaffolding for clot formation. **Microfibrillar collagen (Avitene)** serves a similar function.

    **2. Generalized disorders**

        **a. Underlying disorders.** Bleeding during surgery may be the result of any of the previously described congenital or acquired disorders of platelets or of the coagulation system (e.g., hemophilia A, hypoprothrombinemia, or disseminated intravascular coagulation).

        **b. Transfusion complications** (see sections VI C 2 c and VI C 3)

## VI. TRANSFUSION THERAPY IN SURGERY* (see also Chapter 2, section I C 4 e)

    **A. Blood components** of several types are available for transfusion therapy.

        **1. Whole blood** is collected in citrate phosphate dextrose (CPD) or citrate phosphate double-dextrose adenine (CP2D-adenine) and is stored at 4° C for up to 28 days.

        **a. Banked blood** undergoes several **changes during storage**.

            **(1) Red blood cells** progressively lose their ability to survive. For example, if blood is transfused after it has been stored for 28 days, only 25% of its red cells will still be viable by 60 days after the transfusion. Stored red cells also lose their deformability and become more spherical. Oxygen transport is also reduced because of a decrease in cellular 2,3-diphosphoglycerate (2,3-DPG); this shifts the oxygen-hemoglobin dissociation curve to the left.

            **(2) Clotting factors V and VIII** rapidly deteriorate in banked blood, and **platelets** do not remain active past 24 hours.

            **(3) Changes in chemistry** also take place: The **pH** of stored blood gradually decreases, reaching about 6.7 after 4 weeks of storage. The **potassium** concentration may be 25 to 30 mEq/L at this time. **Ammonia** also steadily rises.

        **b.** Probably the only **indication for the transfusion of whole blood** is hypovolemia secondary to acute hemorrhage. Fresh whole blood (not more than 24 hours old) would be ideal for this purpose, since platelets and clotting factors would still be active and many of the adverse biochemical effects of stored blood would be avoided.

        **2. Packed red blood cells** are prepared by removing most of the plasma, leaving a packed cell volume of 70%. Packed cells are indicated for most transfusions in which the goal is to increase the patient's oxygen-carrying capacity. Packed cells present less volume and a lower electrolyte load for the patient.

        **3. Frozen red cells** are said to reduce the risk of hepatitis transmission, although this has been disputed.

        **4. Fresh frozen plasma (FFP)** contains all of the coagulation factors lacking in banked blood, including factors V and VIII. It is used to replace clotting factors during massive transfusion of packed red cells or to correct the factor abnormalities found in conditions such as liver disease or disseminated intravascular coagulation.

        **5. Cryoprecipitate**, a plasma derivative, contains high concentrations of factor VIII and fibrinogen, along with smaller amounts of other factors. It is used in factor VIII–deficient states such as hemophilia and von Willebrand's disease, and in other states of uncontrolled bleeding such as disseminated intravascular coagulation.

---

*Authors: R. Anthony Carabasi, III, and John S. Radomski

6. **Albumin** is available in 5% and 25% concentrations. It is used as a volume expander.

7. **Specific factor concentrates** provide replacement therapy for inherited deficiency states; several commercial products are available.

B. **Blood substitutes.** Fluorocarbon emulsions have been found to possess oxygen-carrying capacity. They are being evaluated as blood substitutes for patients who refuse blood transfusion or who are difficult to crossmatch. Since blood transfusion is associated with some risk of transmitted disease [e.g., hepatitis, acquired immune deficiency syndrome (AIDS)], a suitable blood substitute would be desirable.

C. **Complications of transfusions**

1. **Disease transmission**
   a. **Hepatitis** is estimated to occur in about 0.2% of transfusions. The incidence is higher with pooled products such as factor concentrates. It is also higher when paid donors are used as suppliers of blood. Effective screening can detect hepatitis B surface antigen; however, most cases of post-transfusion hepatitis are now due to non-A, non-B hepatitis, for which no effective screen exists. Using frozen red cells may decrease the risk.
   b. **Acquired immune deficiency syndrome (AIDS)** is a severe defect in the immune system which leaves its victim susceptible to opportunistic infections and rare neoplasms such as Kaposi's sarcoma. This disease may be transmitted via blood obtained from affected individuals.
   c. **Other diseases.** Syphilis, brucellosis, and cytomegalovirus infection can also be transmitted in transfused blood.

2. **Immediate transfusion reactions**
   a. **Allergic reactions** are the most common type, occurring in up to 2% of transfusions.
      (1) Fever, chills, urticaria, and itching typically occur after at least half of a unit of blood or packed cells is transfused. Respiratory symptoms such as wheezing or stridor occur in severe cases.
      (2) Usually an antihistamine such as diphenhydramine will control the minor symptoms, with epinephrine and steroids reserved for more serious cases.
      (3) If the reaction is typically allergic and responds to treatment it is not necessary to stop the transfusion. However, if there is concern about a hemolytic reaction the transfusion is stopped immediately.
   b. **Febrile reactions** are caused by antigens, on white cells or platelets, to which the patient is sensitive. They occur almost as frequently as allergic reactions. Fever, alone or with chills, occurs after half of a unit of blood has been transfused. Urticaria and respiratory symptoms do not occur. Antipyretics are given to reduce the fever.
   c. **Hemolytic reactions**
      (1) **Early fulminant reactions** are usually due to the transfusion of incompatible blood because of errors in cross-matching, typing, labeling, or patient identification.
         (a) Typically, early reactions appear after only 50 to 100 ml of blood have been given. The patient may develop fever and chills with complaints of chest, back, or flank pain and dyspnea. Hypotension and shock may also occur.
         (b) **Intraoperative hemolytic reactions** in anesthetized patients may be atypical, with unexplained, generalized bleeding as the only manifestation.
      (2) **Delayed hemolytic reactions** are considered to be anamnestic responses to prior transfusions or pregnancies. They may take the form of jaundice that appears several days after the transfusion.
      (3) **Treatment of hemolytic reactions**
         (a) The transfusion is immediately stopped when any patient is suspected of having a hemolytic reaction.
         (b) The remaining transfusion blood and a fresh sample of the patient's blood are sent to the laboratory for retyping and crossmatching. A urine sample should also be sent so that it can be examined for hemoglobin.
         (c) A Foley urinary catheter is inserted and diuresis is established rapidly by giving 25 g of mannitol and infusing lactated Ringer's solution at a rate that should ensure a urine output of at least 100 ml/hr. Sodium bicarbonate may also be given to alkalinize the urine and help prevent tubular damage.

3. **Complications of massive transfusions of banked blood.** Rapid transfusion (within 12 hours) of an amount of stored blood equal to or greater than the patient's blood volume can lead to problems, due primarily to the changes that occur in stored blood (see section VI A 1 a).
   a. **Decreased oxygen-carrying capacity.** Because the 2,3-DPG level gradually falls in stored blood, the hemoglobin affinity for oxygen increases, so that oxygen release to the tissues is less efficient.

**b. Coagulation defects.** These result primarily from a dilutional effect, since blood stored longer than 24 hours has virtually no platelets and no factor V or factor VIII activity. Platelets and fresh frozen plasma must therefore be given in addition to banked blood.

**c. Hypothermia.** This rapidly develops if several units of blood are transfused without being warmed. Arrhythmias will commonly occur at body temperatures of 30° C. During a transfusion, the blood is warmed by immersing an in-line coil in a water bath that is near body temperature—never by warming the container of blood.

**d. Metabolic effects**

   **(1) Hyperkalemia.** Because the plasma potassium concentration rises in banked blood, rapidly administering large amounts of old stored blood can cause transiently dangerous levels of serum potassium. Therefore, when massive transfusions are required, blood less than 2 to 3 days old should be preferentially used or at least alternated with older blood to minimize this problem.

   **(2) Acidosis and citrate toxicity**

   **(a)** Normally, citric acid (from transfused blood) and lactic acid (from poorly perfused tissue) are rapidly metabolized. However, in the hypovolemic patient or the patient in shock with reduced hepatic blood flow, this will be slowed and severe acidosis can occur.

   **(b)** Some authorities advocate giving sodium bicarbonate routinely with extensive transfusions, in an attempt to minimize these changes in pH. One must proceed cautiously, however, since alkalosis acts synergistically with hypothermia and low 2,3-DPG levels to decrease the delivery of oxygen to the tissues. Also, alkalosis can lower the level of ionized calcium, which can cause serious cardiac arrhythmias.

   **(c)** For these reasons, alkalinization is probably not routinely advisable and should be used only if indicated by blood gas analysis.

   **(3) Hypocalcemia**

   **(a)** In citrate overload, the excess citrate will bind ionized calcium. The decrease in ionized calcium can have a detrimental effect on myocardial performance. Thus, some authorities advocate routine administration of calcium in proportion to the number of units of blood transfused. However, the hypothermic patient's heart is very sensitive to the calcium ion.

   **(b)** Giving calcium gluconate 1 g/L of blood is probably safe, but, ideally, replacement should be guided by direct information from a calcium ion–sensing electrode.

**e. Respiratory insufficiency.** Degenerating platelets and white cells in stored blood can lead to microembolization when large amounts of banked blood are transfused, causing pulmonary damage and respiratory insufficiency. This complication is best prevented by transfusing the blood through a micropore filter.

# VII. SURGICAL INFECTIONS.* Surgical infections are either infections that require surgical intervention in order to resolve completely, or infections that develop as a complication of surgery. Some, of course, are in both categories.

**A. General considerations.**

   **1.** Surgical infections generally have the following **characteristics:**

   **a.** They usually involve either a penetrating injury (e.g., from trauma), a perforating injury (e.g., a perforated ulcer), or an operative site such as the surgical wound.

   **b.** Often, multiple organisms are present.

   **c.** Treatment requires surgical drainage of the infection and debridement of necrotic or grossly contaminated tissue; antibiotics alone will not resolve the infection.

   **2. Surgical wound infections** form the major type of surgical infections among hospitalized patients.

   **a.** The incidence of wound infections is directly related to the nature of the surgical procedure being performed. The classification of wounds by extent of contamination is described in section IV D 6 b.

   **(1)** A **clean operative site** from an elective procedure carries a 1% to 2% risk of wound infection. Because the risk is low, the skin edges are closed primarily. A typical example is a hernia repair.

   **(2) Clean contaminated operative sites** (e.g., from a hysterectomy or cholecystectomy) have an infection rate of 5% to 15%, and the skin edges may or may not be closed.

   **(3) Contaminated operative sites**, such as a colectomy, a gastrectomy for a bleeding ulcer, or a cholecystectomy in the presence of infected bile, have an infection rate of 10% to 20% when the wound is closed.

   **(4)** A **dirty operative site** occurs when a perforated viscus or penetrating trauma has al-

*Author: Bruce E. Jarrell

lowed bacteria to contaminate the region prior to surgical intervention. The incidence of wound infection is greater than 50%, and therefore the operative wound is usually left open to heal by second intention.

  **b.** Wound infection often presents as a spiking fever at about the fifth to eighth postoperative day. There may be localized wound tenderness, cellulitis, drainage from the wound, or dehiscence.

  **c.** Simple incision and drainage will resolve most postoperative wound infections. Deeper wound infections, extensive necrosis, or wound breakdown may require open debridement.

**3. Prophylactic antibiotics** are antibiotics given shortly before, during, or shortly after surgery (i.e., during the perioperative period) in an attempt to combat any bacterial invasion into the tissues that occurs during the operative procedure. The general rules for the use of prophylactic antibiotics are as follows:

  **a.** The operation must carry a significant risk of a postoperative wound infection. Thus, a clean procedure would not call for prophylactic antibiotics but the following situations would:

   **(1)** Colon or rectal surgery (the patient is given oral nonabsorbable antibiotics plus intravenous antibiotics)

   **(2)** A procedure (e.g., vascular surgery) in which prosthetic material is to be used

   **(3)** A gynecologic procedure in which the vagina is opened

   **(4)** Gross contamination of the operative site

  **b.** The antibiotics used should be effective against the pathogens likely to be present in the operative site. Narrow-spectrum antibiotics should be used.

  **c.** The antibiotics must have reached an effective tissue level at the time of the incision. Thus, they should be given 1 to 2 hours prior to surgery.

  **d.** The antibiotics should be given for only 6 to 24 hours after surgery. Longer-lasting regimens carry a higher risk of superinfection and offer no additional protection.

  **e.** The benefits of the prophylactic antibiotic should outweigh its potential dangers, such as allergic reactions or the stimulation of bacterial or fungal superinfections from overgrowth of pathogens such as gram-negative bacteria or candida.

**4. Tetanus prophylaxis**

  **a. Active immunization** almost always results when tetanus toxoid injections are given in the recommended schedule. This is usually done in infancy (with DPT shots) or during military induction. A booster dose every 10 years is recommended by the American College of Surgeons.

  **b. Prophylaxis at the time of an injury**

   **(1)** Any person with a penetrating injury must receive tetanus prophylaxis if previous immunization was not recent or cannot be documented.

    **(a)** A previously immunized person should be given a booster dose if none has been given within the past 5 years.

    **(b)** A patient with a clean injury who has never been immunized may be given the first of three immunizing doses, but it is important to be certain that the patient does receive the subsequent two doses.

    **(c)** A patient with a dirty wound who has never been immunized should be given **passive immunization** with homologous (human) tetanus immune globulin. It is always given intramuscularly.

     **(i)** The protection period has a half-life of 1 month.

     **(ii)** The first dose of tetanus toxoid may be given at the same time, but it should be given at a totally separate intramuscular site.

   **(2)** Adequate debridement of devitalized tissue and removal of all foreign matter is also essential.

   **(3)** The value of antibiotics, particularly penicillin, for the prophylaxis of tetanus-prone wounds is unproven. However, for patients who have a suspected *Clostridium tetani* infection or extensive necrosis, prophylactic penicillin should be given in high doses.

**B. Abscesses**

  **1. Causative organisms**

   **a. Staphylococcal organisms** (*Staphylococcus epidermidis, Staphylococcus aureus*) frequently infect cutaneous lesions (such as sebaceous cysts) or intracavitary locations (such as the pleural space), to form abscesses. They may also be blood-borne, resulting in multiple abscesses. Staphylococci usually produce **pus**, which must be drained to allow healing of the infection.

   **b. Other organisms**, including anaerobic and gram-negative organisms, can also cause both cutaneous and deep abscesses. Coliform organisms are often present in inguinal and perineal cutaneous abscesses.

**2. Cutaneous abscesses**

    **a.** The usual **types** are as follows:

        **(1) Furuncles (boils)** are cutaneous staphylococcal abscesses. They are frequently seen with acne and other skin disorders. The bacterial colonization begins in hair follicles and can cause both local cellulitis and abscess formation.

        **(2) Carbuncles** are cutaneous abscesses that spread through the dermis into the subcutaneous region. They may then spread over a larger area, often with a resultant sepsis. Diabetes should be suspected in these cases.

        **(3) Hidradenitis suppurativa** is an infection involving the apocrine sweat glands in the axillary, inguinal, and perineal regions. The infection results in chronic abscess formation and scarring, and often requires complete excision of the apocrine gland–bearing skin to prevent recurrence.

    **b.** The **microbiologic diagnosis** is made by incising the abscess, then culturing and Gram-staining the pus, usually revealing gram-positive cocci. Subsequent culture will reveal the bacterial type as well as its antibiotic sensitivity. Most staphylococcal organisms are resistant to penicillin, and one of the semisynthetic penicillins, erythromycin, or a cephalosporin should be used.

    **c.** The **treatment** includes:

        **(1)** Immobilizing the infected area, applying local heat, and elevating the affected part when the infection is localized to the immediately surrounding tissue

        **(2)** Drainage of pus

        **(3)** Appropriate antibiotic therapy

        **(4)** Wound care, with irrigation and debridement when necessary

        **(5)** Excision of the involved area when it contains multiple small abscesses, sinus tracts, or necrotic tissue

**3. Intra-abdominal (peritoneal) abscesses**

    **a. Causes.** Peritoneal abscesses are common infections and can result from either extrinsic or, more often, intrinsic causes.

        **(1)** The most common **extrinsic causes** are penetrating trauma and surgical procedures.

        **(2) Intrinsic causes** include perforation of a hollow viscus such as the appendix, duodenum, or colon, seeding of bacteria from a source outside the abdomen, or ischemia and infarction of tissue within the abdomen, such as bowel ischemia.

    **b. Sites**

        **(1)** The most common sites are the:

            **(a)** Subphrenic space

            **(b)** Subhepatic space

            **(c)** Lateral gutters along the posterior peritoneal cavity

            **(d)** Pelvic area

            **(e)** Periappendiceal or pericolonic areas

        **(2)** Multiple abscesses are present in up to 15% of cases.

    **c.** Abscesses in the abdominal location produce the **signs and symptoms** of any abscess, such as fever, pain, and leukocytosis.

        **(1)** These abscesses are frequently large and may produce spiking fevers followed by generalized sepsis with hypotension.

        **(2)** Postoperative abscesses usually produce fever during the second postoperative week.

        **(3)** Gastrointestinal bleeding or pulmonary, renal, or hepatic failure may occur.

    **d. Diagnosis.** The key to an expeditious **diagnosis** of an intra-abdominal abscess is a high index of suspicion.

        **(1)** The patient may have tenderness or an abdominal mass, particularly with a pelvic abscess, but often no physical findings are present.

        **(2)** Computed tomography (CT scanning) and ultrasonography are very useful and also can be used to guide the successful drainage of an abscess.

    **e. Treatment**

        **(1)** The mainstay of intra-abdominal abscess treatment is surgical intervention. This is particularly true when blood or debris is present in the abscess.

        **(2)** Deep infections usually require irrigation and drainage.

            **(a)** Classically, this has been performed as an open operative procedure.

            **(b)** More recently, ultrasound techniques and CT scanning have allowed precise localization of abscesses, and percutaneous drainage has been successful.

        **(3)** Ideally, drainage is performed without contaminating the general peritoneal cavity.

            **(a)** Pelvic abscesses may be drained transrectally or through the superior vagina.

            **(b)** Subphrenic abscesses may be drained posteriorly through a twelfth rib approach.

**C. Cellulitis** is an inflammation of the dermal and subcutaneous tissues secondary to nonsuppurative bacterial invasion. It may be the result of a puncture wound or any other type of skin infection.

1. Cellulitis produces redness, edema, and localized tenderness. Fever and leukocytosis are usually present.

2. The cellulitis-causing bacteria may also infect the regional lymphatics, resulting in red, tender streaks on an extremity.

3. The usual organism is a streptococcus which is almost always sensitive to penicillin.

4. A deep abscess can result in an overlying cellulitis and should be suspected when a patient does not rapidly respond to antibiotics.

**D. Necrotizing fasciitis** is a rapidly progressive bacterial infection in which several different organisms invade the fascial planes. The infection travels rapidly along a fascial plane and causes vascular thrombosis as it progresses. This results in necrosis of the tissue involved. However, the overlying skin may appear normal, leading the clinician to greatly underestimate the severity of the infection.

1. Necrotizing fasciitis may **result from** a small puncture wound, a surgical wound, or any open trauma.

2. **Symptoms and signs**
   a. Hemorrhagic bullae, edema, and redness may develop on the skin and crepitus may be present, although many times the skin appears normal.
   b. The patient shows signs of progressive toxicity (fever, tachycardia) and may have localized wound pain.
   c. The necrotic wound or tissue involved usually has a foul serous discharge.

3. **Gram-staining** usually reveals multiple organisms:
   a. Microaerophilic streptococci
   b. Staphylococci
   c. Gram-negative bacilli and anaerobes

4. These organisms usually act synergistically, giving the fasciitis its rapidly progressive and destructive character.

5. **Treatment** is largely surgical, and early diagnosis is extremely important.
   a. It is critical to remove all infected or devitalized tissue at the first debridement because any remaining necrotic tissue will continue the rapidly progressing necrosis.
   b. This may require the removal of large amounts of skin and surrounding tissue and occasionally requires amputation of an extremity.
   c. Daily debridement may be needed.
   d. Antibiotics in high doses are required. Penicillin and an aminoglycoside are the usual drugs used.

**E. Clostridial myositis and cellulitis (gas gangrene)**

1. Gas gangrene is most commonly caused by *Clostridium perfringens* (*Clostridium welchii*).

2. The condition is most likely to develop in wounds with the following characteristics.
   a. Extensive tissue destruction has occurred.
   b. There is marked impairment of the local blood supply, either from the injury itself, from complications of the injury such as vascular thrombosis, or from iatrogenic causes such as an orthopedic cast.
   c. The wound is grossly contaminated.
   d. There has been a delay in treatment (usually greater than 6 hours).
   e. Surgical debridement has been inadequate.
   f. The patient has a preexisting condition that leads to immunologic incompetence, such as corticosteroid drug therapy.

3. **Clinical manifestations**
   a. The average time of onset of symptoms is 48 hours after injury, but onset may be as early as 6 hours after.
   b. The most common complaint, severe pain at the site of injury, is due to the rapidly infiltrating infection. Unfortunately, this pain may be missed because the patient is already receiving narcotics. Any surgical patient who requires an increase in narcotics should be suspected of having a clostridial infection and should be examined before the narcotics dosage is changed.

**c.** A rapid weak pulse is usually present and the patient appears diaphoretic, pale, and weak. There may be mental changes, including delirium or confusion. The temperature is often, but not always, elevated.

**d.** The wound is more tender to the touch than the usual postoperative wound is. The skin may appear normal, but the wound usually drains a serous fluid with a brownish discoloration and a foul odor. There may be crepitus around the wound edges but this is often a late sign.

**e.** Blood studies may reveal a dropping hematocrit and a rising bilirubin due to hemolysis. The white blood count may be mildly elevated but this is often an unreliable indicator.

**f.** Gram-staining of the wound discharge will reveal large gram-positive bacilli. Numerous red blood cells will be present but few white cells.

**g.** A plain roentgenogram of the wound area may reveal air in the soft tissues.

**4. Management**

**a.** Adequate debridement at the time of initial injury is important for **prophylaxis**.

**b. Treatment** for established clostridial infection includes extensive debridement within the tissue planes involved, and antibiotics, especially penicillin. If extensive soft tissue necrosis is present in an extremity, amputation is performed.

  **(1)** Hyperbaric oxygen therapy is used but its value is unproven.

  **(2)** Human tetanus immune globulin will not prevent or treat gas gangrene.

  **(3)** Delay in treatment to consider further diagnostic procedures or to observe the patient's course is usually catastrophic.

**F. Infections after gastrointestinal surgery**

**1. Upper gastrointestinal tract infections**

**a.** The usual rate of serious infections after operations on the upper gastrointestinal tract is 5% to 15%.

**b.** The **oral cavity** is usually colonized by high numbers of aerobic and anaerobic bacteria. These bacteria are generally killed in the low pH environment of the **stomach**, resulting in sterile cultures. Gastric cultures become positive when obstruction (or blood) is present.

**c.** Thus, prophylactic antibiotics are not necessary with elective gastric surgical procedures but should be used when obstruction, hemorrhage, or perforation is present.

**d.** In addition, patients with gastric malignancy, achlorhydria, or a chronic illness should be given prophylactic antibiotics to cover both aerobes and anaerobes.

**e.** The usual antibiotics employed are a cephalosporin or a penicillin–aminoglycoside combination.

**2. Infections in the biliary tree**

**a.** The biliary tree is rarely colonized with bacteria in the normal individual. The colonization rate rises to 15% to 30% for patients with chronic calculous cholecystitis and to over 80% in patients with common duct obstruction.

  **(1)** *Escherichia coli* is present in over one-half of the cases, while other gram-negative organisms account for the remainder.

  **(2)** *Streptococcus fecalis*, the aerobic gram-positive enterococcus, is also sometimes present, and *Salmonella* strains occasionally are. Anaerobic organisms, especially *C. perfringens*, are present in up to 20% of cases.

**b.** No antibiotic prophylaxis is recommended for elective cholecystectomy.

**c.** Therapeutic antibiotics are recommended in patients with cholangitis, with empyema or gangrene of the gallbladder, or with liver abscesses. A cephalosporin or aminoglycoside should be given for 5 to 7 days.

**d.** Prophylactic antibiotics should be used in patients over 70 years of age and in those with common duct stones, a history of fever or chills, or a gram-positive stain of the bile.

**3. Infections of the colon and rectum**

**a.** Surgery performed on these segments of the bowel is frequently followed by wound infection, the risk ranging from 6% to over 60%.

**b.** The normal human colonic microflora is composed of both aerobes and anaerobes.

  **(1) Aerobes** are present at levels of about $10^9$ bacteria per g of stool. *E. coli*, the most common aerobe, is the organism most often found in wound infections after surgery on the colon.

  **(2) Anaerobes** are present at levels of about $10^9$ bacteria per g of stool. Many types are present, but *Bacteroides fragilis* is the most common and is the usual cause of anaerobic wound infection.

  **(3)** Clostridial infections and mixed aerobic or anaerobic infections are not uncommon.

**c.** An effective **preoperative regimen** combines the removal of gross feces (mechanical preparation of the bowel) with the use of oral antibiotics.

(1) Mechanical removal of the feces is the most important factor in lowering the bacterial counts and the incidence of wound infections. Most regimens include aggressive purgation with potent oral agents, such as mannitol or magnesium sulfate, and with multiple enemas.

(2) Antibiotic prophylaxis will only reduce bacterial counts enough to lower the incidence of wound infection after adequate mechanical preparation. Single antibiotics or combinations of antibiotics are not effective unless they inhibit both aerobic and anaerobic organisms simultaneously.

 (a) Oral antibiotics, such as neomycin and erythromycin base, started 10 to 22 hours prior to surgery, will result in maximal bacterial suppression at the time of surgery. Longer treatment periods will allow bacterial overgrowth, with resistant forms emerging.

 (b) Intravenous antibiotics may further lower the incidence of wound infection when given concomitantly with an oral antibiotic combination, but this is controversial.

(3) Preparation of the colon and rectum should be carried out before all elective operations unless a high-grade (complete) obstruction is present. The presence of obstruction calls for a preliminary colostomy to remove the feces mechanically. After adequate purgation, the elective procedure is performed under oral antibiotic "cover."

(4) In emergency procedures (e.g., after trauma) when no bowel preparation is possible, intravenous antibiotics should be given and the wound should not be closed primarily. In these situations, colonic anastomoses should be avoided.

## G. Infections after gynecologic surgery

1. The organisms involved usually arise from the vagina and can include both aerobes and anaerobes.

2. Prophylactic antibiotics can be useful in the premenopausal woman undergoing vaginal hysterectomy.

## H. Infections after urologic surgery

1. Although the normal urinary tract is sterile, the most common pathogen encountered is *E. coli*, followed by other gram-negative rods and enterococci.

2. The general principle that elective surgery should be postponed until any infection has been successfully treated is especially true for urologic surgery.

3. Chronic indwelling tubes (such as suprapubic bladder catheters) and nephrostomies do not call for antibiotic therapy unless the patient has a symptomatic local infection or generalized sepsis, the catheter becomes obstructed, or a urea-splitting organism such as *Proteus* is present.

4. When transurethral prostatectomy, cystourethroscopy (especially in males), or urethral surgery is planned, a urinary tract infection should be sought.
 a. If cultures are positive, the patient should be prophylactically treated with an antibiotic that is specific for the infecting organism.
 b. The procedure should not be performed until cultures are negative.

## I. Infections after vascular surgery

1. The rate of infection when **vascular prosthetic grafts** are employed varies between 1% and 6%. The infection may develop early (within months after surgery) or as late as 7 years after.

2. The source of infection may be direct contamination from the skin or surrounding tissues, or blood-borne organisms. The most common infecting organism is *S. aureus*, followed by coagulase-negative *S. epidermidis*. Coliform organisms are becoming more common.

3. There is strong evidence that giving prophylactic antibiotics at the time of surgery will lower the incidence of graft infection from the high of 6% down to 1%.

4. Prophylactic antibiotics should also be used when a patient with a prosthetic graft undergoes a procedure associated with a transient bacteremia (such as dental extraction).

5. The recommended prophylactic antibiotic is a cephalosporin given pre- and postoperatively for 48 hours or until all intravenous lines and other tubes have been removed.

## J. Infections after cardiac surgery. 
The extracorporeal circulation used for aortocoronary bypass surgery and for prosthetic valve insertion can be contaminated by *S. epidermidis* and *S. aureus*. Infections are severe and life-threatening and include sternal dehiscence and endocarditis. The recommended prophylactic antibiotic therapy is similar to that for vascular surgery.

**K. Infections after noncardiac thoracic surgery.** Lung surgery is particularly associated with infection when the lung is already infected or when a significant volume of lung is removed, as in a pneumonectomy, and a large dead space remains. The usual organisms are gram-positive cocci, but it has not been definitively demonstrated that prophylactic antibiotics are useful.

**L. Infections after orthopedic surgery.** Postoperative sepsis has serious consequences in orthopedic surgery, especially when a prosthesis has been implanted. Several studies have suggested a beneficial effect from prophylactic antibiotics. The appropriate antibiotic is usually one directed toward staphylococcal organisms.

**M. Infections after trauma**

1. **Burns** (second- and third-degree) are prone to develop group A *Streptococcus pyogenes* infection during the first 5 days. Many burn centers recommend using penicillin G or a penicillinase-resistant synthetic penicillin during this phase. In order to reduce the colonization of injured tissues, topical antibiotics should also be applied. These antibiotics should be effective against both gram-negative rods and gram-positive cocci. Purulent infections of intravenous catheter and cutdown sites should be treated by excision of the vein.

2. **Penetrating abdominal trauma** should be treated with an antibiotic regimen that covers both anaerobic and aerobic organisms.

3. **Penetrating chest wounds** should be treated with antibiotics that are effective against organisms commonly found in the respiratory tract.

4. **Human bites** should be treated with penicillin because they are likely to contain mixed anaerobic and aerobic organisms. **Animal bites** warrant prophylactic antibiotics if there is extensive injury.

5. **Other soft tissue injuries** involving a large surface area should be treated with antibiotics effective against normal residents of the skin (gram-positive cocci). If extensive contamination from environmental pathogens is present, antibiotics providing coverage against anaerobic and gram-negative bacilli should be added.

# VIII. POSTOPERATIVE COMPLICATIONS*

**A.** Postoperative complications can be associated with any operation or can be related to a specific kind of surgery. The latter type are discussed in the relevant chapters, and only the general types of complications are discussed here. Thrombophlebitis and pulmonary embolus, which are common postoperative complications, are discussed in Chapter 14.

**B.** Most surgical complications develop in relation to some event that occurs in the operating room, emphasizing the fact that prevention is the best form of management.

**C. General principles of management** during the postoperative period are important both in preventing potential complications and in allowing early detection of problems that do develop. These principles include:

1. Daily or more frequent examination of the patient, including the surgical wound

2. Removal of all surgical tubes as soon as possible

3. Early mobilization of the patient to minimize pulmonary problems

4. Close monitoring of fluid balance and electrolyte levels

5. Adequate but not excessive pain medication

6. Good nursing care

**D. Common postoperative problems** typically occur on certain postoperative days. Most of these problems produce **fever** and can be diagnosed by physical examination and simple laboratory tests.

1. **Pulmonary complications** are the most common cause of fever during the first postoperative days.
   a. Most pulmonary problems develop because of prolonged mechanical ventilation, or because of inadequate ventilation and a poor cough effort. They are made worse by oversedation, preexisting chronic pulmonary disease, or abdominal distention.

---

*Author: Bruce E. Jarrell

    **b. Atelectasis** is the usual problem, but **pneumonia** can supervene if the atelectasis is not quickly treated.

    **c.** Nasotracheal aspiration or bronchoscopy will help to resolve atelectasis by removing secretions and inflating a collapsed lung. Antibiotics should not be given unless evidence of infection is present.

  **2. Urinary tract infection** is the typical cause of fever that develops on postoperative day 3 through 6.

    **a.** An indwelling catheter or preexisting vesical outlet obstruction is often the cause.

    **b.** Also, postoperative pain can cause patients to empty the bladder incompletely when voiding; the residual urine predisposes to infection.

    **c.** Urinary tract infection is best treated by:

      **(1)** Inducing diuresis via adequate hydration

      **(2)** Giving appropriate antibiotics

      **(3)** Relieving any obstruction that is present

      **(4)** Removing the catheter, if feasible

  **3. Wound infections**, including intra-abdominal abscesses, are discussed in section VII.

**E.** Surgical procedures often affect **body fluids**.

  **1. Dehydration** is common after surgery because of third-space sequestration of fluids in the operative site.

    **a.** Oliguria, tachycardia, and orthostatic hypotension may result.

    **b.** Treatment is rehydration.

    **c.** On the third or fourth postoperative day, the body begins to mobilize the third-space fluid, which increases the intravascular volume until the fluid is excreted by the kidneys.

  **2. Overhydration** may occur in patients with impaired cardiac or renal function.

    **a.** Congestive heart failure or pulmonary congestion and impaired oxygenation may result.

    **b.** Salt replacement, attention to fluid balance, and weighing the patient daily should prevent this problem.

    **c.** In addition, the intravascular volume increase that results from the mobilization of third-space fluid should be anticipated.

## IX. SURGICAL TREATMENT OF TUMORS*

**A. Background**

  **1.** The surgeon has historically served as the primary physician in the diagnosis and therapy of solid tumors.

  **2.** In the past 20 years, radiation oncologists and cancer chemotherapists have found their roles in cancer treatment increasing, but the surgeon still cures more cancers (particularly colon cancer, melanoma, and breast cancer) than other oncologic specialists.

  **3.** Cancer patients are now treated by a number of modalities, offered by several kinds of specialists, and the physician must understand the capabilities and limitations of the various modes of treatment.

**B. Diagnostic techniques**

  **1. Biopsy** is the taking of a sample from a lesion for microscopic examination to determine a pathologic diagnosis. There are several common **ways of taking a biopsy specimen**.

    **a.** In **aspiration biopsy**, a narrow-gauge needle is inserted into the lesion and a group of cells is drawn up into a syringe. The procedure may be used for palpable lesions or, with radiographic guidance, for deeper lesions. Its accuracy depends on the skill of the cytopathologist. Aspiration biopsy is typically used for identifying lesions of the thyroid, pancreas, or breast.

    **b.** A **needle biopsy** also involves a needle inserted into a lesion, but here a core of tissue is removed for histologic examination. Complications (bleeding, spread of the tumor) are more likely than with needle aspiration.

    **c.** An **excisional biopsy** is used for small lesions that can be removed entirely, usually with local anesthesia. An example is excision of a 1-cm cutaneous melanoma.

    **d.** In an **incisional biopsy**, a scalpel is used to remove a portion of a lesion for examination. Incisional biopsy is usually performed if a lesion is too large for simple excision.

---

*Author: Stephen M. Weiss

**2. Operative staging** is a reliable method of defining the extent of certain tumors. Its purpose is to guide further treatment and to predict results. The size of the primary tumor, its fixation to adjacent organs, and the involvement of lymph nodes can be learned at operation.

    **a.** In the staging of **breast cancer**, axillary lymph node dissection is done primarily to determine the likelihood that systemic metastases will develop.

        **(1)** Patients with lymph nodes negative for tumor have a 75% likelihood of being free of tumor for 10 years.

        **(2)** Those with malignant lymph nodes have only a 25% chance of being free of tumor for 10 years. Patients with positive lymph nodes are candidates for adjuvant chemotherapy to decrease the chance of recurrent cancer.

    **b.** In **Hodgkin's disease**, a staging laparotomy is performed. This includes biopsies of numerous lymph node chains (para-aortic, splenic, mesenteric, iliac, porta hepatis, celiac) and a splenectomy, as well as liver and bone marrow biopsies.

        **(1)** Patients with lymph node disease only are usually treated with radiation to involved nodes and contiguous normal nodes.

        **(2)** If Hodgkin's disease is found in the liver or other viscera (except the spleen), chemotherapy is required.

**C. Operative treatment of tumors.** The value of resection for a given tumor depends on a variety of factors, including histologic findings, the location and size of the tumor, its fixation to adjacent tissues, and the patient's age and underlying health.

    **1. Curative resection** generally combines the removal of a grossly evident tumor, plus a margin of apparently normal tissue, with removal of the lymph nodes draining the tumor. Curative resection is not appropriate for patients with distant metastases, since the presence of residual tumor precludes cure.

        **a.** A **margin of grossly normal tissue** (i.e., tissue that appears normal on gross inspection) is removed along with the tumor because microscopic cancer cells are likely to extend well beyond a palpable or visible tumor.

        **b. Lymph nodes** are removed because they often harbor cancer cells. Also, a search for the presence of tumor cells in lymph nodes can be used in predicting the prognosis.

    **2. Palliative resection** is used to relieve or prevent a specific symptom of a cancer patient, but not to effect a cure. Palliative surgery can often provide excellent patient comfort for many months. Examples of uses for palliative resection include:

        **a.** Removal of an obstructing colon cancer in a patient with liver metastases

        **b.** A "toilet mastectomy" to remove ulcerating, necrotic, infected breast cancer tissue

**D. Multimodality treatment of cancer** involves combinations of chemotherapy and radiotherapy with surgery.

    **1. Specialized procedures** used in chemotherapy and radiotherapy include the following:

        **a.** In **isolation perfusion**, the artery and vein to an extremity are isolated and cannulated to allow intensive, short-term chemotherapeutic drug perfusion without systemic toxicity.

            **(1)** An example is the treatment of sarcoma of the left leg with phenylalanine mustard administered via the femoral artery.

            **(2)** The efficacy of isolation perfusion can be increased even further by increasing the temperature of the drug (**hyperthermic perfusion**).

        **b. Infusion chemotherapy**, by contrast, provides continuous, long-term regional chemotherapy via a catheter implanted into a blood vessel.

            **(1)** An example is the hepatic artery infusion of liver metastases by means of an implantable catheter and pump.

            **(2)** The advantages of infusion chemotherapy over more traditional methods of drug administration are that a higher dose of the chemotherapeutic agent can be supplied to a specific site, with less systemic toxicity.

        **c. Brachytherapy** involves the implantation of a radioactive source into a cancer for local tumoricidal effect. For example, iodine 125 ($^{125}$I) "seeds" may be implanted into a prostatic or a pancreatic cancer. This allows relatively large amounts of radiation to be delivered precisely to the tumor, with less radiation to surrounding organs.

    **2. Radiation therapy** can be used **in combination with surgery** to improve local tumor control.

        **a.** Many large soft tissue sarcomas, such as a sarcoma involving two muscle compartments of the lower extremity, have traditionally been treated by amputation. Comparable tumor control, with better functional results, may be obtained when preoperative or postoperative irradiation is combined with more limited tumor resection.

        **b.** Combined radiation and resection can also be used for cancers of the esophagus, rectum, stomach, and other sites.

3. **Tumor "debulking"**, or **cytoreduction**, is the removal of a large portion of a tumor, but it is less than complete removal.
    a. Debulking is usually done with the intent of improving response to adjunctive therapy. The rationale is that by removing the many tumor cells in the resting phase (and thus less sensitive to chemotherapy), debulking should leave a much smaller population of cells that are more susceptible to chemotherapy or radiation. (However, the usefulness of this approach has not been established.)
    b. For example, in ovarian cancer stage II, III, or IV, survival time may be increased if little residual tumor is left after laparotomy, since the response to chemotherapy may be improved by the reduction in tumor volume.

4. **Resection of isolated metastases** may be of benefit in some forms of cancer, if the primary tumor is controlled. For example, the resection of solitary liver metastases in colon cancer patients with no other evidence of tumor is reported to provide 2-year survival in 67% of the patients.

**X. HERNIA.*** A **hernia** is the abnormal protrusion of intra-abdominal tissue through a defect in the abdominal wall.

A. **General aspects**

1. In both males and females, hernias occur most commonly in the inguinal region (75% to 80% of all hernias). Incisional ventral hernias occur next in frequency (8% to 10%), followed by umbilical hernias (3% to 8%).

2. **Etiologic factors.** Hernias can occur as a result of various factors.
    a. **Congenital defects** in the abdominal wall, such as in indirect inguinal hernia, are common.
    b. A normal anatomic **foramen that becomes pathologically enlarged** can allow an organ to pass through the defect (e.g., the stomach passing into the chest through the esophageal hiatus is a **hiatal hernia**).
    c. **Loss of tissue strength and elasticity**, especially due to aging, may result in herniation, as in direct inguinal hernia.
    d. **Trauma**, especially **operative trauma** in which normal tissue strength is destroyed surgically, can lead to the development of hernia. Infection in the wound greatly increases the risk of hernia following surgery.
    e. Any cause of **increased intra-abdominal pressure** can result in hernia, such as:
        (1) Heavy lifting
        (2) Coughing, asthma, and chronic obstructive pulmonary disease (COPD)
        (3) Vesical outlet obstruction (e.g., benign prostatic hypertrophy)
        (4) Constipation or difficulty moving one's bowels, as occurs in carcinoma of the colon or rectum
        (5) Pregnancy
        (6) Ascites, intra-abdominal tumors, and abdominal distention
        (7) Obesity

3. **Descriptive terms.** Hernias may be described according to physical or operative findings.
    a. **Complete.** Both the hernia sac and its contents extend through the defect (e.g., in a complete inguinal hernia, both the sac and its contents extend into the scrotum).
    b. **Incomplete.** A defect is present but the sac and its contents do not yet pass through (e.g., in an incomplete inguinal hernia, the sac has not extended through the external inguinal ring).
    c. **Reducible.** The hernia contents can be pushed back into the abdomen.
    d. **Irreducible (incarcerated).** The hernia contents are adherent to the hernia defect and cannot be pushed back.
    e. **Obstructing.** The hernia contains a loop of bowel that is kinked and, therefore, obstructed.
    f. **Strangulated.** The tissue contained in the hernia is ischemic due to interruption of its blood supply.
    g. **Sliding.** The wall of the hernia sac, rather than being formed completely by peritoneum, is in part formed by the wall of another intra-abdominal structure such as the colon or the bladder.
    h. **Richter's hernia.** One side of the bowel wall is trapped in the hernia rather than the entire loop of bowel.

---

*Author: Bruce E. Jarrell

i. **Littre's hernia.** A Meckel's diverticulum is incarcerated in the hernia. Other structures, such as an ovary or the appendix, may also become incarcerated in a hernia.

4. **Complications.** Hernias should be repaired electively to prevent the development of major complications.

   a. **Intestinal obstruction** may occur when a loop of bowel passes through the abdominal wall defect and becomes mechanically obstructed. This was the most common cause of intestinal obstruction in the early 1900s.

   b. **Intestinal strangulation** with **perforation** or **gangrene** may occur if the vascular pedicle to the herniated loop of bowel is also interrupted.

**B. Inguinal hernias**

1. **Anatomy of the inguinal region** (Figs. 1-2 and 1-3)

   a. The **internal inguinal ring** is an opening in the transversalis fascia lateral to the inferior epigastric artery.

   b. The **external inguinal ring** is an opening in the external oblique aponeurosis through which the spermatic cord passes into the scrotum.

   c. The **inguinal canal** is the communication between the internal and external rings. In females the inguinal canal contains the round ligament.

      (1) The anterior wall of the canal is formed by the external oblique aponeurosis.

      (2) The floor of the canal is formed by the inguinal ligament (**Poupart's ligament**) and its reflection.

         (a) Within the floor of the inguinal canal is **Hesselbach's triangle**.

         (b) It is formed laterally by the inferior epigastric artery, inferiorly by the inguinal ligament, and superomedially by the transversalis fascia and portions of the rectus sheath.

      (3) The roof of the inguinal canal is made up of fibers of the internal oblique and transversus muscles, forming a structure termed the **conjoint tendon**.

      (4) The posterior wall is formed by the conjoint tendon structure, containing a strong reinforcing band of transversalis fascia.

   d. The **spermatic cord structures** pass into the internal ring, traverse the inguinal canal, and pass through the external ring into the scrotum. The following structures are contained within the cord:

      (1) **Arteries**: testicular and cremasteric

      (2) **Nerves**: ilioinguinal, genital branch of the genitofemoral, and sympathetic nervous supply

      (3) **Veins**: pampiniform plexus

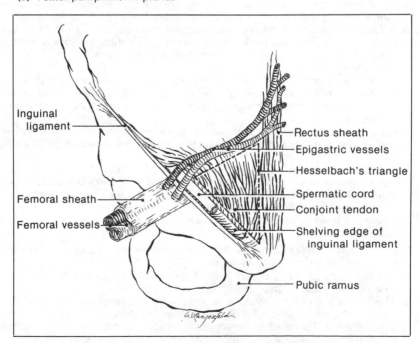

**Figure 1-2.** Anatomy of the inguinal region.

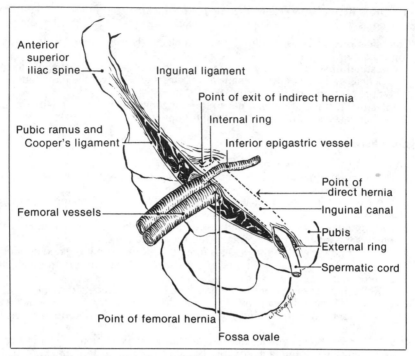

**Figure 1-3.** Sites of direct, indirect, and femoral hernias and their relationship to anatomic structures.

    **(4) Vas deferens**
    **(5) Processus vaginalis**: an invagination of peritoneum that accompanies the descent of the testicle and gubernaculum through the abdominal wall. Normally obliterated, it remains patent in an indirect hernia and forms the hernia sac.

**2. Indirect inguinal hernias**
    **a.** An indirect inguinal hernia passes through the internal inguinal ring and down the inguinal canal (see Fig. 1-3). It may, on occasion, extend into the scrotum (complete hernia).
    **b.** An indirect inguinal hernia occurs as a result of a congenitally patent processus vaginalis, which allows free communication between the peritoneal cavity, inguinal canal, and scrotum. It may also result in a spermatic cord hydrocele.
    **c. Incidence**
        **(1)** Indirect inguinal hernias are five to ten times more common in men than in women. Approximately 5% of men develop an inguinal hernia during their lifetime and require an operation. Indirect inguinal hernias are the most common type of hernias in women.
        **(2)** Indirect inguinal hernias are five times more common than direct hernias.
    **d.** Indirect hernias may occur from infancy to old age but generally occur by the fifth decade of life.
    **e.** A **pediatric inguinal hernia** (see also Chapter 33, section II) is almost always indirect and has a high risk of incarceration. It is more common on the right (75%) and is often bilateral.
    **f. Potential indirect hernias** are associated with an undescended testis, a testis in the inguinal canal, and a testicular or spermatic cord hydrocele.
    **g.** There is a bilateral patent processus vaginalis in up to 10% of patients with an indirect inguinal hernia.

**3. Direct inguinal hernias.** The inferior epigastric vessels are the anatomic landmarks that distinguish indirect and direct inguinal hernias.
    **a.** A direct inguinal hernia occurs in the floor of the inguinal canal, at Hesselbach's triangle (see Fig. 1-2), due to an acquired weakness in the tissue.
    **b.** The hernia is a direct protrusion of abdominal structures into the floor of the canal posterior to the spermatic cord. It is not contained in the cord as the indirect hernia is, and it generally does not pass into the scrotum. The sac is a broadly based defect: it is much less often associated with strangulation than an indirect inguinal hernia is.
    **c.** Direct inguinal hernia increases in occurrence with age and is related to physical activity.

**d.** A **recurrent inguinal hernia** usually occurs as a direct hernia. Generally the defect occurs in the most medial aspect of the repair of the floor of the inguinal canal,

**4.** A **pantaloon hernia** is a combination of a direct and an indirect hernia in which the hernia sac passes around the inferior epigastric vessels both medially and laterally.

**5. Femoral hernia**
  **a.** A femoral hernia occurs when intra-abdominal contents protrude along the femoral sheath in the femoral canal (see Fig. 1-3).
  **b.** The hernia contents usually protrude posterior to the inguinal ligament, anterior to the pubic ramus periosteum (i.e., **Cooper's ligament**), lateral to the **lacunar ligament** (which is composed of fascial attachments medially located above the inguinal ligament), and medial to the femoral vessels.
  **c.** The hernia traverses the femoral canal and may present as a mass at the level of the foramen ovale. It may also turn cephalad once it has exited through the foramen ovale and has crossed anterior to the inguinal ligament.
  **d.** The sac frequently has a narrow neck, and 30% to 40% of femoral hernias become incarcerated or strangulated.
  **e.** Femoral hernias are more common in females than in males.
  **f.** Femoral hernias are related to physical exertion, and to pregnancy in the female.

**6.** The **diagnosis** of an inguinal hernia is based on history and physical examination.
  **a.** The **history** may include the sudden appearance of a lump in the groin. The mass may be intermittently present and may be painful. Its appearance may be associated with strenuous activity. In some patients, it may extend into the scrotum (complete hernia).
  **b. Physical examination** should be performed with the patient in both the recumbent and upright positions.
    **(1)** A mass may be visible, and its size or visibility may depend on its position.
    **(2)** The mass may be tender, may feel like bowel or other intra-abdominal tissue such as fat or omentum, and may be reducible with gentle pressure. Bowel sounds may be audible.
    **(3)** The mass may be small or nonpalpable, but may become palpable as an impulse at the tip of the examining finger upon a sudden increase in the intra-abdominal pressure, as occurs with a cough.
    **(4)** The examining finger should be placed along the spermatic cord at the scrotum and passed into the external ring along the canal.
      **(a)** A **direct hernia** causes a bulge forward low in the canal.
      **(b)** An **indirect hernia** lightly touches the tip of the examining finger during a maneuver that increases intra-abdominal pressure.
  **c.** The **differential diagnosis** includes other causes of an inguinal mass, such as a hydrocele, a varix, a lipoma of the spermatic cord, an inflamed or enlarged lymph node, an undescended testicle, or an abscess or tumor.

**7. Repair of inguinal hernias**
  **a. General principles** for the operative repair of inguinal hernias include:
    **(1)** Return of the hernia contents into the peritoneal cavity
    **(2)** Ligation of the base of the hernia sac
    **(3)** Repair of the abdominal wall defect to prevent recurrence
  **b.** The **repair of indirect inguinal hernia** involves:
    **(1)** Ligation of the hernia sac at the level of the peritoneal cavity—the sac is usually anteromedial to the cord at the level of the internal ring
    **(2)** Tightening of the internal ring
    **(3)** Repair of the inguinal canal floor in adults
  **c.** The **repair of direct inguinal hernia** is based upon reinforcement of the inguinal canal floor after reinvaginating the hernia sac.
  **d.** In the **repair of femoral hernia**, the femoral sheath defect is usually approached suprainguinally.
    **(1)** The space is closed by apposing Cooper's ligament and the inguinal ligament posterior reflection.
    **(2)** The femoral sheath is sutured to these structures.
    **(3)** Often the floor of the inguinal canal is also reinforced, using the transversalis fascia.
  **e.** For **repair of the abdominal wall defect**, many different techniques are used, some of which are discussed below.
    **(1)** The **Bassini repair**
      **(a)** The transversalis fascia and conjoint tendon are sutured to the reflection of the inguinal ligament (i.e., the shelving edge of Poupart's ligament).

        **(b)** The spermatic cord is returned to its normal anatomic location between the reinforced inguinal canal floor and the external oblique aponeurosis.

        **(c)** In women, the round ligament may be ligated and the internal ring closed.

    **(2) Cooper's ligament repair (McVay's method)**

        **(a)** This is similar to the Bassini repair except that the transversalis fascia is sutured to Cooper's ligament, which is the periosteum of the pubic ramus.

        **(b)** Because Cooper's ligament is more inferoposterior than the inguinal ligament, a "relaxing" incision is often made in the anterior rectus sheath adjacent to the reflection of the external oblique aponeurosis. This allows the transversalis to be sutured to the ligament without undue tension.

    **(3)** The **Shouldice repair** is also similar to the Bassini repair except that the transversalis fascia is divided longitudinally and the subsequent two layers are imbricated to the inguinal ligament. The internal oblique muscle and conjoint tendon are then sutured over the initial closure into the external oblique fascia.

  **f.** **Recurrence rates** after surgical repair vary, depending on the type of hernia, but hernias generally recur in about 1% of cases.

  **g.** **Special situations**

    **(1)** When **strangulation or necrosis of the incarcerated bowel** is suspected but the bowel returns to the peritoneal cavity spontaneously prior to visual examination by the surgeon, the abdomen should be opened and explored and any necrotic bowel should be resected.

    **(2) Recurrent hernias** or **hernias with large defects** may require the insertion of prosthetic material such as polypropylene to obliterate the defect adequately.

    **(3)** Simple high ligation of the hernia sac is employed for hernias occurring in the **pediatric age group** when no other defect is present.

    **(4)** A **truss** is a device that exerts external compression over the hernia defect, keeping the space obliterated. It is generally used only when surgery cannot be safely performed or when the patient refuses surgery.

**C. Other types of abdominal wall hernias**

  **1. Umbilical hernias** occur in the region of the umbilicus, usually in relation to a defect where the umbilical structures passed through the abdominal wall.

    **a.** Umbilical hernias occur ten times more often in females than in males.

    **b.** The defect is common in children but usually closes by age 2 years, and fewer than 5% of umbilical hernias persist into later childhood and adult life.

    **c.** In adults, umbilical hernias are often associated with increased intra-abdominal pressure, especially pressure caused by ascites or pregnancy.

    **d.** Management of an umbilical hernia is through a simple transverse repair of the fascial defect.

  **2. Epigastric hernias** result from a defect in the linea alba above the umbilicus.

    **a.** They occur more commonly in males (in a 3 to 1 ratio).

    **b.** Some 20% of epigastric hernias are multiple at the time of repair.

    **c.** Repair (simple suturing) is associated with a recurrence rate as high as 10%.

  **3. Ventral hernias** occur in the abdominal wall in areas other than the inguinal region.

    **a.** An **incisional hernia**, the most common type of ventral hernia, results from poor wound healing in a previous surgical incision.

      **(1)** Common etiologic factors include wound infection or hematoma, advanced age, obesity, general debilitation or malnutrition, surgical technique, or a postoperative increase in abdominal pressure, as occurs with ileus, ascites, or pulmonary complications of surgery.

      **(2)** Incisional hernias are repaired after the patient has recovered from the surgical trauma. The wound must be epithelialized prior to repair in order to prevent recurrent sepsis.

    **b.** **Spigelian hernias** protrude through the abdominal wall along the spigelian line, which is at the lateral edge of the rectus sheath where the transversus muscle becomes an aponeurosis.

# Trauma and Burns

Jerome J. Vernick

## I. TRAUMA

### A. General considerations

1. Trauma is the leading cause of death in people under 35 years of age.
   a. Over 120,000 persons die from trauma per year.
   b. One-half of these deaths result from motor vehicle accidents.

2. Some 10% to 15% of traumatized patients have serious multisystem injuries.

3. Mortality can be greatly reduced by efficient handling of the injured. This involves three major components:
   a. A **trauma center** with professional personnel who are trained in delivering rapid care and with facilities capable of handling a number of patients at one time
   b. A **transportation system** capable of rapid transport to a trauma center
   c. **Emergency medical technicians** who are capable of maintaining vital functions until the trauma surgeon can take over

4. The management of trauma requires adherence to an established **order of priority**.
   a. This ensures that the most life-threatening injuries will be treated first, but less serious injuries will not be neglected following resuscitation.
   b. The **order of priority** is as follows:
      (1) Initial assessment, including an "AMPLE" history (Table 2-1)
      (2) Provision of airway control and establishment of respiration
      (3) Establishment of venous access and restoration of tissue perfusion
      (4) Diagnosis of immediately life-threatening injuries, followed by rapid treatment
      (5) Reassessment of the patient's status
      (6) Diagnosis of other significant injuries
      (7) Definitive treatment, including surgery

5. Prophylactic antibiotics should be given to all patients with major trauma, and tetanus prophylaxis should be administered (see Chapter 1, section VII).

**Table 2-1.** Points Covered in the "AMPLE" History

| |
|---|
| **A**llergies |
| **M**edications |
| **P**revious illnesses |
| **L**ast meal |
| **E**vents surrounding injury |

### B. Mechanisms of injury

1. Knowing the mechanism of injury is helpful in allowing one to:
   a. Anticipate lesions that otherwise remain undiagnosed
   b. Decide on the appropriate management for lesions that may be more extensive than they might at first appear

2. **Acceleration–deceleration injuries** are typically caused by falls from heights, blunt trauma, or vehicular accidents.
   a. Obvious injuries result from direct contact with the landing site (the ground, the vehicle)
   b. More subtle injuries result from shearing forces produced by the momentum when heavy organs are suddenly halted or accelerated by a crash.

**(1)** Heavy organs include fluid-filled loops of bowel, the blood-filled thoracic aorta, and mobile parenchymal organs such as the liver and spleen.

**(2)** The momentum of these organs is maintained after the motion of the victim has been stopped.

**(3)** Damage occurs because force is exerted on the tethered portion of the viscus by the still-moving, mobile portion of the viscus.

  **(a)** The aortic arch shears at the fixed ligamentum arteriosus.

  **(b)** The small bowel tends to pull away from its mesenteric attachments, creating a "bucket-handle" tear with massive bleeding from mesenteric vessels.

  **(c)** Avulsion of the spleen at its hilus or peritoneal reflections is common.

  **(d)** Renal pedicle avulsion is another example of the type of injury that can occur.

**3. Missile wounds**

  **a.** Injury from **low-velocity missiles** includes most civilian gunshot injuries.

  **(1)** Missiles fired from handguns have a velocity in the range of 600 to 1100 feet per second.

  **(2)** Wounds from this type of missile are generally restricted to the path and the residual cavity created by the missile as it penetrates tissues such as blood vessels and organs.

  **(3)** However, secondary injuries can occur.

  **(a)** External articles (clothing, buttons, keys) may be driven into the wound by the missile.

  **(b)** Bone fragments, produced when the missile strikes a large bone, can also cause secondary injury.

  **b.** The shocking, "knock-down" effect of a missile depends on factors that influence the energy transferred to the victim by the impact.

  **(1)** Striking energy is directly proportional to the weight of a missile and the square of its velocity.

  **(2)** Missiles that completely penetrate the victim expend much of their energy on the objects beyond. Maximum energy transfer results from the missile's remaining within the victim.

  **c.** The penetration is diminished when a bullet is used that expands or tumbles after impact.

  **d. Shotgun wounds** are common.

  **(1)** They cause devastating injuries at **close range.**

  **(a)** Large soft-tissue defects are created, with widespread damage.

  **(b)** Close-range shotgun wounds often introduce nonopaque foreign material which originates from the wadding or packing used in the manufacture of the shotgun shell.

  **(2)** **Longer-range** shotgun wounds consist of multiple low-velocity pellet injuries. These cause widespread penetration but are generally not severe unless the missile happens to strike a major blood vessel or organ.

  **e. High-velocity missile injuries** can be recognized by a small entrance wound and a large exit wound with severe underlying tissue damage.

  **(1)** High-velocity wounds cause damage remote from the apparent tract of the missile.

  **(2)** This is due to a large temporary cavity created by the tissue's recoiling from the path of the bullet as it passes through (see section I C 6 e).

  **f.** All missile tracts should be debrided.

  **g.** Missiles need not be sought and removed unless they are symptomatic or are in close proximity to a vital structure where body movements or tissue erosion could cause further injury.

**C. Management of trauma victims**

  **1.** The **initial assessment** of the patient's state, performed when the patient arrives in the emergency room, is intended to determine rapidly the extent of injury and the need for immediate care.

  **a.** This assessment can be performed by an experienced physician within seconds.

  **b.** The following three questions should be answered.

  **(1)** Is ventilation adequate?

  **(2)** Is tissue being perfused?

  **(3)** Is significant neurologic injury present?

  **2.** Alcohol on the patient's breath does not relieve the trauma team of the responsibility of applying sound judgment.

  **3. Airway assessment and control**

  **a. Assessment**

  **(1)** The patient should be examined for chest wall motion and asymmetry, cyanosis, and evidence of air exchange.

**(2)** The chest should be examined for subcutaneous emphysema or fractures and auscultated for breath sounds.

**(3)** The mouth and upper airway should be inspected for foreign bodies or other causes of obstruction.

**b. Establishing ventilation.** If ventilation is unsatisfactory, then rapid corrective measures are necessary.

  **(1)** Early **intubation** is important, since potentially unstable patients quickly become apneic.

    **(a)** Oxygen is needed for all severely injured patients.

    **(b)** Intubate rapidly in the presence of:

      **(i)** A decreased level of consciousness

      **(ii)** Hypotension

      **(iii)** Major head, face, or neck injury

      **(iv)** Chest trauma

      **(v)** Cyanosis

    **(c)** Any patient with major trauma may have a cervical spine injury.

      **(i)** Therefore, the neck should not be extended during intubation unless it is definitely known that no such injury exists.

      **(ii)** When this is not known, either a nasotracheal tube should be used or a tracheostomy or cricothyroidotomy should be performed.

  **(2) Ventilation** should be performed with either a hand-held bag or a volume respirator.

    **(a)** The **adequacy of ventilation** should be assessed by auscultation of the chest, followed by arterial blood gas measurement.

    **(b)** The most common causes of inadequate ventilation are:

      **(i)** Incorrect placement of the endotracheal tube into either the esophagus or the right main stem bronchus

      **(ii)** The presence of a pneumothorax

    **(c)** The thorax should be assessed when ventilation is started.

      **(i)** After auscultation, if breath sounds are absent in one or both hemithoraces, aspiration with a large-bore needle followed by insertion of a chest tube is an acceptable diagnostic and therapeutic maneuver.

      **(ii)** A tension pneumothorax produces a high-pressure condition in the pleural space, compressing the pulmonary parenchyma and impairing venous return to the heart. It must be treated rapidly with a chest tube and should not wait for confirmation by chest x-ray.

    **(d) Signs of tension pneumothorax are:**

      **(i)** Inadequate ventilation, with cyanosis and absent breath sounds

      **(ii)** Hypotension

      **(iii)** A shift of the mediastinum and trachea away from the pneumothorax

      **(iv)** Impaired venous return, with elevated central venous pressure

**4.** Once adequate ventilation has been established, the physician should rapidly proceed to the next critical stage of resuscitation, namely, **establishment of tissue perfusion**, or **circulatory support**.

  **a. Cardiac resuscitation**

    **(1)** If the patient is asystolic or demonstrates evidence of poor cardiac function, closed chest cardiac massage should be performed while fluid resuscitation is begun.

    **(2) Immediate emergency-room thoracotomies are rarely indicated.**

      **(a)** They should be done only by personnel trained to do them, and should not be done unless trained personnel are present to finish the procedure begun in the emergency room.

      **(b)** The major indications for emergency-room thoracotomy are:

        **(i)** Hypovolemic cardiac arrest despite vigorous blood volume replacement plus closed-chest massage and defibrillation

        **(ii)** Cardiac arrest with penetrating injury to the chest

      **(c)** Relative contraindications include:

        **(i)** Major, obvious injuries to the central nervous system

        **(ii)** Failed external cardiac massage lasting more than 10 minutes

        **(iii)** Major blunt-chest trauma

  **b. Assessment of the circulatory status** in a patient with a beating heart should include the following items, which can be rapidly appraised:

    **(1) Character of the pulse**

      **(a)** A rapid, faint pulse suggests profound hypovolemia in most cases.

      **(b)** A slow, full pulse may be indicative of severe neurologic injury, with increasing intracranial pressure or hypercarbia.

    **(2) Peripheral perfusion**, as indicated by level of consciousness, rate of capillary refilling, and body temperature

    **(3) Blood pressure.** The presence of a mild hypotension may be associated with inadequate tissue perfusion.

  **c.** The condition of patients with major injury and seemingly stable vital signs is dangerous and deceptive.

    **(1)** Previously healthy trauma patients, especially if young, are able to maintain pulse and blood pressure, despite a continuing occult hemorrhage, until vasomotor response fails.

    **(2)** When this occurs, the patient "crashes." This is manifested by a rapid loss of blood pressure, vomiting, and unconsciousness.

    **(3)** These patients maintain stable hemodynamic parameters and may remain quietly pale, or become excitable with progressive mental deterioration, until overt shock develops.

    **(4)** At this stage, they may not respond to further volume replacement.

  **d. Venous access**

    **(1)** Lines should be inserted by a reliable method that the physician is comfortable with. Subclavian catheterization should be learned in controlled settings, not on unstable trauma patients.

    **(2)** Usually two lines are inserted simultaneously.

      **(a)** It is best to keep one on each side of the diaphragm so that volume replacement will be effective in case of vena caval or subclavian venous trauma.

      **(b)** Shock patients often require four separate lines for volume replacement in order to raise the blood pressure above 100 mm Hg in under 10 minutes.

    **(3)** The first intravenous insertion should include the withdrawal of 100 ml of blood for crossmatching and for laboratory studies, including a toxicology profile.

    **(4)** Femoral artery punctures should be done early for blood gas analyses.

    **(5)** In general, subclavian lines and a saphenous cut-down are the quickest for venous access.

      **(a)** The saphenous vein will not look like a typical vein in a hypovolemic patient, and should be recognized rather than divided.

      **(b)** It is often empty and may look pale and tendon-like.

    **(6)** All resuscitation lines should be replaced in 12 to 24 hours. The urgent insertion of these lines leaves sterility in question, and catheter sepsis can become a serious problem after 24 hours.

  **e. Blood components** (see also Chapter 1, section VI)

    **(1) Plasma**

      **(a) Pooled plasma** carries a relatively high risk of transmitting hepatitis and other viral syndromes.

      **(b) Fresh-frozen plasma** has a lower risk of transmitting viral syndromes. It should be included in massive volume replacement because it contains important clotting factors.

    **(2) Whole blood** is generally not available nor indicated.

    **(3) Packed red cells**

      **(a)** These are given urgently if the initial hematocrit is less than 25%.

      **(b)** They are also started if the patient is obviously bleeding vigorously or if volume replacement of more than 1000 ml will be required.

      **(c)** Fresh-frozen plasma, 2 units, and platelets, 8 units, should be given with each 10 units of red cells.

    **(4)** All rapidly infused fluids should be warmed during infusion.

    **(5) Use of unmatched blood**

      **(a)** Profound shock is an indication for the use of type-specific but uncrossmatched blood cells.

      **(b)** If there is no time even for blood typing, then O-negative blood cells can be used.

      **(c)** O-positive blood cells are generally safe for young males who have never had a previous blood transfusion. They can be used if O-negative cells are not available.

      **(d)** If the patient receives over 4 units of unmatched type O cells, the physician should not revert to the native blood type during resuscitation.

      **(e)** Legal liability for a transfusion reaction is not a serious problem if the patient faces a 100% mortality risk without red cell replacement.

  **f. Maintenance of circulating blood volume** (see also Chapter 1, section I)

    **(1) Fluid replacement** at first is based on judgments made during the initial assessment concerning shock and visible sources of blood loss.

    **(2)** Continuing fluid replacement, after an initial 2 to 3 L of lactated Ringer's solution, is based on the patient's urine output and central venous pressure.

      **(a) Urine output**

        **(i)** Monitoring the trends in the patient's urine output provides an important guideline to the accuracy of fluid resuscitation and the changing needs of the patient.

(ii) Renal perfusion disappears early in shock. A urine output in excess of 30 ml/hr implies adequate perfusion to all vital organs, and indicates that the patient is not in shock.

**(b) Central venous pressure** is usually monitored via a subclavian vein puncture.

(i) Central venous pressure reflects the available blood volume, which is not necessarily the same as the absolute amount of circulating blood.

(ii) The available blood volume will be decreased if the absolute volume has decreased due to external or internal losses.

(iii) The available blood volume may also be decreased if the vascular system has dilated so that the normal volume no longer fills it.

(iv) An inadequate circulating volume, as implied by diminished central venous pressure, generally indicates inadequate venous return to the heart. If venous return is inadequate, the cardiac chambers cannot distend to their normal filled volumes and cardiac output therefore diminishes.

(v) The trends in a series of central venous pressure measurements are sometimes more informative than the absolute magnitude on a single reading.

(vi) Moreover, in assessing circulating volume, the central venous pressure must be interpreted in conjunction with urine output, pulse rate, and other vital signs. Coexisting pulmonary and cardiac derangements can influence central venous pressure readings, and account for the wide variations in initial readings seen in different patients.

(vii) Readings are falsely raised by pressure ventilation. It is often advisable to slow the volume replacement when an initially negative central venous pressure reading rises above zero during resuscitation.

**(3)** Further replacement should be based on continued assessment.

**(4)** The use of **fluid challenges** can provide valuable guidance in judging the adequacy of volume resuscitation. Examples include:

**(a)** Rapid infusion of 200 ml of colloid solution (e.g., albumin, Plasmanate, hydroxyethyl starch) in a patient with progressive tachycardia

(i) If the central venous pressure rises beyond normal limits (15 cm $H_2O$), it signifies overload or failure, pericardial tamponade, or tension pneumothorax.

(ii) If the central venous pressure falls or remains low, it indicates inadequate volume replacement or continued volume loss.

**(b)** Infusion of 200 ml of colloid solution in a patient with a slowing pulse rate: If the central venous pressure rises, it indicates adequate or improving volume status.

**g. Control of hemorrhage** must accompany fluid resuscitation.

**(1) External bleeding**

**(a)** Applying direct pressure on bleeding wounds with manually held gauze pads is safe and usually effective.

**(b)** Proximal and distal digital compression of bleeding superficial vessels may allow visualization of the bleeding point and accurate clamping. Blind clamping is never indicated.

**(c)** Pressure dressings may be used to control diffuse bleeding from abrasions and avulsions that involve large areas.

**(d)** Temporary packing of missile tracts and stab wounds can slow the blood flow until surgical exposure is obtained.

**(e)** Pneumatic splints and medical antishock trousers (MAST) help in tamponading bleeding and increasing peripheral resistance in order to raise the blood pressure. The antishock trousers provide increased peripheral resistance without the pharmacologic effects of pressor agents.

**(2) Internal bleeding** requires early diagnosis and prompt treatment by appropriate surgical intervention.

**5. Neurologic injury** (see also Chapter 31). After adequate ventilation and tissue perfusion have been restored, immediate attention must be given to the patient's neurologic condition.

**a. Assessment of head trauma**

**(1)** Loss of consciousness signifies a head injury until such an injury has been ruled out.

**(2)** Intracranial trauma cannot be adequately assessed while the patient is in shock.

**(3)** If hypotension is present in a patient with a head injury, it is rarely secondary to the head trauma, and the physician must look for another cause of the hypotension.

**(4)** The neurologic evaluation should assess the following factors rapidly:

**(a)** Level of consciousness—is the patient alert, lethargic and disoriented, comatose but responsive to pain, or unresponsive?

**(b)** Motor activity and tactile sensation

        **(c)** Obvious head trauma, such as a depressed skull fracture or gunshot wound, or leaking cerebrospinal fluid

        **(d)** Pupil size and response to light

        **(e)** Oculocephalic ("doll's eye") reflex—since testing involves rotating the patient's head, it should only be done after spinal cord injury has been proven absent

     **(5)** Evolving hypertension and bradycardia (Cushing's phenomenon) indicate increasing intracranial pressure and indicate a worsening neurologic problem.

  **b. Treatment of head trauma**

     **(1)** A neurosurgeon is imperative for proper management of patients with head injuries. If one is not available, then a telephone consultation should be obtained and initial treatment begun, followed by rapid transfer of the patient to a center where a neurosurgeon is available.

     **(2)** Initial management includes the following considerations.

        **(a)** Sterile saline-soaked gauze should be placed over open injuries.

        **(b)** Steroids, mannitol, and other drugs to lower intracranial pressure should be given after consultation with the neurosurgeon.

        **(c)** Hypotension and hypoventilation will seriously injure brain cells. It is therefore important to be certain that fluid requirements have been adequately assessed and ventilation secured.

        **(d)** Overhydration will increase intracranial pressure and should be avoided once fluid requirements have been met and the patient is stable.

  **c. Assessment of spinal cord trauma**

     **(1)** Until proven otherwise, the spine should be considered unstable, and the cord therefore liable to injury, in all patients with major blunt trauma.

     **(2)** The **cervical spine** should be considered unstable in the following patients:

        **(a)** Every unconscious patient

        **(b)** Every patient with face and head contusions

        **(c)** Every patient with decreased mentation which precludes adequate neurologic examination

     **(3)** X-ray films showing all seven cervical vertebrae intact should be obtained before one allows the patient's neck to be extended for any reason.

     **(4)** Evidence for injury to the spinal cord should be sought.

        **(a)** It should be recognized that the cord may not yet be injured even though the spine is unstable. A negative neurologic examination does not prove absence of injury to the cervical spine.

        **(b)** These unknowns must be considered and appropriate spinal stabilization must be performed until proper studies have been done.

        **(c)** The following findings should be sought:

           **(i)** Absence of motor or sensory function below the injury

           **(ii)** Loss of muscle tone

           **(iii)** Loss of anal sphincter tone

        **(d)** Hypotension may be present if there is a loss of vascular tone (arterial and venous) within the affected region.

  **d. Treatment of spinal cord injuries.** The required stabilization and reduction of the injury must be done under the supervision of a neurosurgeon or an orthopedic surgeon experienced in treating these injuries.

**6. Other serious injuries** can be attended to once the immediately life-threatening crises have been cared for and the patient has been stabilized.

  **a.** It is important to attempt to obtain information about the following, from the patient or from others:

     **(1)** Events surrounding the injury

     **(2)** Allergies that the patient may have

     **(3)** The patient's past medical history, including significant major illnesses

     **(4)** Medications that the patient is currently taking

  **b. Thoracic injuries** (see also Chapter 27, section II)

     **(1)** Upright chest x-rays should be obtained:

        **(a)** To detect fluid collections or a pneumothorax which may have been missed in the initial assessment

        **(b)** To search for the presence of great vessel injury, a tracheal shift, or other injuries.

     **(2)** The electrocardiogram and central venous pressure should be monitored for clues regarding cardiac contusions or tamponade, such as elevated ST segments and a rising central venous pressure.

     **(3)** A continuing large air leak through a chest tube in a patient with a lung that fails to expand with suction may call for urgent bronchography or bronchoscopy to determine if a bronchus is ruptured.

**(4)** Penetrating wounds that traverse the mediastinum are an indication for contrast esophagography and great vessel aortography to rule out esophageal perforation or aortic injury.

**(5)** X-ray findings that suggest the need for angiography include:
  **(a)** Lateral deviation of the nasogastric tube in the esophagus
  **(b)** A widened mediastinum (greater than 8 cm)
  **(c)** Loss of visualization of the aortic knob
  **(d)** Hematoma of the left cervical pleura ("pleural cap")
  **(e)** A depressed left main stem bronchus
  **(f)** Right lateral deviation of the trachea
  **(g)** Forward displacement of the trachea on the lateral chest film
  **(h)** Fracture of the first or second rib
  **(i)** Massive chest trauma with multiple rib fractures
  **(j)** Fracture or dislocation of the thoracic spine

**(6)** A history of a major deceleration injury, such as a fall from a height or an airplane crash, indicates the need for angiography.

**(7) Events requiring surgical intervention**
  **(a) Thoracic cavity hemorrhage.** The patient should undergo urgent thoracotomy in the operating room if either of the following events occur:
    **(i)** More than 1500 ml of blood are found in the chest
    **(ii)** Bleeding continues at a rate of 100 ml/hr after the initial hemothorax is evacuated via a chest tube
  **(b) Pericardial tamponade**
    **(i)** If a patient with chest trauma develops hypotension with an elevated central venous pressure, pericardial tamponade should be suspected after a tension pneumothorax has been ruled out.
    **(ii)** The principal diagnostic test is a pericardial tap, usually performed by inserting a catheter through the subxiphoid space.
    **(iii)** If tamponade is present, the catheter should be left in place and the patient taken to the operating room for exploratory thoracotomy.

**c. Abdominal injuries**
  **(1)** These injuries may be subtle or overt.
  **(2)** Evidence of trauma may be visible on the abdominal wall or pelvis.
  **(3)** Early tense abdominal distention usually indicates severe bleeding.
  **(4)** An abdomen that progressively becomes scaphoid suggests herniation of the abdominal contents through a traumatic diaphragmatic hernia.
  **(5)** The critical step for the physician is to recognize the presence of an abdominal injury and establish its degree of urgency.
  **(6) Peritoneal lavage** should be used when the need for abdominal exploration is not clear. It is also useful when physical assessment is not productive; for example, when the patient is unconscious or neurologically impaired.
    **(a)** The best **technique for peritoneal lavage** is the "semiopen" technique.
      **(i)** The bladder is first emptied with a bladder catheter.
      **(ii)** The peritoneal dialysis catheter is inserted through a small incision made in the midline fascia below the umbilicus.
      **(iii)** One L of crystalloid solution is infused in adults.
    **(b)** The lavage is positive if any of the following are found:
      **(i)** Gross blood or more than 100,000 red blood cells per ml
      **(ii)** Vegetable fibers or other fecal matter
      **(iii)** Bacteria
    **(c)** It is helpful to leave the dialysis catheter in place in the case of a negative lavage if the patient will be undergoing a lengthy orthopedic, neurologic, or thoracic surgical procedure.
      **(i)** Hypovolemia sometimes occurs during these procedures, and may be due to delayed abdominal bleeding.
      **(ii)** If the peritoneal lavage catheter is in place, lavage can be repeated during the procedure.
  **(7) Imaging techniques** that aid in the diagnosis of abdominal injury include:
    **(a) Intravenous pyelography**
      **(i)** A unilateral delay or absence of excretion is the major finding noted on a positive emergency intravenous pyelogram.
      **(ii)** A knowledge of bilateral renal function is essential for the surgeon operating on a patient with multiple, massive intra-abdominal injuries.
    **(b) Retrograde pyelography.** This provides morphologic evidence of extravasation of urine or disruption of a ureter or collecting system.

    (c) **Cystourethrography.** This is indicated in pelvic fractures when urethral bleeding is evident.
  (8) **Surgical treatment of abdominal injuries**
    (a) A generous midline incision has been found to be the most expeditious.
    (b) **Hemostasis** is the major priority in surgery for abdominal trauma.
      (i) A bleeding aorta can be temporarily clamped for hemostasis while resuscitation is carried out.
      (ii) Rapid methods of temporary hemostasis, such as packing and direct pressure, are applied while fluid resuscitation is carried out.
      (iii) Meticulous exploration and repair should wait until volume replacement is complete and the patient is stable.
    (c) **Retroperitoneal hematomas** in the pelvic and lower abdominal regions are best not explored unless they are actively expanding or an arterial source has been demonstrated on angiography. Many of these are associated with pelvic fractures and are not controllable by surgical means.
    (d) Retroperitoneal hematomas in the upper abdomen, particularly those in proximity to the duodenum, pancreas, and renal pedicles, should be explored.
      (i) The **pancreas and duodenum** should be immobilized and then thoroughly palpated to rule out pancreatic disruption.
      (ii) The duodenum can be patched or repaired if the injury is diagnosed very early. Delayed diagnosis of duodenal disruption is associated with tissue of poor quality that is not safely repaired.
      (iii) Pancreatic transections are best treated by distal resection. Most pancreatic injuries can be handled by simple sump drainage if transection or major duct damage has not occurred.
    (e) **Liver injuries** should be treated as conservatively as possible.
      (i) Resective debridement of detached or almost-detached portions is carried out.
      (ii) Hemostasis is accomplished under direct vision, if possible. Packs can be used for a 24-hour period, and then reexploration is accomplished when required.
**d. Genitourinary injuries** (see also Chapter 29, section VI)
  (1) **Urethral injury**
    (a) Blood at the meatus is an indication for urethrography. Even gentle insertion of a Foley catheter can disrupt a partially divided urethra.
    (b) Major injuries should be repaired surgically.
  (2) **Bladder injuries** will usually heal spontaneously if adequate urinary drainage is established.
  (3) **Kidneys** are commonly injured organs.
    (a) Most renal injuries can be managed nonoperatively.
    (b) Renal pedicle disruption or major parenchymal damage with hemorrhage are the primary indications for surgery.
    (c) Intravenous pyelography provides a good test of renal function, but it is not adequate for determining anatomic continuity of the organ. Extravasated contrast is an indication for drainage of the area where the leakage occurred.
**e. Soft tissue injuries** (see also Chapter 30)
  (1) **Debridement** is the key to avoiding infection and promoting rapid healing.
    (a) All devitalized tissue must be removed during debridement.
    (b) It is helpful to understand how different tissues respond to injury. The degree of injury often depends on the density of the tissue and its water content.
      (i) The lung, for example, tends to receive relatively minor degrees of damage remote from the missile tract.
      (ii) By contrast, muscle or liver, due to their greater density and water content, develop large temporary cavities and require extensive debridement beyond the apparent missile tract.
  (2) **Muscle**
    (a) Wide areas of devitalized tissue occur in high-velocity wounds and require debridement.
    (b) Viable muscle tissue will contract visibly when touched with an electrosurgical instrument set on a low power. It will also contract when gently pinched with a forceps.
    (c) Muscle that does not react must be removed even though weakness and deformity can be anticipated.
  (3) **Arteries**
    (a) Palpable pulses do not rule out arterial injury.
    (b) Grossly injured vascular areas that exhibit intramural bleeding or disruption, require removal. It is not necessary to remove apparently normal areas of arteries.

(c) Repair should be done with autogenous material if at all possible. There is an increased incidence of infection and failure when prosthetic material is used.

(d) Fasciotomies are almost always required in conjunction with vascular repair. It is far better to anticipate swelling and tension in muscle compartments, and to do a fasciotomy early, than to wait until tissue loss has occurred.

(e) Any stab wound or missile tract in proximity to major vascular structures requires either surgical exploration or, at a minimum, emergency arteriography.

(f) Major **veins** should be repaired when injured.

**(4) Nerves**

(a) It is not necessary to debride nerves that are injured.

(b) Exposed nerves should be covered with normal muscle or fat, leaving definitive repair for a future time.

**(5) Bone.** Contaminated small pieces of bone that are not attached to soft tissue may be removed. Attached bones should generally be left in situ to speed healing.

**(6) Lung tissue** is usually resistant to remote damage. Because of its spongy nature, the lung absorbs shock without injury, so that a missile tract generally contains all of the injury.

**(7) Parenchymal organs** such as the **liver** and **kidney**

(a) Bleeding is the major problem. Devitalized tissue should be removed, with as much functional tissue left as possible.

(b) An effort should be made to salvage an injured **spleen**, particularly in a child. There is evidence that a small spleen slice, reimplanted in the omentum, will grow and will provide some splenic function.

**(8) Genitalia.** Very conservative debridement is indicated. Exposed testicular tissue should be covered with scrotal skin or reimplanted under attached skin, if possible.

**f. Fractures** (see also Chapter 32, section III B, C, D)

**(1)** A fracture is seldom a major priority in the presence of other, life-threatening injuries.

(a) Hemorrhage or vascular compromise associated with a fracture gives it a higher priority, as does a threat to the viability of an extremity.

(b) It is important to remember that bleeding associated with a fracture can account for a large portion of a patient's circulating blood volume, and that hypovolemic shock is commonly associated with bilateral femoral fractures.

**(2)** Early fractures that are open can be treated in accordance with the associated soft tissue injury.

(a) Debridement, vascular repair, and other soft tissue surgery should be done prior to stabilization of the fracture.

(b) However, adequate splinting and stabilization should be accomplished because it decreases the risk of fat-embolism syndrome.

(c) Internal fixation devices are generally hazardous in the presence of extensive soft tissue injury and should be avoided if possible.

**(3)** Fractures that are more than 6 to 8 hours old should be allowed maximal spontaneous recovery before any attempt is made to stabilize them surgically.

**g. Tendon injuries** require conservative debridement only. Tendons should be covered with normal tissue or they will become devitalized and useless.

**h. Neck injuries.** All penetrating neck injuries and all hematomas in the neck should be surgically explored.

**(1)** Arteriography is recommended for penetrating injuries above the angle of the mandible or in the supraclavicular area.

**(2)** Bronchoscopy, esophagoscopy, and x-rays with oral diatrizoate meglumine as contrast agent can help to rule out tracheal or esophageal injuries.

## II. BURNS

### A. General considerations

1. The initial treatment of burns is based on the same principles and priorities as for other forms of trauma. The same "AMPLE" history must be taken; the same resuscitation priorities are in order (see section I A 4 b).

2. One **special priority** in burn care involves the need to stop the continued burn injury caused by smoldering clothes or corrosive chemicals. All garments should be flushed away from the injured area with neutral solutions.

3. The management of the burned patient depends, obviously, on the **severity of the burns**. This, in turn, is dependent on the depth, extent, and location of the burned area.

**a. Depth of burns**
  **(1) First-degree burns.** Clinical findings are limited to erythema.
  **(2) Second-degree (partial-thickness) burns**
    **(a)** Clinical findings include vesicles, swelling, and a moist surface.
    **(b)** Partial-thickness burns are painful and are hypersensitive to a light touch or even the movement of air.
  **(3) Third-degree (full-thickness) burns**
    **(a)** These burns have a charred or waxen appearance and may be white or grayish in color. They usually appear dry.
    **(b)** The burn surface is pain-free and is anesthetic to a pin-prick or to touch.
**b. Extent of burns.** This is determined by the **"rule of nines"** (Fig. 2-1).
  **(1)** In-patient treatment is required for a patient with either:
    **(a)** Full-thickness burns extending over 2% or more of the body surface area (BSA)
    **(b)** Partial-thickness burns extending over 10% or more of the BSA
  **(2)** Intravenous fluid resuscitation is required for all partial- or full-thickness burns extending over 20% or more of the BSA.
**c. Location of burns**
  **(1)** In-patient treatment is required for second- or third-degree burns of the face, hands, feet, or genitalia.
  **(2)** Second- or third-degree burns involving major flexion creases usually require hospital treatment to minimize contractures and other late problems.

**4.** Transfer of the burn patient to a burn center, or consultation with the center, should be considered for all but minimal burn injuries.

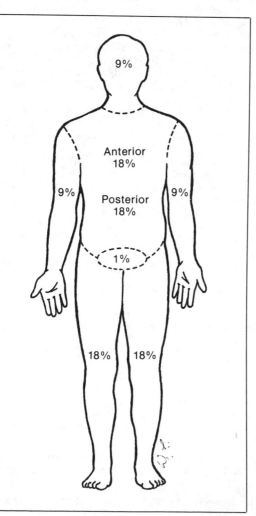

**Figure 2-1.** The "rule of nines." The body surface area (BSA) is divided into anatomic areas, each of which is 9% (or a multiple thereof) of the total BSA. This is a simple method of estimating the total burn surface.

**B. Airway control and ventilation**

1. **Airway obstruction** may develop rapidly after inhalation injury or may be delayed.

   a. **Delayed airway obstruction** is due to progressive swelling and is apt to develop 24 or 48 hours after the injury.

   b. The possibility should be suspected if any of the following conditions are present:

   (1) A history of being burned in a confined space

   (2) A facial burn or singed facial hair

   (3) Charring or carbon particles in the oropharynx

   (4) Carbonaceous sputum

   (5) Circumferential burns of the trunk, especially those with a thick eschar (which may require emergency excision—see section II D 7)

2. Early measurement of arterial blood gases is indicated.

3. Endotracheal intubation should be done before the patient develops respiratory problems. Intubation is preferable to a tracheostomy in the patient with burns of the face, neck, or respiratory tract, since tracheostomy through a burn carries a high mortality risk.

**C. Circulatory support and fluid resuscitation**

1. Major burns—those involving 20% or more of the BSA—call for fluid resuscitation.

2. Intravenous fluids should be administered through a 14-gauge or 16-gauge intravenous catheter.

   a. The catheter may be placed through the burn wound, if required.

   b. Intravenous fluids should not be given via a lower extremity, since the site is prone to sepsis and its increased mortality risk.

3. Fluid resuscitation should begin with lactated Ringer's solution.

   a. The **volume to be given** is calculated as follows:

   (1) **For adults:**

   % BSA burned $\times$ kg of body weight $\times$ 2–4 ml of electrolyte solution

   (2) **For children:**

   % BSA burned $\times$ kg of body weight $\times$ 3 ml of electrolyte solution

   (3) The percentage of the body surface area that is burned (% BSA) is estimated by the **rule of nines** (see Fig. 2-1).

   b. One-half of the calculated amount of fluid is given in the first 8 hours, and the remaining one-half is distributed over the succeeding 16 hours.

   c. The volume and rate of fluid administration should be varied, if necessary, depending on the central venous pressure, urine output, and other vital signs.

   (1) **Optimal urine output** is 30 ml to 50 ml per hour in adults, and 1 ml per kg of body weight per hour in children.

   (2) To aid urine flow, and to allow monitoring of output, an indwelling urethral catheter should be inserted early, even in children.

**D. Burn wound care**

1. Cold compresses may be applied to relieve the pain of partial-thickness burns if the burns cover less than 10% of the BSA.

2. If burns cover a large area, cold compresses or immersion in water will cause unacceptable lowering of the body temperature, with associated problems.

3. Maintenance of body temperature is important, especially in children, who have a high evaporative heat loss and may rapidly become hypothermic.

4. Shielding the burn from air movement by covering it with a clean, warm linen dressing will help to relieve the pain of partial-thickness burns.

5. Topical antimicrobial treatment with agents such as silver nitrate solution is usually recommended for deep second-degree and for third-degree burns.

6. No ointments should be applied to the burn except for specific antibacterial burn wound medications.

7. Debridement and escharectomy are often required, but are best done in specialized centers. However, escharotomy may be urgently required:

**a.** In circumferential extremity wounds causing distal circulatory impairment

**b.** In circumferential trunk or neck wounds causing respiratory impairment

**E. Other considerations** in the care of burn patients

1. Nasotracheal intubation is indicated for any patient with nausea or vomiting and for most patients with burns covering 25% or more of the BSA.

2. Analgesia should be confined to conservative use of intravenous narcotics in small, frequent doses.

3. Systemic antibiotics are usually not indicated. However, in some situations, particularly in the early treatment of patients with partial-thickness burns, prophylaxis against $\beta$-hemolytic streptococci is warranted.

**4. Chemical burns**
   **a.** Alkali burns are generally deeper and more serious than acid burns.
   **b.** All chemical burns should be treated by thorough flushing with neutral solutions.
      **(1)** Immediate drenching in a shower or with a hose is helpful.
      **(2)** Burns of the eye require extensive flushing over an 8-hour period.

**5. Electrical burns**
   **a.** These are usually deeper and more severe than indicated by the surface appearance.
   **b.** Surface burns occur at both the entrance and the exit points of the current.
   **c.** Oliguria is common, as is acidosis.
      **(1)** It is necessary to maintain urine output at high levels—at least 100 ml/hr in adults. Mannitol administration is usually needed to maintain this level.
      **(2)** The arterial blood pH should be monitored and maintained with intravenous bicarbonate, given as 50 mEq every half hour until the pH reaches normal levels.

# 3
# Medical Risk Factors in Surgical Patients

Bruce E. Jarrell

**I. GENERAL ASPECTS.** Even though the natural history of each medical disorder has a pattern of its own, certain considerations apply to most disease processes in evaluating and minimizing operative risk.

**A.** The operative risk is a function of many **factors**:

    **1.** The **natural history** of the acute process that precipitated the need for surgery

    **2.** The general **status of the patient** prior to the acute process

    **3.** The **skill of the physicians** caring for the patient and the level of **current medical expertise** in the relevant areas

    **4.** The **patient's mental outlook**

**B.** The **history** is the most helpful parameter in alerting the physician to certain risk factors. These include:

    **1.** A history of **familial disorders**, such as bleeding disorders

    **2. Prior difficulties** with surgical procedures or anesthetics

    **3.** The presence of **allergies** or **asthma**

    **4.** The effects of **current medications**, such as steroids, diuretics, anticoagulants, or over-the-counter products such as aspirin that a patient might not consider a drug

**C.** Attention to certain **physiologic parameters** in all preoperative patients will lower the operative risk.

    **1. Electrolyte abnormalities** (see Chapter 1, section I) should be corrected.

    **2.** The patient's **fluid status** should be assessed.
      **a.** Factors to consider include:
        **(1)** A comparison of past and current weight
        **(2)** Skin turgor, mucous membrane moistness, axillary sweat, and vital signs such as blood pressure and heart rate
      **b.** The hourly **urine output** should be determined if time permits.
      **c.** A comparison of the supine and the upright blood pressures will indicate the presence of **orthostatic blood pressure changes**.
      **d.** Even in semiemergencies such as perforated ulcer it is beneficial to wait several hours in order to attain improved hydration and urine output prior to surgery.
      **e.** Electrolyte levels in the peripheral blood may not reflect the true fluid status.
        **(1)** Therefore, they should be appraised in conjunction with other factors.
        **(2)** For example, the presence of nausea, vomiting, diarrhea, bleeding, chronic anorexia, or bowel obstruction should be expected to result in dehydration.

    **3. Red blood cell mass** should be evaluated.
      **a.** Most physicians will accept a **hemoglobin level** of 10 g/dl of blood prior to major surgery.
      **b.** Acute blood loss may not alter the peripheral blood hematocrit for up to 24 hours. Thus the need for red cell replacement should be determined from other variables, such as obvious blood loss sites.
      **c.** Chronic anemia is usually well compensated by an increase in plasma volume.

    **d. Preoperative blood replacement** is recommended in the following situations:
      **(1)** When excessive blood loss during surgery is anticipated
      **(2)** When the patient has significant coronary artery disease or a history of congestive heart failure. In these cases, replacement of red blood cells should be slow in order to avoid acute overhydration
      **(3)** In hypoxia
      **(4)** After preoperative hemorrhage
      **(5)** In the presence of sepsis or malnutrition

**D.** In certain acute conditions, such as acute appendicitis or an ischemic or perforated viscus, the operative risk depends principally on how quickly the diagnosis is made and treatment is begun.

    **1.** Therefore, a basic surgical axiom in these conditions is to establish the diagnosis before a complication such as perforation has developed, even if this requires a surgical diagnostic procedure such as a laparotomy.

    **2.** Clearly, expeditious management in such cases can keep a patient in a lower-risk category.

**E. Malnutrition** (see Chapter 1, section II) can increase the operative risk.

**F. Infection** (see Chapter 1, section VII) should be controlled prior to surgery whenever possible.

    **1.** Elective procedures should be postponed until infections are under control. For example, a urinary tract infection or a skin carbuncle should be treated prior to hernia repair.

    **2.** In emergency conditions that involve potential contamination, such as a perforated viscus or penetrating trauma, the patient should be given appropriate antibiotics at the earliest possible time.

    **3.** Prophylactic antibiotics (see Chapter 1, section VII A 3) should be used only in situations where controlled studies have documented a benefit.

    **4.** Preoperative shaving of the operative area may produce superficial nicks that predispose to infections which can appear overnight. Many surgeons therefore shave patients in the operating room or use a depilatory agent to remove hair.

**G.** Finally, making sure that the patient has a realistic understanding of the prognosis and the expected outcome of the operative procedure will ensure the patient's cooperation postoperatively and thus improve the operative risk.

## II. CHRONIC LUNG DISEASE

**A. Chronic lung disease** is a common disorder affecting surgical patients of all ages and diagnoses. It may be symptomatic in the form of dyspnea or totally asymptomatic. There may be an acute infectious process superimposed upon a chronic disorder.

    **1.** Chronic lung disease is associated with **multiple risk factors.**
      **a.** There is a slight decrease in pulmonary function with **age.**
      **b. Obesity** increases the work of ventilation and impairs the function of the chest wall.
      **c. Cigarette smoking** is toxic to respiratory epithelium and cilia, and it results in impaired mucus transport with consequent impaired resistance to infection.
      **d.** Exposure to **environmental toxins**, such as air pollution and industrial toxic agents, increases the risk of lung disease.
      **e.** Other **systemic diseases,** such as thromboembolic disease, cystic fibrosis, and tuberculosis, are factors leading to lung disease.

    **2.** Chronic lung disease should be **suspected preoperatively** in any patient with:
      **a.** Any of the **risk factors** mentioned in section II A 1
      **b.** A **history of lung disorders,** including dyspnea, sputum production, recurrent bronchitis or pneumonia, emphysema, or previous lung surgery
      **c. Abnormal** results of **physical examination** including:
        **(1)** Anatomic abnormalities, such as scoliosis or chest wall abnormalities
        **(2)** Abnormal findings on auscultation of the chest, including decreased breath sounds, wheezing, and rhonchi or rales
        **(3)** Signs of inadequate oxygenation, such as cyanosis, finger clubbing, and use of accessory muscles for breathing
      **d.** Abnormal findings on **chest roentgenogram,** including blebs, a flattened diaphragm, or pneumonitis

**e. Abnormal arterial blood gases,** especially hypoxemia or retained carbon dioxide
**f. Secondary polycythemia**

**B. Pulmonary complications** occur in the perioperative period in up to 50% of patients with chronic lung disease. Patients with **obstructive lung disease** have the **highest risk,** but patients with restrictive lung disease, neuromuscular disorders, or pulmonary vascular disease also are at increased risk.

1. The most **common complication** is atelectasis followed by pulmonary infection, both of which lead to pulmonary failure. These are usually due to retained tracheobronchial secretions. Other significant complications include:
   **a.** Bronchospasm
   **b.** Pulmonary edema
   **c.** Aspiration of gastric contents
   **d.** Pneumothorax

2. **Intraoperative factors** are associated with increased complications. These factors include the following:
   **a. Type of surgery.** Procedures performed on the lung have complications more often than nonpulmonary procedures.
   **b. Length of surgery.** Procedures lasting longer than 2 hours have an increased complication rate.
   **c. Site of surgical incision**
      **(1)** In general, incisions that transect muscle groups rather than splitting them in the direction of the fibers result in increased pulmonary complications.
      **(2)** Thoracic and upper abdominal surgery have the highest complication rate.
         **(a)** Chest wall and diaphragmatic excursion mechanics are altered.
         **(b)** Pain results in hypoventilation and a poor cough reflex.
   **d. Anesthesia.** Both the anesthetic itself and techniques employed in its use may have an adverse effect on postoperative function.
      **(1) Mechanical ventilation** impairs many protective mechanisms, such as ciliary function and mucus action. It also increases the risk of pneumothorax from ruptured pulmonary blebs.
      **(2)** The venous admixture may be altered with an increase in the ventilation-perfusion mismatch.
      **(3)** Chest wall mechanical properties may be altered due to muscle relaxation and impaired diaphragmatic excursion.
      **(4)** Anesthesia may decrease functional residual capacity (FRC), resulting in hypoxemia; both may persist for up to 1 week postoperatively.
      **(5)** The mortality rate among patients receiving anesthesia is as high as 1 in 1500, and 50% die with hypoxia.
   **e. Postoperative narcotics.** These result in impaired function with a suppressed cough reflex and decreased sighing as well as hypoventilation due to respiratory center depression.

**C.** Pulmonary risk may be **evaluated preoperatively** in many ways. The optimal methods are controversial and are affected by the patient's disease and the contemplated type of surgery. The best method of determining the effectiveness of pulmonary ventilation is with blood gas analysis.

1. **Chronic obstructive pulmonary disease (COPD)** patients have the highest risk. They may not be able to generate enough force to cough. To evaluate the severity of COPD, **spirometry** is used to measure the **total forced expiratory volume (FEV)** and the **forced expiratory volume during the first second (FEV$_1$).** FEV$_1$ is usually expressed as a percentage of FEV.
   **a.** A patient with an FEV$_1$ greater than 2 L has no increased risk.
   **b.** A patient with an FEV$_1$ equaling 1 L to 2 L has mild increased risk.
   **c.** A patient with an FEV$_1$ equaling 0.5 L to 1 L (or FEV$_1$/FEV less than 40%) has a moderate increased risk.
   **d.** A patient with an FEV$_1$ less than 0.5 L (or FEV$_1$/FEV less than 25%) has a very high risk.
   **e. Carbon dioxide retention,** especially in the resting state, indicates severe pulmonary impairment and a resultant increased risk.

2. Patients with **restrictive lung disease, neuromuscular disorders,** or other **chest wall abnormalities** have an impaired ventilatory reserve as a result of weak muscles or abnormal mechanics of ventilation. The **vital capacity (VC), maximal inspiratory flow (MIF),** and **maximal expiratory flow (MEF)** are decreased. Muscular strength may be indirectly evaluated by measuring the maximal static inspiratory (or expiratory) pressure that is generated.
   **a.** A patient whose MIF is greater than 25 cm H$_2$O has minimal risk.
   **b.** A patient whose MIF equals 15 cm to 25 cm H$_2$O has a high risk.

**c.** A patient whose MIF is less than 15 cm $H_2O$ has a very high risk.
**d.** A patient whose VC is greater than 50% of the predicted value has minimal risk.
**e.** A patient whose VC is less than 25% of the predicted value has a very high risk.

**3.** Patients undergoing **pulmonary resection** must also be evaluated to determine if they will tolerate removal of part or all of a lung. In addition to the previously mentioned factors, **pulmonary vascular measurements** should be made.
   **a. Pulmonary artery pressure** should be measured with a **Swan-Ganz catheter.**
      **(1)** Pulmonary artery pressure that is elevated at rest or that becomes elevated with exercise is associated with a significant increase in risk.
      **(2)** If the pulmonary artery pressure rises significantly when the pulmonary artery of the affected lung is occluded with a balloon catheter, it indicates an inability to tolerate the resection.
   **b.** A **perfusion** or **ventilation lung scan** may be helpful in predicting the ability to tolerate a resection. If the affected lung tissue lacks ventilation or perfusion preoperatively, resection probably will be tolerated because the patient is currently surviving without the functional use of that tissue.

**D.** Certain **pre- and postoperative maneuvers** may improve pulmonary function and reduce the number of postoperative complications.

  **1. Preoperative maneuvers** include the following:
   **a. Cigarette smoking should be stopped** at least 2 to 3 weeks preceding surgery. Although the optimal time period is unknown, the acute effects of smoking on respiratory epithelium are probably gone in that amount of time.
   **b.** Preoperative **respiratory muscle conditioning** may improve function that was initially impaired.
   **c.** Use of a **bronchodilator** may improve function in patients with asthma or COPD.
   **d.** Appropriate **antibiotics** should be used in patients with acute bronchitis or purulent sputum production prior to proceeding with surgery.
   **e.** Use of **aerosols** and **mucolytic drugs** such as acetylcysteine may help to liquefy and mobilize retained secretions. Postural drainage also expedites this.
   **f. Steroids** should be used preoperatively only when absolutely necessary because of their adverse effects on wound healing and resistance to infection.
   **g.** Preoperative instruction in the **methods of pulmonary toilet** to be used postoperatively is helpful. Instruction should include methods of coughing and deep breathing, postural drainage, and other pulmonary therapy.

  **2. Postoperative care** of respiratory patients includes the following:
   **a. Extubation** should be performed only after the patient is awake and has full respiratory muscle strength. After extubation, respiratory sufficiency should be carefully observed and evaluated. If there is doubt, arterial blood gases should be measured and chest roentgenography should be performed, but a **physical examination** should be done first.
   **b. Oxygen** should be administered if necessary but cautiously in patients with COPD. It should be heated and humidified.
   **c.** Patients should be out of bed and upright as much as possible. This allows gravity to assist more in respiration and also helps to minimize secretion retention.
   **d.** Pulmonary aspiration of gastric contents should be prevented by the use of a **nasogastric tube** if an ileus is present.
   **e. Pneumothorax** should always be suspected if sudden respiratory insufficiency occurs.

## III. CHRONIC RENAL FAILURE

**A. The preoperative condition of patients with chronic renal failure** is strongly dependent upon the residual **glomerular filtration rate (GFR)** and the presence of other major disease processes.

  **1. As the GFR approaches 25% of normal**, the kidney loses its ability to correct many different abnormalities.
   **a. Fluid and electrolyte homeostasis** is altered.
     **(1)** This results in
       **(a)** Hypertension
       **(b)** Peripheral edema
       **(c)** Hyponatremia as a result of fluid retention
       **(d)** Salt retention
       **(e)** Metabolic acidosis as a result of failure to excrete organic acids such as phosphates and sulfates
       **(f)** Hyperkalemia

        **(2)** Certain renal diseases such as chronic pyelonephritis, medullary cystic disease, and other interstitial diseases may result in salt wasting and subsequent dehydration.

    **b. Nutritional status** is impaired, because of:

        **(1)** Proteinuria, which may be as high as 25 g/day

        **(2)** Decreased body stores of nitrogen, which is catabolized more often as uremia progresses

        **(3)** Decreased dietary intake as a result of anorexia, nausea, or malabsorption; it may also be the result of dietary restrictions placed by the physician

    **c. Metabolism of or excretion of medications**, especially many antibiotics and radiopaque iodinated angiographic dye, is impaired.

    **d. Immune function** is affected.

        **(1)** This results in

            **(a)** Increased urinary tract infections as a result of oliguria

            **(b)** Impaired mucocutaneous barriers, which may be secondary to pruritus or epidermal atrophy

            **(c)** Increased pulmonary infections, which are related in part to decreased pulmonary clearance mechanisms

            **(d)** Increased incidence of malignancies

            **(e)** Impaired phagocytosis

        **(2)** The response to vaccines may be normal or mildly impaired.

        **(3)** The elimination of certain viruses, such as hepatitis B virus, is impaired. This becomes a major problem in dialysis patients, with as many as 60% becoming chronic antigen carriers once they contract the infection.

    **e. Hematologic functions are altered.**

        **(1)** Anemia occurs as the GFR drops and becomes profound as the GFR approaches zero.

        **(2)** Coagulation defects occur as a result of altered platelet adhesion and aggregation and abnormalities in the coagulation cascade (see Chapter 1, section IV A).

    **f. Cardiac and other vascular abnormalities** develop, including:

        **(1)** Increased incidence of atherosclerosis

        **(2)** Pericarditis and pericardial effusions

    **g. Altered calcium metabolism and parathyroid hormone metabolism** result in secondary hyperparathyroidism and bone disease with hypocalcemia and hyperphosphatemia.

  **2.** When the GFR is less than 5% of normal, **dialysis** is required for maintenance of bodily functions.

    **a.** Dialysis corrects or improves many of the uremic symptoms and abnormalities, such as fluid and electrolyte problems, hypertension, and nutritional problems related to dietary intake.

    **b.** Dialysis is, however, related to several other complications.

        **(1) Peritoneal dialysis** is associated with an increased risk of peritonitis.

        **(2) Hemodialysis** requires systemic heparin levels that may worsen the coagulopathy of chronic renal failure. In addition, the vascular access necessary for dialysis is associated with blood-borne infections, especially staphylococcal infections.

  **3.** Patients with renal failure are susceptible to appendicitis, cholecystitis, diverticulitis, and peptic ulcer disease. In addition, they may require surgery for problems related specifically to their disease, such as vascular access procedures and urologic procedures.

**B. Preparation for surgery**

  **1. Residual renal function may be adversely affected** by a surgical procedure. It is best protected by the following maneuvers:

    **a.** Correction of overhydration or dehydration and any accompanying electrolyte disorders, either by medical management or by the use of dialysis

    **b.** Proper treatment of infections, especially urinary tract infections

    **c.** Avoidance of nephrotoxic drugs

  **2. Dialysis patients with no preservable renal function** should be treated similarly. Nephrotoxic drugs may be used safely if blood levels are followed and other side effects such as ototoxicity are monitored.

  **3.** The **general medical preparation** of patients with chronic renal failure is important.

    **a. Anemia** is well tolerated by these patients. A hematocrit of 20% to 25% is adequate for most major surgical procedures.

    **b. Hyperkalemia** must be treated expeditiously. A reading of the potassium level must be obtained immediately preceding surgery, and dialysis must be instituted if the level is greater than 5.0 mEq/L. Exchange resins such as Kayexalate also control potassium levels and may be given as an enema.

      **c. Acidosis** should be corrected by either bicarbonate administration or dialysis therapy.

      **d.** The **coagulopathy** of chronic renal failure is best controlled preoperatively by adequate dialysis. Bleeding tendencies during or after surgery may also be controlled by the administration of cryoprecipitated plasma.

      **e. Pericarditis** and **pericardial effusion** should be resolved prior to the administration of a general anesthetic because of impaired cardiac output and the risk of pericardial tamponade.

      **f.** A **urinary bladder catheter** should not be used in patients with no preservable renal function or with oliguria.

      **g.** Supplemental **steroids** should be given in the perioperative period to patients on long-term steroid therapy.

      **h.** Elective surgery should be postponed for patients with **malnutrition** until the nutritional status improves. In emergency surgery, the nutritional requirements should be supplied intravenously postoperatively until adequate oral intake is possible.

      **i. Systemic disorders**, such as diabetes mellitus or a thyroid disorder, should be controlled.

      **j.** Patients manifesting **signs and symptoms of uremia** such as asterixis, hemorrhagic disorders, and seizures should be dialyzed prior to surgery.

**C. Intraoperative management** follows the same basic principles as those for any surgical patient. The effects of uremia, however, require special consideration.

    **1. Fluid management** must be closely monitored.

    **2.** The altered metabolism and excretion in chronic renal failure must be taken into consideration with the use of **anesthetics.** This is particularly true in the use of muscle-relaxing drugs, since prolonged drug action or recurrent paralysis postoperatively may cause catastrophic problems.

    **3.** In patients with preservable renal function, maintaining a **diuresis** with osmotic or diuretic agents may protect against further renal insult.

    **4.** Operative decisions are similar to those for normal patients. It is probably wise, however, to make conservative decisions when dealing with **gastrointestinal pathology.** Patients with chronic renal failure have delayed healing of serosal surfaces and a higher anastomotic disruption rate.

**D. Postoperative complications** are more common in patients with chronic renal failure.

    **1. Hyperkalemia** is common due to blood transfusions, operative trauma, hematomas, and the patient's catabolic state. It occurs in 25% of patients, but is nearly twice as common (44% ) if the patient receives transfusions intraoperatively.

    **2. Wound healing is impaired** and results in complications in up to 40% of cases. Wound infections are very common (occurring in up to 33% of cases) when the gastrointestinal tract is opened.

    **3.** Postoperative **hematomas** in the operative site are common (occurring in up to 15% of cases) and frequently become secondarily infected.

    **4. Gastrointestinal complications** postoperatively are also common and may result in nausea, vomiting, anorexia, hiccups, or prolonged ileus. Upper gastrointestinal bleeding, esophagitis, and stomatitis may also occur.

**IV. LIVER DISEASE.** Hepatic insufficiency increases the risk of complications and death in the postoperative period. The recognition and management of liver disease preoperatively can minimize the postoperative problems.

    **A. Recognition**

      **1.** The **history** can alert one to the possibility of liver disease if it includes any of the following items:

        **a.** Jaundice, pancreatitis, hepatitis, biliary stone disease, malignancy (e.g., gastrointestinal or breast cancer), or enzyme deficiencies (e.g., $\alpha_1$-antitrypsin deficiency)

        **b.** Hemolytic or parasitic disease

        **c.** Drug or alcohol abuse

        **d.** Upper gastrointestinal bleeding, delirium tremens, or encephalopathy

        **e.** Possible contact with infectious hepatitis agents (e.g., via tattoos or blood transfusions)

        **f.** Environmental or other exposure to hepatotoxins, particularly hepatotoxic anesthetic agents

2. The **physical examination** may reveal findings suggestive of liver disease:
   a. Jaundice, ascites, peripheral edema, muscle wasting, testicular atrophy, palmar erythema, gynecomastia
   b. Evidence of portal hypertension, including caput medusae (dilated periumbilical vessels) or splenomegaly
   c. Evidence of bleeding disorders, encephalopathy, asterixis, or spider angiomas
   d. Hepatomegaly or a shrunken liver, especially with a rounded edge or with palpable nodules upon its surface; also, hepatic tenderness to percussion.

3. **Laboratory tests** may confirm the diagnosis but are normal in some cases, even in the presence of moderate liver disease.
   a. Most useful are the serum bilirubin, serum glutamic oxaloacetic and pyruvic transaminases (SGOT and SGPT), serum alkaline phosphatase, serum albumin, and prothrombin time.
   b. Hepatitis B surface antigen should be sought if its presence is suspected, particularly since the hospital staff may be exposed.

4. A **liver biopsy** may be necessary preoperatively if an acute hepatitis, particularly acute alcoholic hepatitis, is suspected.

B. **Management** of risk factors during surgery in patients with preexisting liver disease has not been fully defined, but several generalizations are useful.

1. It is advisable to delay elective surgery in the patient with **acute hepatitis** until the hepatitis has resolved.
   a. Use of a general anesthetic in patients with **acute alcoholic hepatitis** has been associated with an operative mortality rate of 50% or more when portal decompressive surgery is performed.
   b. In **acute drug-induced hepatitis**, results of studies have ranged from no increase in risk to as high as a 20% morbidity and mortality rate.

2. The presence of **coagulopathy**, especially if secondary to vitamin K deficiency or thrombocytopenia, should be corrected.

3. Severe **malnutrition**, with its attendant increased risks of infection and wound complications, should be improved by adequate nutrition and treatment of current infections.

4. Patients with **chronic liver failure from cirrhosis** will tolerate most surgical procedures well if they are in a relatively compensated state preoperatively. The risk would seem to be related to the Child classification level (see Chapter 9, Table 9-1), as it is for patients undergoing portal decompressive procedures.

5. The optimization of the patient's preoperative cardiovascular and pulmonary status is obviously also useful. Avoidance of narcotics (which may precipitate hepatic encephalopathy), correction of hypokalemia and alkalosis, and use of nonhepatotoxic agents during surgery are all advisable.

V. **CARDIAC DISEASE.** The evaluation and perioperative management of a surgical patient with preexisting cardiac disease require the analysis and regulation of many complex factors to minimize the risk of complications or death. These may be divided into general factors and specific cardiac diagnoses.

A. **General factors affecting cardiac mortality**

1. **Increasing age** increases the surgical risk of death from cardiac disease. The risk of perioperative cardiac death is increased 10 times in patients over 70 years of age.

2. The **type of surgery** performed has an effect on perioperative cardiac mortality; the **duration of surgery** is less important.
   a. Major abdominal, thoracic, and aortic surgery have a cardiac mortality rate of 2% to 6% versus 0.5% to 2% for head and neck or extremity procedures.
   b. Emergency procedures have a mortality rate that is up to four times greater than the rate for elective procedures.

3. **Hemodynamic factors**
   a. **Hypertension**, if stable and controlled, does not have a major role in cardiac mortality.
      (1) Medication for hypertension should be continued until the morning of surgery and reinstituted as soon as possible.
      (2) Patients taking propranolol, however, should continue taking this drug.
         (a) Withdrawal may result in rebound hypertension and tachycardia.

    **(b)** Normal compensatory mechanisms for maintaining blood pressure remain effective despite continuing levels of the drug (the half-life of the drug is about 4 hours).

  **b. Hemodynamic monitoring** and careful control of blood pressure, both during and after surgery, are extremely important in any patient, but especially the cardiac patient. Such monitoring is largely responsible for recent improvements in the mortality rate in cardiac patients.

    **(1) Nonhypertensive patients** develop hypertension in the operating room in 8% of cases, and they develop hypotension in 19% of cases.

    **(2) Hypertensive patients** develop significant intraoperative hypertension in 25% of cases, and they develop hypotension requiring vasopressors or fluid supplementation in 25% of cases.

    **(3)** The risk of significant cardiac complications rises if the blood pressure drops by 50% at any time or by 33% for 10 minutes or longer.

  **c. Postoperative hypertension** has a multitude of causes, such as hypoxia, hypothermia, pain, and fluid overload. It is especially common after vascular procedures.

    **(1)** It is best managed acutely by intravenous administration of nitroprusside.

    **(2)** At the same time, therapy with more long-acting drugs should be started.

 **4.** The **overall medical status** of the patient also affects cardiac mortality. The risk is improved if electrolyte and pH abnormalities, hypoxia, anemia, and sepsis are corrected.

 **5. Postoperative surgical complications**, such as sepsis and venous thromboembolic episodes, may precipitate cardiac complications.

 **6. Anesthesia considerations** are important but are best left to the anesthesiologist. There is probably little difference between spinal and general anesthesia with respect to the risk of hypotension. There may be less myocardial depression with spinal anesthesia.

 **7.** Risk factors for atherosclerotic coronary artery disease, such as a history of smoking or hyperlipidemia, in and of themselves are not associated with cardiac risk at the time of surgery.

**B. Specific cardiac conditions** are highly likely to increase the risk of death from cardiac complications in patients undergoing noncardiac surgical procedures.

 **1. Angina**

  **a.** Patients with **stable angina** have either no or a slightly increased (up to three times that of age-matched controls risk of perioperative myocardial infarction.

  **b.** Patients with a history of **crescendo angina** have a very high perioperative risk of myocardial infarction, similar to that of patients with a recent myocardial infarction (see section V B 2 d).

    **(1)** These patients should be evaluated by cardiac catheterization to determine the need for bypass surgery prior to other elective surgery.

    **(2)** Prior **coronary artery bypass surgery** greatly reduces the perioperative cardiac mortality rate for noncardiac surgery to 1% or 2%. The rate of myocardial infarction is also low.

 **2. Myocardial infarction**

  **a.** The overall risk of myocardial infarction in American adults undergoing a major surgical procedure with general anesthesia is about 0.1% to 0.2%.

  **b.** The risk of death when a perioperative myocardial infarction does occur is as high as 50%.

  **c.** Most perioperative myocardial infarctions (i.e., 60%) occur during the first 3 postoperative days, and the remaining 40% occur in the next 3 days.

  **d.** A myocardial infarction in the recent past carries a high risk of a perioperative recurrence. Therefore, elective surgery should be postponed until 6 months following a myocardial infarction. Emergency procedures require careful operative management if surgery cannot be avoided.

  **e.** Patients who have had a previous myocardial infarction have an increased risk of perioperative arrhythmias.

  **f.** There is probably little difference in the operative risk factor between transmural and subendocardial myocardial infarction.

 **3. Congestive heart failure** from valvular or ischemic heart disease is associated with a high risk of cardiac death in the perioperative period.

  **a.** The presence of congestive heart failure is determined in several ways:

    **(1)** A history of shortness of breath, dyspnea, or pulmonary edema

    **(2)** Physical signs, such as an S3 gallop, jugular vein distention, and pulmonary edema on chest roentgenogram

  **b.** In general, patients over 40 years of age undergoing major surgery have a less than 2% risk of developing **pulmonary edema** perioperatively.

(1) However, the risk becomes 15% to 35% in patients with preoperative findings of congestive heart failure.
(2) Certain other factors also increase the risk of pulmonary edema in the perioperative period:
    (a) Age over 60 years
    (b) Poor preoperative condition
    (c) Hemodynamically significant valvular heart disease, especially aortic stenosis

c. The **mortality rate associated with pulmonary edema** in the perioperative period depends on the etiology.
    (1) It is as high as 40% in patients with cardiac failure.
    (2) It is much lower (up to 17% of the patients) if the pulmonary edema develops as a result of excessive fluid administration.
    (3) It is as high as 87% if pulmonary edema follows a thoracotomy.
d. Postoperatively, congestive heart disease and pulmonary edema occur principally during two periods:
    (1) Immediately postoperatively when positive pressure ventilation has been discontinued
    (2) One to four days postoperatively during periods of rapid mobilization of tissue fluid

4. Certain **arrhythmias** lead to increased risk during surgery.
    a. **Atrial fibrillation**, especially in connection with coronary artery disease, is associated with a mortality rate as high as 18% for major surgical procedures.
    b. **Supraventricular tachycardias** are associated with a slightly increased mortality rate (as high as 4% to 8%), especially when occurring with coronary artery disease.
    c. **Premature ventricular contractions (PVCs)** increase the risk.
        (1) Patients with five or more PVCs per minute on the preoperative electrocardiogram have a mortality rate as high as 14%.
        (2) This arrhythmia is even more serious if any of the following factors are present:
            (a) More than 12 PVCs per minute
            (b) Two or more consecutive PVCs
            (c) Multifocal PVCs
            (d) PVCs occurring on the T wave of the preceding beat
        (3) **Lidocaine** should be used with caution preoperatively for the prophylactic treatment of PVCs, because general anesthesia lengthens the activity of lidocaine and masks its central nervous system toxicity.

5. **Electrocardiographic changes** suggestive of ischemia are associated with an increased mortality rate. Even nonspecific ST-T wave changes are associated with an increased risk.

6. **Valvular heart disease** of most types has a high perioperative mortality rate. The risk is related to the severity of valvular dysfunction and the presence of associated cardiac disorders.
    a. The risk in significant **aortic stenosis** is especially high (as high as 13%).
    b. The risk inherent in **mitral stenosis** is lower, at 5% to 7%, but rises to as high as 18% with atrial fibrillation.
    c. **Mitral valve prolapse** causes little increase in the mortality rate unless congestive heart failure is present.

7. The presence of **prosthetic replacement valves** also carries an increased perioperative cardiac mortality risk, principally related to anticoagulant therapy.
    a. If anticoagulants are discontinued 1 to 5 days preoperatively, the mortality rate is as high as 6% as a result of thromboembolic phenomena.
    b. If anticoagulants are continued, the mortality rate is as high as 11%, a problem related to hemorrhagic diathesis.

C. **Prophylactic maneuvers** may be helpful in some cardiac patients.

1. **Antibiotics** should be used in patients with valvular heart disease when major surgery—or, indeed, any procedure associated with bacteremia—is undertaken. Thus, patients with prosthetic valves should also be treated with antibiotics for endoscopic procedures.
    a. The antibiotics used should include those effective against enterococci and gram-negative rods. The current recommendations include:
        (1) Either penicillin G or ampicillin (vancomycin for allergic patients), plus
        (2) Either gentamicin or streptomycin
    b. Doses are given 1/2 hour preoperatively and for two doses postoperatively.

2. **Digitalis therapy** should be continued perioperatively in patients with congestive heart failure or certain arrhythmias. **Prophylactic digitalis**, although not of proven value, may be useful in the following patients:
    a. Elderly patients undergoing pulmonary surgery

  **b.** Patients with subcritical valvular heart disease
  **c.** Patients with a history of paroxysmal tachycardia

  **3. Cardiac pacemakers** should only be used perioperatively in patients with indications for long-term pacemaker use. These indications include sick sinus syndrome, bifascicular block, a prolonged P-R interval, and atrial fibrillation.

**VI. DIABETES MELLITUS** affects 2% to 5% of the general population. As many as one-half of these patients have no symptoms until a stressful situation such as sepsis or surgery results in overt manifestations of hyperglycemia.

  **A.** The diabetic patient frequently requires surgery for a complication of the diabetes as well as for nondiabetic surgical problems.

   **1.** The diabetic patient is generally **older physiologically** than the chronologic age would suggest and thus should be treated as an older patient.

   **2.** The **mortality rate for emergency surgical procedures** in diabetics is several times higher than that for elective procedures.

   **3.** The **overall mortality rate for surgery** in diabetics is approximately 2%. Close to 30% of deaths are a direct result of **cardiovascular complications,** and 16% are related to **sepsis,** particularly from staphylococcal infections.

  **B.** The **patient history** should give particular reference to the diabetes and its management, and the **physical examination** should include an assessment of the preoperative risk.

   **1.** The **type of diabetic control** used, **dosage schedules,** and the **adequacy of control** should be determined.

   **2.** The propensity to develop ketosis, ketoacidosis, and hyper- or hypoglycemia and a history of **"brittleness"** (unpredictable wide swings in blood glucose level) should be assessed.

   **3.** The patient's **fluid and electrolyte status** should be assessed, especially in relation to the acuteness of the disease requiring surgery and to associated vomiting and diarrhea.

   **4.** Specific questions related to the **complications of diabetes,** such as nephropathy, neuropathy, peripheral vascular and coronary artery disease, and retinopathy, should be answered.
    **a. Retinopathy** is associated with diffuse small vessel disease.
    **b. Autonomic neuropathy** occurs as a result of diabetic degeneration of the autonomic nervous system. This may be manifested as the following conditions:
     **(1)** Postural hypotension
     **(2)** Bladder emptying problems
     **(3)** Impaired intestinal motility
     **(4)** Gastroparesis
     **(5)** Impotence
    **c. Cardiac autonomic dysfunction** is an uncommon but serious form of autonomic neuropathy.
     **(1)** It may be associated with postural hypotension, nocturnal diarrhea, or sweating. There is no change in the heart rate with changes in posture. There may be an abnormal carbon dioxide ventilatory response curve.
     **(2)** Cardiac autonomic dysfunction may be **diagnosed on electrocardiogram** by comparing the longest and shortest R-R intervals during a Valsalva maneuver. The **normal ratio** is greater than 1.21%. The test is **abnormal** if the ratio is less than 1.11%.
     **(3)** This diagnosis increases the risk of cardiorespiratory arrest.
     **(4)** The overall **mortality rate** is as high as 50% over 2½ years. This rate should be considered carefully when assessing the need for elective surgery.
    **d. Diabetic neuropathic cachexia** is a form of neuropathy associated with anorexia, profound weight loss, mental depression, impotence, and a painful peripheral neuropathy. This entity may be associated with an occult malignancy.

  **C. Preoperative management** of the diabetic patient depends upon the severity of the diabetes and the severity of the acute disease.

   **1.** The **serum glucose level** should be monitored.

   **2.** The **anion gap** should be followed, and if it is elevated, arterial blood gases should be tested. The usual finding is low serum bicarbonate and a decreased pH. This may be due to:
    **a.** Diabetic ketoacidosis
    **b.** Lactic acidosis

    **c.** Retained organic acids containing phosphates and sulfates secondary to chronic renal failure

**3. Radiopaque dye studies** performed on diabetics increase the risk of acute renal failure. This is especially true in patients over 40 years of age or with a creatinine level greater than 2 mg/dl.

**4.** Patients who are managed by orally administered **hypoglycemic agents** should usually have the drug discontinued on the day of surgery. The sulfonylurea drugs, however, have a prolonged half-life (e.g., the half-life of chlorpropamide is 38 hours) and should be withheld on the day prior to surgery.

**5.** Patients who are on **insulin therapy** usually are given **one-half of the daily dose of insulin** on the morning of surgery to prevent hypoglycemia; an intravenous drip of glucose-containing solution should be maintained.

**6.** Patients with **diabetic ketoacidosis** are acidotic, are dehydrated as a result of a massive osmotic diuresis, have decreased body stores of potassium and sodium, and are ketotic. They may have Kussmaul's respirations, which are rapid deep breaths.
    **a.** There is a drop in serum sodium levels of 1.35 mEq/L to 1.6 mEq/L for each 100 mg/dl that the glucose is elevated.
    **b.** Surgery should be withheld until the ketoacidosis is partially resolved, as measured by improvement in pH, hydration, and correction of electrolyte abnormalities and serum glucose levels. Ketoacidosis is best corrected by administration of IV fluids, insulin, bicarbonate, and potassium.

**7.** The stress of surgery, infection, or the high glucose load of hyperalimentation may induce a nonketotic, hyperglycemic, hyperosmolar coma in patients with adult-onset diabetes.

# Part I
# Study Questions

## QUESTIONS

**Directions:** Each question below contains five suggested answers. Choose the **one best** response to each question.

1. Which of the following studies is most helpful in evaluating a patient's risk for a routine operative procedure?

(A) History
(B) Physical examination
(C) Chest x-ray
(D) Electrocardiogram
(E) Liver function profile

2. Following active immunization with tetanus toxoid injection, how often should a tetanus toxoid booster be given?

(A) Every year
(B) Every 2 years
(C) Every 5 years
(D) Every 10 years
(E) Never

3. Surgery is contraindicated in patients with

(A) serum creatinine levels of 2.5 mg/dl
(B) atrial fibrillation
(C) chronic obstructive lung disease with a $P_{CO_2}$ of 45 mm Hg
(D) a history of subendocardial myocardial infarction (4 weeks ago)
(E) a history of a stroke (6 months ago)

4. The most important aspect in treating disseminated intravascular coagulation (DIC) is to

(A) administer heparin
(B) administer platelets
(C) treat the underlying disease process
(D) achieve normal levels of fibrinogen
(E) transfuse with fresh frozen plasma and cryoprecipitate

5. In elderly patients undergoing major surgery, the highest operative risk is associated with which of the following disorders?

(A) Pulmonary vascular disease
(B) Asthma
(C) Chronic obstructive lung disease
(D) Carcinoma of the lung
(E) History of a pulmonary embolus

6. A patient with normal renal function has a serum sodium concentration of 120 mEq/L and does not appear to be dehydrated. This patient most likely has

(A) a total body sodium deficit
(B) dilutional hyponatremia
(C) a contracted blood volume
(D) diabetes insipidus
(E) Cushing's disease

7. Patients with chronic renal failure are likely to present with all of the following clinical manifestations EXCEPT

(A) overhydration and overnourishment, resulting in an increased weight gain
(B) impaired immune function, resulting in an increased incidence of infection
(C) altered platelet function, resulting in an increased incidence of wound hematomas
(D) anemia with the ability to tolerate a hematocrit of 25%
(E) pericarditis, resulting in pericardial effusion

8. There are three basic phases in wound healing that ultimately lead to the return of tissue strength. All of the following statements about these phases are true EXCEPT

(A) there is no increase in wound strength during the lag phase
(B) capillaries migrate into the wound during the proliferative phase
(C) an uncomplicated wound has good resistance to infection from surface contamination in the earliest phase
(D) wounds attain breaking strength equivalent to normal tissue during the maturation phase
(E) neutrophils and macrophages are the predominant cell types during the early phases

9. Which of the following statements best characterizes a cutaneous abscess?

(A) Hidradenitis suppurativa is an infection of the exocrine glands
(B) *Streptococcus* is the most common infecting organism in an upper extremity furuncle
(C) Gram-negative cocci are most apt to be present in an abscess in the inguinal area
(D) The most effective treatment for a cutaneous abscess is penicillin
(E) A carbuncle is a cutaneous abscess that burrows through the dermis into subcutaneous tissue

10. Alveolar hypoventilation in an overweight patient is caused principally by

(A) retention of carbon dioxide
(B) impaired chest wall expansion and contraction
(C) bronchospasm
(D) increased pulmonary dead space
(E) increased pulmonary arterial resistance

11. Palliative resection for breast cancer consists of

(A) axillary lymph node dissection
(B) toilet mastectomy
(C) lumpectomy
(D) internal mammary lymph node biopsy
(E) incisional biopsy

12. The hernia most frequently seen in women is the

(A) femoral hernia
(B) indirect inguinal hernia
(C) epigastric hernia
(D) direct inguinal hernia
(E) pantaloon hernia

13. The most common cause of pulmonary insufficiency in the early postoperative period following major abdominal surgery is

(A) aspiration of gastric contents
(B) bronchospasm
(C) atelectasis
(D) pneumothorax
(E) pulmonary edema

14. Important components of collagen synthesis and wound strength and contraction include all of the following EXCEPT

(A) fibroblasts
(B) myofibroblasts
(C) vitamin C
(D) lysine
(E) normal $PO_2$

15. What anatomic landmark is used to distinguish an indirect hernia from a direct hernia?

(A) Femoral artery and vein
(B) Inferior epigastric vessels
(C) Spermatic cord
(D) Transversalis fascia
(E) Processus vaginalis

**Directions:** Each question below contains four suggested answers of which **one or more** is correct. Choose the answer

A if **1, 2, and 3** are correct
B if **1 and 3** are correct
C if **2 and 4** are correct
D if **4** is correct
E if **1, 2, 3, and 4** are correct

16. A young man is brought to the emergency room with multiple injuries following an automobile accident. Management of his thoracic injuries would involve

(1) upright chest x-rays obtained as soon as possible
(2) monitoring the electrocardiogram and central venous pressure for evidence of cardiac contusion or tamponade
(3) contrast studies of the esophagus to look for perforation
(4) thoracotomy if bleeding from a chest tube exceeds 100 ml per hour

17. Uses of 5% sodium chloride solution include which of the following?

(1) It provides normal daily sodium requirements
(2) It is ideal for maintenance or replacement therapy
(3) It can correct hyperosmolar dehydration
(4) It can correct symptomatic body sodium deficits

18. Characteristics of hemophilia A include which of the following?

(1) Prolonged bleeding time
(2) Normal prothrombin time
(3) Autosomal recessive transmission
(4) Prolonged partial thromboplastin time

19. A 60-year-old woman with moderately advanced chronic obstructive lung disease and mild wheezing requires an exploratory laparotomy. Which of the following maneuvers will reduce complications postoperatively?

(1) Corticosteroid administration
(2) Preoperative pulmonary therapy instruction
(3) Discontinuance of cigarette smoking several days before surgery
(4) Use of a bronchodilator such as aminophylline

20. Correct statements concerning intra-abdominal infections include which of the following?

(1) A common cause of intra-abdominal infections is perforation of a hollow viscus
(2) Treatment usually includes surgical exploration with drainage and debridement of the abscess
(3) A high index of suspicion is essential for the diagnosis because there may be no physical signs of infection
(4) Ultrasonography or computed tomography (CT) can be used to direct surgical drainage

21. Certain steps are essential during the early management of trauma victims, including

(1) airway assessment and control
(2) cardiac resuscitation
(3) insertion of venous access lines
(4) suturing of all facial lacerations

22. Statements that characterize intraperitoneal abscesses or their treatment include which of the following?

(1) Staphylococcal abscesses are often seen postoperatively
(2) The most effective treatment is surgical drainage
(3) They are rarely associated with fever
(4) Computed tomography (CT) is useful in locating these abscesses

23. Correct statements concerning lactated Ringer's solution include which of the following?

(1) It can correct body water deficits in isosmolar dehydration
(2) It is isosmolar with extracellular fluid
(3) It contains 130 mEq sodium per L of solution
(4) It contains 2.5 g albumin per dl of solution

24. Many postoperative problems can be anticipated, provided that the physician knows that

(1) urinary tract infection can cause fever on postoperative days 3 through 6
(2) wound infection can cause fever on postoperative days 5 through 8
(3) pulmonary complications are the most common cause of fever in the first few postoperative days
(4) the body accumulates third-space fluid by postoperative day 3, making fluid supplementation necessary

25. Patients with chronic liver failure and acute alcoholic hepatitis undergoing surgery may have which of the following difficulties?

(1) Lethargy and hepatic coma due to continued doses of narcotics
(2) Acute liver failure and death
(3) Coagulopathy due to impaired absorption of vitamin K or thrombocytopenia
(4) Esophageal variceal bleeding if a prophylactic shunt is not used

26. When a trauma patient is in profound shock, management involves

(1) subclavian lines and saphenous vein cutdowns
(2) crystalloid solutions, followed by packed red blood cells if the hematocrit is less than 25%
(3) uncrossmatched type-specific blood cells
(4) initial use of type O-negative blood, if available, if there is no time for blood typing

27. Correct statements concerning hypertrophic scar formation include which of the following?

(1) Most of these scars have completed remodeling by 3 months
(2) These scars are more common in black and Oriental patients than in white patients
(3) Invasion of nearby normal tissue is unusual
(4) Histologically, these scars appear as large, swollen, eosinophilic collagen bundles

28. Which of the following statements characterizes necrotizing fasciitis or its treatment?

(1) Surgical debridement is the primary treatment
(2) High doses of antibiotics are required for treatment
(3) The skin overlying the infection site often appears normal
(4) The organisms likely to be involved are staphylococci, microaerophilic streptococci, and gram-negative anaerobes

29. General endotracheal anesthesia results in which of the following alterations in pulmonary function?

(1) Impaired ciliary function
(2) Pneumothorax
(3) Altered chest wall mechanical properties
(4) Increased functional residual capacity

30. Causes of vitamin K deficiency include

(1) malnutrition
(2) total parenteral nutrition
(3) obstructive jaundice
(4) antibiotic therapy

31. True statements concerning postoperative drainage tubes include which of the following?

(1) An underwater-seal drain is necessary when draining the pleural space
(2) Rigid drains may erode through the wall of a hollow viscus or blood vessel, resulting in a gastrointestinal fistula or local hemorrhage
(3) A T tube is used to drain bile following common duct exploration until spasm of the sphincter of Oddi resolves
(4) Open drains reduce the risk of bacterial wound infection

32. True statements concerning peritoneal lavage of the trauma patient with abdominal injuries include

(1) it is useful for unconscious patients
(2) the best technique is the semiopen technique
(3) the lavage is positive if gross blood or more than 100,000 red blood cells per ml are found in the lavage aspirate
(4) the patient's bladder need not be empty prior to lavage

33. Correct statements concerning inguinal hernias include which of the following?

(1) Pediatric inguinal hernias are usually indirect
(2) Femoral hernias are more common in women than in men
(3) Recurrent inguinal hernias following repair usually recur as direct hernias
(4) Femoral hernias rarely become incarcerated

34. Failure to obliterate a patent processus vaginalis completely may result in

(1) a femoral hernia
(2) an indirect inguinal hernia
(3) a direct inguinal hernia
(4) a spermatic cord hydrocele

35. Characteristics of granulation tissue include which of the following?

(1) It contains large numbers of capillaries
(2) It contains small numbers of phagocytes
(3) It has a beefy, red, moist appearance
(4) It poses a high risk of infection

36. A normal bleeding time is maintained by a normal

(1) vascular response to injury
(2) platelet quantity
(3) platelet function
(4) intrinsic coagulation mechanism

37. A patient with multiple injuries is brought to the hospital. Which of the following management procedures in the emergency room would control the hemorrhage?

(1) Applying pressure on the wounds with gauze pads
(2) Hemostats used proximally and distally to control arterial-type bleeding in the base of deep puncture wounds
(3) Pneumatic splints and medical antishock trousers to tamponade bleeding and increase peripheral resistance
(4) Suturing closed actively bleeding missile tracts or stab wound sites

38. Which of the following principles may apply to the proper repair of an indirect inguinal hernia?

(1) The abdominal wall defect is repaired
(2) The external oblique aponeurosis contributes significantly to the strength of the repair
(3) The hernia sac is ligated at its base
(4) The spermatic cord is placed deep to transversalis fascia to eliminate the internal ring

39. Correct statements concerning prophylactic antibiotics include which of the following?

(1) They should be administered for 24 hours before and at least 48 hours after surgery
(2) They are useful when there is a risk of infection at the operative wound site
(3) Broad-spectrum antibiotics are the treatment of choice
(4) They are beneficial when used during insertion of prosthetic devices

40. Protein intake should be reduced in patients with which of the following conditions?

(1) Uremia
(2) Sepsis
(3) Hepatic encephalopathy
(4) Multiple long bone fractures

41. Which of the following structures accompany the spermatic cord through the inguinal canal in the normal male?

(1) Vas deferens
(2) Ilioinguinal nerve
(3) Pampiniform plexus
(4) Poupart's ligament

**Directions:** The groups of questions below consist of lettered choices followed by several numbered items. For each numbered item select the **one** lettered choice with which it is **most** closely associated. Each lettered choice may be used once, more than once, or not at all.

**Questions 42–45**

For each serum abnormality listed below, select the metabolic or fluid and electrolyte disorder most likely to be associated with it.

(A) Compensated respiratory acidosis
(B) Respiratory alkalosis
(C) Hypotonic dehydration
(D) Hypochloremic alkalosis
(E) Metabolic acidosis

42. $\dfrac{HCO_3^-}{H_2CO_3}$ of $\dfrac{10}{1}$

43. $K^+$ concentration of 3.5 mEq/L

44. $Na^+$ concentration of 120 mEq/L

45. $P_{CO_2}$ of 30 mm Hg

**Questions 46–50**

For each condition listed below, select the treatment that would be most appropriate.

(A) Cryoprecipitate
(B) Factor VIII concentrate
(C) Fresh frozen plasma
(D) Albumin
(E) Fresh whole blood

46. Volume expansion

47. Acute hemorrhage

48. von Willebrand's disease

49. Replacement of clotting factors

50. Fibrinogen deficiency

## ANSWERS AND EXPLANATIONS

**1. The answer is A.** (*Chapter 3 I B*) The history is the most helpful study in evaluating a patient's operative risk because it gives a complete profile of the patient and how he or she has reacted to stress and to other adverse conditions in the past. A history of familial disorders, prior illnesses, prior difficulties with surgical procedures or anesthetics, the presence of allergies or asthma, and the effects of medications, including over-the-counter products, should be included. Physical examination, chest x-ray, electrocardiogram, and a liver function profile are useful, but an alert physician will suspect problems from the history alone.

**2. The answer is D.** (*Chapter 1 VII A 4 a*) Active immunization results when tetanus toxoid injections are given on the recommended schedule, usually in infancy (with DPT shots) or during military induction. A follow-up booster every 10 years is recommended by the American College of Surgeons. However, any person with a penetrating injury must receive tetanus prophylaxis if previous immunization cannot be documented or if more than 5 years have passed since the last immunization.

**3. The answer is D.** (*Chapter 3 V B 2*) A myocardial infarction within 3 to 6 months of surgery carries a much higher operative mortality risk due to the perioperative recurrence. The mortality rate of a perioperative myocardial infarction is as high as 50% and usually occurs in the first postoperative week. There is little difference in the risk factors for a subendocardial and for a transmural myocardial infarction. Emergency procedures that cannot be avoided require careful operative management.

**4. The answer is C.** [*Chapter 1 V C 3 c (1)*] Disseminated intravascular coagulation (DIC) results from the simultaneous activation of the coagulation and fibrinolytic systems as a consequence of a severe underlying disorder, such as sepsis, malignancy, trauma, shock, or serious obstetrical complications. Platelets and clotting factors are consumed, and fibrin split products are released. Clinically, there is widespread hemorrhage. The consumptive coagulopathy of DIC cannot be interrupted until the underlying pathologic process that precipitated the disorder has been controlled. Until this is accomplished, administration of platelets, fresh frozen plasma, and cryoprecipitate are helpful adjuncts. Heparin administration, although advocated by some, probably is inadvisable in the profusely bleeding patient with DIC.

**5. The answer is C.** (*Chapter 3 II B*) Although patients with pulmonary vascular disease, asthma, carcinoma, or a history of pulmonary embolus are at increased operative risk, the highest operative risk is for patients with chronic obstructive lung disease. These patients may not be able to generate enough force to cough and clear their airways postoperatively. Atelectasis, pneumonia, and other infections can lead to acute pulmonary decompensation and an inability to be weaned from the respirator.

**6. The answer is B.** [*Chapter 1 I B 2 a (3)*] If a patient with hyponatremia (i.e., a deficiency of salt in the blood) does not show signs of dehydration, then it is likely that he or she is overhydrated, resulting in dilutional hyponatremia, which is not a true sodium deficit. The blood volume would be overexpanded, and the total body sodium would be normal. Diabetes insipidus produces hypernatremia and dehydration. Cushing's disease can cause overhydration due to salt retention, but this is much less likely.

**7. The answer is A.** [*Chapter 3 III A 1 b (3), d, e, f (2), B 3 a*] Although patients with chronic renal failure are often overhydrated and as a result overweight, the weight gain is due to peripheral edema not to an increased food intake. Patients with renal failure have decreased body stores of nitrogen, which is catabolized more often as uremia progresses. There is usually decreased dietary intake as a result of anorexia, nausea, malabsorption, or perhaps dietary restrictions by the physician. Immune function is affected, resulting in more infections; hematologic functions are impaired, resulting in anemia and altered platelet adhesion and aggregation, and cardiac and vascular abnormalities develop, including pericarditis and atherosclerosis.

**8. The answer is D.** (*Chapter 1 IV A 2 a, B 1–3*) The lag phase of wound healing occurs during the first several days. Neutrophils predominate for the first 48 hours, after which the macrophages become active. There is no increase in wound strength at this time; however, an uncomplicated wound has good resistance to infection from surface contamination in this phase. The proliferative phase is characterized by the migration of fibroblasts and capillaries into the wound, although neutrophils and macrophages continue to be abundant. The maturation phase of wound healing occurs when the cellular activity in the wound diminishes. Wounds rarely attain the same breaking strength that was present in the tissue prior to injury. Some wounds reach 80% of the original strength, but this may require years.

**9. The answer is E.** (*Chapter 1 VII B 2 a–c*) Cutaneous abscesses are of three types: furuncles, carbuncles, and hidradenitis suppurativa. Furuncles are cutaneous staphylococcal abscesses that are frequently seen with acne. Carbuncles are cutaneous abscesses that spread through the dermis into the subcutaneous region. Hidradenitis suppurativa is an infection involving the apocrine sweat glands. Staphylococci are the most likely causative organisms. The microbiologic diagnosis is made by incising the abscess, then culturing and Gram-staining the pus, which usually reveals gram-positive cocci. Most staphylococcal organisms are resistant to penicillin; thus, one of the semisynthetic penicillins, erythromycin or cephalosporin, should be used.

**10. The answer is B.** (*Chapter 3 II A 1*) Because obesity markedly increases the work of respiration and impairs the bellows function of the chest wall, the obese surgical patient is at increased risk for respiratory failure postanesthesia as a result of alveolar hypoventilation. As a result of the failure to move enough air in and out of the lungs, carbon dioxide retention and inadequate oxygenation of blood occur. Bronchospasm and increased pulmonary dead space and pulmonary resistance have no particular association with obesity.

**11. The answer is B.** (*Chapter 1 IX B 1 c, d, 2, C 1, 2*) Palliative resection is used to relieve or prevent a specific symptom of a cancer patient but not to effect a cure. Palliative surgery can provide comfort for a patient for months. Palliative resection for breast cancer would consist of a toilet mastectomy to remove large, ulcerating, necrotic, breast cancer tissue. Removal of lymph nodes is effective in defining or limiting the extent of certain tumors. Lumpectomy is used either for diagnosis or as part of combined treatment involving radiotherapy. Incisional biopsy is performed to remove a portion of a lesion for examination, usually if the lesion is too large for simple excision.

**12. The answer is B.** (*Chapter 1 X B 2–5*) Although indirect inguinal hernias are five to ten times more common in men than in women, they are still the most common type of hernias seen in women. They may occur from infancy to old age but generally occur by the fifth decade of life. An indirect inguinal hernia passes through the internal inguinal ring and down the inguinal canal. It occurs as a result of a congenitally patent processus vaginalis, which allows free communication between the peritoneal cavity and inguinal canal.

**13. The answer is C.** (*Chapter 3 II B 1*) The most common complication in the postoperative period after abdominal surgery is atelectasis (i.e., collapse of a segment or a lobe of the lung), which leads to pulmonary insufficiency. Atelectasis is thought to be the result of insufficient ventilation during anesthesia. Because it is quite common following major surgery, it should always be the diagnosis of exclusion. Aspiration of gastric contents, bronchospasm, pneumothorax, and pulmonary edema are also significant, albeit less common, complications of the postoperative course and thus should be suspected and excluded.

**14. The answer is D.** (*Chapter 1 IV A 1, 3*) Collagen, which is formed by fibroblasts, is responsible for binding tissues together and ultimately is a major determinant of wound strength. Proline, hydroxyproline, and glycine are very important in collagen synthesis as are adequate tissue oxygen, ferrous iron, $\alpha$-ketoglutarate, and ascorbic acid. Contraction occurs in the tissue of a wound, helping it to close by decreasing its surface area; the myofibroblasts are responsible for wound contraction.

**15. The answer is B.** (*Chapter 1 X B 1–3*) The inguinal canal is the communication between the internal and external rings. The anterior wall of the canal is formed by the external oblique aponeurosis. The floor of the canal is formed by the inguinal ligament and its reflection. Within the floor of the canal is Hesselbach's triangle, which is formed laterally by the inferior epigastric artery, inferiorly by the inguinal ligament, and superomedially by the transversalis fascia and portions of the rectus sheath. An indirect inguinal hernia passes through the internal ring and down the inguinal canal. A direct inguinal hernia occurs in the floor of the inguinal canal at Hesselbach's triangle due to an acquired weakness of tissue. The inferior epigastric vessels are the anatomic landmarks that distinguish the indirect and direct hernias.

**16. The answer is E (all).** (*Chapter 2 I C 6 b*) Upright films of the chest should be obtained as soon as possible after a patient with chest injuries arrives in the emergency room. A significant finding would be pneumothorax, fluid in the chest cavity, or evidence of widening of the mediastinum. Penetrating injuries that traverse the mediastinum are an indication for contrast studies of the esophagus and arteriography of the great vessels to rule out injury to these vital structures. If significant fluid or pneumothorax is present, a chest tube should be inserted. If there is a continuing massive air leak and the lung fails to re-expand, a ruptured or lacerated bronchus should be suspected. Bleeding through a chest tube at a rate greater than 100 ml per hour is an indication for a thoracotomy for control of the bleeding.

**17. The answer is D (4).** (*Chapter 1 Table 1-5*) Five percent sodium chloride solution is a very hyperosmolar solution that contains 80 mEq of sodium chloride per dl or 800 mEq of sodium chloride per L of solution. Because of its severe hyperosmolarity, this solution is indicated only for correcting symptomatic sodium deficits in the body and not for maintenance or replacement therapy. It is contraindicated in hyperosmolar states and indicated only in the treatment of symptomatic hypo-osmolar states.

**18. The answer is C (2, 4).** [*Chapter 1 V C 3 a (1)*] Hemophilia A is an X-linked recessive disorder of the procoagulant activity of factor VIII. As factor VIII is a component of the intrinsic coagulation system, the partial thromboplastin time is usually prolonged, but the prothrombin time is normal. The bleeding time also is normal, because there is no defect in platelet aggregation. Severity depends on the degree of deficiency of factor VIII. Spontaneous bleeding can be avoided by plasma activity levels of at least 5%.

**19. The answer is C (2, 4).** (*Chapter 3 II D 1–2*) Certain pre- and postoperative maneuvers may improve pulmonary function and reduce the number of postoperative complications. Preoperative instruction in the methods of "pulmonary toilet" to be used postoperatively is helpful to ensure patient compliance. Cigarette smoking should be stopped at least 2 to 3 weeks preceding surgery to eliminate the acute effects of smoking on the respiratory epithelium. Bronchodilators can improve, to some degree, wheezing in patients with lung disease. Steroids should never be used prophylactically before surgery because of their association with impaired wound healing and decreased resistance to infection.

**20. The answer is E (all).** (*Chapter 1 VII B 3 a, d, e*) Intra-abdominal abscesses can result from penetrating trauma, surgical procedures, perforation of a hollow viscus, seeding of bacteria from outside the abdomen, or ischemia and infarction of tissue within the abdomen. Although abscesses in the abdominal region produce the signs and symptoms of any abscess—fever, pain, and leukocytosis—a high index of suspicion is essential as there may be no physical signs of infection. The mainstay of treatment is surgical intervention with drainage and debridement of the abscess. Ultrasonography and computed tomography (CT) have recently proved useful in localizing the abscess and guiding the drainage procedure.

**21. The answer is A (1, 2, 3).** (*Chapter 2 I C*) The initial assessment of the critically injured patient will most likely determine the ultimate outcome. The patient should be examined for chest wall motion and cyanosis. If ventilation is unsatisfactory, corrective measures must be quickly taken. Early intubation is important and should be carried out without neck extension, since the status of the cervical spine often is not known. Ventilation can then be performed. Cardiac resuscitation may be required if the patient is asystolic or severely hypovolemic. Venous access lines should be placed rapidly, and the two most effective means for doing so are subclavian puncture and saphenous vein cut-down. Lacerations of the face can cause bleeding; however, these are not high-priority injuries during the initial evaluation of the critically injured patient.

**22. The answer is C (2, 4).** (*Chapter 1 VII B 3 c–e*) Surgical drainage is the treatment of choice for peritoneal abscesses. Both computed tomography (CT) and ultrasonography are useful in locating the abscesses and in guiding precise drainage. Multiple abscesses occur in about 15% of cases. Most abscesses, regardless of location, are associated with fever, pain, and leukocytosis. Usually, an enteric type of organism is found.

**23. The answer is B (1, 3).** (*Chapter 1 Table 1-5*) Lactated Ringer's solution is a balanced electrolyte solution that contains 274 mOsm. It is slightly hyperosmolar to extracellular body fluid, which contains essentially 310 mOsm. However, lactated Ringer's solution is an excellent fluid for correction of isosmolar body water deficits, and the addition of 5% dextrose makes it slightly hyperosmolar. The solution contains 130 mEq of sodium, 4 mEq of potassium, and 3 mEq of calcium per L with 109 mEq of chlorine and 28 mEq of bicarbonate per L. It is strictly a crystalloid solution and contains no albumin. It can also be used as a replacement solution for gastrointestinal losses because of its similar electrolyte constitution.

**24. The answer is A (1, 2, 3).** (*Chapter 1 VII A 2 c; VIII D, E*) Common postoperative problems typically occur on certain postoperative days. Urinary tract infection, triggered by an indwelling catheter or pre-existing vesical outlet obstruction, is the typical cause of fever that develops on postoperative days 3 through 6. Wound infection often presents as a spiking fever on postoperative days 5 through 8. Pulmonary complications, the most common cause of fever in the first few postoperative days, develop as a result of prolonged mechanical ventilation or because of inadequate ventilation and a poor cough effort. Dehydration is common after surgery because of third-space sequestration of fluids in the operative site; however, on the third or fourth postoperative day, the body begins to mobilize third-space fluid, making fluid restriction or renal diuresis necessary.

**25. The answer is A (1, 2, 3).** (*Chapter 3 IV B 1–5*) Management of surgical patients with preexisting liver disease and alcoholic hepatitis has not been fully defined, but several important generalizations should be considered. It is advisable to delay elective surgery in a patient with acute alcoholic hepatitis until the hepatitis has resolved, as use of a general anesthetic in these patients is associated with an operative mortality rate of 50% or more. Coagulopathy, especially if due to a vitamin K deficiency or thrombocytopenia, should be corrected temporarily with a transfusion of blood products. Any central nervous system depressant should be avoided in patients with liver failure as it may precipitate hepatic encephalopathy. It has been shown that prophylactic shunts carry a higher mortality risk than just simple observation.

**26. The answer is E (all).** (*Chapter 2 I C 4 d, e*) The subclavian vein is useful for percutaneous placement of large-bore venous catheters. In addition, the saphenous vein can be quickly isolated at the ankle and is similarly useful. It is important to remember that the saphenous vein will be flaccid and empty in a hypovolemic patient and may resemble a tendon during the cut-down. This vein can almost always be cannulated and will provide a conduit for the rapid administration of fluid. Crystalloid solutions should be started as soon as the patient reaches the emergency room when shock is present. If the hematocrit is low, packed cells are indicated, and usually these can be obtained within a matter of minutes. If the patient is in profound shock and there is no time even for blood-typing, O-negative blood can be used. If the patient initially responds to the saline infusion, uncrossmatched type-specific blood is preferred, particularly if the patient has no history of prior transfusion.

**27. The answer is C (2, 4).** (*Chapter 1 IV F 1, 2*) Most scars continue to remodel for more than 1 year. Hypertrophic scars, which result from wounds that heal with excessive collagen synthesis, are unsightly and have a raised surface. They occur most commonly in black, Oriental, and dark-skinned white patients, and in relatively younger patients. An ordinary hypertrophic scar lies entirely within the confines of the wound, but a keloid invades nearby normal tissue that was not previously involved in the wound. Histologially, these scars are large, swollen, eosinophilic collagen bundles, the treatment of which is very difficult as excision often results in recurrence.

**28. The answer is E (all).** (*Chapter 1 VII D 1–5*) Necrotizing fasciitis is a rapidly progressive bacterial infection in which several different organisms—staphylococci, microaerophilic streptococci, and gram-negative anaerobes—invade the fascial planes. The infection results in necrosis of the tissue involved; however, the overlying skin may appear normal, leading the physician to underestimate the severity of the infection. On the other hand, the patient with necrotizing fasciitis often is critically ill with a high fever, leukocytosis, and severe pain in the affected area. Treatment is largely surgical: It is critical to remove all infected or devitalized tissue at the first debridement so that the rapidly progressive necrosis does not continue. Daily debridement may be needed, and antibiotics in high doses are required.

**29. The answer is A (1, 2, 3).** (*Chapter 3 II B 2 d*) Both the anesthetic and the technique employed in its use can have adverse effects on postoperative function. Anesthesia markedly interferes with the normal clearing mechanisms of the tracheobronchial tree by impairing ciliary action, mucus function, cough reflexes, sighs, and other reflex actions. The chest wall dynamics are altered due to muscle relaxation and impaired diaphragmatic excursion, and the risk of pneumothorax is increased by positive pressure ventilation. Anesthesia may decrease functional residual capacity, resulting in hypoxemia.

**30. The answer is E (all).** [*Chapter 1 V C 3 c (2)*] Vitamin K, a fat-soluble vitamin, is acquired both from diet and as a product of metabolism of some of the gastrointestinal bacterial fluids. Malnutrition and total parenteral nutrition without vitamin K supplements will lead to deficiency. Obstructive jaundice will block the passage of bile salts to the gut; these are necessary for the absorption of fat-soluble vitamin K. Antibiotic therapy can alter the normal flora of the gut, resulting in a deficiency. Thus, a deficiency of vitamin K is common in surgical patients because of all of the above reasons.

**31. The answer is A (1, 2, 3).** [*Chapter 1 III A 1 a (2), b, 3 d, 4 c (1)*] Various types of tubes are used in surgery to permit drainage that is either abnormal, such as pus, or is a normal body fluid that cannot be handled normally by the body. An underwater-seal drain, a type of closed drain, is useful for draining the pleural space because it prevents air and fluid from reentering the body. A T tube is used to drain bile following common duct exploration until spasm of the sphincter of Oddi resolves. Rigid drains may erode through the wall of a blood vessel or a hollow viscus, a complication that may be minimized by using soft drains or removing drains early. Open drains allow free movement of bacteria because they are not sealed at either end, and as a result carry a high risk of deep wound infection.

**32. The answer is A (1, 2, 3).** (*Chapter 2 I C 6 c*) Peritoneal lavage is used when the need for abdominal exploration is unclear. It is especially useful if the patient is unconscious or neurologically impaired, as that patient will not be able to give information regarding abdominal pain. With the semiopen technique, a small incision is made below the umbilicus and the fascia is visualized directly, so that the catheter is placed under direct vision. One L of saline is infused and then aspirated. If gross blood is found or if there are more than 100,000 red cells per ml, the lavage is considered to be positive. It is essential to empty the patient's bladder prior to doing the lavage, as a distended bladder may be inadvertently entered.

**33. The answer is A (1, 2, 3).** (*Chapter 1 X B 2, 3*) A pediatric inguinal hernia is almost always indirect and has a high risk of incarceration. It is more common on the right (75%) and is often bilateral. A femoral hernia occurs when the intra-abdominal contents protrude along the femoral sheath in the femoral canal; often 30% to 40% become incarcerated. Femoral hernias are more common in females than males; they are often related to physical exertion and to pregnancy. A recurrent inguinal hernia usually occurs as a direct hernia. Generally, the defect occurs in the most medial aspect of the repair of the floor of the inguinal canal.

**34. The answer is C (2, 4).** [*Chapter 1 X B 1 d (5), 2 b*] The processus vaginalis is an invagination of peritoneum that accompanies the descent of the testicle and gubernaculum through the abdominal wall. Normally obliterated, it remains patent in an indirect hernia and forms the hernia sac. Thus, a patent or incompletely obliterated processus vaginalis allows free communication between the peritoneal cavity and the scrotum, resulting in an indirect inguinal hernia and sometimes in a spermatic cord hydrocele.

**35. The answer is B (1, 3).** (*Chapter 1 IV C 2 a–c*) Granulation tissue forms on wound surfaces when healing is by second intention. It is beefy, red, moist tissue that contains a high number of inflammatory cells and capillaries. Granulation tissue is not sterile, but the large number of phagocytes act as a barrier to invasive infections. A bacterial count of $10^4$ organisms per mm$^3$ is necessary to allow the ingrowth of epithelial cells.

**36. The answer is A (1, 2, 3).** (*Chapter 1 V B 3 c*) The upper limit of a normal bleeding time is 5 minutes, which implies an adequate number of platelets, normal platelet function, and a normal vascular response to injury. Neither the intrinsic nor the extrinsic coagulation system has an effect on bleeding time.

**37. The answer is B (1, 3).** (*Chapter 2 I C 4 g*) When a patient presents with hemorrhage in the emergency room, the application of direct pressure on bleeding wounds with manually held gauze pads is usually effective and safe. No attempt should be made to clamp blindly arterial bleeders in the emergency room. Compression of the wound should be carried out until the patient can be moved to the operating room, where definitive repair of these injuries can be accomplished. Pneumatic splints and antishock trousers are useful in tamponading bleeding and increasing peripheral vascular resistance. One advantage of these devices is that they increase peripheral vascular resistance without the pharmacologic effects of pressor agents. Stab wounds and missile tracts should never be sutured in the emergency room, but should be packed until definitive repair of the underlying injury can be accomplished in the operating room.

**38. The answer is B (1, 3).** (*Chapter 1 X B 7 a, b*) Operative repair of inguinal hernias includes a return of the hernia contents into the peritoneal cavity, ligation of the base of the hernia sac, and repair of the abdominal wall defect to prevent recurrence (about 1% recur). To repair the abdominal wall defect the transversalis fascia and conjoint tendon are sutured to either the inguinal ligament or Cooper's ligament. This procedure is responsible for the strength of the repair. The spermatic cord is returned to its normal anatomic location within the inguinal canal in almost all repairs.

**39. The answer is C (2, 4).** (*Chapter 1 VII A 3 a–e*) Prophylactic antibiotics should be given 1 to 2 hours preceding surgery and for only 6 to 24 hours postoperatively. Longer periods increase the risk of superinfection with resistant organisms. Narrow-spectrum antibiotics aimed at the usual infecting organism for a particular type of operation are the treatment of choice. Broad-spectrum antibiotics often select for resistant organisms, which are then more difficult to treat than the original organism. Prosthesis insertion carries a significant risk of infection, which is very difficult to eradicate and may result in loss of life or limb. Many studies have demonstrated the usefulness of prophylactic antibiotics in prosthetic surgery.

**40. The answer is B (1, 3).** (*Chapter 1 II B 2*) Patients with impaired ability to excrete nitrogen, such as those with uremia and hepatic encephalopathy, usually do not tolerate intravenous protein administration well and should receive a reduced amount of amino acids. Patients with sepsis and multiple injuries are often highly catabolic and require increased amounts of calories, including excess protein.

**41. The answer is A (1, 2, 3).** (*Chapter 1 X B 1 d*) Spermatic cord structures—testicular and cremaster arteries, the ilioinguinal nerve, the genital branch of the genitofemoral nerve, the pampiniform plexus, and the vas deferens—pass into the internal ring, traverse the inguinal canal, and pass through the external ring into the scrotum. Poupart's ligament forms the floor of the inguinal canal; it does not traverse the canal.

**42–45. The answers are: 42-E, 43-D, 44-C, 45-B.** (*Chapter 1 I B 1 b, C 1–4*) A decrease in serum bicarbonate ($HCO_3^-$) concentration with a normal carbonic acid ($H_2CO_3$) concentration results from $HCO_3^-$ loss and is associated with metabolic acidosis. In hypochloremic alkalosis, there is always an accompanying decline in serum potassium, as it exchanges for hydrogen ion at the cellular level and in the renal tubule in an attempt to restore normal pH. By definition, hypotonic hypohydration is associated with a low serum sodium concentration, while plasma pH and serum potassium concentrations may be normal. Respiratory alkalosis is caused by hyperventilation, with a loss of carbon dioxide and a reduction in $P_{CO_2}$. Compensated respiratory acidosis is associated with an increase in $P_{CO_2}$ and an increase in plasma $HCO_3^-$.

**46–50. The answers are: 46-D, 47-E, 48-A, 49-C, 50-A.** [*Chapter 1 V C 3 a (2) (c), (11); VI A 1 b, 4–6*] Albumin, which is available in concentrations of 5% and 25%, is obtained by fractionating blood from humans. It is used as a volume expander as are whole blood and fresh frozen plasma; however, the latter two should not be used unless there has been a significant blood loss or loss of clotting factors.

Probably the only indication for the transfusion of whole blood is hypovolemia secondary to acute hemorrhage. Fresh whole blood (not more than 24 hours old) would be ideal for this purpose, since platelets and clotting factors would still be active, and many of the adverse biochemical effects of stored blood would be avoided.

Purified factor VIII concentrates do not contain the von Willebrand factor (factor VIII R:WF) and are therefore ineffective for treatment. Cryoprecipitate provides both portions of the factor VIII complex and corrects the bleeding disorder of von Willebrand's disease.

Fresh frozen plasma contains all of the coagulation factors lacking in banked blood, including factors V and VIII. It is used to replace clotting factors during massive transfusion of packed red cells or to correct factor abnormalities found in conditions such as liver disease or disseminated intravascular coagulation (DIC).

In addition to high concentrations of factor VIII, cryoprecipitate contains high concentrations of fibrinogen; thus, it is used appropriately to correct afibrinogenemia.

# Part II
# Gastrointestinal Disorders

# 4
# Common Life-Threatening Disorders
Bruce E. Jarrell

**I. ACUTE ABDOMEN** is the term used for an episode of severe abdominal pain that lasts for several hours or longer and requires medical attention. Prompt diagnosis is important because an acute abdomen is caused by an intra-abdominal emergency in most patients.

**A.** The history obtained from the patient should elicit both general, nonspecific symptoms and items typical of a specific disease process.

  **1. Nonspecific symptoms.** Pain is usually the initial symptom and is often followed by nausea, anorexia, and vomiting.

    **a. Pain**

      **(1)** A **gradual periumbilical pain** indicates visceral peritoneal irritation, such as appendicitis, diverticulitis, or other inflammatory conditions. The pain may become more specifically localized as the disease process progresses.

      **(2)** **Pain that is explosive and severe in onset** indicates a process that immediately soils the parietal peritoneum, such as perforation of a hollow viscus. The pain may be either localized or generalized.

      **(3)** **Progressively more severe pain** suggests a progressively worsening intra-abdominal condition, such as occurs with ischemic necrosis of the bowel or other organs.

      **(4)** **Localized pain that disappears but then recurs as a generalized pain** suggests that the inflamed organ has perforated. Acute appendicitis, for example, causes right lower quadrant pain, which then becomes generalized if perforation occurs.

      **(5)** **Crampy pain** indicates an obstruction in the gastrointestinal tract. This type of pain has a crescendo component, building up to intense pain, followed by a decrescendo component; the patient may then have an interval with no pain.

        **(a)** Distinguishing between crampy pain versus constant or other types of pain is very important when determining whether a bowel obstruction is present.

        **(b)** If crampy pain develops into constant severe pain, it suggests that the involved bowel segment is now ischemic or gangrenous.

    **b. Anorexia, nausea, and vomiting** are common accompanying symptoms in acute inflammatory abdominal processes. Although they are reliably present when a problem is surgical, they also accompany nonsurgical diseases, in which case they often precede the pain (as in gastroenteritis).

    **c. A change in bowel habits** is so common that it is seldom helpful unless a very specific type of change occurs. For example:

      **(1)** Bloody diarrhea suggests colitis, salmonella infestation, or colonic ischemia.

      **(2)** Patients with intestinal obstruction will usually pass no flatus or bowel movement per rectum for 1 to 2 days prior to seeking medical attention.

    **d. Symptoms of sepsis**, such as **chills and fever**, may be nonspecific, although certain patterns are typical of certain diseases. For example:

      **(1)** The fever of uncomplicated appendicitis rarely exceeds 101° F, whereas that of perforation often exceeds 101° F.

      **(2)** Cholangitis with choledocholithiasis is often accompanied by a shaking chill.

  **2. Specific symptoms and facts** should be elicited as clues to specific diseases.

    **a.** A history of **previous surgery** yields important information:

      **(1)** Adhesions may have formed within the peritoneal cavity, leading to intestinal obstruction.

      **(2)** If the surgery was for malignant disease, the malignancy may have recurred, causing pain, sepsis, intestinal obstruction, and other symptoms.

      **(3)** Previous removal of any organ (most likely the appendix, the gallbladder, or the uterus, ovaries, and fallopian tubes) eliminates that organ from consideration.

        **(4)** The previous surgery may point to a specific problem; for example, suppurative cholangitis in a patient with previous choledocholithiasis and retained common duct stone.

    **b.** A previous episode of similar pain warrants questions about the subsequent disease course and about the results of any diagnostic studies that were performed.

    **c.** Questions specifically directed toward other body systems may be very useful.

        **(1) Urinary tract.** Symptoms such as dysuria, hematuria, or changes in urinary habits should be sought.

        **(2) Reproductive tract in the female.** The patient should be asked about a past or present vaginal discharge, dysmenorrhea, a history of pelvic inflammatory disease, time of last menstrual period, and so forth.

        **(3) Cardiovascular system.** Atrial fibrillation of recent onset or digitalis therapy might suggest intestinal ischemia.

        **(4) Diabetes mellitus** is associated with sepsis.

    **d.** In certain diseases, a characteristic maneuver will provide temporary relief of pain.

        **(1)** A patient with acute peritonitis will lie very still; any movement results in excruciating pain.

        **(2)** A patient with a common duct stone or a kidney stone will pace the floor, unable to get into a comfortable position.

        **(3)** The pain of an acute peptic ulcer may be relieved by food or antacids, whereas pain from acute cholecystitis or pancreatitis may be exacerbated by food.

**B.** The **physical examination** of the patient with acute abdominal pain yields new information that one hopes will reinforce the impressions obtained from the history. As with the history, there are both specific and nonspecific findings.

  **1. A complete physical examination** must be performed so that an important related or unrelated extra-abdominal diagnosis will not be missed. Points requiring particular attention include the following:

    **a.** Changes in vital signs, particularly fever, tachypnea, hypotension, or cardiac rhythm irregularities

    **b.** Inspection for jaundice, dehydration, feculent breath, pneumonia, or mental disorientation or obtundation

    **c.** Examination of the extremities for loss of pulses

  **2. The abdominal examination**

    **a.** This should begin with an **overall inspection**. For example:

        **(1)** A distended abdomen with visible peristalsis suggests small bowel obstruction.

        **(2)** Prominent muscle guarding or rigidity will be visible, particularly if it is localized to one area of the abdomen.

        **(3)** A scaphoid abdomen may suggest herniation of the abdominal contents through the diaphragm and into the thoracic cavity.

        **(4)** Hernias are frequently visible, particularly when the patient is standing.

    **b. Palpation of the abdomen** should be done gently and should begin away from the area of maximum tenderness.

        **(1)** The inguinal area should be examined for hernias or inflammatory conditions.

        **(2)** The abdomen should be examined to determine the points of maximum tenderness or the presence of referred tenderness.

        **(3) Rebound tenderness** is tenderness that occurs when the examining hand is quickly removed from the abdominal wall. It is indicative of acute peritoneal irritation.

        **(4) Spasm** is determined by gently depressing the abdominal wall muscles.

            **(a)** Comparing two areas with one another simultaneously will allow the examiner to distinguish an abnormal area from a normal one.

            **(b)** A spasm is **voluntary** if the patient is tensing the muscle in response to pain; **involuntary** if the muscle is taut secondary to the underlying inflammatory process.

        **(5) Palpation for abdominal masses** should be done systematically. A mass in a particular abdominal quadrant suggests a specific diagnosis.

            **(a) Right upper quadrant:** Acute cholecystitis or a complication of this diagnosis, such as subhepatic or intrahepatic abscess

            **(b) Left lower quadrant:** Acute diverticulitis or peridiverticular abscess

            **(c) Right lower quadrant:** Acute appendicitis or appendiceal abscess

            **(d) Left upper quadrant** (uncommon in the acute abdomen): Complication of gastric or colonic malignancy, subphrenic abscess, or some acute inflammatory process related to the spleen, such as infarction

            **(e) Midabdominal area:** Pancreatic malignancy or abscess, complication of a perforated ulcer, or leaking abdominal aortic aneurysm

    **c. Percussion of the abdomen**

          **(1)** This is useful in that it confirms areas of maximum tenderness and the presence of rebound tenderness.

          **(2)** On rare occasions the hollow sound of **tympany** indicates free intraperitoneal air, but it usually is present because of air in the intestine.

          **(3)** A large area of tympany in the right upper quadrant suggests acute gastric dilation, a condition that can lead to hypotension through vagal pathways.

     **d. Auscultation** is useful in many acute abdominal problems.

          **(1) A silent abdomen** indicates the absence of peristalsis, suggesting diffuse peritonitis, which occurs with major abdominal sepsis, intestinal ischemia or gangrene, or prolonged (longer than 3 days) mechanical obstruction with marked distention of the bowel. Absent peristalsis may also indicate an ileus resulting from some other process, such as pneumonia, a renal stone, or trauma.

          **(2) Intermittent peristaltic rushes** that have a crescendo followed by silence suggest an intestinal obstruction. This sign is particularly useful when the peristaltic rush coincides with the onset of episodic abdominal pain.

          **(3)** Certain nonsurgical inflammatory conditions, such as gastroenteritis, produce **high-pitched intermittent peristaltic rushes**. The pain pattern is usually not synchronous with the rushes.

  **3. A rectal examination** should be performed routinely in patients with acute abdominal pain.

     **a.** Rectal palpation may localize the tenderness. In acute appendicitis, if the patient's appendix is located in the pelvis, the only physical finding may be a right pelvic tenderness found on rectal examination.

     **b.** The presence of blood in the stool suggests either a malignancy, hemorrhoids, or an acute inflammatory gastrointestinal process such as an ulcer or colitis.

     **c.** A mass palpable on rectal examination may be a pelvic abscess secondary to a perforated viscus, a sign of pelvic inflammatory disease, or a metastatic malignancy.

     **d.** Acute prostatitis in the male is diagnosed rectally even though it may present with vague abdominal pain.

  **4. A gynecologic examination** should be performed in all females with abdominal pain. (The patient's bladder should be empty.)

     **a.** Cervical or parauterine tenderness suggests pelvic inflammatory disease.

     **b.** A uterine, ovarian, or pelvic mass suggests:

          **(1)** Intrauterine pregnancy

          **(2)** Ectopic pregnancy with rupture and hemorrhage

          **(3)** Pelvic, ovarian, or tubal inflammatory disease, with or without abscess formation

          **(4)** Pelvic or gynecologic malignancy

     **c.** Cervical discharges should be examined microscopically for gonococci.

  **5.** Certain **special signs** are useful in diagnosing acute abdominal pain.

     **a.** Tenderness to percussion over the liver or the kidney suggests acute hepatitis or pyelonephritis.

     **b.** The **iliopsoas sign** is pain in the lower abdomen and psoas region that is elicited when the thigh is flexed against resistance. It suggests that an inflammatory process such as appendicitis or perinephric abscess is in contact with the psoas muscle. Patients may also limp while walking and may lie with the ipsilateral hip flexed to minimize psoas muscle use.

     **c.** The **obturator sign** is pain elicited when the thigh is flexed and then rotated internally and externally. It suggests an inflammatory process in the region of the obturator muscle, such as an obturator hernia.

     **d. Murphy's sign** is elicited by palpating the right upper quadrant during inspiration: as the gallbladder descends during inspiration, acute pain is elicited. It suggests acute cholecystitis.

     **e. Cough tenderness** occurs in the area of maximum tenderness when the patient coughs. The tenderness may also be elicited by shaking the patient or by any other sudden jarring movement.

     **f. Ecchymosis** in the flank, periumbilical region, or back suggests a retroperitoneal hemorrhage. Possible causes include trauma, acute hemorrhagic pancreatitis, a leaking abdominal aortic aneurysm, and intestinal gangrene.

     **g.** Subcutaneous, subfascial, or pelvic **crepitus** suggests a rapidly spreading gas-forming infection. These infections must be rapidly diagnosed and explored surgically if they are to be cured.

**C.** Certain **medical illnesses** can cause an acute abdomen, and these, particularly life-threatening ones, should be sought.

  **1.** These include lower lobe pneumonias, acute myocardial infarction, diabetic ketoacidosis, and acute hepatitis.

**2.** Acute polyserositis (occurring with collagen vascular diseases), rheumatic fever, porphyria, and chronic lead intoxication are uncommon causes of acute abdominal pain that can be exceedingly difficult to diagnose preoperatively. A careful history and physical examination may, however, raise them as possibilities.

**3.** Musculoskeletal problems, particularly vertebral compression of abdominal wall nerves, can also mimic acute general surgical conditions.

**D. Laboratory tests** provide important information in many diseases.

**1. Complete blood count (CBC)**
   **a.** A **red cell count** may reveal anemia or suggest hemoconcentration secondary to dehydration.
   **b.** The **white cell differential count** is usually shifted to the left.
      **(1)** A leukocytosis in the 20,000 to 40,000 range suggests a major septic process in need of rapid surgical intervention.
      **(2)** Profound leukopenia, particularly with a lymphocytic predominance, suggests a viral illness.
   **c.** The white cell count may be misleading. For example, a normal white cell count in an elderly or diabetic patient may in fact accompany a major septic episode because advanced age can bring on an inability to generate a leukocytosis.
   **d.** Other conditions, such as leukemia or lead intoxication, may also be diagnosed from the CBC.

**2. Urine examination** will generally rule out urinary tract infection or kidney stone disease. Pelvic inflammatory processes in contact with the ureter or bladder may produce a few white cells and red cells in the urine. If there is doubt, intravenous pyelography should be performed prior to surgery.

**3. Serum amylase** should be measured in all patients with acute abdominal pain. In general, if the level is high, it usually indicates acute pancreatitis, although other surgical illnesses such as mesenteric thrombosis and perforated ulcer should not be overlooked.

**4. Arterial blood gases** may be very helpful in identifying a profound metabolic acidosis. This suggests either septic shock or severely ischemic or necrotic tissue. It is evidence that argues strongly in favor of surgery if no other obvious cause, such as diabetic ketoacidosis, can be found.

**E.** A **plain roentgenogram of the abdomen** should be obtained in most cases of acute abdominal pain. The following items should be specifically noted:

**1. Bony structure abnormalities.** These frequently overlooked clues may be important in trauma or malignant disease.

**2. Gastrointestinal gas pattern**
   **a.** Air is commonly present in the stomach and colon. However, air in the small intestine is abnormal and suggests an intra-abdominal process.
   **b. Paralytic ileus** (see section II B)
      **(1)** Air that is **evenly distributed** throughout the small and large intestine usually signifies paralysis of the bowel secondary to another process that is not primarily gastrointestinal.
      **(2)** Ileus may be **localized** to a specific area, such as the "sentinel" loop, an area of localized duodenal ileus adjacent to the pancreas in acute pancreatitis.
   **c. Acute gastric dilation** is indicated by a **markedly dilated gastric bubble**. (This condition can result in severe abdominal pain and vasovagal hypotension but is easily treated by nasogastric tube decompression.)
   **d. Mechanical obstruction of the intestine** (see section II A) is revealed by the presence of **distended air- and fluid-filled loops of bowel proximal** to the obstruction and **decompressed intestine distally**. This air may be absent in the distal tract, particularly the rectum, unless air has been introduced by an enema given in the past 24 hours.
      **(1)** Mechanical bowel obstruction is an important diagnosis because it may be associated with strangulation of the bowel, with resultant ischemia and necrosis.
      **(2)** Postoperative adhesions, carcinoma of the colon, and inguinal hernias are the three most common **causes of bowel obstruction**, in that order.
      **(3)** Several specific causes may be diagnosed by the intestinal gas pattern.
         **(a) Hernias** may result in intestinal air located in a nonanatomic location. For example, an inguinal hernia may show gas-filled intestine extended below the inguinal ligament.
         **(b)** A **volvulus** is a segment of bowel that has twisted upon itself, resulting in both

mechanical obstruction and vascular compromise. It may appear on the plain film as an isolated distended loop of bowel with tapered (''bird-beak'') margins. A sigmoid volvulus is treated by sigmoidoscopy and decompression. Other types of volvulus are treated operatively.

**(c)** An **ischemic or gangrenous bowel** may produce few radiologic findings. If the colon is affected, however, the mucosal edema may be seen as ''thumb-printing'' on the wall of a dilated colon.

**(d)** Isolated **distention of the colon by large amounts of air** may be seen on x-ray. It may be due to any of the acute processes:

**(i)** **Distal colonic obstruction** may be secondary to malignancy, profound constipation, stricture, or volvulus.

**(ii)** **''Toxic megacolon,''** a massive colonic dilation, is associated with acute colitis.

**(iii)** **Colonic ileus**, a condition of obscure etiology, results in marked distention of the cecum. If the cecum enlarges past 10 cm or 12 cm in diameter, there is a significant risk of perforation.

**3. Abnormal air collections outside the intestinal lumen**

**a. Free air within the peritoneal cavity** signals a perforation of a hollow viscus and should be interpreted as indicating a surgical emergency.

**(1)** It is present in over 80% of gastroduodenal perforations but in fewer than 25% of colonic perforations.

**(2)** Free peritoneal air is rarely secondary to other causes. However, it may be present in patients undergoing peritoneal dialysis and for up to 1 week following a laparotomy.

**b. Air collections within the wall of the colon**, a condition termed **pneumatosis cystoides intestinalis**, generally indicate an isolated, walled-off intestinal perforation.

**c. Air stippling within soft tissue structures** may indicate the dissection of air into the tissues from a thoracic source such as a pneumothorax. It may, however, be due to a rapidly progressive, catastrophic gas-forming infection (see Chapter 1, section VII), which is a true surgical emergency.

**d.** A subphrenic or subhepatic abscess may be associated with an air-fluid level in a location outside the intestinal tract.

**e. Air within the biliary tree** indicates an abnormal communication between the biliary tree and the intestinal tract.

**(1)** The usual causes are either

**(a)** A surgical connection created to provide biliary drainage (e.g., choledochoduodenostomy)

**(b)** A gas-forming infection within the biliary tree (**cholangitis**). Cholangitis is associated with biliary obstruction and should be treated with antibiotics followed by surgery to drain the biliary tract.

**(2)** Large gallstones, particularly in the elderly, can erode into the adjacent intestine (usually the duodenum), allowing air to enter the biliary tract and the gallstone to enter the bowel. Usually this produces transient symptoms initially, until several days later when the gallstone impacts upon and obstructs the distal ileum, producing small bowel obstruction.

**f. Air within the portal vein** is seen when a gas-forming infection affects the portal system (**pylephlebitis**). The infection usually derives from necrotic tissue, particularly from the small intestine, appendix, or left colon.

**4. Abnormal calcifications**

**a. Renal stones** are calcified in up to 85% of cases and appear along the path of the ureter.

**b.** A **fecalith** (calcified material within the appendix) is strong evidence for acute appendicitis in a patient with abdominal pain.

**c. Pancreatic calcification** suggests chronic pancreatitis.

**d. Gallstones** are calcified in 15% of cases.

**e. Heavily calcified vessels** may be present in mesenteric ischemia.

**f.** Masses such as teratomas or malignant neoplasms may calcify.

**5. Soft tissue shadows**

**a. Peritoneal fat lines** and **psoas muscle shadows** may be lost in rapidly spreading infections, hematomas, or abscesses.

**b. The margins of solid organs** (liver, kidney, spleen) may be displaced from their normal locations by an abnormal mass.

**c. A distended bladder** may be visible and may be responsible for marked abdominal pain.

**F. Contrast roentgenography** can be highly useful in patients with an acute abdominal process that remains undiagnosed after other studies.

**1.** An **intravenous pyelogram (IVP)** should be obtained if a renal stone is suspected. It is also useful in identifying acute pyelonephritis, perinephric abscess, or renal infarction. When a patient suspected of having appendicitis has microscopic hematuria, the IVP is particularly useful to verify that the hematuria is due to the periappendiceal inflammation rather than to a renal stone.

2. A **"barium swallow"** is helpful if it is suspected that the patient's esophagus has ruptured during a violent episode of vomiting. Known as **Boerhaave's syndrome**, this unusual accident may result in a left pleural effusion which communicates with the esophageal rent, as demonstrated by the barium swallow.

3. An **"upper GI series"** using diatrizoate meglumine (Gastrografin), a water-soluble radiopaque dye, should be performed if a perforation of the stomach or duodenum is suspected but cannot be proven because free air is not visible on the plain film.

4. Placing contrast materials into the colon and rectum should be done very cautiously when an inflammatory condition or a perforation is suspected, because even a small increase in pressure could easily convert friable tissue into a frank perforation.
   a. This procedure is best used when the diagnosis of colon perforation is suspected and especially in a patient taking anti-inflammatory or immunosuppressive drugs, particularly corticosteroids.
   b. In such cases, Gastrografin should be used because barium sulfate, when it mixes with stool and detritus from an infection, becomes firmly attached to the peritoneal cavity. Extensive abscess formation results, even after the surgeon attempts to irrigate the area thoroughly.

5. A **"small-bowel follow-through"** contrast study tracks the barium through the small intestine after an upper GI series. It is useful in identifying a point of small bowel obstruction when either the history, the physical examination, or plain roentgenography fails to verify the diagnosis of small bowel obstruction.

G. **Abdominal ultrasonography** is usually of little diagnostic value in the patient with abdominal distention and severe pain, but it can be helpful when acute cholecystitis, cholelithiasis, biliary obstruction, or an abscess is suspected. **Computed axial tomography** may also be helpful but is generally reserved for the patient who remains undiagnosed after other studies have been exhausted.

H. Certain **general principles** should be employed in the approach to the patient with acute abdominal pain.

1. Most important is **routinely to follow a careful and systematic evaluation** of the patient. The overwhelming majority of patients will have a well-documented diagnosis if this principle is fulfilled.

2. The second most important principle is to remember that, **statistically** speaking, **certain diagnoses are very common**, such as appendicitis and gastroenteritis, while **other diagnoses are quite rare**, such as pylephlebitis. The physician should not be misled into searching for an occult diagnosis when a common diagnosis is far more likely to be the correct one.

3. In cases **where the diagnosis is not initially clear**, continuing observations and repeated blood studies (complete blood count, arterial blood gases, amylase, and electrolytes) may lead the physician to the correct diagnosis as the disease process evolves.
   a. However, although this practice might be desirable in a patient with gastroenteritis, the **delay can be catastrophic** in diseases such as acute appendicitis, ischemic bowel, small bowel obstruction, volvulus, or incarcerated hernia.
   b. Thus it is a surgical principle that if the diagnosis is not certain but the patient may have a potentially lethal condition that could be cured by an early operation, then an early operation should be performed.
   c. This means that a small percentage of negative laparotomies can be justified in patients with acute abdomen.
   d. This premise is best illustrated by the case of a patient with acute appendicitis. Here, a policy of watchful waiting may convert a simple appendicitis into a perforated appendicitis with generalized peritonitis and septic shock. The risk of death from this complication is many times higher than the risk from a small right lower quadrant incision in a patient who proves to have a normal appendix and mesenteric adenitis.

4. Analgesics, particularly **narcotics, should be withheld** from the patient until the diagnosis is established or until the decision to proceed to surgery has been made. Serial physical examinations will be totally useless if the patient has been given narcotics.

5. **Antibiotics should also be withheld** until a diagnosis has been made and the antibiotic

therapy is known to be needed. The only exception to this is the patient who presents in septic shock from an unknown cause. In that situation, broad-spectrum antibiotics should be part of the patient's resuscitation.

6. Both **fluid deficits and electrolyte imbalances should be corrected** before surgery. The few **exceptions** are:
   a. Conditions that threaten immediate exsanguination, such as a ruptured abdominal aortic aneurysm
   b. Conditions in which the fluid or electrolyte abnormality cannot be corrected in a reasonable amount of time. In particular this is limited to conditions causing profound acidosis, such as necrotic bowel, where the acidosis cannot be corrected until the bowel is surgically removed.

7. A **nasogastric tube** should be put in place before the induction of anesthesia in order to empty the stomach and thus minimize the risk of pulmonary aspiration.

## II. INTESTINAL OBSTRUCTION. 
The normal flow of intestinal contents can be blocked by a mechanical obstruction or by a functional obstruction that occurs because of impaired intestinal motility. An acute abdomen often ensues.

A. **Mechanical obstructions** are common and have various benign and malignant causes. If not treated expeditiously (usually by surgical removal of the cause), mechanical obstructions can rapidly become lethal.

1. **Acute obstruction** occurs over hours to days and has a rapidly evolving course, whereas **chronic obstruction** may have a slow course with malnutrition, constipation, and other signs of chronic illness.

2. **Types of mechanical obstruction**
   a. **Simple obstruction:** There are no complicating factors such as ischemia or perforation.
   b. **Strangulating obstruction:** The blood supply to the involved segment of bowel is significantly impaired. The ischemia may result from a twisting of the intestinal blood supply upon itself (**volvulus**) or from a constriction of the blood flow by a tight band or hernial opening.
   c. **Closed loop obstruction:** The colon is obstructed but the ileocecal valve remains intact, permitting intestinal contents to enter the obstructed region and greatly distend the cecum. This may result in cecal perforation if not treated expeditiously.
   d. **Intussusception:** The bowel invaginates itself, causing a narrowing of the lumen and subsequent obstruction. It may result from either viral infections or intraluminal polypoid tumors.
   e. **Perforating obstruction**: The bowel proximal to the obstruction overdistends and perforates. The most common area of perforation when the colon is obstructed is the cecum.

3. **Causes and their management**
   a. **Intestinal adhesions** are the most common cause of obstruction.
      (1) They may result from a previous surgical exploration, particularly when talc was used to lubricate the surgeon's gloves, or their etiology may be obscure.
      (2) They may be diffuse, involving all peritoneal structures, or solitary, blocking only one area of the intestine.
      (3) The **management** is surgical lysis of the obstructing bands.
   b. **Hernias** (see Chapter 1, section X, and Chapter 33, section II) are a second very common cause of intestinal obstruction.
      (1) A segment of intestine migrates through a defect in the abdominal wall (**external hernia**) or through a mesenteric or omental defect (**internal hernia**) and becomes blocked by the narrow ring that is usually present at the peritoneal communication of the hernia.
      (2) The **management** is reduction of the hernia contents and repair of the hernia. The bowel must always be examined for necrosis.
   c. **Intestinal tumors** are the third most common cause of obstruction.
      (1) The most common obstructing tumor is an adenocarcinoma of the colon or rectum. Benign lesions of the small bowel and colon, such as lipomas, can become the leading point of an intussusception. Other malignant tumors such as carcinoid or lymphoma can obstruct the intestinal lumen.
      (2) The **treatment** of these lesions is surgical removal.
   d. **Other intrinsic lesions** within the bowel wall or the lumen can cause acute obstruction; their treatment depends upon the lesion.
      (1) **Congenital lesions:** Webs, malrotations, atresias

       **(2) Inflammatory lesions:** Crohn's disease, diverticulitis, ulcerative colitis, infections such as tuberculosis

       **(3) Luminal foreign bodies:** bezoars, parasites, gallstones

       **(4) Radiation injury**, other **trauma**, or **endometriosis**

     **e. Other extrinsic lesions** can compress the intestinal lumen, such as large intra-abdominal tumors or abscesses.

**B. Functional obstructions** are blockages in the intestinal flow that result from impaired motility **(paralytic** or **adynamic ileus)**. These are usually **treated** by observation and by fluid and nutritional support until the causal agent resolves. Possible **causes** include:

    **1. Direct irritation of the intestine**, such as generalized peritonitis. Irritation may also be a factor in the postoperative adynamic ileus that can last for 3 to 7 days following surgery.

    **2. Extraperitoneal causes**, such as a retroperitoneal hematoma or nerve root compression. Retroperitoneal dissections, such as a nephrectomy or sympathectomy, can cause a prolonged ileus.

## III. UPPER GASTROINTESTINAL HEMORRHAGE

**A.** The **causes** of massive upper gastrointestinal hemorrhage as shown by endoscopy are given in Table 4-1.

**Table 4-1.** Causes of Upper Gastrointestinal Hemorrhage

| Cause | Incidence |
| --- | --- |
| Duodenal ulcer | 40% |
| Gastric ulcer | 10% to 20% |
| Diffuse erosive gastritis | 15% to 20% |
| Esophageal varices | 10% |
| Mallory-Weiss tear of the gastro-esophageal junction | 10% |
| Gastric carcinoma | Lower than 5% |

**B.** The diagnosis of hemorrhage is generally obvious, but **locating the site of bleeding** may be difficult. The **type of gastrointestinal bleeding** may give a clue to its source.

    **1. Hematemesis** is the vomiting of blood, either bright red or resembling coffee grounds in appearance. Hematemesis usually indicates a bleeding source proximal to the ligament of Treitz. **Coffee-grounds hematemesis** indicates that the blood has been in contact with gastric acid long enough to become converted from hemoglobin to methemoglobin.

    **2. Hematochezia** is the passage of bright red blood by rectum. Although it indicates gastrointestinal bleeding, it does not specify the level within the gastrointestinal tract.

    **3. Melena** is the passage of black, usually tarry, stools. Although the melena signifies a longer time within the gastrointestinal tract than bright red blood, it does not guarantee that the bleeding is from the upper tract.

    **4. Cranberry-colored stool**, or **"currant-jelly" stool**, is typically a jelly-like stool that may originate from a Meckel's diverticulum, particularly in children.

**C.** The **history** should include information about previous episodes of gastrointestinal bleeding, current medications (e.g., aspirin or Coumadin use), and related diseases (e.g., hematologic disorders, alcoholism, peptic ulcer disease, and recent episodes of vomiting).

**D.** The **physical examination** should specifically include a search for evidence of nasopharyngeal bleeding, portal hypertension, weight loss, malignancy, or systemic diseases such as chronic hepatic or renal failure.

**E.** The cause and the location of the bleeding must be confirmed unless imminent exsanguination calls for immediate measures (see Chapter 2, section I C 4). In less urgent circumstances, once the patient has been stabilized, one may continue with **diagnostic procedures**.

    **1. Fiberoptic endoscopy** of the upper gastrointestinal tract has become the optimal diagnostic procedure because it allows direct visualization of the lesion in over 80% of cases.
      **a.** Endoscopy allows:
       **(1)** Determination of the size and number of lesions in most cases (lesions are multiple in 15% of cases)

**(2)** Assessment of which site is actively bleeding
**(3)** Assessment of the rate of bleeding. If, for example, an arterial vessel is visibly bleeding in the base of a large duodenal ulcer, then there is a good chance that it will not stop bleeding.
**(4)** Distinction between an ulcer, varices, gastritis, and a tear in the esophagus (Mallory-Weiss syndrome) that follows forceful vomiting
**(5)** Determination of whether a lesion is benign or malignant
  **b.** Endoscopy is only safe if the patient's vital signs are relatively stable. Sedation is dangerous because it increases the risk of vomiting followed by aspiration of the gastric contents into the pulmonary bed.

**2.** An **upper GI series** helps to define anatomy or pathology more completely, but unfortunately it sheds little light on the relationship of a particular lesion to the hemorrhage.

**3. Passage of a nasogastric tube** aids considerably in determining that the source of bleeding is proximal to the ligament of Treitz.

**4. Angiography** and **radionuclide scanning** may occasionally help to locate the site of bleeding, but both procedures are more useful in lower gastrointestinal hemorrhage.

**F.** If **treated** expeditiously in a systematic fashion, the patient with upper gastrointestinal hemorrhage has an excellent chance for recovery. Treatment is aimed at supporting the patient's vital signs as well as stopping the hemorrhage.

**1. Resuscitation measures** should begin immediately when the patient is first seen.

**2. Medical treatment** of aggravating factors can then begin.
  **a.** A nasogastric tube is inserted, and the residual thrombus in the stomach is removed with an iced saline solution.
  **b.** Any clotting abnormalities are corrected with appropriate factors (see also Chapter 1, section V C 3).
    **(1)** Fresh frozen plasma if the prothrombin time is abnormal
    **(2)** Platelets if thrombocytopenia is present
    **(3)** Vitamin K if bleeding is from esophageal varices
  **c.** An aggressive antacid regimen is begun.
    **(1)** Hourly antacid therapy with gastric pH monitoring is probably the most effective method of stopping hemorrhage.
    **(2)** Histamine$_2$ (H$_2$) receptor antagonists such as cimetidine are less effective than antacids in stopping a hemorrhage. They are useful, however, for preventing the development of secondary erosive gastritis.
  **d.** Vasopressin, a powerful vasoconstrictor, may be useful.
    **(1)** It can be infused through a peripheral vein at a rate of up to 1 unit per minute.
    **(2)** Alternatively, it can be infused directly into the bleeding vessel by means of angiography.
    **(3)** Vasopressin temporarily controls bleeding in 75% of patients; by contrast, bleeding was stopped in 30% of patients treated conventionally without vasopressin.
    **(4)** Vasopressin is contraindicated in patients with significant coronary artery disease. It reduces cardiac output, an effect that can be partially corrected by isoproterenol (given with caution in patients with portal hypertension).

**3.** Other procedures are often helpful.
  **a. Fiberoptic endoscopy**, in addition to being a diagnostic procedure, may also be useful when esophageal varices are to be sclerosed (see Chapter 9, sections I E 6 and 7) or small bleeding sites are to be coagulated.
  **b. Angiography** similarly may be a therapeutic aid. It allows bleeding from small vessels to be controlled either by embolization of the bleeding vessel or by intra-arterial administration of vasopressin.
  **c. Balloon tamponade** (see Chapter 9, section I E 7 c) can be important in controlling bleeding from varices.

**4. Surgery for upper gastrointestinal hemorrhage**
  **a.** The patient's cardiovascular status, as well as the amount and duration of bleeding, is particularly important. For example, a patient with heart disease may tolerate continued bleeding only poorly, and thus may need early surgery.
  **b.** Only about 10% of patients will require surgery.
  **c.** The **general indications** for surgery are as follows:
    **(1) Exsanguinating hemorrhage.** A patient with uncontrollable hemorrhage who is losing blood faster than it can be replaced should go straight to the operating room for direct control of the site of bleeding.

        **(2) Profuse bleeding**, especially in association with **hypotension**. Patients should be treated with surgery

          **(a)** If more than 4 units of blood are required for initial resuscitation

          **(b)** If bleeding continues at a rate greater than 1 unit per 8 hours

          **(c)** If a brief hypotensive episode could have catastrophic results, as in patients with coronary artery disease or cerebrovascular disease, or in those more than 60 years old

        **(3) Continued hemorrhage** despite resuscitation and other treatment

          **(a)** The mortality rate of upper gastrointestinal bleeding is low among patients who need less than 6 to 7 units of blood.

          **(b)** The rate rises dramatically with requirements above 7 units. Thus, surgery should be undertaken before the blood loss reaches that point.

        **(4) Recurrent bleeding** after its initial cessation. About one-fourth of patients rebleed, and the mortality rate for these patients is as high as 30%, in contrast to a mortality rate of about 3% among patients who do not rebleed.

     **d.** Certain **pathologic features** of the bleeding site **increase the risk** of recurrent bleeding and so perhaps should be considered as indications for early surgery. Examples include:

        **(1)** A posterior duodenal ulcer with the gastroduodenal artery visible in its base

        **(2)** A giant gastric ulcer

        **(3)** Esophageal varices

     **e.** Erosive gastritis is more likely to respond to medical management.

   **5. Special situations** may call for a modification of the usual routines of management.

     **a.** A patient with a rare or hard-to-find blood type should be operated upon while blood is still available.

     **b.** A patient who refuses blood transfusion for any reason should be explored earlier.

     **c.** A patient with a coagulopathy should have the disorder corrected, if possible, prior to surgical exploration.

   **6.** The **type of surgery** performed is discussed in Chapter 5.

  **G.** The **prognosis** for patients who are bleeding from a source other than esophageal varices is as follows:

   **1.** Some 25% to 50% will have a recurrence of bleeding during the next 5 years, and about 20% will require surgery.

   **2.** The mortality rate is low (about 3%) if the bleeding stops spontaneously, whereas it is as high as 33% in patients who soon rebleed.

## IV. LOWER GASTROINTESTINAL HEMORRHAGE

  **A.** Acute lower gastrointestinal hemorrhage is managed initially in much the same way as upper gastrointestinal hemorrhage.

   **1.** The patient is **resuscitated** with blood and intravenous fluids.

   **2.** The **history** is taken and a **physical examination** is performed.

   **3.** Studies are begun to **identify the site and cause** of the bleeding.

   **4.** Vasopressin may be used as in upper gastrointestinal bleeding (see section III F 2 d).

  **B.** **Initial studies** include the following steps:

   **1.** An **anorectal examination** is performed to determine if the source of bleeding is a hemorrhoid, anal fissure, anal carcinoma, or other anorectal lesion.

   **2.** Studies are done to **rule out a bleeding site in the upper gastrointestinal tract.**

     **a.** A **nasogastric tube** is passed to ascertain that no bleeding site is present in the gastroduodenal region.

        **(1)** On occasion, however, duodenal bleeding will not reflux into the stomach because of a closed pyloric sphincter.

        **(2) Endoscopy** (see section III E 1) is therefore required to rule out upper gastrointestinal bleeding with absolute certainty.

     **b.** Most physicians will withhold endoscopy when a highly probable source of the bleeding is found in the lower gastrointestinal tract. However, if surgery is anticipated, particularly when one is not sure of the diagnosis, endoscopy of the upper gastrointestinal tract should be performed to exclude any bleeding site there.

**3.** Once the upper tract has been eliminated as a source of bleeding, the **lower tract** should be investigated, including the distal small bowel, colon, and anorectal area.

    **a. Sigmoidoscopy** should be performed.

        **(1)** The presence of a mass lesion, such as rectal carcinoma, is visualized in about 3% of patients with massive lower gastrointestinal bleeding.

        **(2)** Discrete bleeding sites from ulcers or hemorrhoids may be seen.

        **(3)** A diffusely hemorrhagic mucosa suggests colitis, a platelet deficiency, or a hematologic disorder.

        **(4)** Even if no lesion is visualized, it is important to make certain that the lower 15 cm of the rectum is normal, because this region is inaccessible intraperitoneally if laparotomy is necessary. Additionally, if it is normal it gives presumptive evidence that the bleeding is coming from a more proximal site.

    **b. Anoscopy** is frequently overlooked, but should be routinely performed because bleeding lesions in the anal canal may be missed on sigmoidoscopy.

**C.** The choice of **subsequent diagnostic tests** will depend upon whether the bleeding stops or continues.

    **1.** About 75% of the patients will spontaneously stop bleeding without further intervention. **If bleeding stops**, the following steps are taken.

        **a.** A "barium enema," a **colonoscopy**, or both procedures should be performed

        **(1)** To identify or rule out diverticulosis or colon carcinoma

        **(2)** To provide indirect evidence for colonic mucosal ischemia

        **b.** The patient should be monitored thereafter.

    **2. If the bleeding continues**, further diagnostic studies should be done in an attempt to identify the source more precisely in preparation for surgery if it becomes necessary.

        **a.** If bleeding continues slowly, a barium enema may be useful to determine the presence, number, and location of diverticuli. However, if bleeding is more rapid, the residual barium in the colon may make subsequent angiography difficult or impossible.

        **b.** If bleeding is profuse, angiography and radionuclide scanning are useful.

        **(1)** The **selective mesenteric angiogram** will identify the bleeding site (or sites) in up to 80% of patients when the rate of bleeding exceeds 0.5 ml per minute. Angiography is also highly useful for identifying angiodysplastic lesions of the colon.

        **(2)** The **radionuclide scan**, which uses red blood cells labeled with technetium-99m ($^{99m}$Tc), is sensitive enough to detect a bleeding site when the rate is as low as 0.05 ml per minute.

        **c. Colonoscopy** is unsatisfactory and may be dangerous when lower gastrointestinal bleeding is rapid: Visualization is poor and there is a risk of colon perforation.

**D.** Persistent bleeding is the principal **indication for surgery**.

    **1.** The patient's cardiovascular status and amount and duration of bleeding are taken into consideration, as for upper gastrointestinal hemorrhage (see section III F 4).

    **2.** The surgical procedure is aimed at removing the underlying cause of the bleeding.

    **3.** On occasion, the precise point of bleeding cannot be established.

        **a.** In these instances, the stomach, duodenum, and small intestine should be carefully examined. Meckel's diverticulum, Crohn's disease, and other inflammatory or malignant lesions should not be overlooked.

        **b.** A "blind" total colectomy may be necessary if no other source of the bleeding is found.

**E.** The **mortality rate** for lower gastrointestinal bleeding is currently about 10%.

# 5

# The Stomach and Duodenum

R. Anthony Carabasi, III
Martha Shenot Matthews

## I. ANATOMY

**A.** The **stomach** is a muscular organ that functions in food storage and digestion.

    **1.** The stomach has four **parts** (Fig. 5-1).
        **a.** The **cardia** is the area near the gastroesophageal junction.
        **b.** The **fundus** is the extension of the stomach above the gastroesophageal junction.
        **c.** The **body** is the area between the fundus and the antrum.
        **d.** The **antrum** is the distal quarter of the stomach. It begins at the incisura angularis and ends at the pylorus.

    **2.** The stomach is bounded by two **sphincteric mechanisms**.
        **a.** The **gastroesophageal sphincter** is a high-pressure zone of muscular activity in the distal esophagus. It relaxes with swallowing to allow food to enter the stomach. When contracted, it prevents the reflux of food from the stomach into the esophagus.
        **b.** The **pylorus** is a well-defined muscular sphincter that controls the movement of food out of the stomach. It also prevents the reflux of duodenal contents into the stomach.

    **3.** The **nervous supply** of the stomach is via parasympathetic and sympathetic fibers.
        **a.** The **parasympathetic supply** is through the **vagus nerves**. The anterior or left vagus supplies the anterior portion of the stomach. The posterior or right vagus supplies the posterior stomach. The vagi contribute to gastric acid secretion both by direct action on parietal cell secretion and by stimulating the antrum to release gastrin. They also contribute to gastric motility.
        **b.** The **sympathetic innervation** is via the **greater splanchnic nerves**. These terminate in the **celiac ganglion**, and postganglionic fibers travel with the gastric arteries to the stomach. The sympathetic afferent fibers are the pathway for perception of visceral pain.

    **4.** The **arterial supply** to the stomach is via the right and left gastric arteries, the right and left gastroepiploic arteries, and the vasa brevia.
        **a.** The **right gastric artery** is a branch of the common hepatic artery and supplies the lesser curvature.
        **b.** The **left gastric artery** is a branch of the celiac axis and supplies the lesser curvature.
        **c.** The **right gastroepiploic artery** is a branch of the gastroduodenal artery and supplies the greater curvature.
        **d.** The **left gastroepiploic artery** is a branch of the splenic artery and supplies the greater curvature.
        **e.** The **vasa brevia** arise from either the splenic artery or the left gastroepiploic artery and supply the fundus.

    **5.** **Venous drainage** of the stomach is both portal and systemic.
        **a.** The right and left **gastric and gastroepiploic veins** accompany their corresponding arteries. They drain into the portal system.
        **b.** The **left gastric vein** also has multiple **anastomoses** with the **lower esophageal venous plexus**. These drain systemically into the azygous vein.

    **6.** **Lymphatic drainage** of the stomach is extensive. Lymph nodes draining the stomach are found at the cardia, along the greater and lesser curvatures, and near the pylorus.

**B.** **Microscopically**, the stomach has four layers and three distinct mucosal areas.

    **1.** The four **layers of the stomach wall** are **serosa, muscularis, muscularis mucosae**, and **mucosa**. There are three **layers of muscle fibers: longitudinal, oblique**, and **circular**.

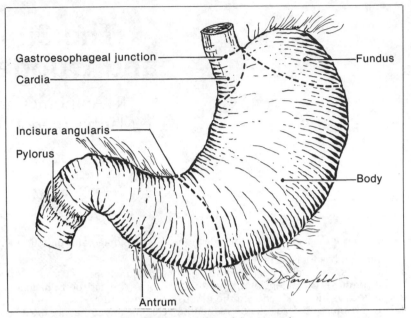

**Figure 5-1.** Anatomy of the stomach.

2. There are three **divisions of the mucosa** that correspond to the gross divisions of cardia, body, and antrum.
    a. The **cardiac gland area** is a ½- to 4-cm zone beginning at the cardia. These shallow glands secrete mucus.
    b. The **parietal cell area** comprises the proximal three-quarters of the stomach. Four **types of cells** are found **in its glands:**
        (1) **Mucous cells** secrete an alkaline mucous coating for the epithelium. This 1-mm–thick coating primarily facilitates food passage. It also provides some mucosal protection.
        (2) **Zygomatic** or **chief cells** secrete pepsinogen. They are found deep in the fundic glands. **Pepsinogen** is the precursor to **pepsin**, which is active in protein digestion. Chief cells are stimulated by cholinergic impulses, by gastrin, and by secretin.
        (3) **Oxyntic** or **parietal cells** produce **hydrochloric acid** and **intrinsic factor**. They are found exclusively in the fundus and body of the stomach.
        (4) **Argentaffin cells** are scattered throughout the stomach. Their function is unclear.
    c. The **pyloroantral mucosa** is found in the antrum of the stomach.
        (1) Parietal and chief cells are absent here.
        (2) **G cells**, which secrete gastrin, are found in this area. They are part of the **APUD (amine precursor uptake and decarboxylase) system** of endocrine cells. **Gastrin** is a hormone that causes the secretion of hydrochloric acid and pepsinogen in the stomach. It also influences gastric motility.

C. The **duodenum** is the first portion of the small intestine.

    1. The duodenum is divided into four **portions** (Fig. 5-2).
        a. The **first portion** of the duodenum, the **duodenal cap**, is the horizontal portion distal to the pylorus. It is approximately 5 cm in length and is partially retroperitoneal at its distal margin.
        b. The **second** or **descending portion** of the duodenum is approximately 7 cm in length. The **common bile duct** and **pancreatic duct** empty into the duodenum here.
        c. The **third** or **transverse portion** of the duodenum is 12 cm long. It runs horizontally to the left and ends to the left of the third lumbar vertebra.
        d. The **fourth portion** of the duodenum runs superiorly and to the left for 2½ cm. At its terminal portion, the **duodenojejunal flexure**, it changes direction sharply and becomes the **jejunum**. This area of the duodenum is fixed in position by the **ligament of Treitz**.

    2. The **arterial supply** of the duodenum is via the **superior pancreaticoduodenal artery**, a branch of the hepatic artery, and the **inferior pancreaticoduodenal artery**, a branch of the superior mesenteric artery.

    3. **Venous drainage** is via anterior and posterior **pancreaticoduodenal venous arcades**. These drain into the portal and superior mesenteric veins.

**D.** The **microscopic anatomy** of the duodenum is similar to that of the rest of the small intestine.

  **1.** The **anterior wall** of the duodenum has four **coats**—the **serosa**, the **muscular layer**, the **muscularis mucosae**, and the **mucosa**. The **posterior wall** is retroperitoneal and lacks serosa. The **muscular layer** consists of inner **longitudinal** and outer **circular muscle fibers**.

  **2.** **Specialized glands** of the duodenum, **Brunner's glands**, are found in the proximal duodenum and secrete an alkaline mucus. This mucus is thought to protect the mucosa.

**II. GASTRIC ACID SECRETION** is mediated by a complex interplay of neuronal and hormonal influences. The **secretory response during eating** is divided into three **phases**.

  **A.** The **cephalic phase** is mediated by vagal stimulation. It is provoked by the sight, smell, and thought of food.

  **1.** Vagal stimulation has a direct effect on parietal cells, causing acid secretion.

  **2.** Vagal stimulation also causes release of gastrin from the antrum. **Gastrin** is the most potent stimulator of gastric acid secretion.

  **B.** The **gastric phase** of secretion is provoked by mechanical distention of the antrum by food. This stimulates additional gastrin release.

  **C.** The **intestinal phase** of secretion is not well understood. Intestinal factors such as cholecystokinin are mild stimulators of acid production.

  **D.** **Feedback mechanisms** that inhibit gastric acid secretion include a decline in vagal stimulation. At an antral pH of 2, gastrin release is inhibited. Finally, as acid chyme enters the duodenum, it triggers the release of secretin. This further inhibits gastrin secretion.

**III. ULCER DISEASE.** The most common manifestations of ulcer disease are gastric ulcers and, even more common, duodenal ulcers.

  **A. Gastric ulcers**

  **1.** Gastric ulcers are nearly always **located** in the antrum near the junction of antral and body mucosa. They are frequently found near the incisura angularis. **Pyloric channel ulcers** and gastric ulcers found near the pylorus behave like duodenal ulcers and will be discussed with them (see section III B).

  **2.** Gastric ulcers are more common in men, in the elderly, and in the lower socioeconomic classes. The ratio of gastric to duodenal ulcers is 1 to 4.

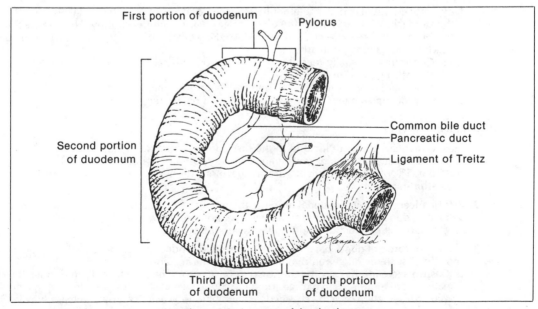

**Figure 5-2.** Anatomy of the duodenum.

3. The **etiology** of gastric ulcer is multifactorial and not completely delineated. Damage to the gastric mucosal barrier appears to be the key.
   a. **Reflux of bile** into the stomach is thought to change the mucosal barrier, allowing gastric acid to enter the mucosa and injure it. This appears to be a major factor in gastric ulcer formation.
   b. **Drugs** can alter the mucosal barrier to hydrogen ion.
      (1) Ethanol, indomethacin, and salicylates are examples, though none has been proven to cause gastric ulcers.
      (2) The combination of smoking and salicylate ingestion is strongly implicated in the development of gastric ulcers.
   c. Persons with gastric ulcer tend to have lower than normal rates of acid secretion. Their serum gastrin levels are approximately twice the normal levels.

4. **Diagnosis**
   a. Gastric ulcer usually presents with a **history** of burning epigastric pain that is relieved by food but recurs ½ to 1½ hours later.
   b. The **"upper gastrointestinal (upper GI) series"** is the usual initial diagnostic test. It can detect about 70% of gastric ulcers.
   c. This is followed by endoscopy if the radiologic examination is positive.
      (1) **To rule out malignancy, multiple biopsies** must be done.
      (2) **Gastric washings** and **cytology** are useful adjuncts in ruling out malignancy.

5. **Gastric ulcers and cancer**
   a. Evidence suggests that gastric ulcer does not degenerate into carcinoma.
   b. However, gastric cancer will ulcerate in 25% of cases, and it is therefore mandatory to prove histologically that suspicious or nonhealing gastric ulcers are not carcinoma.

6. **Initial medical therapy** of gastric ulcer is indicated. Most gastric ulcers will heal within 12 to 15 weeks.
   a. Antacid therapy has not been demonstrated to be superior to placebo.
   b. **Histamine₂ (H₂)-receptor antagonists** such as cimetidine may be effective in speeding the healing of ulcers, particularly in those patients who have a high or normal rate of acid secretion.
   c. **Cytoprotective agents** such as sucralfate have been shown to be effective. **Sucralfate**, when exposed to acid, forms a viscous substance that binds to damaged mucosa. It also can neutralize small amounts of acid.
   d. **Avoidance of** ethanol, tobacco, and **drugs that irritate** the gastric mucosa is important.

7. Gastric ulcer is associated with a high **recurrence rate** of 25% to 60% in 5 years. Most of the recurrences are within 6 months of the first event.

8. **Surgery** is recommended if malignancy cannot be ruled out, if an ulcer fails to heal after 12 to 15 weeks of medical therapy, or if a complication such as perforation or severe hemorrhage occurs.
   a. The procedures of choice are either **hemigastrectomy** (excision of the distal 50% to 60% of the stomach) with **excision of the ulcer**, or **antrectomy and vagotomy**. Hemigastrectomy has historically been the favored procedure. However, the technique of antrectomy and vagotomy is gaining popularity.
      (1) **Continuity** is usually reestablished by gastroduodenal anastomosis. This is known as **Billroth I gastrectomy** (Fig. 5-3 *A*).
      (2) Mortality is approximately 1%, and the recurrence rate is less than 1%.
   b. Other procedures may also be used, but have a higher recurrence rate.

B. **Duodenal ulcers**

1. Most duodenal ulcers are **located** in the first portion of the duodenum.
   a. They are equally frequent on the anterior and posterior walls.
   b. About 5% of duodenal ulcers are in the more distal duodenum; these are known as **postbulbar ulcers.**

2. **Pyloric ulcers** occur in duodenal mucosa, though they are anatomically in the stomach. They behave as duodenal ulcers although they respond poorly to medical therapy. They can lead to gastric outlet obstruction and frequently require surgery.

3. The major **cause** of duodenal ulcer is increased acid production. Duodenal ulcer patients are capable of secreting larger amounts of acid than normal controls.
   a. **Gastrin secretion** has also been shown to be a factor. The parietal cells in duodenal ulcer patients are more sensitive to gastrin and require significantly less gastrin to stimulate the maximal secretion of acid. The feedback inhibition, by acid, of gastrin release may be impaired in some patients.

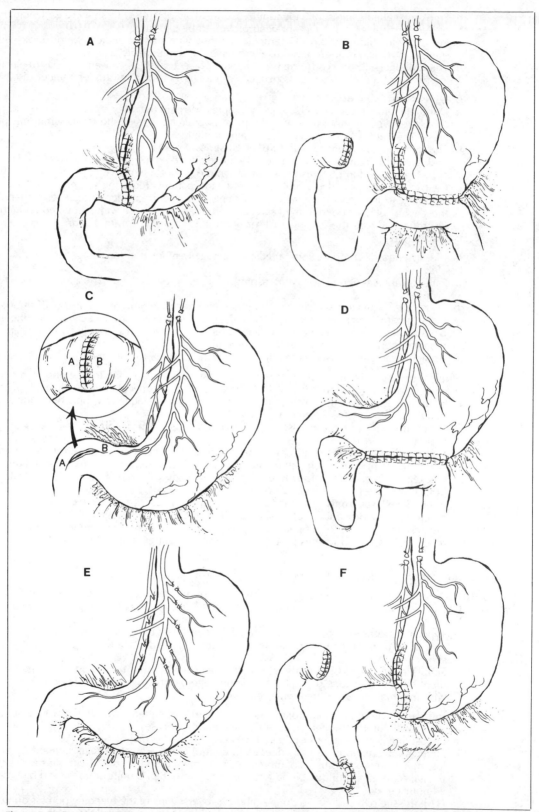

**Figure 5-3.** Common gastric surgical procedures: (*A*) vagotomy and antrectomy (Billroth I), (*B*) vagotomy and antrectomy (Billroth II), (*C*) vagotomy and pyloroplasty, (*D*) vagotomy and gastrojejunostomy, (*E*) parietal cell vagotomy, and (*F*) Roux-en-Y gastrojejunostomy.

      **b.** Smoking, caffeine ingestion, and aspirin use are all associated with an increased incidence of duodenal ulcer, but have not been proven to be causative.

      **c.** Persons with blood group O, particularly those who do not secrete blood group substances in their saliva, are more likely to have duodenal ulcer.

      **d.** The **Zollinger-Ellison syndrome** (see Chapter 22, section II C), caused by a gastrin-secreting tumor of the pancreas, is associated with a virulent form of duodenal ulcer disease.

   **4. Diagnosis and laboratory studies**

      **a.** Duodenal ulcer presents with a **history** of epigastric pain that may radiate to the back. The pain is relieved by food; however, the period of relief becomes shorter as symptoms progress. The pain typically wakes the patient at night.

      **b.** The **mainstay** of diagnosis is the **upper GI series**.

      **c. Endoscopy** is not necessary routinely, as the incidence of carcinoma is very small. Endoscopy is indicated in patients with typical symptoms but a negative barium study.

      **d. Gastric analysis** provides useful baseline data in patients requiring surgery.

      **e. Serum gastrin levels** are obtained in patients with recurrent ulceration after surgery, in those who fail to respond to medical management, and in those with suspected endocrine disorders, such as the Zollinger-Ellison syndrome. Normal serum gastrin levels are less than 200 pg/ml.

   **5.** In the absence of complications, **medical management** of duodenal ulcer is usually successful.

      **a.** Patients are cautioned to **avoid** aspirin, coffee, and smoking. Stress should also be avoided.

      **b. $H_2$-receptor antagonists** (cimetidine, ranitidine) have become the **mainstay** of duodenal ulcer therapy. The majority of duodenal ulcers will heal with 4 to 6 weeks of such therapy. Because there is a high recurrence rate after discontinuation of medical therapy, maintenance therapy is often advised following ulcer healing.

      **c. Antacids** can also be used as an adjunct to help control gastric pH and to promote healing.

   **6. Surgical therapy** of duodenal ulcer is reserved for patients who fail to respond to medical therapy or who have complications. There are a number of surgical options. The **goal** of each is to reduce acid secretion; therefore, most approaches concentrate on abolishing vagal stimulation, antral gastrin secretion, or both.

      **a. Vagotomy with antrectomy** (see Fig. 5-3 *A* and *B*) is the procedure associated with the lowest recurrence rate.

      **b. Vagotomy and drainage** is associated with a recurrence rate of 6% to 7%. After vagotomy, the motility of the stomach and pylorus is impaired, creating a functional obstruction. For this reason a drainage procedure such as a **pyloroplasty** (see Fig. 5-3 *C*) or **gastrojejunostomy** (see Fig. 5-3 *D*) is added.

      **c. Parietal cell vagotomy** (see Fig. 5-3 *E*), also known as **superselective vagotomy**, is a relatively new procedure. Only the gastric branches of the vagus nerves are divided. Because innervation to the pylorus is retained, no drainage procedure is needed. Recurrence rates reported for this procedure are variable but average around 10%.

**C. Complications of ulcers** include perforation, hemorrhage, and obstruction.

   **1. Perforations** occur most commonly with ulcers on the anterior surface of the duodenum. Gastric perforations are less common. Occasionally, ulcers can perforate posteriorly into the lesser sac.

      **a.** Typical **symptoms of perforation** include sudden onset of severe abdominal pain, radiation of pain to the shoulder, nausea, and vomiting. **Signs** include a rigid abdomen and shock.

      **b.** Simple operative closure of the perforated ulcer is the usual **treatment**. Definitive treatment of the ulcer (e.g., by antrectomy and vagotomy) is reserved for good-risk patients with minimal soilage of the peritoneal cavity.

   **2. Hemorrhage** will occur in approximately 15% to 20% of patients with ulcers. Medical management will control the hemorrhage in the majority of cases.

      **a.** Endoscopy is necessary to evaluate the site of the hemorrhage.

      **b.** Surgical intervention is usually needed to control **massive hemorrhage**, defined as blood loss that requires transfusion of more than 1500 ml of blood products without stabilization of vital signs, or continued blood loss requiring more than 6 units of transfused blood in a 24-hour period.

         **(1)** If the site of bleeding is a **duodenal ulcer**, oversewing of the bleeding point is done via a longitudinal opening through the pylorus. If this fails to control the vessel, it is necessary to isolate and ligate the gastroduodenal artery. The incision through the pylorus is then closed transversely. This is known as a **pyloroplasty**, or **widening of the pylorus**. A **truncal vagotomy** (division of the two main vagal trunks) is also done (see Fig. 5 3 C).

(2) **Vagotomy and antrectomy** is another option in good-risk patients.

3. **Gastric outlet obstruction** can be caused by **prepyloric ulcers** and by chronic **scarring of the pyloric channel**. Patients respond poorly to medical therapy.

   a. **Obstruction** causes symptoms of crampy abdominal pain, nausea, and vomiting. The stomach is usually markedly dilated.

   b. **Initial treatment** consists of several days of nasogastric suction to allow the stomach to return to normal size.

   c. After this, **vagotomy and antrectomy** or **vagotomy and drainage** is done.

## IV. GASTRITIS AND DUODENITIS are both mucosal lesions. Gastritis is classified as acute or chronic.

### A. Acute gastritis

1. **Acute diffuse gastritis** can be due to a number of irritating agents, chief among them being aspirin and ethanol. Hemorrhage can occur and can be massive. Removal of the inciting agent and antacid therapy will usually result in prompt healing.

2. **Stress ulceration**, also known as **acute hemorrhagic gastritis**, is another form of acute gastritis. Ischemia of the gastric mucosa is the inciting event. The injury is compounded by the effect of intraluminal acid.

   a. Affected patients frequently have sepsis, multiple organ systems failure, severe trauma, or a complicated postoperative course. Stress ulceration that occurs in burn patients is known as **Curling's ulcer**.

   b. Stress ulcers are characteristically shallow mucosal lesions that start in the fundus. They then spread distally and can involve the entire stomach.

   c. Antacid therapy that raises the gastric pH to greater than 5 is effective **prophylaxis** against stress ulceration. Cimetidine alone is not effective.

   d. In cases of uncontrolled hemorrhage, the **surgical approach** is a near-total gastrectomy. Mortality in this situation is very high—54% in one series.

### B. Chronic gastritis (atrophic gastritis)

1. Atrophy of the gastric tubules and inflammatory infiltration of the lamina propria are the **lesions found** in atrophic gastritis. Intestinal metaplasia may occur.

2. There are two **types** of chronic gastritis. Both are associated with an increased risk of cancer. Their etiology is unknown.

   a. **Type A gastritis** involves the proximal stomach diffusely but spares the antrum. This gastritis is associated with parietal cell antibodies in the serum. Acid secretion is markedly reduced and vitamin $B_{12}$ absorption is impaired.

   b. **Type B gastritis** is the more common type. It is found in association with duodenal and gastric ulcers, and its incidence increases with age. No parietal cell antibodies are found, and acid production is only slightly reduced.

## V. MALIGNANT TUMORS OF THE STOMACH constitute 90% to 95% of all tumors of the stomach, and 95% of all malignant tumors of the stomach are carcinomas.

### A. Gastric carcinoma

1. The **incidence** of carcinoma of the stomach has been decreasing; however, the **prognosis** still remains poor. Only about 40% of patients have potentially curable disease at the time of diagnosis.

2. Gastric carcinoma becomes symptomatic late in its course. Pain, anorexia, and weight loss are common **symptoms**.

3. **Diagnosis** can be made with an upper GI series and confirmed with endoscopic biopsy.

4. **At operation**, the presence of nodal and liver metastases is assessed. The extent of the operation is determined by the site of the cancer. If the procedure is done for cure, removal of the lymph nodes of the greater and lesser omentum is done. For lesions in the fundus or cardia, the spleen is also removed with the tumor.

5. **Radiation therapy** is not effective for carcinoma of the stomach. **Chemotherapy** with a combination of doxorubicin, fluorouracil, and either mitomycin or semustine appears to be an effective accompaniment to surgery.

**B. Gastric lymphoma** can be primary or can occur as part of disseminated disease. The stomach is the most common site of **primary intestinal lymphoma**.

   **1.** The tumors are bulky, with central ulceration.

   **2.** Surgical excision, combined with radiation therapy if excision is not curative, is the treatment of choice.

   **3.** The 5-year survival rate is over 50%.

**C. Leiomyosarcomas** are bulky, well-localized tumors. They are slow to metastasize and can be treated with partial gastrectomy.

## VI. BENIGN TUMORS OF THE STOMACH are uncommon.

**A. Leiomyomas** are the most common benign gastric tumors. They are usually asymptomatic but may undergo hemorrhage or cause a mass effect. They are submucosal and well encapsulated.

**B. Gastric polyps** are usually hyperplastic, but may be adenomatous. Most are asymptomatic. They can be excised via an endoscope.

**C. Other benign tumors** are fibromas, neurofibromas, aberrant pancreas, and angiomas.

## VII. TUMORS OF THE DUODENUM, both benign and malignant, are rare.

**A. Malignant tumors** are usually adenocarcinomas. Treatment of resectable lesions is pancreatico-duodenectomy (**Whipple's procedure**).

**B. Benign tumors** include lipomas, leiomyomas, and adenomas. They can be locally excised.

## VIII. ACQUIRED OBSTRUCTIVE DISORDERS OF THE STOMACH AND DUODENUM

**A. Gastric outlet obstruction** (see section III C 3)

**B. Gastric volvulus** is an uncommon entity.

   **1.** There are several **types of volvulus.**
   **a. Organoaxial volvulus** is a rotation around the cardiopyloric line, a line drawn along the length of the stomach between cardia and pylorus.
   **b. Mesentericoaxial volvulus** occurs around a line perpendicular to the cardiopyloric line.
   **c.** Volvulus may also occur as a combination of these two types.

   **2.** The volvulus may be intermittent. It is caused by laxity of the ligaments supporting the stomach and is frequently associated with diaphragmatic hernias.

   **3.** Surgical treatment includes reducing the torsion and fixation of the stomach.

**C. Superior mesenteric artery syndrome**

   **1.** Especially in young, thin females, the third portion of the duodenum can be obstructed by the superior mesenteric artery, which takes a sharp angle from the aorta and courses over the duodenum.

   **2.** This anatomic configuration is combined with **predisposing factors** such as a lack of the retroperitoneal fat cushion, prolonged immobilization, and pressure (e.g., from a body cast). The syndrome is also known as **cast syndrome** because of its association with patients in body casts.

   **3.** The usual **symptoms** are vomiting and postprandial pain.

   **4. Treatment** consists of eliminating all contributing factors, such as casts, girdles, and lying in the supine position. Weight gain may alleviate symptoms.

   **5. Surgical treatment** includes either:
   **a.** Releasing the ligament of Treitz (which moves the duodenum out from beneath the superior mesenteric artery)
   **b.** Bypass of the obstruction

## IX. MISCELLANEOUS DISORDERS OF THE STOMACH AND DUODENUM

**A. Mallory-Weiss tears** are linear mucosal lesions found at the gastroesophageal junction. They are caused by repeated forceful vomiting and can result in profuse hemorrhage, requiring surgery. Diagnosis is made by endoscopy. Surgical therapy consists of oversewing the mucosal tear.

**B. Bezoars** are agglutinated masses of hair (**trichobezoars**), vegetable matter (**phytobezoars**), or a combination of the two that form within the stomach.

  **1.** Most **trichobezoars** occur in young, neurotic women. **Phytobezoars** are seen after a partial gastric resection and tend to be more common in older males.

  **2. Symptoms** of a bezoar include nausea, vomiting, weight loss, and abdominal pain. **Complications** include obstruction and ulceration.

  **3. Treatment** generally requires surgical removal, although enzymatic dissolution of some bezoars has been successful.

**C. Menetrier's disease** is an abnormality of the gastric mucosa with an unknown etiology.

  **1.** Several **distinctive features** are associated:
    **a.** A hypertrophic gastric mucosa is seen on x-ray.
      **(1)** Giant rugal folds are characteristic; these spare the antrum.
      **(2)** Mucous cells are increased in number, and parietal and chief cells are decreased.
    **b.** There is gastric hypersecretion of mucus with a high protein and low acid concentration; systemic hypoproteinemia is the result.

  **2.** Total gastrectomy is required in patients with severe hypoproteinemia.

**D. Duodenal diverticula** are frequently asymptomatic. The most common location is opposite the ampulla of Vater.

  **1.** These are **pulsion diverticula**, caused by "pulling" of muscles.

  **2.** Severe hemorrhage or perforation can occur, but in the absence of such complications, no treatment is indicated.

**X. COMPLICATIONS SPECIFIC TO GASTRIC SURGERY.** These symptom complexes, known as **postgastrectomy syndromes**, can be disabling.

**A. Alkaline reflux gastritis** is the most common problem after a gastrectomy, occurring in about one-quarter of all patients.

  **1. Symptoms** are postprandial epigastric pain, nausea, vomiting, and weight loss. **Endoscopy** demonstrates the gastritis and a free reflux of bile.

  **2. Treatment** is conversion of the Billroth I or II gastrectomy (see Fig. 5-3 *A* and *B*) to a Roux-en-Y anastomosis (see Fig. 5-3 *F*).

**B.** The **afferent loop syndrome** is caused by intermittent mechanical obstruction of the afferent loop of a gastrojejunostomy.

  **1. Symptoms** include early postprandial distention, pain, and nausea, which are relieved by vomiting of bilious material not mixed with food.

  **2. Treatment** consists of providing good drainage of the afferent loop, usually by conversion to a Roux-en-Y anastomosis.

**C. Dumping syndrome** affects most postgastrectomy patients, but is a significant problem in only a few.

  **1.** Dumping syndrome is **caused** by the release of hypertonic chyme into the small bowel. This in turn causes rapid accumulation of fluid and consequent jejunal distention.

  **2. Symptoms** may include epigastric fullness or pain, nausea, palpitations, dizziness, and diarrhea. **Signs** include tachycardia and elevated blood pressure.

  **3. Conservative measures** control most patients' symptoms. They are advised to avoid a high carbohydrate intake, and not to drink fluids with meals.

  **4.** Various **surgical approaches** are used to delay gastric emptying, including interposition of an antiperistaltic jejunal loop between the stomach and small bowel.

**D. Postvagotomy diarrhea** is common in its mild form, but seldom is a disabling problem. Symptoms usually improve during the first year after surgery.

# 6
# The Small Intestine

R. Anthony Carabasi, III
Michael J. Moritz

## I. ANATOMY

**A.** The **small intestine** is the length of bowel extending from the distal end of the pylorus to the cecum.

   **1.** The area extending from the pylorus to the ligament of Treitz is the **duodenum**.

   **2.** The remainder of the small intestine is made up of the **jejunum** (the proximal 40%) and the **ileum**.

      **a.** The caliber of the jejunum is larger than that of the ileum, and the mucosal folds (**valvulae conniventes** or **plicae circulares**) are more prominent proximally.

      **b.** The lymphoid tissue (**Peyer's patches**) found in the submucosa becomes more prominent distally in the ileum.

**B.** The **wall** of the small intestine is made up of four **layers**.

   **1.** The **mucosa** is composed primarily of columnar epithelium with goblet cells. The absorption of nutrients takes place through the mucosa. The mucosa covers the intestinal villi and has an absorption area of approximately 500 m². Mucosal cells proliferate rapidly and have a life-span of 5 days.

   **2.** The **submucosa** is the strongest layer and provides strength to an intestinal anastomosis. It contains nerves, blood vessels, and fibrous and elastic tissue.

   **3.** The **muscularis**—the muscle layer—is composed of an outer longitudinal layer and an inner circular layer.

   **4.** The **serosa** is the outermost layer and derives embryologically from the peritoneum.

**C.** The **blood supply** to the small intestine is primarily from the superior mesenteric artery.

## II. PHYSIOLOGY

**A.** The **primary functions** of the small intestine are **digestion** and **absorption**. All ingested food and fluid, and also secretions from the stomach, liver, and pancreas, reach the small intestine. The total volume may reach 9 L per day, and all but 1 L to 2 L will be absorbed.

**B. Motility**

   **1.** Following a meal, two **types of contractions** are found.

      **a.** A **to-and-fro motion** mixes chyme with digestive juices and provides prolonged exposure to the absorptive mucosa.

      **b.** A **peristaltic contraction** moves food more rapidly in an aboral direction.

   **2.** In the fasting state, a strong contraction beginning in the duodenum occurs every 2 hours. This completes the emptying of residual food from previous meals.

   **3.** Parasympathetic stimulation promotes contractions while sympathetic stimulation inhibits them.

**C. Absorption.** Vitamins, fat, protein, carbohydrates, water, and electrolytes are all absorbed in the small intestine.

   **1. Water** is absorbed throughout the small intestine although the majority is absorbed in the jejunum. Passive absorption is the mechanism.

2. Of the **electrolytes, calcium** is actively transported (regulated by vitamin D). **Potassium** is absorbed by passive diffusion. **Sodium** is actively transported, and once a gradient is established **chloride** follows passively.

3. **Fat** absorption occurs chiefly in the duodenum and jejunum. Fat is digested by lipase and becomes emulsified in bile acid micelles. The micelles release fatty acids and monoglycerides to the mucosal cells. After absorption, the fatty acids are synthesized into triglycerides, which are assembled into chylomicrons and transported into the lymphatics.

4. **Carbohydrates** are digested by salivary and pancreatic amylase. Enzymes of the brush border further reduce sugars to fructose, galactose, and glucose. These are absorbed into portal blood by active transport.

5. **Protein** digestion is started in the stomach and is continued by pancreatic enzymes. The process is completed at the brush border, yielding tripeptides, dipeptides, and amino acids. All are absorbed by active transport.

6. **Vitamins** A, D, E, and K are fat-soluble and are absorbed in micelles as described in section II C 3. Most water-soluble vitamins are absorbed by passive diffusion. Vitamin $B_{12}$ is complexed with intrinsic factor and absorbed by pinocytosis at the distal ileum. Vitamin C, thiamine, and folic acid are actively transported.

7. **Iron** is absorbed as the ferrous (reduced) ion $Fe^{2+}$. Conversion of the ferric to the ferrous ion is enhanced by the presence of reducing substances in the diet, such as vitamin C (ascorbic acid). Absorption is via active transport and occurs primarily in the proximal small bowel.

## III. TUMORS OF THE SMALL INTESTINE

A. **Benign neoplasms** are usually asymptomatic. They are 10 times more common than malignant tumors.

1. **Polyps**
   a. **Adenomatous polyps** are rare in the small intestine. They may be seen in the **familial polyposis** syndromes and have malignant potential in this setting.
   b. **Hamartomatous polyps** are found in patients with **Peutz-Jeghers syndrome** (mucocutaneous pigmentation accompanied by widespread intestinal polyposis). There is virtually no malignant potential in this syndrome.
   c. **Juvenile (retention) polyps** are benign hamartomas, and not true neoplasms. They are more common in the rectum and usually autoamputate. They may cause bleeding or obstruction, and are resected if symptoms occur.

2. **Other benign tumors** include lipomas, leiomyomas, hemangiomas, fibromas, and neurofibromas (in descending order of frequency), any of which require resection if symptomatic.

B. **Malignant neoplasms**

1. **General information**
   a. Malignant tumors constitute 75% of symptomatic small bowel tumors, and usually present with bleeding, perforation, or obstruction (which may be due to intussusception).
   b. The most common tumors are adenocarcinoma (40%), carcinoid (30%), lymphoma (20%), sarcoma, and metastases from distant malignancies.
   c. Preferred **treatment** is segmental resection. This should include margins of 6 inches proximally and distally and as much mesentery as possible without compromising the blood supply to the remaining small intestine.

2. **Adenocarcinoma** is most common in the proximal jejunum. Metastases are present in a large percentage of patients at operation. Patients with resectable tumors have a 25% 5-year survival rate.

3. **Carcinoid tumors** are derived from enterochromaffin cells. These cells are part of the amine precursor uptake and decarboxylation system (APUD cells), and hence carcinoid tumors are classified as **apudomas**. Carcinoid tumors are most common in the appendix, then the small bowel (usually the ileum), then the rectum. Other sites are uncommon.
   a. **Prognosis** is related to size; if tumors are less than 1 cm in diameter, metastases are unusual, but if they are greater than 2 cm in diameter, metastases are present in over 80%. The tumors are slow-growing.
   b. **Carcinoid syndrome**—flushing, bronchoconstriction, diarrhea, and tricuspid and pulmonic valvular disease—is caused by serotonin and other vasoactive substances secreted by the tumor.

**(1)** These substances are cleared by the liver, so only liver metastases, which drain into the systemic veins, or primary carcinoids that drain similarly (e.g., bronchial carcinoids), cause the syndrome.

**(2)** About 10% of patients with small bowel carcinoids present with the syndrome. **Diagnosis** is made by finding elevated levels of 5-hydroxyindoleacetic acid (5-HIAA), the breakdown product of serotonin, in the urine.

**(3)** **Treatment** includes resection of the primary tumor and resection or ''debulking'' of metastases. Liver metastases can be resected (when solitary) but usually require palliative therapy with intra-arterial chemotherapy or embolization of the hepatic artery (which is performed by a radiologist using angiographic methods) to decrease the blood flow to the metastases.

**(4)** The overall 5-year survival rate for small bowel carcinoid patients is 70%. If liver metastases are present, the 5-year survival rate is 20%.

4. Primary small bowel **lymphomas** usually arise in the ileum.
   **a.** Perforation is a frequent presentation; however, lymphomas can present instead with fever of unknown origin or with malabsorption.
   **b.** Biopsies of lymph nodes and the liver are necessary for staging.

5. **Leiomyosarcoma** is the most common of the small bowel sarcomas.

6. **Metastases** to the small bowel are present in 50% of malignant melanoma patients at autopsy. Many other carcinomas can also metastasize to the small bowel.

**IV. CROHN'S DISEASE (regional enteritis; granulomatous ileitis)** is a chronic, transmural granulomatous inflammatory disease that can involve any area of the gastrointestinal tract. Its cause is unknown.

**A. Distribution.** The small bowel alone is involved in 25% of the patients, both the small and the large bowel in 50%, and the colon alone in almost 25%. The distal ileum, the most common site, is involved in 70% of all cases, which accounts for the older name, **terminal ileitis**.

**B. Diagnosis**

1. **Symptoms** include diarrhea (usually not bloody), abdominal pain, lethargy, fever, weight loss, and anorectal disease. Anal fissures, fistulas, or ulcers, or pararectal abscesses, are seen in 20% of patients with colonic involvement.

2. **Signs** include an abdominal mass, anemia, and malnutrition. Extraintestinal manifestations are similar to those found in ulcerative colitis.

3. **X-ray findings** characteristically include segmental areas of stricture separated by ''skip areas'' of uninvolved bowel, cobblestone appearance of the mucosa, and fistulas.

**C. Differential diagnosis** includes ulcerative colitis, lymphoma, and infectious enteritides (tuberculosis, amebiasis, and *Yersinia, Campylobacter*, and *Salmonella* infections).

**D. Medical treatment** is preferred and can include rest, a low-residue diet, prednisone and oral antibiotics (sulfasalazine or metronidazole), sedatives, antispasmodics, and, when necessary, total parenteral nutrition. Although antibiotics and steroids are helpful in acute active disease, their effectiveness in preventing relapse of symptoms has not been established.

**E. Surgical treatment**, which is reserved for **complications** of the disease, ultimately becomes necessary in most cases.

1. The complication seen most often is **intestinal obstruction**, usually due to stricture and inflammation.

2. **Abscesses** and **fistulas** are also common. Abscesses may be intra- or retroperitoneal. Fistulas (see Chapter 8) form from bowel to skin, to bladder, to vagina, to urethra, or to other loops of bowel.

3. **Perianal disease** likewise is common, and oral metronidazole has been found to be helpful in its treatment.
   **a.** Perirectal abscesses require drainage. Anal fistulas or fissures may need surgery if they are multiple or severe.
   **b.** In general, **surgery** for perianal disease should be as limited as practical, because wound healing in these patients is quite poor and recurrences are common.

4. Perforation, hemorrhage, and intractable symptoms are less common indications for surgery.

     **5.** Surgical therapy is conservative—resecting as little bowel as necessary. If resection is hazardous, bypass or exclusion of the involved segment may be necessary.

  **F. Prognosis** is only fair. Roughly 50% of patients who require surgery will require it again within 5 years. The likelihood of recurrence after each reoperation is again approximately 50%.

**V. SMALL BOWEL FISTULAS** (see Chapter 8)

**VI. RADIATION INJURY TO THE SMALL BOWEL** occurs in two phases.

  **A. Acute-phase injury** is due to mucosal injury. Symptoms include nausea, vomiting, and diarrhea and are transient. Rarely, bleeding or perforation occurs and requires surgery.

  **B. Chronic effects** appear months to years later and are due to an obliterative vasculitis. The symptoms and signs are similar to those associated with recurrent malignancy, and, indeed, this possibility must always be fully evaluated.

     **1.** Relatively **minor symptoms**—abdominal pain, malabsorption, and diarrhea—require symptomatic therapy only.

     **2. Major complications** that require surgery include bowel obstruction (unrelieved by decompression with a nasogastric or long tube), perforation, abscess, fistula, and hemorrhage. Hemorrhage may be from mucosal erosion or an enteroarterial fistula.

     **3.** Surgery is technically difficult due to fibrosis and scarring.

     **4.** Resection or bypass is the surgical treatment of choice. Unirradiated bowel must be used for any anastomosis. Even so, the anastomosis or other surgical wound is likely to break down, with subsequent fistula formation or other complications.

  **C. Prognosis.** The perioperative mortality rate is less than 15%, but long-term mortality rates are high. The 5-year survival rate is less than 50%.

**VII. SHORT BOWEL SYNDROME** is a complication of massive small bowel resection.

  **A.** It is **characterized** by malabsorption with diarrhea and an excessive loss of fat and protein in the stool. Inadequate absorption of water, electrolytes, minerals, and vitamins also invariably occurs.

  **B.** The length of bowel necessary to avoid the syndrome is variable, but patients with less than 100 cm (3.5 feet) of small bowel are susceptible.

  **C.** Postoperatively, total parenteral nutrition (TPN; see Chapter 1, section I E 3) is essential. The small bowel will hypertrophy with time, and most patients can be weaned from parenteral nutrition gradually.

  **D.** Ensuring that **oral nutrition** is adequate requires attention to several points.

     **1.** The total calories ingested must increase, to compensate for that portion not absorbed.

     **2.** A low-residue or elemental diet is needed. An **elemental diet** contains only components that are directly absorbed by the intestinal mucosa without any enzymatic digestion (medium-chain and short-chain triglycerides, mono- and disaccharides, and mono- and dipeptides), plus vitamins and minerals. It contains *no* residue (undigestible material).

     **3.** Antiperistaltic agents should be given.

     **4.** Reflex gastric hypersecretion should be controlled with $H_2$ receptor antagonists.

     **5.** Fat- and water-soluble vitamin supplementation is needed.

     **6.** Parenteral vitamin $B_{12}$ is needed if the distal ileum has been resected.

     **7.** Calcium and magnesium supplementation should be given.

     **8.** Medium-chain triglycerides should replace dietary fats because they do not require micelles for absorption.

  **E.** If adequate oral nutrition cannot be attained, **surgical therapy** is available, consisting of reversal of a short segment of distal small bowel to slow the intestinal transit time.

  **F.** For refractory cases, long-term total parenteral nutrition (**home TPN**) is available.

# 7
# The Colon, Rectum, and Anus

Anthony V. Coletta

## I. GROSS ANATOMY

**A.** The **large intestine** is divided into **five parts.**

1. The division is based on the mesenteric attachments:
   **a.** Ascending colon
   **b.** Transverse colon
   **c.** Descending colon
   **d.** Sigmoid colon
   **e.** Rectum

2. The **colon** is that part of the large intestine extending from the cecum to the rectum.

3. Scattered throughout the surface of the colon are fat-filled appendages, **appendices epiploicae**.

4. The outer longitudinal muscle layer of the colon is restricted to three bands, the **teniae coli**.

**B.** The **cecum** is the first part of the ascending colon. Its mesenteric attachments, and thus its relation to the retroperitoneum, vary.

**C.** The **vermiform appendix** averages 9 cm in length.

1. The appendix most often arises at the convergence of the teniae coli on the cecum, a most useful landmark at operation.

2. The **location** of the **tip of the appendix** varies. It is most often pelvic, but it may be subcecal, retrocecal, retrocolic, ileocecal, or, rarely, subhepatic.

**D.** The **ascending ("right") and descending ("left") portions of the colon define**, in their retroperitoneal course, **the right and left paracolic gutters**, respectively. These gutters form dependent regions of the abdominal cavity where fluid may collect.

**E.** At the pelvic brim, the colon again becomes intraperitoneal, forming the **sigmoid colon**.

1. The **sigmoid colon** is suspended from the **sigmoid mesocolon**, and its position and configuration are variable.

2. Here the teniae coli become indistinct as they fuse to form the single longitudinal outer muscular layer of the rectum.

**F.** The **rectum** begins where the sigmoid mesocolon ends. The lower limit of the rectum is the point at which it pierces the pelvic floor, formed here by the levator ani muscle group.

1. At the **rectosigmoid junction**, the rectum turns posteriorly to follow the curve of the sacrum.

2. In the **male**, anterior to the rectum, the peritoneum reflects upward along the posterior wall of the bladder, forming the **rectovesical pouch**.

3. In the **female**, the peritoneum reflects in a similar fashion along the posterior wall of the uterus and vagina, forming the **rectouterine pouch**.

4. The **ampulla of the rectum**, the part that lies just above the pelvic floor, is the widest segment and is capable of substantial distention.

**G.** The **anal canal** extends posteriorly and inferiorly, from the pelvic diaphragm to the opening of the

**anus**, for a distance of 3 cm to 4 cm. The angle that the canal makes with the pelvic floor is known as the **carrying angle of the rectum**, and it is the site of rectal prolapse (see section XVIII F).

1. The mucosa of the upper two-thirds of the anus forms longitudinal folds that are 1 cm long. These folds are called the **anal columns of Morgagni**.

2. The base of the columns, along with the semilunar folds of tissue that join them, the **anal valves**, form the **pectinate (dentate) line**. This line separates the upper two-thirds of the anal canal, the visceral portion, from the lower one-third, the somatic portion. An understanding of these anatomic variations is essential to a proper surgical approach to the region.
   a. The **visceral anus** is an extension of the rectum with respect to mucosa, blood supply, venous drainage, and innervation. The epithelium here is insensitive to touch.
   b. The **somatic anus** is distinct from its visceral counterpart in that it derives its mucosa, blood supply, and innervation from the surrounding perineum. The epithelium here is extremely sensitive.
   c. Behind the anal valves and between the bases of the anal columns lie the **anal sinuses**, into which the **anal glands** empty.

3. The opening of the anus is surrounded by the **anal sphincter**.
   a. The **internal sphincter** is a continuation of the inner circular smooth muscle of the wall of the anal canal. This muscle is under **involuntary control**.
   b. The **external sphincter** is composed of striated muscle and is under **voluntary control**. It surrounds the anus and is subdivided into subcutaneous, superficial, and deep portions.

## II. HISTOLOGIC ANATOMY. Several aspects are of considerable clinical importance.

A. Histologically, the colon is composed of **four layers**:

1. **Mucosa**, which contains goblet cells, glands, and absorptive cells

2. **Submucosa**

3. **Muscularis**, which is composed of inner circular and outer longitudinal smooth muscle layers (i.e., teniae coli; see section I A 4)

4. **Serosa** (i.e., the visceral peritoneum). (The rectum lacks a serosa.)

B. In the region of the **pectinate line**, there is an abrupt **transition** from the simple columnar mucosal epithelium of the rectum to the stratified squamous epithelium of the lower anal canal. At the level of the anus, this surface layer assumes the histologic structure of skin.

## III. ARTERIAL VASCULAR SUPPLY

A. The three **branches of the superior mesenteric artery** that are described below have ample anastomotic connections.

1. The **ileocolic artery**, which is the terminal branch of the superior mesenteric artery, supplies blood to the **appendix**, via the **appendicular artery**, and to the **cecum** and the proximal **ascending colon**.

2. The **right colic artery**, which may originate from the superior mesenteric artery or the ileocolic artery, supplies the remainder of the **ascending colon** and the **hepatic flexure**. Its presence and course are variable.

3. The **middle colic artery**, originating from the proximal superior mesenteric artery, supplies the **transverse colon**.

B. The **left colic** branch of the **inferior mesenteric artery** supplies the **splenic flexure** and the **descending colon**. It communicates with the **middle colic artery** (and thus the superior mesenteric artery) via the **marginal artery of Drummond**. This anastomosis may be variable in the region of the splenic flexure.

C. The **sigmoid colon** receives its blood supply from the **sigmoid** and **rectosigmoid arteries**. These are branches of the inferior mesenteric artery, which communicate with the left colic artery via the marginal artery.

D. The **rectum** is supplied by branches of the **superior rectal (hemorrhoidal) artery**, which is a branch of the inferior mesenteric artery, by the **middle rectal (hemorrhoidal) artery**, a branch of the **internal iliac artery**, and by the **inferior rectal (hemorrhoidal) artery**, a branch of the **internal pudendal artery**. There is a rich submucosal anastomotic network between these vessels.

    **E.** The **anus** receives its blood supply mainly from the **internal pudendal artery**.

**IV. VENOUS DRAINAGE.** The veins that drain the colon and rectum in general parallel the arteries, are similarly named, and ultimately drain into the portal venous system.

    **A.** The veins draining the middle and lower thirds of the **rectum** communicate directly with:

        **1.** The **systemic venous system** via the **internal iliac veins** and via rich **venous collaterals** in the rectal submucosa

        **2.** The **portal venous system** via the **inferior mesenteric vein**

    **B.** Below the pectinate line, the **lower anal canal** is drained via the **inferior rectal veins**, a rich submucosal network of veins, which communicate with the submucosal veins *above* the pectinate line and, when varicose, are known as **hemorrhoids** (see section XVIII B).

## V. LYMPHATIC DRAINAGE

    **A.** In general, the lymphatic pathways follow the arterial blood supply, with lymph nodes interspersed along these channels.

        **1.** Understanding this concept is essential to a proper surgical approach to cancer of the large intestine.

        **2.** For example, recalling the complex blood supply to the rectum, it may be seen that carcinoma may spread via the lymphatic system both inferiorly and superiorly.

    **B.** Above the pectinate line, the lymphatic drainage is into the **internal iliac nodes**. Below this line, lymph drains into the **superficial inguinal nodes**.

**VI. INNERVATION.** The two main neural pathways are the **autonomic** and the **visceral afferent** systems.

    **A. The autonomic system**

        **1. The parasympathetic division**
            **a.** The **vagus nerve** provides parasympathetic innervation of the lower gastrointestinal tract to the level of the splenic flexure.
            **b.** From the splenic flexure to the pectinate line, parasympathetic innervation arises from the **nervi erigentes** (i.e., the **pelvic splanchnic nerves**), which originate from levels $S_2$, $S_3$, and $S_4$ of the spinal cord.
            **c.** The parasympathetic nerves provide motor innervation to the wall of the bowel.

        **2. The sympathetic system**, via the **greater and lesser splanchnic nerves**, innervates the blood vessels of the lower gastrointestinal tract.

    **B. The visceral afferent system**

        **1. Parasympathetic nerves** carry **afferent reflex arcs** along the vagal and splanchnic pathways.

        **2. Sympathetic nerves** for the most part carry pain and pressure afferents along sympathetic pathways and are responsible for referred pain.

## VII. PHYSIOLOGY

    **A.** The major function of the colon is the **absorption of water and electrolytes**.

        **1. Sodium, chloride**, and **water** are actively absorbed.

        **2.** The absorptive capacity is about 2 L/day, and diarrhea may result if the ileum delivers more than this amount.

    **B. Excretion**

        **1.** The colonic mucosa secretes **potassium** and **bicarbonate** into the colonic lumen.

        **2.** Excessive diarrhea may result in potassium and bicarbonate losses and metabolic acidosis.

    **C. Motility** is under **parasympathetic control** via the vagus and pelvic splanchnic nerve plexus.

        **1. Transit time** through the colon normally is slow (5 cm/hr) to allow time for absorption of water and electrolytes.

    **2.** Following a meal, colonic contraction increases, causing a net increase in the transit time to 11 cm/hr. This movement often distends the rectum with feces, creating the primary stimulus for defecation.

**D.** The **defecation reflex** is initiated by rectal distention, which stimulates receptors in the rectal wall, causing the rectum to contract and the internal sphincter to relax. Simultaneously, the external sphincter contracts—a major factor in the maintenance of continence.

**E. Colonic gas** may come from one of several different sources.

    **1. Swallowed air** that reaches the distal colon is often composed primarily of **nitrogen**.

    **2. Fermentation** produces gas by the action of bacteria on the slowly moving contents of the colon. **Hydrogen** is produced in the greatest quantity. **Methane** and **hydrogen sulfide** may also be produced.
        **a.** The quantity of gas produced via fermentation depends on the composition of the colonic residue, which is controlled both by food intake and by mucosal function.
        **b.** For example, a milk-drinker with **lactase deficiency** can have a substantially increased gas volume, because this common disorder allows large quantities of lactose to reach the colonic flora following the ingestion of milk.

    **3. Carbon dioxide** is produced in the colon by the reaction of secreted bicarbonate with organic acids.

    **4.** Colonic gas travels rapidly through the gut due to its relatively low viscosity. Hence, **flatus** may often be the first obvious sign of returning intestinal function.

## VIII. DIAGNOSTIC PROCEDURES

**A.** The **patient's history** should always include a description of the following:

    **1.** A characterization of pain, if present

    **2.** Recent and past bowel habits

    **3.** Conformation and consistency of the stool

    **4.** Patterns of bleeding, if applicable

**B. Physical examination**

    **1.** The standard techniques for **examination of the abdomen** are followed.

    **2. A proper rectal examination should *always* be performed.**
        **a.** The anatomic relationships of structures surrounding the rectum (see section I F) should be kept in mind during the examination. For example, the tip of the examining finger may reach the upper rectum, where anteriorly there is a peritoneal covering, thus allowing assessment of inflammation or nodularity of the peritoneum at this point.
        **b.** The patient may be **positioned** either standing, with the hips flexed and the upper body resting across the examining table or bed, or in the left lateral decubitus position, with the right knee and hip flexed and the buttock close to the edge of the examining table.
        **c.** In women, the rectal examination often follows a pelvic examination, with the patient remaining in the lithotomy position.
        **d.** The **sacrococcygeal and perianal regions** are inspected initially. **Palpation** of any abnormal external area follows.
        **e.** As the patient strains, inspection of the anus is carried out, followed by insertion of a gloved, lubricated index finger, directed towards the umbilicus. The sphincter tone of the anus should be noted, as should any tenderness or irregularities of the anal canal.
        **f.** The finger is then inserted further into the rectum and the lateral and posterior walls are palpated, and irregularities are again noted.
        **g.** The hand is turned so that the finger can palpate anteriorly, allowing examination of the prostate gland and seminal vesicles in the male and the vagina and cervix in the female.
        **h.** The finger is withdrawn gently, and a fecal sample is taken for occult blood testing.

**C. Roentgenologic studies**

    **1. Plain abdominal x-rays** can assess patterns of air and fluid, such as free intra-abdominal air and small bowel gaseous distention. Colonic (and cecal) diameter may be determined also.

    **2. Barium enema.** Properly performed, this study is invaluable to the diagnosis of colorectal disease.

**a. Colon preparation.** Incomplete cleansing of the colon is a major source of diagnostic error.
  **(1)** Colon preparation usually involves:
    **(a)** A clear liquid diet for 24 hours
    **(b)** Ingestion of an **oral cathartic** on the evening before examination (except in patients with evidence of colonic obstruction)
    **(c)** **Enemas** on the morning of examination
  **(2)** Care must be taken to **avoid dehydration** secondary to colon preparation in the predisposed patient.
**b. Fluoroscopy** is essential in all phases of the examination, with spot films of any suspicious or redundant regions.
**c.** The examination usually involves three phases.
  **(1)** The **barium-filled phase**. Films are taken with the patient in both prone and supine positions.
  **(2)** The **postevacuation phase**. Films are taken with the patient in the prone position. These films are especially useful in diagnosing diffuse inflammatory disorders.
  **(3)** The **air contrast phase** is performed by insufflation of air after barium evacuation. This phase provides excellent mucosal detail and is most useful in detecting small polypoid lesions.
**d. Anticholinergics or glucagon** may be administered in evaluating spastic regions of the colon.
**e. Complications of barium enema studies**
  **(1) Perforation**, the most serious complication, may be due to mechanical factors such as overdistention or tube insertion. Acute inflammation and diminished bowel wall integrity may be contributing factors, and call for the use of extreme caution.
  **(2) Barium impaction** results from incomplete evacuation of the barium, followed by inspissation.
  **(3) Barium granulomas**, nonspecific ulcerative or polypoid lesions, which are often subclinical, are caused by tearing of the rectal mucosa during administration of the barium.

## D. Endoscopic studies

**1. Rigid proctosigmoidoscopy**
  **a.** When properly performed, examination with a rigid sigmoidoscope can evaluate approximately 20 cm to 25 cm of the rectum and sigmoid colon.
  **b. Indications for its use** include any condition that requires colonic evaluation, such as blood in the stool, persistent diarrhea, or abnormal findings on barium enema. Routine use for cancer screening is advocated by some authorities, but its necessity is not universally accepted.
  **c.** Although recent studies have indicated an increase in the number of more proximal colon cancers, many authorities still believe that 60% to 70% of colorectal cancers lie within the reach of the 25-cm rigid sigmoidoscope.
  **d.** The **morbidity rate** associated with the procedure is quite low. Fewer than 0.1% of patients experience **perforation**, the most worrisome complication. The **mortality rate** approaches zero.
  **e.** Proper **preparation of the bowel** is essential for adequate visualization and a productive examination.
    **(1)** If the physician chooses, preparation may include a clear liquid diet on the night before and the morning of the examination, and use of a gentle **oral cathartic**.
    **(2)** Two **Fleet enemas** are routinely administered within 2 hours before the examination.
  **f. Complications can be minimized** by using the proper technique and taking certain **precautions**, which include:
    **(1)** Reassuring the patient
    **(2)** Proper positioning of the patient, using either the prone, jackknife, head-down, or left lateral Sims's position.
    **(3)** Performing a digital examination while the patient strains, which may relax the external sphincter, allowing the adequately lubricated scope to be introduced with minimal difficulty
    **(4)** Slowly and gently advancing the scope under direct vision, minimizing insufflation of air, and never using force, especially when stricture or excessive spasm is encountered

**2. Flexible proctosigmoidoscopy**
  **a.** Flexible fiberoptic sigmoidoscopes are now available. These are 35 cm or more in length and 14 mm in diameter, have the ability to bend in four directions, and are equipped with suction-biopsy chambers. These features give the new scopes advantages over the rigid instrument.
    **(1)** The average length of colon that can be examined is 50 cm and may be as much as 75 cm

with the newer, longer scopes. This has significantly improved the detection of polyps and cancer of the left side of the colon.

(2) The patient's discomfort is minimized in many cases.

b. In general, the examination takes longer with the flexible instrument than with the rigid one.

c. The morbidity and mortality rates are comparable for the two types of scope; however, the flexible sigmoidoscope requires more training and should not be used by individuals unfamiliar with it.

d. Bowel preparation is similar to that for rigid proctosigmoidoscopy.

3. **Colonoscopy**

a. The flexible fiberoptic colonoscope is 165 cm to 185 cm long and provides capability for examining the entire colon. The instrument is about 12 mm in diameter and has various chambers that allow suction, irrigation, and passage of instruments for biopsy or polypectomy.

b. **Indications** for colonoscopy include:

(1) Abnormal findings on barium enema

(2) Abnormal findings on sigmoidoscopy

(3) Unexplained symptoms

(4) A history of lower gastrointestinal bleeding (but see Contraindications, below)

(5) Assessment of inflammatory bowel disease

(6) Polypectomy

(7) Extraction of a foreign body

c. **Contraindications** include:

(1) Active, acute inflammation:

(a) Fulminant colitis

(b) Peritonitis

(c) Acute diverticulitis

(2) Severe ischemic bowel disease

(3) Acute, severe radiation colitis

(4) Massive, active lower gastrointestinal bleeding

(5) Pregnancy

d. **Bowel preparation** is necessarily more rigorous than it is for proctosigmoidoscopy.

(1) The usual preparation is as follows.

(a) A clear liquid diet is started 48 hours prior to examination.

(b) An oral cathartic (usually 10 oz of magnesium citrate) is taken the evening before the examination.

(c) Tap water or saline enemas are given on the morning of the examination, repeated until the effluent is clear.

(2) Alternatively, 1 L of 10% mannitol orally, with additional oral fluids ad lib, can be given on the morning of the examination, preceded by a 48-hour clear liquid diet. This will cause an osmotic purging of the colon.

(3) None of the above vigorous methods should be used in the face of obvious hazards (e.g., dehydration or impending obstruction) without proper precautions, including a longer preparation time and use of milder cathartics, given in divided doses.

e. **Complications** related to colonoscopy vary according to the indications. **Bleeding and perforation are the most common problems**.

(1) **Diagnostic colonoscopy** has an overall complication rate of approximately 0.1%.

(2) **Therapeutic colonoscopy** (which is most often a polypectomy) has a somewhat higher incidence of complications, in the range of 3%.

(a) Pedunculated polyps are easier to manage endoscopically and have an overall complication rate of 1.9% in contrast to that of sessile polyps, which is 4.9%.

(b) Larger polyps are associated with greater risks. In general, sessile polyps that are larger than 2 cm in diameter should not be removed via the colonoscope.

(3) The mortality rates are quite low.

4. **Anoscopy**, using any one of a number of commercially available anoscopes, is a simple office procedure.

a. When properly performed it causes little discomfort, and it can be done with little, if any, bowel preparation.

b. Anoscopy is invaluable for evaluating various anal disorders, and it is the first step in evaluating rectal bleeding.

## IX. DISORDERS OF MOTILITY

A. **Constipation.** Several aspects are of importance to the surgeon.

1. When prolonged, constipation progresses to obstipation with obstruction of the colon (see section IX B).

2. The postoperative use of narcotics can aggravate constipation, prolonging the return to normal bowel function.

3. Constipation with constant straining at bowel movements can precipitate or aggravate hemorrhoidal disease.

4. In management, stool softeners and **gentle cathartics** used judiciously are often helpful.

### B. Fecal impaction

1. Feces that are impacted within the rectal ampulla cause functional obstruction.

2. The disorder is seen most often in the elderly, the mentally ill, and the bedridden patient.

3. Frequently, fecal impaction **presents clinically** as watery diarrhea, as very liquid fecal matter passes around the obstruction. The disorder is considered by some authorities to be the most frequent cause of watery diarrhea in the elderly.

4. **Treatment** is by means of **digital disimpaction** followed by mineral or olive oil retention enemas or saline enemas. Rectal dilation under general anesthesia may be necessary.

5. The key to **prevention** is to recognize the patients at risk and to treat them with stool softeners and cathartics.

### C. Incontinence

1. Fecal incontinence is loss of control of the anal sphincter with subsequent uncontrolled bowel movements. It may be **complete** (loss of control of both the internal and external sphincters) or **partial** (loss of control of either the internal or the external sphincter).
   a. **Complete incontinence** with uncontrolled defecation is most often **due to a loss of muscle mass or innervation**. Central nervous system disease may also be causative.
   b. **Partial incontinence**, with involuntary passage of flatus, intermittent soiling, or both, may be caused by local inflammatory disorders, carcinoma, rectal prolapse, trauma, obstetrical procedures, or anal surgery.

2. **Treatment** is directed towards the specific etiology.
   a. **Operative intervention** is indicated only when a muscle defect is present. Eradication of the defect by sphincteroplasty or muscle transposition may solve the problem.
   b. **Colostomy** may be indicated in severe incontinence that is not amenable to other forms of therapy, allowing for easier management of fecal flow.

### D. Diarrhea

1. Excessive loose stools that are rapidly evacuated may be due to a number of causes, including infectious, inflammatory, metabolic, neural, gastric, pharmacologic, organic, and motility disorders.
   a. When diarrhea is associated with a disorder of motility, the diagnosis of "irritable bowel," "spastic colon," or "mucous colitis" is often applied.
   b. Irritable bowel syndrome is a poorly understood disorder that probably has multiple etiologies. The diagnosis is one of exclusion, and is too often applied without proper evaluation.
   c. The **proper evaluation of diarrhea**, whether acute or chronic, is vital to proper diagnosis and therapy. Evaluation may involve not only the patient's history, physical examination, and laboratory evaluation (e.g., stool culture), but also a barium enema and, when indicated, endoscopy.

2. **Treatment** is directed towards the etiology. **Pharmacologic therapy**, using one of a host of agents, is often indicated.

### E. Colonic ileus and pseudo-obstruction (Ogilvie's syndrome)

1. Adynamic colonic ileus, causing the picture of colonic obstruction (hence the term pseudo-obstruction), is most often seen in the seriously ill patient with multisystem pathology.
   a. The fundamental **etiology remains obscure**, however.
   b. Conditions that cause ileus of both the small and large bowel may also be associated with colonic ileus alone. These conditions include sepsis, shock, renal failure, and electrolyte imbalance.

2. The **clinical features** are similar to those associated with mechanical colonic obstruction (see section IX G 3), although pain is not often present.

3. **Plain x-rays of the abdomen** may be the most useful **diagnostic maneuver**, with the characteristic findings of segmental colonic distention (most marked proximally) out of proportion to small bowel distention. Obviously, organic mechanical colonic obstruction must be ruled out.

4. **Treatment**
   a. Therapy is conservative initially, with restoration of fluids and electrolytes, maintenance of nutrition, continuous nasogastric suction, and gentle enemas. The response to therapy may be monitored by serial abdominal x-rays.
   b. **Operative therapy** may be indicated if the colon (especially the cecum) fails to decompress within 72 hours after the institution of the above maneuvers.
      (1) A cecum that is distended beyond 9 cm to 11 cm or right lower quadrant tenderness are causes for concern that may require immediate operative intervention (see section IX G 6 a).
      (2) Decompression of the cecum is the operative goal, and this may be achieved via tube cecostomy performed under local anesthesia.

5. The **prognosis** is directly related to associated systemic disorders.

F. **Megacolon** involves dilatation of the colonic lumen, increased length and tortuosity of the large bowel, and, with chronicity, hypertrophy of the bowel wall. It is seen most often with chronic partial colonic obstruction and constipation.

1. **Congenital megacolon (Hirschsprung's disease)** is primarily a disease of infants and children, but occasionally it goes undiagnosed until adult life (see also Chapter 33, section VIII).

2. **Acquired megacolon**
   a. Acquired megacolon may result from partial mechanical obstruction of the lower colon, rectum, or anus. The causes are many, and treatment is aimed at relief of the obstruction, after which the colon reverts towards, but not completely to, normal.
   b. It may also result from destruction of innervation, with resultant loss of peristalsis and subsequent obstipation.
      (1) **Chagas' disease** may cause megacolon from destruction of the intramural nervous system by the offending protozoan, *Trypanosoma cruzi*. Surgical therapy with resection of the chronically dilated, obstipated colon is sometimes necessary.
      (2) **Neurologic diseases** such as paraplegia may result in constipation and megacolon as well. The key to prevention is a bowel regimen that includes stool softeners, enemas, and suppositories.

3. **Idiopathic megacolon** is frequently seen in institutionalized psychotic patients, with no definable organic causes. Severe constipation secondary to extreme inactivity and psychogenic causes (such as voluntary inhibition of defecation) are the presumed etiologies.
   a. Again, prevention is important. Surgical therapy with subtotal colectomy may be indicated in extreme cases.
   b. Elongation associated with the megacolon is a prominent cause of volvulus (see section XVI B) in this population.

G. **Large bowel obstruction** affects males and females with equal frequency, most often after 50 years of age. The left colon is the most common site of obstruction, followed by the cecum.

1. **Etiology. Carcinoma** is by far the most common cause of large bowel obstruction. Other causes include volvulus, adhesions, diverticulitis, hernia, and intussusception.

2. **Pathophysiology**
   a. **Left colon obstruction** secondary to cancer, which is the most common presentation of large bowel obstruction, often results from progressive narrowing of the lumen via "napkin-ring" or "apple-core" lesions.
      (1) When the **ileocecal valve is competent**, closed-loop obstruction of the colon is present. In this condition, both proximal and distal bowel are obstructed. Colonic distention progresses as ileal contents continue to be delivered to the obstructed bowel. **Rupture** is a serious **complication** in this setting.
      (2) An **incompetent ileocecal valve** allows for some decompression of the colon by reflux of the colon contents back into the small bowel.
   b. **Right colon obstruction** is most often associated with large bulky tumors that have less of a tendency to encircle the bowel. This, in addition to the fact that the cecal and right colon

diameters are greater and the contents more liquid, may account for the lower incidence of clinical obstruction than is seen in the left colon.

  c. **Volvulus**, which involves the mesentery of the colon, is much more likely to result in ischemia and gangrene of the obstructed colon than is carcinomatous obstruction.

**3. Diagnosis**
  a. **Clinical presentation**
    (1) **Crampy abdominal pain**, obstipation, and, later on, nausea and vomiting constitute the most common form of clinical presentation.
    (2) Abdominal distention, mild abdominal tenderness (with no perforation present), a silent abdomen or high-pitched tinkling bowel sounds, and an empty rectal vault are common **physical findings** with large bowel obstruction. With lower obstructions, a mass may be appreciated on rectal examination.
    (3) Although fluid shifts occur with large bowel obstruction, **major electrolyte imbalances are rare** without prolonged vomiting.
  b. **Abdominal x-rays** may show both large and small bowel distention, with air-fluid levels depending on the level of obstruction and the function of the ileocecal valve.
  c. **Barium enema** may assist in the diagnosis when no signs of peritonitis are present. Caution should be used when there is the possibility of perforation.
  d. **Sigmoidoscopy** is almost routinely used to characterize the type and extent of the lesion, except when there is a possibility of perforation.

**4. Treatment**
  a. **Left colon obstruction**
    (1) **Immediate decompression** is mandatory when there is complete, closed-loop left colon obstruction.
      (a) **Nasogastric intubation** alone is helpful but is not sufficient.
      (b) **Operative intervention** via tube cecostomy or transverse colostomy is indicated, along with proper fluid replenishment, antibiotic therapy, and attention to associated medical disorders (e.g., cardiac or pulmonary disorders).
        (i) Although **tube cecostomy** may be performed under local anesthesia, and the opening usually closes spontaneously on removal of the tube, it is not as effective in decompressing the colon as is transverse colostomy.
        (ii) However, **transverse colostomy** usually requires general anesthesia and a separate surgical procedure for closure.
    (2) Once the colon is decompressed, left colon obstructions can be **resected** in a staged, definitive fashion, with lower morbidity and mortality rates than with primary resection.
  b. **Right colon obstruction**, on the other hand, involves a shorter length of colon and may be managed by **primary resection** with acceptable morbidity and mortality rates.

**5. Prognosis**
  a. The presence of obstruction in a patient with colon carcinoma does not, of itself, worsen the prognosis that is associated with the carcinoma.
  b. The survival rate with other causes of colon obstruction is directly related to the disease process itself, if no complications of obstruction have ensued.

**6. Complications**
  a. **Rupture**
    (1) The **cecum**, having the largest diameter of any section of the colon, is the most common site of colon rupture. Here, according to the law of Laplace, given equal pressure throughout the colon, tension is greatest in the thin wall of the cecum. Cecal distention beyond 11 cm on x-ray may indicate impending rupture.
    (2) Fever, leukocytosis, and peritoneal signs may be present.
    (3) **Treatment** of any rupture is urgent operative therapy, with exteriorization or resection.
      (a) Staged operative therapy is indicated when fecal contamination or infection is present.
      (b) Antibiotics and drainage are also imperative.
  b. **Strangulation**
    (1) **Volvulus with mesenteric infarction** is the usual mechanism of strangulation.
    (2) **Treatment** is urgent operative resection.

## X. LOWER GASTROINTESTINAL BLEEDING (see Chapter 4, section IV)

## XI. POLYPS OF THE COLON AND RECTUM

  **A. Definition.** Colonic or rectal polyps are growths (usually of the mucosa and submucosa) into the lumen of the colon or rectum.

**B. Anatomic classification**

1. **Pedunculated polyps** are suspended from the bowel wall via a stalk.

2. **Sessile polyps** are broad-based with no definable stalk.

**C. Histologic classification.** Polyps are usually classified as inflammatory, neoplastic, hamartomatous, or hyperplastic.

1. **Inflammatory polyps** are outgrowths in response to active inflammation.
   a. When seen in inflammatory bowel disease (either granulomatous or ulcerative colitis), they are referred to as **pseudopolyps**, lesions that are really islands of swollen mucosa surrounded by shallow ulcerations.
   b. Inflammatory polyps may also be nonspecific or benign lymphoid structures.

2. **Neoplastic polyps** (see also section XI D) are characterized by unrestricted cell division and incomplete cellular differentiation. The **malignant potential** of these polyps may be related to:
   a. **Size.** Smaller polyps (< 1 cm) are associated with a much lower incidence (1%) of malignancy.
   b. **Histologic type**
      (1) **Adenomatous polyps** (or **tubular adenomas**) have a 5% incidence of malignancy.
      (2) **Villous adenomas** have a 35% incidence of malignancy.
      (3) **Villoglandular polyps** (i.e., those with mixed villous and adenomatous elements) have a 20% incidence of malignancy.
   c. **Degree of epithelial atypia.** Larger polyps show a more severe atypia and have a greater potential for malignancy.

3. **Hamartomatous polyps** fit the general description of hamartomas; that is, they are normal tissue in an abnormal configuration. **Juvenile polyps** are the **most common type** of hamartomatous colonic polyps.
   a. They occur principally in children.
   b. They usually present as blood-streaked stools.
   c. They are benign, with no malignant potential.
   d. Treatment should reflect the benign behavior. Removal of the polyps is indicated if safe; otherwise, observation is indicated.

4. **Hyperplastic polyps** arise in as many as 50% of adult colons and are often located where colorectal cancers present (see section XII C).
   a. They arise as presumably minor imbalances between cell division and desquamation, are benign, and require removal only to ascertain the diagnosis.
   b. Their clinical importance lies in the need to differentiate them from adenomatous polyps.

**D.** Because of their malignant potential, **neoplastic polyps** deserve further discussion.

1. **Adenomatous polyps**
   a. **General considerations.** These are the most common neoplasias of the adult colon, occurring at one time or another in approximately 5% of the adult population in the United States.
      (1) Eighty percent are located in the rectosigmoid colon.
      (2) Most are pedunculated, with a vascular, connective tissue stalk covered by normal mucosa. The texture is usually firm.
      (3) Two-thirds are smaller than 1 cm in diameter.
      (4) Malignancy is characterized by invasion of the stalk.
      (5) Although they are most commonly asymptomatic and are discovered as incidental sigmoidoscopic findings, adenomatous polyps may present as rectal bleeding.
   b. **Treatment** is directed towards their malignant potential.
      (1) Polyps that can be removed safely via sigmoidoscope or colonoscope [see section VIII D 3 e (2)] should be removed and submitted for histologic evaluation. Evidence of malignant invasion of the stalk calls for formal colonic resection.
      (2) Similar consideration should be given to polyps showing malignant lymphatic invasion or a high degree of undifferentiation.
      (3) When polyps cannot be removed endoscopically, therapy must be individualized, weighing the malignant potential against the patient's overall operative risk. When surgery is indicated, options include colotomy with polypectomy or, especially when malignant potential is high (e.g., for larger polyps), formal colonic resection (i.e., resection including an adequate margin of normal tissue).

**2. Villous adenomas** are far less common than adenomatous polyps and are rarely seen in patients under 45 years of age, the average patient being in the sixth decade of life.
   **a.** Sixty percent of villous adenomas are located in the rectum, thirty percent in the rectosigmoid or sigmoid colon, and ten percent elsewhere.
   **b.** These polyps are characterized by multiple frond-like projections from their surface. Grossly, they are often bulky, sessile, and soft, making detection by palpation sometimes difficult.
   **c.** The incidence of malignancy is the highest of all colorectal polyps, approximately 35%. Invasive malignancy is present in as many as one-third of all specimens.
   **d.** The clinical presentation is usually rectal bleeding, often accompanied by mucus. A rare syndrome includes watery diarrhea, muscle weakness, and weight loss.
   **e. Treatment** is directed towards the malignant potential.
      **(1) Biopsy** is often the initial step.
      **(2)** Small polyps may be removed endoscopically. Removal is sufficient therapy for polyps not showing invasive malignancy.
      **(3)** Larger polyps and those showing evidence of invasive malignancy on biopsy may be removed via formal anterior resection when they are located more than 7 cm above the dentate line.
      **(4)** For lesions located lower than 7 cm above the dentate line, wide local transanal excision is indicated, with abdominoperineal resection for lesions showing invasive malignancy.
         **(a)** Efforts to save the anal sphincter and spare the patient a permanent colostomy are discussed in section XII F 1 d and e.
         **(b)** Recurrence of villous adenomas is common, and thus frequent endoscopic follow-up is recommended after local excision.

**3. Villoglandular polyps** are now more frequently recognized. **Treatment** again is directed towards the malignant potential.

## E. Polyposis syndromes

**1. Familial polyposis** is a rare autosomal dominant disorder, characterized by multiple adenomatous polyps throughout the colon and rectum. Approximately one-half of the children of affected parents are afflicted with the disorder, and only those individuals with polyps transmit the disorder. Left untreated, the disease is uniformly fatal, with carcinoma developing in 100% of affected patients by the age of 50 years.
   **a. Clinical presentation**
      **(1)** Polyps usually present in early adult life.
      **(2)** Early on, the polyps are sessile and are found in the distal colon and rectum. Later, they become pedunculated and diffuse throughout the colon and rectum. The small bowel is not involved.
      **(3)** The disorder usually presents as rectal bleeding, abdominal pain, or both. Anemia and weight loss may be present.
   **b.** The **diagnosis** is confirmed by sigmoidoscopy and barium enema. Once the disorder has been diagnosed in one member of a family, examination of the entire family is indicated.
   **c. Treatment** is surgical, directed towards eradicating the polyps. Surgery should be performed prior to the third decade of life to prevent the development of cancer.
      **(1)** Total colectomy with ileoproctostomy saves the patient a permanent colostomy but demands fulguration of polyps remaining in the rectal stump as well as frequent and regular sigmoidoscopic examinations of the remaining rectum.
      **(2)** Other options include abdominoperineal resection with permanent ileostomy (which is not desirable in such a young age group) and colectomy with removal of rectal mucosa and ileoanal anastomosis.

**2. Gardner's syndrome** is considered by some authorities to be a variant of familial polyposis. It is transmitted by an autosomal dominant gene with varying penetrance.
   **a. Clinical presentation**
      **(1)** Gardner's syndrome is characterized by multiple colorectal polyps which are more scattered than those seen in familial polyposis. Polyps are occasionally present in the small bowel.
      **(2)** As compared to familial polyposis, the polyps often develop later in life but have very similar malignant potential.
      **(3)** Additional features include:
         **(a)** Hard tissue tumors (e.g., osteomas)
         **(b)** Soft tissue tumors (e.g., inclusion cysts)
         **(c)** Desmoid tumors

        **(d)** Mesenteric fibromatosis
        **(e)** Dental anomalies
    **b. Treatment** is surgical and is identical in approach to that for familial polyposis.

  **3. Peutz-Jeghers syndrome** is also an autosomal dominant disorder.
    **a. Clinical presentation**
      **(1)** Melanin spots appear on the buccal mucosa, lips, and digits.
      **(2)** There are polyps throughout the entire gastrointestinal tract. These polyps are hamartomas with no malignant potential.
      **(3) Presenting symptoms** may be those of intussusception with colicky abdominal pain.
    **b. Treatment** is designed to remove symptomatic polyps with minimal intestinal resection.

  **4. Turcot syndrome** is believed to be a variant of Gardner's syndrome. Patients develop central nervous system tumors as well as polyposis coli.

## XII. CARCINOMA OF THE COLON AND RECTUM

  **A. Incidence**

    **1.** Carcinoma of the colon and rectum is the **most common visceral cancer in the United States**. After skin cancer (the most common cancer in both sexes), colorectal cancer ranks second in incidence to lung cancer in men and breast cancer in women.

    **2.** The disease has a peak incidence in the seventh decade of life.

    **3.** Cancer of the colon is slightly more prevalent in women. For rectal cancer, this prevalence is reversed.

  **B. Etiology**

    **1. Genetic.** Although there is no absolute evidence of genetic inheritance, some families do have a very high incidence of colorectal cancer.

    **2. Environmental.** Some regions, such as the United States and Great Britain, have an exceptionally high incidence of colorectal cancer, while others, such as Saharan Africa, have an extraordinarily low occurrence. **Food intake** has been implicated.
      **a.** Diets high in fat and low in fiber may explain the increased incidence in some regions.
      **b.** Increased bile acids and a slow intestinal transit time, the results of a high-fat, low-fiber diet, have been put forth as explanations.

    **3. Inflammatory and polypoid disorders** have been associated with an increased risk of colorectal cancer.

  **C. Pathologic findings**

    **1.** Over 60% of colorectal cancers are located in the distal colon, and more than one-third of these are in the rectum, within reach of the examining finger. Recent reports have indicated an increase in the number of cancers found in the cecum and ascending colon. Colonoscopy has contributed to these recent trends.

    **2. Gross description**
      **a.** Colorectal carcinomas may be
        **(1)** Polypoid (sessile or pedunculated)
        **(2)** Scirrhous
        **(3)** Ulcerated
        **(4)** Nodular
      **b.** Scirrhous lesions are most often left-sided, with "napkin-ring" encirclement of the bowel.
      **c.** Bulky polypoid lesions are most often right-sided.

    **3. Histologic classification**
      **a.** Adenocarcinoma is the predominant type of lesion.
      **b.** The most widely accepted classification is the **Duke-Astler-Coller system**.
        **(1)** Classification is based on the primary mode of spread:
          **(a)** Direct extension through the bowel wall
          **(b)** Lymphatic spread (which is the most common)
          **(c)** Hematogenous spread
        **(2)** Lesions are usually classified grossly at operation and then histologically by the pathologist.
          **(a) Stage A**: Confined to the mucosa
          **(b) Stage $B_1$**: Negative nodes; extension into, but not through, the muscularis propria
          **(c) Stage $B_2$**: Negative nodes; extension through the muscularis propria

      (d) **Stage C$_1$**: Same as stage B$_1$ but with positive nodes
      (e) **Stage C$_2$**: Same as stage B$_2$ but with positive nodes
      (f) **Stage D**: Distant metastases

### D. Prognosis

1. The prognosis does not correlate well with the size of the lesion on gross examination, and it correlates only moderately well with the cell morphology.

2. However, the prognosis does correlate well with the Duke-Astler-Coller classification: 5-year survival rates are lower in patients who have greater penetration into the bowel wall and positive nodes.

3. Rectal cancer has an overall lower survival rate than does colon cancer.

### E. Diagnosis

1. **Clinical presentation** depends upon the location of the tumor, the size of the tumor, and the extent of spread.
   a. **Right-sided lesions**, those associated with midgut origin, often present as anemia from a slow, chronic blood loss. Although pain and a right-sided mass may be present, the large caliber of this part of the bowel and the liquid nature of the stool make obstruction uncommon.
   b. **Left-sided lesions** more often present as a degree of obstruction that begins as a change in bowel habits. A smaller bowel lumen with more solid stool, along with the more frequent occurrence of annular lesions, contributes to this mode of presentation.
   c. **Rectal carcinoma** most often presents as blood in the stool. Obstruction is uncommon.
   d. In addition to obstruction, the complications of hemorrhage, perforation, or both may be presenting symptoms. This is rare, however.

2. **Diagnostic studies** include:
   a. Barium enema
   b. Endoscopy with biopsy
      (1) Sigmoidoscopy
      (2) Colonoscopy
   c. Preoperative determination of baseline carcinoembryonic antigen (CEA) levels (see section XII G 1)

### F. Treatment

1. **Surgery** is the mainstay of treatment.
   a. A properly prepared bowel, cleansed of fecal material and with a diminished microbial flora, is associated with a lower incidence of postoperative complications. Although many regimens exist, there are three major **components to colon preparation**.
      (1) **Mechanical.** Enemas are given after oral cathartics such as magnesium citrate or mannitol.
      (2) **Antimicrobial.** Oral antibiotics are usually administered after cathartics and are not absorbed from the bowel lumen. A basic regimen consists of 1 g of neomycin and 1 g of erythromycin base at 1 P.M., 2 P.M., and 11 P.M., on the day prior to surgery.
      (3) **Dietary.** The diet is restricted to clear liquids for several days prior to surgery.
   b. **Prophylactic use of a broad-spectrum antibiotic** with anaerobic coverage, administered intravenously just prior to operation and for 24 hours postoperatively, has been shown to lower the incidence of postoperative wound infection.
   c. **Surgical resection** involves the removal of the cancerous bowel plus varying lengths of proximal and distal segments of colon, and also the lymph node–bearing mesentery consistent with the arterial blood supply to that segment of colon.
      (1) For example, resection of a cecal lesion would involve removal of a short segment of terminal ileum, the cecum, and the ascending colon up to the midtransverse colon, including mesentery incorporating the ileocolic and right colic arteries and the right branch of the middle colic artery.
      (2) Resection of lesions of the descending colon, sigmoid colon, or upper rectum would involve **coloproctostomy**. This procedure is often referred to as **low anterior resection** when the anastomosis is below the peritoneal reflection.
   d. One of the primary considerations in resection of rectal carcinoma involves **how low in the rectum the lesion is located**.
      (1) In the past, 5 cm of distal rectum beyond the lesion was considered a mandatory margin for adequate resection. Thus, low lesions (i.e., those at or below 5 cm to 7 cm above the dentate line) were routinely treated with abdominoperineal resection (**Miles's operation**), which includes removal of the distal colon, rectum, and anus and a permanent colostomy.

    **(2)** A distal margin of 5 cm is no longer universally mandated. This fact, along with newer surgical techniques (e.g., the use of stapling devices), has allowed low rectal lesions to be treated by resection and reanastomosis to a much smaller rectal cuff or to the anus. The anal sphincter is thereby saved and permanent colostomy is avoided without a decrease in survival rates or an increase in recurrence rates.

  **e.** As is true in all of surgery, operations for colorectal cancer need to be individualized. More limited resection of the bowel, even in the face of widespread disease or distant metastases, is indicated to avoid colonic obstruction. Attempts at sphincter-saving procedures may be more desirable in younger patients to avoid a permanent colostomy.

  **f.** When surgery must be performed in the face of complications (i.e., obstruction, perforation, or hemorrhage), consideration must be given to the increased morbidity associated with an unprepared bowel, an active intra-abdominal infection, or both.

    **(1)** No anastomosis should be performed when there is active, acute infection.

    **(2)** Many surgeons feel that a right-sided lesion can be treated by hemicolectomy with primary anastomosis despite an unprepared bowel.

    **(3)** Left-sided lesions are usually treated in staged procedures, with removal of the lesion if possible, exteriorization of the proximal end of the colon as a colostomy, and either exteriorization of the distal stoma as a mucous fistula or intra-abdominal closure of the distal segment as a Hartmann's pouch, followed by reanastomosis at a later date, again if possible.

    **(4)** A simple diverting colostomy of the proximal end of the colon may be indicated in high-risk patients.

  **2. Adjuvant therapy**

    **a.** The role of **radiation therapy** for colorectal cancer is an evolving one. Presently, many centers are combining this modality with surgical therapy to improve survival rates, local recurrence rates, or both.

    **b. Chemotherapy**, although used, has been ineffective in improving the survival rates.

**G. Recurrences**

  **1. Determination of CEA levels** has become an accepted means of **screening** for the recurrence of colorectal cancer.

    **a.** The CEA level drops after adequate initial resection.

    **b.** An elevated CEA level in the follow-up period should prompt a search for recurrences. Some authorities advocate doing a repeat laparotomy based on an elevated CEA level even when no recurrence of disease is identified by routine diagnostic studies (e.g., endoscopy).

  **2.** Recurrence of colorectal cancer is often painful, debilitating and **difficult to treat**.

    **a. Surgery** to provide palliation and to relieve obstruction may be indicated.

    **b. Chemotherapy** is used with modest success.

    **c. Radiation therapy** may be palliative, especially for recurrences in the perineal area and for isolated bony metastases.

    **d. Hepatic resections** for isolated liver metastases and intrahepatic chemotherapeutic infusions have been associated with improved survival rates.

# XIII. MISCELLANEOUS COLORECTAL NEOPLASIAS

**A. Carcinoid tumors**

  **1.** Carcinoid tumors are rare in the colon.

    **a.** When present, they are usually benign and asymptomatic (i.e., they are not usually associated with carcinoid syndrome).

    **b.** Unlike the case in adenocarcinoma, the malignancy of carcinoid tumors correlates with size: Lesions larger than 1 cm have a high incidence of malignancy.

    **c.** Surgical therapy is identical to that for adenocarcinoma (see section XII F).

  **2. Rectal carcinoids** are usually small and asymptomatic; they are considered incidental findings and are treated with local excision.

  **3.** The **appendix** is the most common location of carcinoid tumors; even here they are rare. They are nearly all benign and are adequately treated by means of simple appendectomy. Right hemicolectomy is indicated for invasive carcinoids of the appendix.

**B. Tumors of the appendix** are extremely rare. There are three recognized histologic types:

  **1.** Carcinoid tumors (see above)

2. Adenocarcinoma, which is treated identically to colonic carcinoma; the prognosis is similar as well

3. Mucoceles, benign cystic dilatations of the appendix containing mucinous material

C. Neoplasia may, although rarely, involve any type of tissue in the colon and rectum, including:

1. **Lymphoid** (e.g., lymphoma, lymphosarcoma)

2. **Adipose** (e.g., lipoma, liposarcoma)

3. **Muscle** (e.g., leiomyoma, leiomyosarcoma)

## XIV. INFECTIOUS DISORDERS

A. **Pseudomembranous colitis**

1. **Etiology**
   a. Pseudomembranous colitis is a severe diarrheal disorder that follows **prolonged antibiotic administration**.
   b. Clindamycin and ampicillin are the antibiotics that are implicated most frequently, although incidence reports vary.

2. Overgrowth of *Clostridium difficile* has been reported as the **pathogenesis**.

3. **Diagnosis** is confirmed by:
   a. **Endoscopy**, which usually shows whitish raised plaques and a pseudomembrane
   b. **Testing the stool** for the presence of *C. difficile* exotoxin

4. **Treatment** consists of discontinuing the offending antibiotics and administering **vancomycin** in 500-mg doses four times a day for a least 4 days.

B. **Amebic colitis**

1. **Etiology.** Amebiasis is caused by the protozoan *Entamoeba histolytica*.

2. The infection primarily involves the colon (other organs, such as the liver, are involved secondarily), and it is seen in both acute and chronic forms.
   a. **Acute amebic colitis** is rare and is associated with high fever, severe abdominal pain, and diarrhea. **Diagnosis** is confirmed by endoscopy and identification of the offending organism in the stool.
   b. **Chronic amebic colitis**, the more common form of the infection, results in a prolonged, less severe diarrhea. The most common serious **complication** is amebic abscess of the liver.

3. **Treatment** is with metronidazole.

## XV. INFLAMMATORY DISORDERS

A. **Acute appendicitis** is the most common acute condition requiring acute abdominal surgery.

1. The peak **incidence** of this disease is in the second and third decade of life. It is rare in the very young.

2. **Etiology**
   a. **Obstruction of the lumen of the appendix** is the principal cause.
      (1) **Fecaliths** (inspissated stool) are the **most common cause** of the obstruction.
      (2) Less common causes include:
         (a) Lymphoid hypertrophy
         (b) Barium
         (c) Intestinal worms
   b. Obstruction of the lumen is followed by persistent appendiceal mucosal secretions, gradual distention with inflammation of the appendix, bacterial overgrowth, and, if the condition is allowed to progress, ischemia, gangrene, and perforation.

3. **Diagnosis** is based on history, physical examination, laboratory findings, and, when necessary, x-rays.
   a. The **classic history** includes **pain** as the prime symptom.
      (1) The pain begins in the epigastrium, gradually moves to the periumbilical region, and finally, over a period of 1 to 12 hours, localizes in the right lower quadrant.
      (2) This pain sequence is not invariable, and may differ considerably from the above de-

        scription, especially in light of the varied anatomic locations of the appendix (see section I C).

    **b.** **Anorexia** is a second prominent symptom and is nearly always present to some degree. **Vomiting** occurs in about three-fourths of the patients.

    **c.** The **sequence of symptoms** is important in contributing to the diagnosis. Anorexia followed by pain and then by vomiting (when it occurs) is the classic course. Vomiting preceding pain should call the diagnosis into question.

    **d.** **Physical findings** depend primarily on the stage of the disease and the location of the appendix.

        **(1)** Temperature and pulse are only slightly elevated early in the disease. Higher elevations may indicate a complication such as perforation or abscess.

        **(2)** Physical examination usually reveals pain on palpation over **McBurney's point** (two-thirds of the distance from the umbilicus to the anterior iliac spine) when the appendix is located anteriorly. When it is located in the pelvis, abdominal findings may be minimal and only rectal examination may yield significant findings.

        **(3)** Abdominal muscle guarding and rebound tenderness reflect the stage of the disease, since progression is associated with peritoneal irritation.

    **e.** Several **signs**, if present, assist in the diagnosis.

        **(1)** **Rovsing's sign** is pain in the right lower quadrant on palpation of the left lower quadrant.

        **(2)** **Psoas sign** is pain on extension of the right thigh with the patient lying on the left side.

        **(3)** **Obturator sign** is pain on internal rotation of the flexed right thigh with the patient supine.

    **f.** **Laboratory findings**

        **(1)** A moderate leukocytosis (10,000 to 16,000 white blood cells) with a predominance of neutrophils is usual. A normal white blood cell count does *not* rule out appendicitis, however.

        **(2)** Urinalysis may show a few red blood cells.

    **g.** **X-ray studies** are usually used only when the diagnosis is in question.

        **(1)** **Plain abdominal films** may show a localized right lower quadrant ileus or, on occasion, a radiopaque fecalith.

        **(2)** **Barium enema** may be helpful in difficult cases when an accurate diagnosis remains elusive. A filling defect in the cecum is the most reliable indicator of appendicitis with this study.

    **h.** The **differential diagnosis** for right lower quadrant pain includes:

        **(1)** Mesenteric lymphadenitis

        **(2)** Regional ileitis

        **(3)** Pelvic inflammatory disease

        **(4)** Gastroenteritis

        **(5)** Ruptured ovarian cyst (or other ovarian disorders)

        **(6)** Urinary tract disorders (infection, calculus)

        **(7)** Meckel's diverticulitis

        **(8)** Cecal or sigmoid diverticulitis

**4.** The accuracy of diagnosis is generally in the range of 80% to 85%. Thus, at operation, surgeons will encounter disorders other than appendicitis in 15% to 20% of the patients with this preoperative diagnosis.

**5.** **Treatment** is surgical.

    **a.** The appendix is usually approached via a transverse (Rocky-Davis) or oblique (McBurney) incision placed over McBurney's point.

    **b.** Appendectomy is performed, with ligation of the mesoappendix, containing the blood supply, followed by ligation and transection of the appendix at its base where it joins the cecum.

    **c.** When a normal appendix is encountered, thorough exploration should be performed to rule out other pathologic processes.

**6.** **Complications**

    **a.** **Clinical course**

        **(1)** Left untreated, an unknown number of cases of appendicitis will proceed to **perforation**.

        **(2)** Following perforation, the contents of the abdominal cavity will attempt to contain the process, forming a **phlegmon**, an inflamed mass of matted intestine and omentum.

        **(3)** A phlegmon may progress to a fibrous walling off of a collection of pus secondary to the rupture, an **appendiceal abscess**.

        **(4)** If the body's attempts to contain the perforation are unsuccessful, the entire abdominal cavity may become contaminated, causing a diffuse **peritonitis**.

        **(5)** Significant temperature and pulse elevation, marked leukocytosis, and findings typical of peritoneal inflammation, with or without a mass (phlegmon or abscess) in the right lower quadrant, indicate **appendiceal rupture**. The mass may sometimes be appreciated only on rectal examination.

    **b.** Abdominal ultrasonography may assist in the differential diagnosis of a right lower quadrant mass.

    **c. Therapy** of appendiceal rupture includes antibiotics and intravenous fluid therapy, with surgical intervention including appendectomy and abscess drainage. The timing of such intervention is individualized to each patient.

    **d.** Rupture of the appendix significantly increases **postoperative morbidity and mortality rates**. The approach to acute appendicitis should be timely intervention in order to prevent progression to this complication.

**7. Antibiotics in appendicitis**

    **a. Preoperatively**, broad-spectrum intravenous antibiotics are indicated to lessen the incidence of postoperative wound infection.

    **b. Postoperatively**, antibiotics are continued for 24 hours for patients with uncomplicated appendicitis.

        **(1)** Antibiotics are usually continued for 5 to 7 days postoperatively for cases of appendiceal rupture with abscess formation.

        **(2)** Antibiotics are usually continued for 7 to 10 days for cases of appendiceal rupture with diffuse peritonitis.

**8. Appendicitis in the child**

    **a.** Though rare in infants and young children, appendicitis does occur in this age group.

    **b. Perforation** is more common, and usually results from misdiagnosis and consequently delayed treatment.

    **c.** In general, the disease progresses more rapidly, and when perforation occurs, it results in a diffuse peritonitis, as the immature omentum is not successful in containing the process.

**9. Appendicitis in the elderly**

    **a.** Signs and symptoms may be deceptively mild in this age group, making the diagnosis more difficult.

    **b.** Despite its mild presentation, appendicitis in the elderly has a significantly higher morbidity and mortality rate.

    **c.** The frequency of perforation and diffuse peritonitis is significantly higher. This, along with the higher number of concomitant diseases (e.g., cardiopulmonary disorders), accounts for the severity of the disease in the elderly.

**B. Ulcerative colitis** is an uncommon inflammatory disorder primarily involving the mucosa and submucosa of the large bowel.

**1. Incidence**

    **a.** In the United States, the incidence is higher among Jews than among non-Jews.

    **b.** Females are affected more often than males in a ratio of 5 to 4.

    **c.** There is a bimodal age incidence, with peaks at ages 15 to 30 years and 50 to 80 years.

**2. Etiology.** The true etiology is unknown, but infectious, immunologic, genetic, and environmental causes have all been implicated.

**3. Pathologic findings**

    **a.** The colitis involves the rectum in almost all cases and then spreads proximally. When the rectum alone is involved, the disorder is termed "**ulcerative proctitis**." Spread is continuous, with no skip areas of normal bowel.

    **b.** The mucosa is involved initially, and spread to the submucosa with abscess formation in the crypts of Lieberkühn is common. The muscle layers are rarely involved.

    **c.** Pseudopolyps of the mucosa may be seen.

    **d.** In 30% of the patients, the entire colon is involved (**pancolitis**).

**4. Diagnosis**

    **a. Clinical presentation**

        **(1)** The onset may be acute or insidious.

        **(2)** The patient commonly presents with watery diarrhea, mixed with blood, pus, and mucus and accompanied by tenesmus and urgency.

        **(3)** Pain, fever, weight loss, and dehydration occur to varying degrees.

        **(4)** Extraintestinal manifestations may occur, including arthropathy, skin or mucosal lesions, uveitis, and pericarditis.

    **b.** The results of **physical examination** vary and depend on the acuteness and severity of the condition. There may be few abdominal findings or severe abdominal tenderness.

c. **Endoscopy**, with biopsy when safe, should be performed for diagnosis.
   (1) Findings include a mucosa that is friable and reddish, with no normal intervening areas.
   (2) Pseudopolyposis may be seen.
   (3) Endoscopy should be performed without cathartics, especially in fulminant cases. It should not be performed in the face of toxic dilatation of the colon because of the risk of perforation.
d. **Barium enema**
   (1) Mucosal irregularity is demonstrated, with shortening of the colon and loss of haustral markings in advanced cases.
   (2) Barium enema should not be done in the presence of megacolon.
e. **Laboratory findings**
   (1) Anemia and leukocytosis may be present to varying degrees.
   (2) Stool cultures are usually negative.
f. **Differential diagnosis**
   (1) Ulcerative colitis must be differentiated from other inflammatory or infectious disorders of the colon, especially Crohn's disease (see section XV C).
   (2) Malignancy and diverticular disease may also mimic ulcerative colitis in some ways.

5. **Complications**
   a. **Anorectal complications** including abscess with fistula formation may occur, although they are less common and less severe than in Crohn's colitis.
   b. **Toxic megacolon** is present in 3% to 5% of cases, with the transverse colon exceeding 6 cm. It is associated with severe prostration, and often the disease involves the muscular coats.
   c. **Colonic perforation**, often fatal, occurs in 3% of cases, especially in those with toxic megacolon. The sigmoid colon and the splenic flexure are the most common sites of perforation.
   d. **Massive hemorrhage** may occur, although this is rare.
   e. The incidence of **carcinoma** increases with the length of time that the disease exists, reaching 30% to 40% after 30 years.
      (1) Carcinomas tend to be multicentric and highly malignant when they occur.
      (2) Colonoscopic surveillance with mucosal biopsies is advocated by some authorities. Finding severe epithelial dysplasia warrants prompt proctocolectomy.

6. **Treatment**
   a. **Medical therapy** is the mainstay for uncomplicated disease, which includes 70% to 80% of all cases. It involves:
      (1) Antidiarrheal agents
      (2) Sulfasalazine, which is the anti-inflammatory agent of choice and probably should be tried in all patients
         (a) Sulfasalazine (salicylazosulfapyridine) combines a sulfa molecule with a salicylate molecule.
         (b) Apparently, the sulfa molecule acts as a carrier, delivering the therapeutic anti-inflammatory salicylate molecule to the colonic mucosa.
      (3) Steroids
         (a) Their role is controversial but steroids have been shown to control symptoms in many cases.
         (b) Maintenance steroid therapy does not prevent exacerbation of the disease.
      (4) Diet: A milk-free diet may be of benefit.
      (5) Supportive therapy, including physical and emotional rest
      (6) Immunosuppression, which is still under investigation
   b. Initial therapy for **toxic megacolon** is medical, and it is intensive. It involves nasogastric decompression, antibiotics, and intravenous administration of fluids and nutrition with discontinuation of anticholinergic and antidiarrheal agents.
   c. **Surgical therapy** is indicated when medical therapy fails or a surgically treatable complication ensues, such as hemorrhage, perforation, obstruction, or carcinoma. Long-standing ulcerative colitis, because of the increased risk of carcinoma, may be an indication for surgical intervention.
      (1) **Total proctocolectomy with permanent ileostomy** is the definitive procedure for cure. It is curative in 90% to 95% of the patients.
      (2) Various procedures have been devised to maintain "continence" of the ileostomy and thus dispense with external devices (e.g., Kock's "continent" ileostomy). These have had limited success.
      (3) Subtotal colectomy with ileoproctostomy may be attempted in patients with less severe rectal involvement, no perianal complications, and adequate sphincter function. As many as 60% of these patients will do well if properly selected.

**(4)** Subtotal colectomy with mucosal proctectomy and ileoanal anastomosis is now being performed in some centers. This may be done with or without an ileal reservoir and, when successful, spares the patient a permanent abdominal ileostomy. Again, patients should be selected carefully, and the operation should not be performed if the rectum is extensively involved or if the diagnosis of ulcerative colitis is in doubt.

**(5)** The morbidity and mortality rates are high in patients requiring emergency surgery.

**C. Crohn's disease** (see also Chapter 6, section IV)

    **1.** The major **diagnostic** consideration is differentiation of Crohn's disease (granulomatous colitis) from ulcerative colitis. Among the **characteristics of Crohn's colitis that distinguish it from ulcerative colitis** are:

        **a.** A greater likelihood of proximal colon involvement

        **b.** Transmural inflammation

        **c.** Skip areas of normal mucosa

        **d.** A higher incidence of fistulas

        **e.** More severe perianal disease

        **f.** X-rays demonstrating less shortening of the colon and increased preservation of haustral markings

        **g.** A lower incidence of severe acute complications (e.g., hemorrhage or perforation)

    **2. Treatment**

        **a.** Medical therapy is less effective than it is for ulcerative colitis. It includes the use of:

            **(1)** Steroids

            **(2)** Sulfasalazine

            **(3)** Azathioprine: Therapy with immunosuppressive agents is more successful in Crohn's disease than in ulcerative colitis.

        **b. Surgical therapy.** There is disagreement over the surgical procedure of choice.

            **(1)** Subtotal colectomy with ileoproctostomy can be performed either primarily or as a subsequent procedure.

            **(2)** Recently developed procedures being used for ulcerative colitis (see section XV B 6 c), are associated with unacceptable complications and recurrence rates in Crohn's disease.

    **3. Prognosis.** In general, the long-term outlook is not as favorable as that for ulcerative colitis. The recurrence rate in Crohn's disease is as high as 30%.

**D. Ischemic colitis**

    **1.** Individuals with ischemic colitis are usually elderly and have complicating medical disorders.

    **2.** The onset is usually characterized by acute abdominal pain, followed by a bloody bowel movement. Clinical presentation and course depend primarily on the extent, duration, and location of vascular occlusion.

        **a. Transient ischemia**

            **(1)** The affected area of the bowel receives some vascular compensation from the collateral circulation, and the associated symptoms are mild.

            **(2)** Barium enema may reveal "thumbprinting."

            **(3)** The ischemia may result in mucosal sloughing followed by mucosal regeneration with or without subsequent stricture formation.

        **b. Persistent ischemia** is due to a more prolonged impairment in blood flow.

            **(1)** The symptoms do regress, but slowly.

            **(2)** "Thumbprinting" as well as stricture may be seen on barium enema.

            **(3)** Secondary invasion by intestinal bacteria induces an inflammatory cycle that ends in healing by fibrosis, often with subsequent obstruction by stricture formation.

        **c. Total arterial occlusion**

            **(1)** The symptoms progress rapidly to peritonitis and septic shock.

            **(2)** Barium enema is contraindicated.

            **(3)** Gangrene and perforation are grave complications warranting immediate surgical intervention.

    **3. Treatment**

        **a.** When symptoms progress, indicating total arterial occlusion with gangrene of the large bowel, resection of the involved segment is performed as soon as the patient has been stabilized by rapid resuscitation.

        **b.** Transient and persistent ischemia may often be treated conservatively, with surgery performed subsequently for late complications (e.g., fibrotic stricture with obstruction), should they occur.

   **E. Radiation enterocolitis**

      **1.** Radiation enterocolitis is a dose-dependent disorder occurring after the intestines are exposed to more than 4000 rads of radiation.

      **2.** It is primarily an ischemic disorder in which an aggressive vasculitis results in small vessel thrombosis. Thickening of the bowel wall, fibrosis, and ulceration follow. Healing is impaired.

      **3.** Symptomatic **treatment** is desirable. Surgical intervention is difficult and is often unrewarding.

## XVI. VOLVULUS

   **A. General considerations**

      **1.** Volvulus occurs when mobile segments of large bowel rotate on the mesenteric axis, causing luminal obstruction and varying degrees of vascular compromise.

      **2.** This condition is seen most commonly in the sigmoid colon (90% of cases), followed by the cecum (10% of cases). It almost never occurs in the transverse colon.

   **B. Sigmoid volvulus**

      **1. Pathogenesis.** An elongated mobile sigmoid colon on a narrow mesenteric root is the classic setting. This anatomic state is often associated with prolonged chronic constipation, which can cause dilatation and lengthening of the sigmoid colon. Patients with neurologic disorders and elderly patients with prolonged periods of inactivity are therefore frequently at risk.

      **2. Clinical findings.** Symptoms are those of colonic obstruction. Marked abdominal distention and tympany may be present. Strangulation may occur, with concurrent progressive symptoms.

      **3. Diagnosis.** Plain x-rays may be diagnostic, showing a markedly distended sigmoid loop. Barium enema may show the typical **"bird's beak" deformity**.

      **4. Treatment**
         **a.** The **therapy of choice** is decompression. The site of obstruction is first determined by sigmoidoscopy, and a rectal tube is inserted to deflate the distended loop. Elective sigmoid resection then follows. Nonoperative therapy alone is associated with a very high recurrence rate.
         **b.** Signs of **strangulation** should always be looked for, since this complication necessitates early operative intervention. Sigmoidoscopy reveals a bluish or black mucosa when strangulation is present.

   **C. Cecal volvulus**

      **1.** An abnormally mobile cecum and ascending colon, which are usually attached retroperitoneally, are prerequisites for cecal volvulus. Twisting is usually around the pedicle of the ileocolic artery, and thus closed-loop obstruction and ischemia occur earlier in this disease than in sigmoid volvulus.

      **2. Clinical findings** are those of acute small-bowel obstruction with peritoneal signs indicating strangulation (e.g., rebound tenderness, involuntary muscle guarding).

      **3. Diagnosis** may be by plain abdominal x-rays, barium enema, or both.

      **4. Treatment** is immediate surgical intervention.
         **a.** Detorsion with fixation of the cecum to the lateral abdominal wall (**cecopexy**) suffices if the cecum is viable.
         **b.** Right colectomy with ileotransverse colostomy is indicated for a nonviable cecum.

      **5.** Delay in the diagnosis and treatment of cecal volvulus contributes significantly to the mortality rate, which is in the range of 10%.

## XVII. DIVERTICULOSIS

   **A.** The herniated mucosal pouches of diverticulosis occur principally in the left colon. Diverticulosis is a common disorder, seen in up to 35% of adult Americans by the age of 65 years.

   **B. Etiology**

      **1.** The mechanism whereby diverticula occur is not fully clear, although chronic constipation, age, and perhaps familial tendencies do seem to contribute.

2. **Dietary factors** appear to be prominent. Increased intraluminal pressure, hard stools, and constipation may be associated with the low-residue diets that are common in industrial countries. Diverticulosis is rare in Asia and Africa, where diets are high in fiber.

C. **Pathophysiology**

1. In diverticulosis, the mucosa and submucosa herniate through the circular muscle layer. (The herniations are thus strictly "false" diverticula, lacking a muscle layer.)

2. The **sigmoid colon** is involved most frequently, with other portions of the large bowel involved to a greater or lesser extent.

3. Diverticula are usually located between the mesenteric and antimesenteric teniae in regions where blood vessels penetrate the muscle wall into the submucosa.
   a. These penetrating vessels cause areas of weakness where a mucosal-submucosal herniation may occur.
   b. They also remain in close proximity to the neck of the diverticulum, explaining the bleeding that can be a prominent symptom of diverticulosis.

D. **Clinical presentation**

1. Diverticulosis per se causes no symptoms, and thus the majority of affected individuals never receive therapy.

2. Patients present clinically when **complications** ensue, principally bleeding or inflammation (**diverticulitis**).

3. Many authorities believe that dietary management using foods with a high fiber content and stool bulk–forming agents may be a **prophylactic measure**, although this has not been proven.

E. **Complications of diverticulosis**

1. **Bleeding** is associated most often with diverticulosis, as opposed to diverticulitis. (The bleeding is felt to be secondary to thrombosis of the penetrating vessels in diverticulitis.) Such bleeding accounts for as many as two-thirds of the cases of massive lower gastrointestinal hemorrhage.
   a. **Diagnosis**
      (1) Commonly there is **acute and profuse rectal bleeding** without symptoms of inflammation.
      (2) **Diagnostic steps** include endoscopy, radionuclide scanning, arteriography, and barium enema.
   b. **Treatment**
      (1) Most bleeding will stop with **transfusions and supportive care**, ideally allowing a more controlled workup to identify the source of bleeding accurately.
      (2) Unceasing or recurrent hemorrhages are cause for **surgery**.
         (a) In general, all bleeding diverticular areas of the large bowel should be removed.
         (b) When the hemorrhage is massive and the site of bleeding has not been identified preoperatively, management may be difficult.
            (i) Attempts to localize the site intraoperatively are often frustrating.
            (ii) When the site cannot be identified with confidence, **total abdominal colectomy with ileoproctostomy** may be the only alternative.
            (iii) Selective intra-arterial infusion of vasopressin may be a therapeutic and temporizing measure to avoid the higher risk of mortality associated with emergency surgical intervention.

2. **Diverticulitis** is the most common complication of diverticular disease.
   a. **Pathogenesis**
      (1) It is believed that the neck of the diverticulum becomes obstructed by inspissated fecal contents, followed by gradual distention of the diverticulum with bacterial proliferation.
      (2) One diverticulum may set up a process of inflammation and edema that secondarily involves multiple diverticula.
         (a) Extension may be longitudinal, resulting in the formation of intramural fistulas.
         (b) Progression of the inflammation may lead to the most serious complications of perforation (confined or free), abscess formation, and intestinal obstruction.
   b. **Diagnosis**
      (1) **Clinical presentation** usually involves left lower quadrant pain (cramping or dull aching), a change in bowel habits, a low-grade fever (possibly with chills), leukocytosis, anorexia, and nausea (less frequently, vomiting).

(2) **Physical examination** may reveal signs of peritoneal inflammation in the left lower quadrant. A mass may be palpable. Bowel sounds are usually normal.

(3) When done properly, **sigmoidoscopy** and **barium enema** may aid in confirming a diagnosis. However, they should not be performed in the presence of significant peritoneal findings, as the risk of perforation is great.

c. **Treatment**

(1) **Nonoperative therapy** should be the initial approach to uncomplicated diverticulitis.

    (a) This includes bowel rest, with or without nasogastric suction, and administration of intravenous fluids and broad-spectrum antibiotics.

    (b) On this regimen, substantial clinical improvement should occur within 24 to 48 hours.

(2) Patients who do not respond to medical therapy, those with complications of the disease, or those with recurrent attacks should undergo **surgical therapy**.

    (a) Surgical therapy is ideally carried out electively after the acute process has subsided.

    (b) Resection of the properly prepared diverticular colon with primary anastomosis may then be performed.

d. **Complications of diverticulitis**

(1) **Types**

    (a) **Obstruction** results when inflammation and edema narrow the lumen of the large bowel. The small bowel can also become obstructed if it is involved in the inflammatory process.

    (b) **Perforation** occurs when the inflammation and distention disrupt the integrity of the diverticular mucosa and submucosa.

        (i) Early on, the perforation can be walled off, forming a localized abscess and thus preventing a spreading peritonitis.

        (ii) If small, these walled-off abscesses can often be managed nonoperatively until elective resection can be carried out.

    (c) **Fistulas** may form if adjacent organs become involved. Symptoms such as urinary or vaginal drainage of feces should alert one to this complication.

(2) **Treatment**

    (a) Ideally, even these complications of diverticulitis may respond to the aggressive medical management used in uncomplicated diverticulitis, allowing resection of the bowel after the acute infection has subsided.

    (b) **When to intervene surgically** is a matter of clinical judgment that is based on the severity of the patient's disease and the direction of the clinical course.

    (c) When surgical intervention is necessary in the face of acute diverticulitis with associated infection and inflammation, primary anastomosis is dangerous.

        (i) Although operative therapy in this setting remains controversial, the **Hartmann procedure** is commonly performed. All diseased bowel is removed, a proximal diverting colostomy is created, and the distal end of the colon is oversewn (Hartmann's pouch), with drainage.

        (ii) Once the acute process has subsided (which usually takes several months), the patient returns for reanastomosis of the proximal colon to the Hartmann's pouch, restoring continuity.

3. **Cecal diverticulitis**

a. This is a rare entity involving **inflammation of a single**, usually congenital, **diverticulum**. The condition may mimic appendicitis.

b. **Treatment** is dictated by operative findings, with the extent of resection and the question of primary anastomosis based on considerations similar to those for sigmoid diverticulitis [see section XVII E 2 d (2) (c)].

# XVIII. DISORDERS OF THE ANORECTUM

A. **General surgical principles**

1. **Diagnostic considerations.** A principle to remember is that **anorectal symptoms may reflect other systemic diseases**, and thus thorough evaluation, including sigmoidoscopy, is indicated in the workup of patients with anorectal complaints.

2. **Preoperative care**

a. Prior to surgery, the anorectum should be prepared by cleansing enemas.

b. Whether or not to shave the anorectal region prior to surgery is controversial.

c. Depending on the severity of the condition, anorectal procedures may often be performed under local anesthesia in an outpatient setting, or under spinal anesthesia.

**3. Surgical techniques**

    **a.** In general, these involve gentle handling of tissues, sharp dissection wherever possible, the use of absorbable suture material, and closure of wounds whenever possible.

    **b. Proper exposure** is essential. This is aided by the positioning of the patient, the use of anorectal retractors, relaxation of the anal sphincter via anesthesia, and gradual anal dilation.

**4. Postoperative care**

    **a.** An important aspect is **relief of pain**, which includes softening of the stool.

        **(1)** Oral stool softeners, gentle laxatives, warm sitz baths, and the local application of anti-inflammatory agents are all helpful.

        **(2)** Often, when wounds are left open, packing is in place, and gradual removal of the packing after sitz baths helps to minimize discomfort.

    **b. Complications** include **bleeding**, which is common and can usually be managed locally, **stricture**, **incontinence**, and urinary tract symptoms, most commonly **urinary retention**.

## B. Hemorrhoidal disease

**1.** The superior, middle, and inferior rectal veins form a submucosal network in the area of the columns of Morgagni. These veins give rise, upon dilatation, to **internal hemorrhoids**. Dilatation of the most inferior rectal veins, which drain into the systemic circulation, give rise to **external hemorrhoids**.

**2. Etiology**

    **a.** Both **systemic and local factors** are involved, including constipation, increased abdominal pressure on voiding or secondary to straining while moving the bowels, and chronic cough.

    **b. Diet** has been implicated as well.

**3. Clinical presentation** varies according to the location of the dilated hemorrhoidal veins. Hemorrhoids are most commonly located in the left lateral, right anterior, and right posterior anal canal.

    **a. External hemorrhoids** usually are located beneath the dentate line and are covered by squamous epithelium. They are normally asymptomatic except when an external hemorrhoid becomes acutely thrombosed and quite painful.

    **b. Internal hemorrhoids** most often present as painless blood-streaked stool. As internal hemorrhoids enlarge, they may prolapse.

    **c. Diagnosis** of either disorder is relatively simple, involving direct inspection via anoscopy.

**4. Treatment**

    **a.** Recent trends have emphasized **nonoperative therapy**. Most hemorrhoidal disease may be treated with medicated suppositories, sitz baths, and dietary adjustments.

    **b. Acutely thrombosed external hemorrhoids** may be treated by excision under local anesthesia as an outpatient procedure. Incision with evacuation is usually inadequate.

    **c. Small hemorrhoids** that do not respond to medical therapy and that remain a constant concern to the patient may also be treated via **rubberband ligation**. This can also be done as an outpatient procedure.

    **d. Surgical hemorrhoidectomy** is usually reserved for **complications** of hemorrhoidal disease, including persistent prolapse, pain or bleeding, and for **large hemorrhoids** that do not respond to medical treatment. In general, the patient who requires surgical management is suffering from severe symptoms.

        **(1)** Surgery is directed at removing all hemorrhoidal tissue followed by primary closure, if possible, without formation of anal stricture and without disruption of anal continence.

        **(2)** Following adequate removal of hemorrhoidal tissue, recurrence requiring surgery is uncommon.

## C. Anal fissure

**1.** An anal fissure is a tear of the squamous-lined portion of the anal canal. It most commonly results from persistent trauma in the anal canal. It is usually found in the midline and is more often posterior than anterior.

**2. Diagnosis** may be made by direct inspection and palpation, which should be gentle as these lesions are often extremely painful. Severe cases should alert the physician to search for **inflammatory bowel disease**.

**3. Treatment**

    **a.** This is most often **conservative** and involves the use of stool softeners, agents to relax the anal sphincter such as warm sitz baths, and local application of anti-inflammatory agents.

    **b. Operative therapy** is reserved for cases in which conservative measures have failed.
      **(1)** Lateral partial internal sphincterotomy, which can be done under local anesthesia, relieves tension on the fissure and relaxes the anal sphincter, thus allowing the fissured region to heal.
      **(2)** Sphincterotomy is combined with continued local and dietary management.

### D. Anal fistula

1. By **definition**, an anal fistula is an inflammatory tract between the perianal skin and the anal canal.

2. These tracts usually result from intersphincteric abscesses secondary to a chronic anorectal infection, perhaps complicated by anorectal trauma.

3. **Recurrent anorectal** abscesses should alert the physician to the possibility of fistula-in-ano, and a fistula should alert the physician to the possibility of inflammatory bowel disease.

4. **Treatment** is usually surgical.
    **a.** The primary procedure is **fistulotomy**. Identification of the fistula is mandatory before the unroofing of the fistulous tract so that a false tract will not be created when the fistula-in-ano is probed.
    **b. Fistulectomy** with removal of the entire tract is rarely necessary.
    **c.** Following fistulotomy, the wound may heal by second intention.
    **d.** Dietary management and the use of stool softeners, sitz baths, and local agents are combined with the surgical therapy.

### E. Anorectal abscess

1. Acute abscess formation in the perirectal and perianal regions is a common disorder. The abscess most commonly develops by extension of a local traumatic abscess within the anorectal canal.

2. **Clinical presentation** characteristically includes perirectal pain, swelling, and erythema, sometimes with high fever and systemic symptoms.

3. The **diagnosis** is usually apparent when abscesses present in the perianal or ischiorectal regions. Intersphincteric abscesses or abscesses located in deeper regions of the anorectal spaces are more difficult to diagnose.

4. **Treatment** is surgical, with prompt incision and drainage, usually accompanied by antibiotic therapy.
    **a. Adequate drainage** is essential.
      **(1)** The cavity is usually packed open, with removal of the packing over the next several days followed by irrigation of the cavity two to three times a day.
      **(2)** The majority of abscesses treated in this fashion will heal primarily without subsequent formation of a fistula-in-ano.
    **b.** The rapid recurrence of an abscess should alert the observer to the possibility of a fistula-in-ano.
    **c.** Because adequate drainage and adequate visualization of the involved region are mandatory, intersphincteric and supralevator abscesses are drained in the operating room where good relaxation of the anal sphincter may be obtained. Lower abscesses may often be drained in an outpatient setting.

### F. Rectal prolapse

1. In this rare condition, the rectal mucosa or the entire rectal wall prolapses to varying degrees through the anus. Prolapse is most prevalent in inactive elderly or institutionalized patients, and it is associated with irregular bowel habits.

2. The **etiology** is unclear, although theories include both herniation and intussusception in the region of the rectum. Contributing anatomic defects are an elongated and redundant rectosigmoid region, and a loss of muscle tone in the slings that support the pelvic floor and rectum.

3. **Treatment**
    **a.** Surgical intervention is directed towards repair of the anatomic defects, but whether the approach should be transabdominal or transperitoneal remains controversial.
    **b.** Patients with mild and infrequently recurring prolapse may be managed conservatively. Simplified surgical procedures, such as the Thiersch wire procedure, have been devised for elderly patients and for those who are at greater operative risk.

**G. Neoplasms of the anus**

1. **Epidermoid carcinoma** is a rare disorder, comprising 1% to 2% of all colorectal carcinomas.
   a. There are principally two **types**—squamous cell carcinoma and transitional cell or cloacogenic carcinoma.
      (1) **Squamous cell carcinoma** can occur either above or below the dentate line.
      (2) **Cloacogenic carcinoma** usually arises from the transitional zone above the dentate line.
      (3) Both types have a similar clinical course and poor prognosis.
   b. **Clinical presentation** is usually rectal pain and bleeding.
   c. The **diagnosis** is often delayed, contributing to the overall poor prognosis.
   d. **Treatment** is primarily **surgical** and takes into account the common route of spread to the superior rectal nodes, pelvic nodes, and inguinal nodes.
      (1) **Abdominoperineal resection** with wide excision of perineal lymph node–bearing tissue is the **treatment of choice**.
      (2) Newer **radiotherapy** protocols are being investigated and may contribute to the surgical approach.
      (3) **Management of the inguinal lymph nodes** is usually dictated by whether or not clinically palpable nodes are found prior to surgery.
         (a) Prophylactic lymph node dissection is usually not indicated.
         (b) However, the patient may benefit from excision of involved nodes that occur synchronously with the anal lesion, as well as from careful follow-up and excision of subsequently involved nodes.
         (c) The overall incidence of inguinal node involvement at some time during the course of the disease has been as high as 35% to 40%.
         (d) When groin dissection is carried out, it is usually radical in nature, involving both superficial and deep inguinal nodes.

2. **Malignant melanoma**
   a. This is a rare disorder of the anal canal, which represents, however, the third most common site for melanomas following the skin and eyes.
   b. These tumors arise from the epidermal lining of the anal canal and **present** most commonly as **rectal bleeding**.
   c. **Diagnosis** may be difficult, as many of the lesions are lightly pigmented or unpigmented entirely.
   d. **Treatment.** As in melanomas located elsewhere, these lesions are radioresistant and the only hope for cure is **early and radical surgery**.
   e. **Metastases**
      (1) **Lymphatic spread** is to the mesenteric lymph nodes in perhaps 30% of the patients. Inguinal node involvement is less common.
      (2) **Hematogenous spread**, primarily to the liver and lungs, occurs early and is rapid, contributing to the extremely poor **prognosis** for patients with this disorder.

# 8
# Gastrointestinal Fistulas
Stephen M. Weiss

## I. DEFINITIONS

    **A.** A **fistula** is an abnormal communication between two or more hollow organs, or between one hollow organ and a body surface. The variety of fistulas is almost limitless, due to the number of organs and sites that can be involved.

    **B.** Gastrointestinal fistulas are **named** according to the sites that they join. Thus, a **bronchobiliary fistula** connects bile ducts with the bronchial tree; a **gastrocutaneous fistula** communicates between the stomach and the skin.

## II. ETIOLOGIES

    **A. Congenital disorders:** Distal tracheoesophageal fistula with esophageal atresia is the most important congenital fistula (see Chapter 33, section IV).

    **B. Trauma:** Inadvertent operative injury, as well as other trauma, can produce fistulization. Examples include a colocutaneous fistula from an anastomotic leak, or a gastrocutaneous fistula complicating splenectomy.

    **C. Inflammation:** Crohn's disease, for example, can cause fistulas such as ileoilial and ileosigmoid.

    **D. Malignancy:** Fistulas can develop because of the destruction of organs by tumors. A colovesical fistula might occur, for example, in a patient with a large sigmoid colon cancer that erodes into the urinary bladder.

    **E. Radiation damage:** Enterovaginal fistula that develops after pelvic irradiation for cervical carcinoma is an example.

## III. COMPLICATIONS

    **A. Malnutrition** can develop because of

        **1.** Inadequate absorption of nutrients due to the short-circuiting of part of the bowel, or due to external loss of ingested food (examples are gastrocolic fistula and high-output enterocutaneous fistula, respectively)

        **2.** Increased caloric needs due to associated infection or stress

    **B. Fluid and electrolyte imbalances** are frequent complications of fistulas, especially those involving the small bowel, pancreas, or bile ducts. The electrolyte content of various gastrointestinal secretions is shown in Table 8-1. Electrolyte losses can be directly measured from a sample of the fistula drainage.

        **1. High-output fistulas** drain more than 200 ml of fluid per day.

        **2.** A pancreatic fistula developing after distal pancreatectomy might drain 700 ml of bicarbonate-rich fluid per day, producing dehydration and acidosis.

    **C. Sepsis** is a frequent accompaniment of fistulas and occurs because leakage of the enteric contents can produce irritation and contamination.

        **1.** An abdominal abscess or wound infection can result.

Table 8-1. Approximate Electrolyte Content of Gastrointestinal Secretions

| Source | Electrolytes (mEq/L) | | | |
|---|---|---|---|---|
| | Na$^+$ | K$^+$ | Cl$^-$ | HCO$_3$$^-$ |
| Stomach | 60 | 10 | 50–150 | 0–20 |
| Duodenum | 120 | 5 | 100 | 20 |
| Bile duct | 145 | 5 | 100 | 40 |
| Pancreas | 140 | 5 | 75 | 100 |
| Ileum | 100 | 5 | 65 | 30 |

    **2.** Distant infections, such as central venous catheter infections, can develop because of extensive skin contamination or bacteremia.

  **D. Skin excoriation**, often severe, can occur if intestinal secretions drain onto the abdominal skin. This skin disruption can be painful, and can contribute to further sepsis.

  **E. Hemorrhage** is an infrequent but potentially life-threatening complication of enteric fistulas. It occurs because the inflammation associated with a fistula can erode into a blood vessel, causing severe bleeding.

**IV. EVALUATION.** Management of the patient with an enteric fistula requires knowledge of the anatomy, etiology, and physiology of the defect.

  **A. History and physical examination**

    **1.** The **history** can provide useful etiologic information by suggesting whether tumor, trauma, or Crohn's disease may be causative.

    **2. Examining the patient** gives information about the location of an external fistula and the character of its drainage. Dehydration and malnutrition can also be detected by examination.

  **B. Radiographic studies** are vital in determining the dimensions of the fistula tract and what organs are involved. Contrast material may be administered by mouth, by rectum, or directly into the fistula (**fistulogram**).

    **1.** Ultrasonography and computed tomography can be useful in locating an undrained collection (e.g., an abscess) which may be associated with the fistula.

    **2.** Radiographs should also be used to **exclude the presence of intestinal obstruction** distal to the fistula, since such an obstruction prevents spontaneous closure of the fistula.

  **C. Laboratory tests** are useful for evaluating electrolyte and pH disturbances, anemia, and sepsis.

    **1.** Determining the electrolyte content of the drainage is helpful with a high-output fistula.

    **2.** Bacteriologic cultures should be obtained in patients with suspected sepsis.

**V. MANAGEMENT**

  **A. Hydration and correction of electrolyte disturbances** are first in priority.

  **B. Control of infection** also requires immediate attention. Antibiotics and operative drainage of abscesses may be required before patients will improve: A fistula will not heal in the presence of pus.

  **C. Control of external drainage** helps to minimize further morbidity. Suction catheters, drains, collection bags, or operative diversion may be useful in protecting body surfaces from irritation. Bowel rest, provided by prolonged fasting, often diminishes gastrointestinal fluid losses.

  **D. Correction of malnutrition** should begin as soon as the patient is stabilized. Most patients require parenteral nutrition. Occasionally, tube feedings of a low-residue diet, or even oral feedings, will be possible, especially with distal low-output fistulas.

  **E. Spontaneous closure** can occur in many patients. However, spontaneous repair is unlikely, and operative repair is required, when any of the following is present:

    **1.** Distal obstruction beyond the fistula site

    **2.** Pus or foreign body at the fistula site

    **3.** Severe bowel injury, such as radiation damage or extensive inflammatory bowel disease

    **4.** Fistula caused by cancer

    **5.** Epithelialization of the fistula tract

  **F. Operative repair** should be performed electively, in a nonseptic, well-nourished patient. Operation typically involves

    **1.** Identification of the fistula

    **2.** Resection of the fistula and damaged segments of bowel

    **3.** Anastomosis to restore bowel continuity

**VI. RESULTS.** Major improvements in fistula management have occurred in the past 2 decades, with resultant increased survival rates.

  **A.** Until the mid-1960s, mortality rates were in excess of 50% for gastric, duodenal, or small bowel fistulas.

    **1.** Management emphasized early attempts at operative repair before malnutrition developed.

    **2.** Major causes of death were
      **a.** Electrolyte and fluid disturbances
      **b.** Malnutrition
      **c.** Peritonitis

  **B. Present management** should lower mortality rates to between 2% and 10%, depending on the etiology of the fistula.

    **1.** Sepsis and renal failure remain as significant causes of death.

    **2.** Malnutrition and electrolyte disturbances have largely been eliminated as causes of death because of improved techniques of venous access, improved blood chemistry monitoring, and improvements in prolonged parenteral feeding.

# 9

# The Liver and Biliary Tract

Maryalice Cheney
Bruce E. Jarrell

## I. LIVER

### A. Surgical anatomy

1. The liver is composed of two lobes, from a surgical standpoint (Fig. 9-1).
   a. These **two lobes**, the **left and right**, are divided by the **main boundary fissure**, an invisible line between the gallbladder fossa anteriorly and the inferior vena cava fossa posteriorly.
   b. The **falciform ligament** is a visible boundary that marks the **segmental fissure** between the medial and lateral segments of the left lobe.

2. The **vascular supply** to the liver determines lines of hepatic resections.
   a. The **arterial blood supply** is from the common **hepatic artery**, a branch of the celiac axis.
      (1) The common hepatic artery enters the hepatoduodenal ligament medial to the common bile duct.
      (2) The **cystic artery** usually arises from the first branch of the hepatic artery, the right hepatic artery.
      (3) In as many as 25% of the population, the left hepatic artery arises from the left gastric artery. In approximately 15%, the right hepatic artery arises as a branch of the superior mesenteric artery.
   b. The **portal vein** is formed by the confluence of the superior mesenteric, splenic, inferior mesenteric, and coronary veins (Fig. 9-2).
      (1) It enters the liver hilus, where it divides to form a **right and left branch**, which supply the right and left hepatic lobes and upon which the substructure of the liver is based.
      (2) The **hepatic veins** drain directly into the inferior vena cava just caudad to the diaphragm.
   c. Oxygenation of hepatic tissues is shared equally by hepatic arterial and portal venous blood.
      (1) The normal **blood flow** through the portal vein is approximately 1000 ml/min.
      (2) The hepatic artery's contribution to hepatic blood flow is approximately 500 ml/min.
   d. The **biliary system** mimics the portal venous anatomy intrahepatically.

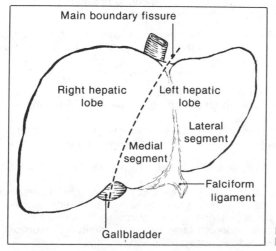

**Figure 9-1.** Surgical anatomy of the liver: left and right lobes.

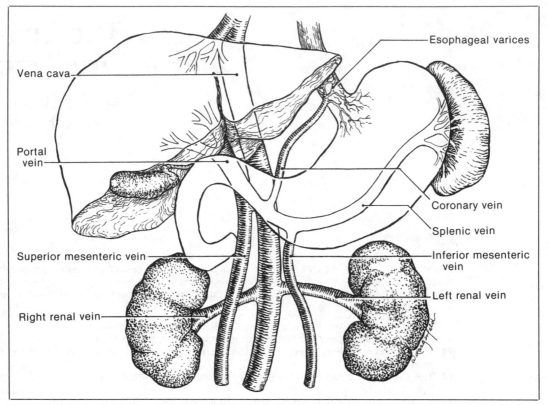

**Figure 9-2.** The portal circulation.

3. **Hepatic resections** are based upon the surgical anatomy. If vascular boundaries are followed, resections can be relatively safe.
   a. **Right hepatic lobectomy** transects the liver along the main boundary fissure through the gallbladder fossa toward the inferior vena cava fossa (Fig. 9-3).
   b. **Left hepatic lobectomy** uses the same guidelines.
   c. **Trisegmentectomy** removes the entire right lobe and the medial segment of the left lobe across the anatomic division of the falciform ligament.
   d. **Left lateral segmentectomy** removes all of the liver to the left of the falciform ligament.
   e. **Left medial segmentectomy** removes the liver between the right lobe and the left lateral lobe. This resection is rarely performed.
   f. **Wedge resections** are performed for small lesions near the liver surface that do not require a full lobectomy. These resections do not adhere to anatomic boundaries but are safe nonetheless because a limited amount of tissue is transected.

B. **Primary tumors of the liver.** In men, 90% of primary liver tumors are malignant; in women, only about 40% are. Oral contraceptive use has increased the incidence of primary liver tumors in women, with up to 75% of those tumors being benign.

1. **Benign tumors**
   a. **Hemangioma**, the most common benign hepatic tumor, is usually asymptomatic. Most commonly it is discovered as a calcification on an abdominal roentgenogram and is managed by simple observation.
      (1) On occasion a hemangioma can be large and can produce symptoms by compressing local structures. In other cases, pain can follow intratumor thrombosis or hemorrhage into the peritoneal cavity.
      (2) Grossly, there may be single or multiple masses, and microscopically, there are vascular lacunae lined with normal endothelial cells.
      (3) Large hemangiomas should be resected to prevent major complications. If the tumor is unresectable or dangerous to resect, radiation therapy or hepatic artery ligation may cause regression, but hepatic transplantation may be necessary if all else fails.
   b. **Hepatocellular adenoma** is a common benign tumor generally limited to women and strongly associated with oral contraceptives, especially prolonged use.

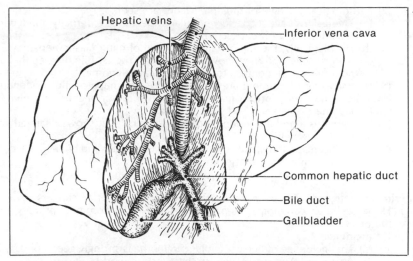

**Figure 9-3.** Plane of resection for right and left hepatic lobectomy.

**(1)** There frequently are no **symptoms** or **physical findings**.
  **(a)** However, approximately 25% of patients have a palpable abdominal mass or abdominal pain.
  **(b)** Up to 30% present with spontaneous rupture and hemorrhage into the peritoneal cavity.
  **(c)** The mortality rate of rupture is as high as 9%.
**(2) Pathologically**, there is a soft solitary tumor with sharply circumscribed edges but not true encapsulation. Histologically, normal hepatocytes are present, and there is no evidence of malignancy.
**(3) Diagnosis**
  **(a)** The tumor is usually suspected when a mass is seen as a "cold" defect on a technetium-99m ($^{99m}$Tc)–sulfur colloid scan of the liver, which is sensitive to tumors as small as 2 cm in diameter.
  **(b)** Angiography is also useful because hypervascularity or arterial splaying is frequently present.
  **(c)** Liver function studies are generally normal.
  **(d)** Open biopsy is needed to determine the precise diagnosis.
**(4) Management.** If the diagnosis is confirmed and the lesion is small, avascular, intrahepatic, and associated with oral contraceptive use, it may be safely observed.
  **(a)** Oral contraceptives, anabolic steroids, and pregnancy should be avoided, and under these conditions the tumor will frequently regress spontaneously.
  **(b)** Occasionally the tumor will be exophytic on a narrow pedicle and is then easily excised.
  **(c)** If the tumor is large and vascular, it should be resected because of the risk of spontaneous rupture and hemorrhage.
**(5)** In cases of **spontaneous rupture with hemorrhage** into the peritoneal cavity, the patient should initially be resuscitated (see Chapter 4, section III F ).
  **(a)** Surgical intervention is indicated when cardiovascular stability is attained.
    **(i)** The procedure most recommended is hepatic artery ligation. This frequently will control the bleeding and is associated with only minor aberrations in liver function when the liver is not cirrhotic.
    **(ii)** Hepatic resection in the presence of acute rupture is not recommended because of a higher mortality rate. Elective resection should, however, be performed at a later date.
  **(b)** If the patient remains very unstable after rupture in spite of major resuscitation efforts, angiographic embolization of the hepatic artery may control the hemorrhage.
**c. Focal nodular hyperplasia** is the third most common benign liver tumor. It also occurs most often in women and is more vascular when associated with prolonged oral contraceptive use.
  **(1) Symptoms and physical findings**, when they occur, are similar to those seen with hepatocellular adenoma, but focal nodular hyperplasia is more commonly asymptomatic and is discovered as an incidental finding. The risk of spontaneous rupture is much lower, reported at less than 9%.

  **(2) Pathologically**, single or multiple lesions are seen.
    **(a)** The lesions have a coarsely nodular appearance externally and a central scar with radiating septa on cut section.
    **(b)** Histologically, the tumors are composed of hyperplastic hepatocytes with inflammatory cells, and they show an inactive cirrhosis. Bile duct epithelium is a prominent finding, in contrast to hepatocellular adenoma.
  **(3) Diagnosis and treatment** are similar to those for hepatocellular adenoma.
  **d. Infantile hemangioendothelioma** is a benign liver tumor of children which has the potential to become malignant.
    **(1)** Grossly, it is a nodular lesion, and microscopically, it shows dilatated vascular spaces lined by endothelium.
    **(2)** Its significance is that it may present as hepatomegaly and high-output cardiac failure in an infant with a large arteriovenous fistula.
    **(3)** Treatment is by excision or hepatic artery ligation.

**2. Primary malignant tumors** of the liver account for 0.7% of all cancers.
  **a. Hepatocellular carcinoma (hepatoma)** is the most common primary malignant liver tumor.
    **(1) Incidence**
      **(a)** The incidence of hepatocellular carcinoma is strongly geographic, being highest in Africa and Asia, and lowest in the Western world.
      **(b)** Males are affected twice as often as females.
      **(c)** The average age of affected individuals is 50 years, but hepatocellular carcinoma may also occur in infants, especially in association with hepatitis B virus (HBV).
    **(2)** The tumor shows an **association** with a number of preexisting diseases and environmental substances. Among these are:
      **(a)** Chronic HBV infection (present in as many as 80% of cases worldwide)
        **(i)** The risk of developing hepatocellular carcinoma is increased up to 200-fold for chronic HBV carriers.
        **(ii)** The risk in male carriers is as high as 50%.
      **(b)** Cirrhosis of the liver (present in approximately 60% to 90% of patients), especially macronodular cirrhosis
      **(c)** In the United States, chronic ethanol abuse
      **(d)** Hemochromatosis due to iron overload and leading to macronodular cirrhosis
      **(e)** Schistosomiasis and other parasitic infestations
      **(f)** Environmental carcinogens
        **(i)** Implicated industrial substances include polychlorinated biphenyls (PCBs); chlorinated hydrocarbon solvents such as carbon tetrachloride; nitrosamines; vinyl monomers and polymers [vinyl chloride and polyvinyl chloride (PVC)]; and organochloride pesticides.
        **(ii)** Other organic materials that show an association are aflatoxins (produced by *Aspergillus flavus* or *A. fumigatus* and found on foodstuffs such as peanuts) and plant pyrrolizidine alkaloids.
    **(3) Clinical findings**
      **(a)** Hepatocellular carcinoma usually presents as a dull aching pain in the right upper quadrant; malaise, fever, and jaundice may be present.
      **(b)** Physical examination reveals hepatomegaly (present in 88% of cases), a tender abdominal mass (in 50%), or findings associated with cirrhosis.
      **(c)** About 10% to 15% of patients present with acute hemorrhage into the peritoneal cavity, with resultant shock.
      **(d)** Paraneoplastic syndromes also may occur, in which tumor cells secrete hormone-like substances that cause unusual syndromes, such as Cushing's syndrome.
    **(4) Laboratory studies** usually reveal mild to moderate abnormalities, but there is no particular diagnostic pattern.
      **(a)** $\alpha$-Fetoprotein, a protein made by embryonal hepatocytes, is present at a level of 400 ng/ml in up to 85% of cases, as compared to 6% in metastatic liver disease, 4% in cirrhosis, and 1% in hepatitis.
      **(b)** Hepatic angiography and computed tomography (CT scanning) are the most reliable studies to determine the presence and operability of the lesions. These studies are positive in up to 90% of cases and can detect lesions as small as 1 cm in diameter.
    **(5) Pathologically**, hepatocellular carcinoma occurs as a solitary mass or multiple masses. Microscopically, malignant hepatocytes are seen in various growth patterns. Local invasion, especially into the hemidiaphragm, is common, as are distant metastases, with the lung being most commonly involved (in up to 45% of cases).
    **(6) Surgical management** includes an operative biopsy to determine the resectability.

**(a)** If lesions are resectable, the average survival time is approximately 3 years; the 5-year survival rate is about 20%.

**(b)** The operative mortality rate is as high as 20% but can be nearly 60% in patients with significant cirrhosis.

**(c)** If lesions are unresectable, patients have a mean survival time of 3 months.

**(d)** Attempts to induce tumor necrosis by hepatic artery ligation have shown poor results, but ligation of the portal venous branch going to the involved area may improve survival.

**(7) Chemotherapy** has been ineffective when given systemically, but administering doxorubicin into the hepatic artery has given some promising preliminary results, improving the survival time in nonresectable patients to between 1 and 2 years.

**b. Hepatoblastoma** is a malignant tumor of epithelial or poorly differentiated mesenchymal cells. Pathologically, 80% are solitary liver masses that microscopically show nests and cords of cells resembling embryonic hepatocytes.

**(1)** Hepatoblastoma is the most common primary malignant liver tumor in children and presents with abdominal distention, failure to thrive, and other symptoms of liver failure. $\alpha$-Fetoprotein is frequently positive.

**(2)** The treatment is surgical excision. Inoperable tumors are treated with irradiation or chemotherapy, but the results are very poor, with most patients dying within 1 year.

**c. Cholangiocarcinoma** is an intrahepatic tumor that arises from the bile duct epithelium; it represents 5% to 30% of all primary hepatic malignancies.

**(1)** The common signs and symptoms include right upper quadrant pain, jaundice, hepatomegaly, and occasionally a palpable mass. The usual patient is aged 60 to 70 years.

**(2)** Pathologically, a hard greyish mass is found within the liver that microscopically shows adenocarcinoma of the tubular biliary epithelium. Metastasis occurs initially to the regional lymph nodes or to liver tissue.

**(3)** The treatment is the same as for hepatocellular carcinoma.

**d. Angiosarcoma**, or **malignant hemangioendothelioma**, is a highly malignant liver tumor composed of irregular spindle cells lining the lumina of hepatic vascular spaces.

**(1)** Most cases (85%) occur in males, and there is a high association with chemical agents, especially vinyl chloride, Thorotrast, and organochloride pesticides.

**(2)** The tumor commonly spreads locally to the spleen (80% of cases) and distantly to the lungs (60% of cases).

**(3)** The treatment is resection when feasible, but patients rarely survive 1 year.

**e. Sarcomas other than angiosarcoma** are rare but are highly malignant and are not curable.

**C. Metastatic tumors to the liver**

**1.** These are much more common than primary tumors.

**a.** The liver is the second most common site of metastasis (exceeded only by regional lymph nodes) for all primary cancers of the abdominal viscera.

**b.** Over two-thirds of all colorectal cancers ultimately involve the liver, and up to 50% of cancers outside the abdomen metastasize to the liver.

**2.** The **diagnosis** may be difficult because liver metastases are frequently asymptomatic.

**a. Laboratory studies**

**(1)** In a recent National Cancer Institute (NCI) study, no single laboratory blood test could predict liver metastases in more than 65% of patients with subclinical disease. This percentage could only be raised using an imaging technique.

**(2)** Liver function studies [serum glutamic oxaloacetic transaminase (SGOT), lactic dehydrogenase (LDH), alkaline phosphatase] are the most useful tests.

**(3)** Testing for carcinoembryonic antigen (CEA) has been valuable for predicting the presence of liver metastasis in colorectal cancer, being positive in over 85% of patients with subsequently proven disease. Unfortunately, this test lacks specificity.

**b. Imaging techniques** are expensive as screening tests but are currently the most reliable nonsurgical method of finding liver metastases.

**(1)** Radionuclide scintiscanning has been of value historically but will miss lesions under 2 cm in diameter.

**(2)** CT scanning is most accurate but is expensive as a screening test.

**(3)** Ultrasonography is almost as reliable as CT scanning and provides a reasonable screening test.

**3.** The **treatment** for metastatic disease to the liver varies greatly and is a function of the type of primary tumor. Colorectal cancer has generated the most reliable statistics, and these are the figures cited here.

**a. Chemotherapy** for liver metastasis from colorectal cancer has been disappointing.

**(1)** Systemic 5-fluorouracil (5-FU) therapy has resulted in a response rate of 9% to 33% and a median survival of 30 to 60 weeks. (A **response** is defined as a 50% decrease in the size of an existing tumor and the development of no new lesions for a period of 1 to 2 months.)

    **(2)** Hepatic arterial infusion of floxuridine (FUDR), using an implantable infusion pump, has shown an increase in response rate but little or no improvement in overall patient survival.

  **b. Radiation therapy** is poorly tolerated by the liver but may be palliative for painful liver metastases.

  **c. Hepatic artery ligation** may cause a dramatic shrinkage in tumor size, but this is usually a transient effect. Although most splanchnic primary cancers metastasize via the portal vein, they quickly become vascularized by the hepatic artery.

  **d. Surgical resection** is perhaps the most effective mode of therapy but is limited, in colorectal cancer, to the few patients who have a solitary, slow-growing liver lesion and no evidence of extrahepatic metastasis.

    **(1)** Experience suggests a 5-year survival rate approaching 30% to 40% in patients with these criteria. The operative mortality rate is generally less than 6%, an acceptable risk.

    **(2)** The incidence of liver metastasis at the time of surgery for primary colorectal cancer is 8% to 25%, and approximately one-fourth of these lesions are solitary and resectable, so that about 5% of patients are potential resection candidates.

**D. Hepatic abscesses and cysts**

  **1.** Infections of the liver or parasitic invasion may result in the formation of an abscess or other space-occupying lesion.

    **a.** These lesions are of surgical importance because of their association with overwhelming sepsis, rupture, generalized debility, and death.

    **b.** They may produce few localizing symptoms (chiefly pain and a mass in the right upper quadrant) while causing major systemic effects (fever, malnutrition, unexplained sepsis, or anemia).

    **c.** The usual signs and symptoms, and the diagnostic tests used, are similar to those associated with tumors of the liver (see sections I B 2 a (3) and I C 2 a).

    **d.** The etiology is strongly dependent upon environmental factors, particularly geographic location and the presence of endemic parasites.

  **2. Bacterial abscesses** are the most common hepatic abscesses in the Western world.

    **a. Etiology**

      **(1)** The abscess is most commonly secondary to an infectious process in the abdomen, particularly appendicitis, diverticulitis, or purulent cholecystitis.

      **(2)** It may also be the result of seeding from a distant infectious focus, such as subacute bacterial endocarditis.

      **(3)** In 10% to 50% of cases, no primary source can be identified.

    **b.** The **infecting organism** is related to the primary source.

      **(1)** When the source is abdominal, the organism is *Escherichia coli*, a *Bacteroides* species, or an anaerobic streptococcus.

      **(2)** When the source is extra-abdominal, gram-positive organisms predominate.

    **c. Clinical findings** are sepsis, with fever and chills, leukocytosis, and anemia.

      **(1)** Liver function studies show elevated enzyme levels, particularly the alkaline phosphatase.

      **(2)** The patient may have right upper quadrant pain, and the liver may be tender or enlarged.

      **(3)** On occasion the sepsis may be overwhelming.

      **(4)** Hemobilia may also occur due to erosion of the abscess into the biliary tree.

    **d. Treatment**

      **(1)** The standard treatment for hepatic abscess is surgical drainage and antibiotic therapy.

        **(a)** Traditionally, drainage is performed as an open surgical procedure and is very effective in controlling the infection.

        **(b)** Recently, hepatic abscesses have been managed by percutaneous drainage using catheter aspiration guided by ultrasonic or CT imaging. This closed procedure may be curative, particularly for abscesses with minimal accompanying necrotic debris.

      **(2)** Periodic sinograms of the abscess cavity are used to monitor healing and the adequacy of drainage.

      **(3)** **Multiple abscesses** are more difficult to manage and rely more heavily on appropriate antibiotic coverage.

      **(4)** It is important in all cases, however, to determine the antibiotic sensitivity of the organism responsible for the abscess and to administer a full course of antibiotics in order to reduce the risk of recurrent or persistent infection.

    **e.** The **mortality rate** for hepatic abscess may be as high as 40% in difficult cases. This high rate is related principally to three factors.

      **(1) Delay in diagnosis.** The possibility of an abscess, whether hepatic, subphrenic, or subhepatic, is frequently overlooked in the critically ill patient. The use of CT scanning and ultrasonography should improve this situation.

      **(2) Multiple abscesses.** These are more difficult to drain properly, and therefore the patient is denied the most effective treatment modality.

      **(3) Malnutrition.** Frequently, catabolism is high in patients with generalized or undiagnosed sepsis. Caloric supplementation, either orally or parenterally, is critical for the patient's well-being, wound healing, and immunocompetence.

**3. Amebic abscess** is the second most common hepatic abscess in the Western world and is more common than bacterial abscess in third-world countries.

    **a. Etiology.** Amebic abscess is due to infestation with the protozoal parasite *Entamoeba histolytica*, which typically reaches the portal vein from intestinal amebiasis.

    **b. Clinical findings** include fever, leukocytosis, hepatomegaly, and right upper quadrant pain. Occasionally, liver enzyme levels are elevated.

      **(1)** The abscess is usually solitary and affects the right lobe of the liver in 90% of patients.

      **(2)** Indirect hemagglutination titers for *Entamoeba* are elevated in up to 85% of patients with intestinal infestation and in 98% of patients with hepatic abscess.

      **(3)** The pus within the abscess is usually sterile and has the appearance of anchovy paste. Trophozoites are occasionally present in the periphery of the abscess.

      **(4)** Abscesses may rupture freely into the peritoneal cavity or into nearby structures such as the pleural or pericardial space.

    **c.** The **treatment** of choice is parenteral metronidazole. The abscess is aspirated if it is large or adjacent to important structures, but surgical drainage is not usually necessary.

**4. Hydatid cysts of the liver**

    **a.** These result from infestation with the parasite *Echinococcus granulosus*.

      **(1)** Man is an intermediate host for the larval colonies, which develop into the fluid-filled hydatid cysts containing **scolices**, the asexual infective parasitic forms.

      **(2)** The cysts are enclosed within a thin fibrous outer layer, the **pericyst**, which enlarges within the liver parenchyma.

    **b.** The **clinical findings** include liver enlargement and right upper quadrant pain in a patient with a history of exposure to an endemic area. Eosinophilia is present in 40% of patients, and the Casoni skin test is positive in many patients. An indirect hemagglutination test is also positive in 80% to 90% of patients.

    **c.** Hydatid cysts may undergo progressive enlargement and rupture.

      **(1)** Close to 50% rupture within the hepatic parenchyma to form daughter cysts.

      **(2)** Cysts may also rupture into a major bile duct, where the debris can result in biliary obstruction.

      **(3)** Occasionally, cysts may rupture into the free peritoneal cavity, resulting in urticaria, eosinophilia, or even anaphylactic shock.

      **(4)** About 20% to 30% of patients develop cysts in the lungs or other extrahepatic organs.

    **d. Treatment**

      **(1)** Because its pericyst is quite fragile and easily ruptured, a hydatid cyst can rarely be removed intact. If the scolices spill into the peritoneal cavity, the parasite will multiply and form new cysts.

      **(2)** Therefore, the current method of treatment is controlled rupture of the cyst, followed by its removal.

        **(a)** This is accomplished by careful isolation of the operative field, followed by trocar aspiration of the cyst.

        **(b)** Once decompressed, the cyst and its contents are peeled off the pericyst lining and removed.

        **(c)** The residual space is then sterilized with 0.5% silver nitrate solution, which is a potent scolicide and relatively nontoxic to humans. (There is no systemic scolicidal agent currently in use.)

      **(3)** When pericystic calcification is visible on an abdominal roentgenogram, it signifies the death of the parasite, a condition which requires no further treatment.

    **e.** The **mortality rate** for patients whose hydatid cysts are surgically removed without complications is up to 4%. If cysts are untreated or if complications develop, the mortality rate rises to as high as 15%.

**E. Portal hypertension**

**1. Anatomic considerations.** (See section I A 2 b and c, and Fig. 9-2.)

2. **Pathophysiology.** Portal hypertension is an abnormal elevation in portal pressure (normal is 10 to 15 cm $H_2O$).
   a. The increase in pressure stimulates the development of numerous venous collaterals in an attempt to decompress the portal system.
   b. These new collateral veins are usually very fragile and have a predilection to form portal-systemic anastomoses that connect the portal system to the inferior vena cava and the azygos system.
   c. With portal pressures over 20 to 25 cm $H_2O$, **dilatated veins**, or **varices**, are likely to develop. When the varices form in a submucosal location, such as at the gastroesophageal junction, they are subject to rupture and hemorrhage.

3. **Etiology**
   a. **Intrahepatic causes** are most common.
      (1) In the United States, **cirrhosis of the liver** causes 85% of portal hypertension cases. The most common etiology of cirrhosis is alcohol abuse, followed by postnecrotic cirrhosis and biliary cirrhosis.
         (a) Cirrhosis, pathologically speaking, produces:
            (i) A progressive narrowing of the sinusoidal and postsinusoidal vessels due to centrilobular collagen deposition
            (ii) Distortion of the local anatomy due to cirrhotic regenerative nodules
         (b) The resultant outflow block in turn causes increased resistance to portal blood flow through the liver and a consequent increase in portal pressure.
      (2) Worldwide, **schistosomiasis** is a common cause. The portal hypertension develops because parasitic ova in the small portal venules cause a presinusoidal block.
      (3) **Acute alcoholic hepatitis** [see section I E 9 a (2)] can cause hepatocyte edema and swelling with a resultant acute portal hypertension.
      (4) Wilson's disease, hepatic fibrosis, hemochromatosis, and idiopathic diseases are occasional causes of portal hypertension.
   b. **Prehepatic causes** of portal hypertension are rare.
      (1) They are associated with portal vein obstruction due to either thrombosis, congenital atresia or stenosis, or extrinsic compression such as occurs with tumors.
      (2) Prehepatic causes are more common in children.
   c. **Postsinusoidal resistance to hepatic flow** is also a rare etiology.
      (1) In the **Budd-Chiari syndrome**, resistance of hepatic venous outflow is secondary to hepatic vein occlusion; hepatomegaly and ascites also occur. This syndrome is associated with tumors, hematologic disorders, use of oral contraceptives, and trauma. In the Orient, inferior vena cava webs are the most common cause of hepatic vein obstruction.
      (2) **Constrictive pericarditis** produces a markedly elevated inferior vena cava pressure, resulting in resistance to hepatic venous outflow. It may be suspected when calcification of the pericardium is present.
   d. **Increased portal venous flow** may result in portal hypertension. It has been associated with Banti's syndrome (primary splenic disease) and kala-azar (tropical splenomegaly).
   e. **Splenic vein thrombosis** may cause hypertension of the veins near the splenic hilus, resulting in varices confined to the gastric fundus. The usual etiology is either a chronic pancreatitis with scar formation around the splenic vein or a pancreatic tumor.

4. **Prognosis**
   a. The overall statistics for cirrhotic patients are as follows.
      (1) Fifteen percent of alcoholics develop cirrhosis.
      (2) Thirty percent of cirrhotics die within the first year after the cirrhosis has been diagnosed; sixty-six percent of cirrhotics with varices die within the first year.
      (3) Forty percent (the range is from thirteen to seventy percent) of cirrhotics develop bleeding varices.
         (a) Fifty to eighty percent of these patients die with their first variceal hemorrhage.
         (b) Sixty-six percent of those who survive the initial hemorrhage bleed a second time, and the mortality rate for the second hemorrhage is again fifty to eighty percent.
   b. Ultimately, in alcoholic patients with cirrhosis, regardless of the type of treatment, hepatic failure and death are intimately related to whether or not the patient continues to consume alcohol.

5. **Clinical findings**
   a. The following are common findings in portal hypertension:
      (1) **Malnutrition**, particularly in alcoholic cirrhosis
      (2) **Encephalopathy**
         (a) This is secondary to impaired portal blood flow (due to shunting of portal blood around the liver) and hepatic insufficiency.

**(b)** It may be related to elevated serum levels of ammonia in some patients, but the correlation is unreliable.

**(3) Hemorrhage**, usually from varices in the gastroesophageal location and complicated by impaired clotting parameters

**(4) Ascites** (see section I F), secondary to hepatic sinusoidal hypertension, hypoalbuminemia, or hyperaldosteronism

**(5) Peripheral edema**, resulting from the previously mentioned factors plus an increase in total body sodium due to increased renal reabsorption of sodium

**(6)** Manifestations of **collateral venous development**, such as a periumbilical caput medusae or hemorrhoids

**b. Splenomegaly** may be present and may be associated with hypersplenism.

**c.** The patient may present with severe abdominal pain, acidosis, and leukocytosis if mesenteric venous gangrene develops secondary to acute portal vein thrombosis.

**6. Acute variceal hemorrhage** is life-threatening and is the principal complication of portal hypertension that necessitates **interventional therapy**.

**a.** The immediate management of acute upper gastrointestinal hemorrhage is described in Chapter 4, section III F.

**b.** Gastroesophagoscopy should be performed as soon as the patient is stable, to determine the site of bleeding and verify the presence of varices. Upper gastrointestinal bleeding in a patient with cirrhosis is not always variceal in origin. Many such patients are bleeding from a gastric or duodenal source.

**(1)** In most series, the cause of an upper gastrointestinal hemorrhage in cirrhotic patients was found to be varices in 20% to 50%, erosive gastritis in 20% to 60%, peptic ulcer disease in 6% to 19%, and esophageal tears (Mallory-Weiss syndrome) in 5% to 18%.

**(2)** In addition, up to 8% of the patients have two bleeding sites.

**7. Measures for controlling proven variceal bleeding** include the following.

**a. Injection sclerotherapy**

**(1)** Injection of a sclerosing agent into a varix will result in thrombosis of the vein.

**(2)** The procedure may be done endoscopically and will control bleeding temporarily in 80% of patients; it carries a mortality rate of 10% to 20%.

**(3)** This is currently the preferred first method of managing variceal bleeding in most centers.

**b. Use of vasopressin** (see Chapter 4, section III F 2 d)

**(1)** This potent vasoconstrictor lowers portal pressure by mesenteric vasoconstriction, with a resultant diminished mesenteric blood flow.

**(2)** It is equally effective whether given intravenously or by infusion.

**(3)** However, vasopressin is useful only for the short-term control of hemorrhage; it does not improve patient survival rates.

**c. Balloon tamponade**

**(1)** Nasogastric tubes with balloons at the lower end may be used to tamponade bleeding varices.

**(2)** These tubes control bleeding in up to 35% of patients, but bleeding may resume when the balloon is deflated.

**(3)** Balloon tamponade has two major complications.

**(a)** Pneumonia, due to the inability to clear salivary secretions, is common unless a tube is left in the esophagus above the balloon.

**(b)** The esophagus may rupture, especially when an esophageal balloon is used. This may be due to either mechanical disruption or ischemia of the esophagus.

**(4)** To minimize these complications, the nasogastric balloon tube should be used for a limited period of time, such as 48 hours, and radiography should be routinely performed to document that the gastric balloon is in the stomach, not the esophagus.

**8. Acute massive bleeding** that fails to respond to nonsurgical maneuvers requires emergency surgery, especially if hypotension is present.

**a.** The **decision to proceed with surgery** is made if bleeding is still continuing despite transfusion of 5 units or more of blood, especially within 24 hours. The risk of death rises dramatically after 10 units of blood have been transfused, due both to sepsis and to the worsening of cirrhotic coagulopathy from the use of banked blood.

**b.** Surgery is not advisable in the presence of pneumonia, moderate or severe encephalopathy, severe coagulopathy, or severe liver failure.

**c.** The **type of surgery** performed may either be to decompress the portal venous system or directly ligate the bleeding varices.

**(1) Emergency portacaval shunting**, although very effective in controlling hemorrhage (over 95% of patients stop bleeding), has an associated operative mortality rate of over 50%.

        **(a)** The usual procedure performed is an end-to-side portacaval shunt or a mesocaval shunt (see section I E 10).

        **(b)** An acute reduction of portal blood flow to the liver following shunting leads to hepatic failure, accounting for two-thirds of the perioperative deaths. Pneumonia, renal failure, and delirium tremens are contributing lethal factors.

    **(2) Ligation of varices** [see section I E 9 b (2) (a)], either directly or by esophageal transection using a stapling device, usually stops the bleeding.

        **(a)** Ligation is associated with an operative mortality rate of up to 30%.

        **(b)** Bleeding recurs within several months in up to 80% of survivors.

  **d.** The possibility of bleeding from sources other than varices should be clearly eliminated before beginning either of the above procedures.

**9. Elective surgery for esophageal varices** is performed when patients are not actively bleeding. The goal of this type of surgery is to prevent bleeding, with its concomitant risk of death, from recurring.

  **a.** The **preoperative evaluation** includes the following:

    **(1)** Proving endoscopically that esophageal varices were the site of bleeding

    **(2)** Ruling out **acute hepatic hyaline necrosis (acute alcoholic hepatitis)**

        **(a)** This syndrome may present with liver failure and a diffusely tender enlarged liver.

        **(b)** Histologically, hyaline necrosis is seen, with discrete hyaline bodies (Mallory's bodies) in hepatic cells.

        **(c)** Liver enzyme levels and liver function will be corrected if the patient survives the acute episode.

        **(d)** If the diagnosis is in question, a liver biopsy should be performed, since the operative mortality rate exceeded 50% in some studies when surgery was performed in the presence of alcoholic hepatitis.

    **(3)** Using the **Child classification** (Table 9-1) to evaluate the operative risk factors

    **(4)** Ruling out active infection

    **(5)** Determining the patient's portal venous anatomy and verifying the presence of a patent portal vein. This may be done by:

        **(a)** Splenoportography, the injection of radiopaque dye into the spleen followed by imaging of the portal system

        **(b)** Splenic and superior mesenteric arteriography followed by delayed venous-phase imaging

        **(c)** Umbilical vein catheterization and subsequent imaging

        **(d)** Transhepatic portal venography (this carries a slightly higher risk of creating portal vein thrombosis, and is not commonly done today)

    **(6)** Measuring the portal venous pressure, although this is not a necessary procedure. It can be done directly, by umbilical vein catheterization or transhepatically, or indirectly, by measuring the wedged hepatic venous pressure.

  **b.** The **type of elective surgery** depends on the surgeon's individual preference and on the patient's pathologic and physiologic status. The choices are as follows:

    **(1) Shunting procedures** (see section I E 10)

    **(2) Direct occlusion of varices**

        **(a) Simple ligation of varices** may be performed by gastrotomy and suture ligation, transthoracic variceal ligation, or esophageal transection and reanastomosis with a stapler.

          **(i)** Simple ligation may temporarily control bleeding, but the incidence of rebleeding is very high.

          **(ii)** It is generally used for the initial control of bleeding, to be followed by some form of portal decompressive surgery.

**Table 9-1.** The Child Classification for Determining the Operative Risk of a Shunting Procedure in a Patient with Portal Hypertension

| | Child Group | | |
|---|---|---|---|
| | **A** | **B** | **C** |
| Serum bilirubin (mg/dl) | < 2 | 2–3 | > 3 |
| Serum albumin (g/dl) | > 3.5 | 3–3.5 | < 3 |
| Presence of ascites | Absent | Easily controlled | Refractory |
| Presence of encephalopathy | Absent | Minimal | Severe |
| Presence of malnutrition | Absent | Mild | Severe |
| Operative mortality rate | 2% | 10% | 50% |

      (b) **Endoscopic variceal sclerosis** is initially effective in up to 80% of patients, and has become the principal initial method of management for esophageal varices.

          (i) However, as many as 33% of patients may require resclerosis procedures because nothing has been done to lower the portal pressure.

          (ii) Major risks include esophageal necrosis in the area of sclerosis, endoscopic perforation of the esophagus, pleural effusion, and esophageal paralysis.

      (c) **Paraesophageal devascularization combined with esophageal transection and re-anastomosis (the Sugiura procedure)** has, in some series, been highly effective in preventing bleeding and has shown a low operative mortality rate.

          (i) The procedure is usually performed in two stages: a transthoracic devascularization, followed in 4 to 6 weeks by a transabdominal proximal gastric devascularization, splenectomy, selective vagotomy, and pyloroplasty.

          (ii) The operative mortality rate has been as low as 5% and the rebleeding rate as low as 4%, although most centers have a limited experience.

**10. Shunting procedures**

    **a.** These are designed to lower the portal venous pressure and therefore decompress esophageal varices and diminish their propensity to bleed.

    **b. Portal-systemic shunts** may be prophylactic or therapeutic, and may be nonselective or selective.

    **c. Prophylactic shunts** are performed on cirrhotic patients with proven varices, but prior to any episodes of esophageal variceal bleeding.

      **(1)** However, only 30% to 40% of this patient group ultimately bleed from their varices, making 60% of the procedures unnecessary.

      **(2)** In addition, by their very nature all nonselective shunts decrease hepatic portal venous flow, thus adding to the risk of hepatic decompensation.

      **(3)** In randomized trials, prophylactic shunts did not improve survival rates. They are therefore currently not advisable.

    **d. Therapeutic shunts** may be performed on cirrhotic patients who have had a variceal hemorrhage.

      **(1)** However, numerous studies have failed to prove convincingly that shunted patients live longer than nonshunted patients following a variceal hemorrhage.

      **(2)** Patients' survival is principally a function of the Child classification (see Table 9-1) prior to surgery. The better the hepatic function, the more likely that a therapeutic shunt will prolong survival. Long-term survival in the alcoholic is principally determined by whether or not the patient returns to alcohol abuse.

    **e. Nonselective portal-systemic shunts** decompress the entire portal venous system into the inferior vena cava, lowering portal pressure.

      **(1)** The **end-to-side portacaval shunt** (Fig. 9-4) is the one most commonly performed, followed by the **mesocaval (mesenteric–caval) shunt** (Fig. 9-5) and the **side-to-side portacaval shunt** (Fig. 9-6).

      **(2)** In the end-to-side shunt, the hepatic limb of the portal vein is ligated, and the remaining portal vein is sutured to the inferior vena cava.

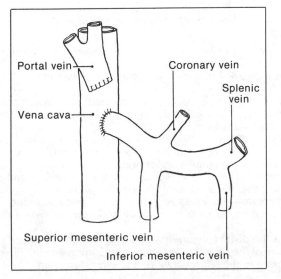

**Figure 9-4.** End-to-side portacaval shunt.

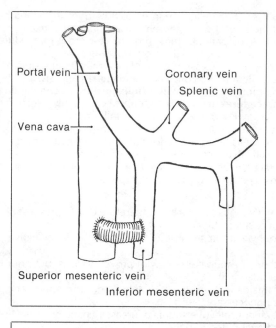

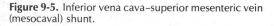

**Figure 9-5.** Inferior vena cava–superior mesenteric vein (mesocaval) shunt.

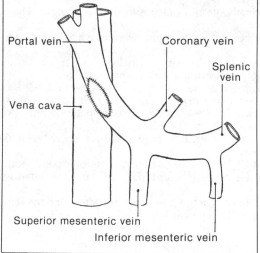

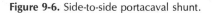

**Figure 9-6.** Side-to-side portacaval shunt.

    **(a)** This results in dramatic lowering of pressure in the portal system and decompression of varices.

    **(b)** The rebleeding rate is less than 5%, but end-to-side shunts have two major side effects.

        **(i)** The portal blood flow into the liver is markedly diminished. Since hepatic function depends on adequate portal blood, reducing the flow increases the risk of hepatic failure and encephalopathy.

        **(ii)** Ligation of the portal vein within the liver does little to lower the intrahepatic sinusoidal pressure, so that the propensity for ascites to develop is greater with end-to-side shunts than with the other types of nonselective shunts.

  **(3)** One difficulty that has been reported with the mesocaval shunt is delayed thrombosis of the shunt. When this occurs, the risk of variceal hemorrhage returns.

 **f. Selective portal-systemic shunts** decrease the pressure in the splenic bed and reduce the risk of gastroesophageal varices by shunting splenic venous blood into the systemic circulation.

  **(1)** Most commonly performed is the **distal splenorenal (Warren) shunt** (Fig. 9-7).

  **(2)** In this procedure, the distal end of the splenic vein (that is, the portion coming directly from the splenic hilus) is sutured to the left renal vein, a low-pressure vein.

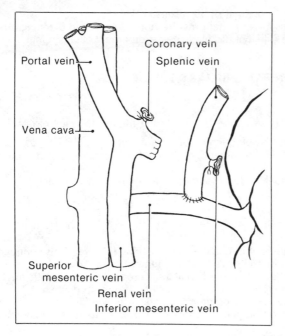

Coronary vein

Splenic vein

Portal vein

Vena cava

Superior
mesenteric vein

Renal vein

Inferior mesenteric vein

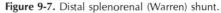

**Figure 9-7.** Distal splenorenal (Warren) shunt.

**(3)** In addition, the coronary vein and other collaterals between the portal system and the gastric and splenic region, including the right gastroepiploic vein, are ligated.
**(4)** As can be seen from Figure 9-7, portal venous flow into the liver is maintained, thus minimizing the problem of hepatic insufficiency and consequent encephalopathy.
**(5)** However, because portal sinusoidal pressure remains high, ascites is common after this procedure.
**(6)** Chylous ascites may also occur as a result of surgical dissection of the retroperitoneum around major lymphatic channels.
  **g.** Prospective trials comparing selective versus nonselective shunts have shown a significant decrease in the incidence of postoperative encephalopathy with the selective type.

  **11. Hypersplenism** is common in patients with portal hypertension.
    **a.** It should be treated medically unless a shunting procedure is necessary for variceal bleeding. Approximately one-half of patients who undergo shunting will show improvement or resolution of the hypersplenism.
    **b. Splenectomy** should be performed rarely for portal hypertension.
      **(1)** It is associated with a variceal hemorrhage recurrence rate as high as 90%.
      **(2)** Sepsis and death may follow splenectomy, especially in children.
    **c.** The best **indication for splenectomy** in a patient with variceal bleeding is radiographic proof of **splenic vein thrombosis**.
      **(1)** This occurs as a result of an obstruction in the vein due to a pancreatic disorder, such as pancreatitis or a neoplasm.
      **(2)** The varices may be limited to the stomach (gastric varices) and therefore curable by splenectomy.

  **F. Ascites** is a complication of hepatic disease.

    **1.** It results from sinusoidal hypertension, hypoalbuminemia, abnormal hepatic and abdominal lymph production, and abnormal salt and water retention by the kidneys.

    **2.** Ascites may be worsened by portal-systemic shunts.

    **3. Medical management** of ascites is most appropriate and involves salt and water restriction and the use of diuretics, especially spironolactone.

    **4. Peritoneal-jugular shunting** may be used to treat ascites that is refractory to medical management.
      **a.** A Silastic tube is implanted surgically, originating in the peritoneal cavity and terminating in the jugular vein. A valve in the tubing circuit controls the direction of flow out of the peritoneal cavity.
      **b.** An abdominal binder helps the flow through the shunt and minimizes shunt thrombosis, which occurs in 10% of cases.

**c.** Diuretics should be continued for optimal shunt results.

**d.** Peritoneal-jugular shunts help to lower portal pressure but may result in bleeding due to the presence of factors in ascitic fluid that stimulate the development of disseminated intravascular coagulation.

## II. THE GALLBLADDER AND EXTRAHEPATIC BILIARY TREE

**A. Embryology**

**1. Development** of the liver and biliary structures begins during the fourth week of fetal life.

**2.** The **hepatic diverticulum** forms as an outpouching of the foregut.
  **a.** The **cranial portion** forms the liver, the larger branches of the intrahepatic ducts, and the proximal extrahepatic biliary tree.
  **b.** The **caudal portion** forms the gallbladder, cystic duct, and common bile duct.

**B. Anatomy** (Fig. 9-8)

**1. Extrahepatic biliary tree**
  **a. Structure**
    **(1)** The **left and right hepatic ducts** join together after leaving the liver. This confluence forms the **common hepatic duct** (3 cm to 4 cm in length).
    **(2)** The common hepatic duct is joined (most often at an acute angle) by the **cystic duct**, to form the **common bile duct** (10 cm in length; 6 mm to 10 mm in diameter).
    **(3)** The common bile duct is lateral to the common hepatic artery and anterior to the portal vein. The distal one-third of the common bile duct passes behind the pancreas to join the **ampulla of Vater**.
    **(4)** The common bile duct joins the **pancreatic duct** in one of three ways.
      **(a)** Most commonly, the ducts unite outside the duodenum and traverse the duodenal wall and papilla as a single duct.
      **(b)** They may join the duodenal wall and have a short common channel.
      **(c)** Least commonly, they enter the duodenum independently.
  **b.** The **sphincter of Oddi** surrounds the common bile duct and controls bile flow.
  **c. Blood supply to the ducts**
    **(1)** The **hilar ducts**, within the liver parenchyma, are supplied primarily from the hepatic arteries.
    **(2)** The blood supply to the **supraduodenal common** bile **duct** is variable. However, an average of eight small arteries (0.3 mm in diameter) supply this portion of the duct. The

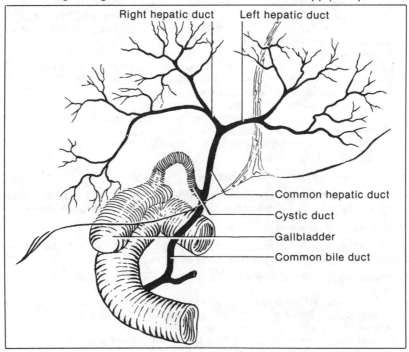

Right hepatic duct    Left hepatic duct

Common hepatic duct
Cystic duct
Gallbladder
Common bile duct

**Figure 9-8.** The gallbladder and extrahepatic biliary tree.

most important vessels (the **"three o'clock"** and **"nine o'clock"** arteries) run along the lateral borders of the duct, as their names imply.

(3) The **retropancreatic portion** of the duct is supplied from the **retroduodenal artery**.

2. The **gallbladder** is located in the bed of the liver and divides the liver anatomically into its right and left lobes.

    a. The gallbladder is divided into four **anatomic portions**:

        (1) The **fundus**

        (2) The **body**, which serves as the storage area

        (3) The **infundibulum (Hartmann's pouch)**, located between the neck and the body

        (4) The **neck**, which connects with the cystic duct

    b. The **wall of the gallbladder** is composed of smooth muscle and fibrous tissue; the lumen is lined with high columnar epithelium.

    c. **Blood supply**

        (1) The gallbladder is supplied by the **cystic artery**, which is nearly always (95% of the time) a branch of the right hepatic artery that passes behind the cystic duct.

        (2) **Venous drainage** is via the cystic vein to the right portal vein and via small veins that drain directly into the liver.

    d. **Lymphatic drainage** from the gallbladder goes to the liver.

    e. **Innervation** is from the **celiac plexus**.

        (1) **Motor innervation** travels via vagal and postganglionic fibers from the celiac ganglia. The preganglionic sympathetic level is $T_8$ to $T_9$.

        (2) **Sensory innervation** travels from sympathetic fibers coursing to the celiac plexus through the right posterior root ganglion at levels $T_8$ and $T_9$.

    f. The **valves of Heister** are mucosal folds in the cystic duct adjacent to the gallbladder. Despite their name, they have no valvular function.

C. **Physiology.** Bile is produced by the liver and transported via the extrahepatic ducts to the gallbladder where it is concentrated and released in response to humoral and nervous control.

1. **Hepatic production of bile**

    a. Approximately 600 ml of bile are produced daily (the normal range is 250 ml to 1000 ml/day).

    b. **Bile secretion by the liver** is under neural, humoral, and pharmacologic control. Vagal and splanchnic stimulation, secretin, theophylline, phenobarbital, and steroids all increase bile flow.

2. **Composition**

    a. **Bile** is composed of:

        (1) Organic and inorganic ions

        (2) Bile pigments

        (3) Protein

        (4) Lipids

            (a) Phospholipids, primarily lecithin

            (b) Cholesterol

            (c) Bile acids; chenodeoxycholic acid and cholic acid conjugate with taurine and glycine

    b. Because the electrolyte concentration of bile approximates that of plasma, **lactated Ringer's solution** is a good replacement fluid for biliary losses.

3. The **functions of the gallbladder** include:

    a. **Storage of bile**

    b. **Concentration of bile**

        (1) The absorption of water and electrolytes by the gallbladder mucosa results in a 10-fold concentration of cholesterol, bile salts, and bile pigments as compared to hepatic bile.

        (2) The **secretion of mucus** protects the gallbladder mucosa from the irritant effects of bile and facilitates the passage of bile through the cystic duct. This mucus secretion represents the **"white bile"** seen with **hydrops of the gallbladder** following cystic duct obstruction.

    c. **Release of bile**

        (1) The coordinated release of bile requires simultaneous contraction of the gallbladder and relaxation of the sphincter of Oddi.

        (2) This process is under predominantly humoral control [via cholecystokinin (CCK)], but vagal and splanchnic nerves also play a role.

D. **Radiologic diagnosis** of biliary tract disease

1. A **plain abdominal film** will demonstrate the 15% of gallstones that are radiopaque.

   **2. Oral cholecystography (OCG)** is the best method of demonstrating biliary calculi.
      **a.** The technique identifies abnormalities (visualization of stones or nonvisualization of the gallbladder) with a 95% to 98% accuracy.
      **b.** The procedure requires the ingestion of iopanoic acid (Telepaque) tablets on the evening before the study. Its chief **disadvantages** lie in its reliance on:
         **(1)** Absorption of the contrast medium from the gastrointestinal tract
         **(2)** Uptake and excretion of contrast medium from the hepatocytes
         **(3)** Uptake and concentration of contrast medium by the gallbladder
         **(4)** Patency of the hepatic and cystic ducts

   **3. CCK stimulation** is used to diagnose gallbladder disease in symptomatic patients with a normal OCG. A **positive study** is represented by either of the following:
      **a.** Failure of the gallbladder to contract by more than 40% at 20 minutes after CCK stimulation
      **b.** Reproduction of the patient's right upper quadrant pain when the CCK is injected

   **4. Real-time ultrasonography** has a 90% to 93% accuracy in identifying calculi, but is limited in detecting small stones. The technique is particularly useful for evaluating pregnant patients.

   **5. CT scanning** is expensive, but delineates dilatated ducts as well as retroperitoneal lymphadenopathy and lesions of the pancreatic head, the liver, or the stomach.

   **6.** A **hepatobiliary iminodiacetic acid (HIDA) scan** makes use of a gamma-emitting radioisotope ($^{99m}$Tc) attached to a substance excreted in the bile.
      **a.** It provides imaging of the liver, the biliary tree, and the intestinal transit of bile.
      **b.** The HIDA scan is the study of choice for the diagnosis of acute cholecystitis secondary to cystic duct obstruction.

   **7. Percutaneous transhepatic cholangiography** (using the Chiba needle) is useful in the evaluation of the jaundiced patient. It localizes disease and allows the preoperative placement of biliary drainage catheters.

   **8. Endoscopic retrograde cholangiopancreatography (ERCP)** is also useful in evaluating the jaundiced patient.
      **a.** The procedure permits evaluation of the stomach, duodenum, ampulla of Vater, pancreatic duct, and common bile duct.
      **b.** If stones are present within the common bile duct, endoscopic papillotomy can be performed.

   **9. Intravenous cholangiography** is no longer performed.

**E. Gallstones (cholelithiasis)**

   **1. Types and their mode of formation.** All gallstones form as a result of biliary solids precipitating out of solution.
      **a. Cholesterol stones** are large, smooth, and solitary.
         **(1)** The **solubility of cholesterol in bile** depends on the concentration of bile salts, lecithin, and cholesterol. Lecithin and cholesterol are insoluble in aqueous solution, but dissolve in bile salt–lecithin micelles.
         **(2)** Failure by the liver to maintain a micellar liquid can be caused by an increase in the concentration of cholesterol or a decrease in the concentration of bile salts or lecithin; either can result in cholesterol stone formation.
         **(3)** Conversely, increasing the biliary concentration of lecithin and bile salts should hinder cholesterol stone formation.
            **(a)** This theory has been investigated in the treatment of patients with cholesterol stones and prophylactically in patients with a predisposition to stone formation.
            **(b)** In the National Cooperative Gallstone Study, patients with known gallstones were treated with chenodeoxycholic acid over a 2-year period. Complete resolution of stones was found in 13% of the patients, and partial dissolution in 41%.
      **b. Pure pigment (bilirubin) stones** are smooth and are green or black in color; they are associated with hemolytic disorders such as sickle cell anemia or spherocytosis.
      **c. Calcium bilirubinate stones** are associated with infection or inflammation of the biliary tree.
         **(1)** Infection results in an increase in biliary calcium as well as an increase in $\beta$-glucuronidase (which converts conjugated bilirubin to the unconjugated form).
         **(2)** The calcium binds to the unconjugated bilirubin and precipitates to form calcium bilirubinate stones.
         **(3)** Normal bile contains glucaro-1,4-lactone, which inhibits the conversion of conjugated to unconjugated bilirubin and thus deters calcium bilirubinate stone formation.

**d.** In the Western world, most stones (70%) are made up of all three elements (cholesterol, bilirubin, and calcium), with cholesterol as the major component.

**2. Clinical findings**
  **a.** The patient may have a variety of **symptoms** ranging from mild right upper quadrant or right scapular pain following a meal to severe, crampy abdominal pain with nausea, vomiting, and other systemic symptoms. Pain in the scapular region is referred along nerve pathways from the gallbladder fossa and is a common occurrence.
  **b.** **Physical examination** may reveal tenderness or guarding in the right upper quadrant or a mass in that area. An elevated temperature suggests infection of the gallbladder **(cholecystitis)**.
  **c.** **Laboratory findings**, in addition to those studies mentioned previously, might include elevated levels of serum phosphatase, bilirubin, or amylase.
    **(1)** Elevation of amylase levels suggests an associated pancreatitis secondary to spasm of the sphincter of Oddi.
    **(2)** An elevated white blood cell count suggests infection.

**3. Treatment**
  **a.** **Cholecystectomy** should be performed, either:
    **(1)** **Electively**, after the patient has improved (usually bed rest and taking nothing by mouth will allow the symptoms to resolve)
    **(2)** **Acutely**, if convenient for the patient and surgeon
  **b.** There is little difference in operative risk between immediate and delayed surgery, with the following exceptions.
    **(1)** If infection is present, surgery should be performed sooner.
    **(2)** If other major medical problems exist (e.g., acute myocardial infarction), the patient should first be treated optimally with medical therapy; then cholecystectomy should be performed.
  **c.** Following cholecystectomy, **operative cholangiography** should be performed, because about 10% to 20% of patients have concomitant **common duct stones**, requiring common duct exploration.
  **d.** Diabetic patients with cholelithiasis or cholecystitis should definitely undergo cholecystectomy because of the higher risk of complications and a mortality rate as high as 15% if acute cholecystitis is present.

**4. Asymptomatic cholelithiasis**
  **a.** The **treatment** of asymptomatic cholelithiasis is controversial.
    **(1)** Excluding diabetics and patients with sickle cell disease, truly asymptomatic cholelithiasis may be amenable to nonoperative management.
      **(a)** In several studies, however, up to 50% of patients developed symptoms and 10% to 20% developed serious complications.
      **(b)** Criticism of the study is based on the assumption that these patients were not truly asymptomatic at the onset or that the symptoms that they developed were not truly biliary symptoms.
    **(2)** The operative mortality rate for cholecystectomy in patients with asymptomatic cholelithiasis is 0.7%, compared to 2.5% for patients with acute cholecystitis.
  **b.** The incidence of carcinoma of the gallbladder is small but present (less than 5%).

**F. Cholecystitis**

**1. Etiology.** Cholecystitis is **acute inflammation of the gallbladder** associated with obstruction of the cystic duct.
  **a.** In 85% to 95% of cases, cholecystitis is associated with calculi. Whether the stones are the cause or the effect has not yet been determined. However, bile stasis, bacteria, and pancreatic juice irritation have all been implicated as causative factors.
  **b.** Cholecystitis is associated with bacterial infection of the tissue in many cases, particularly when complications occur.

**2. Acute cholecystitis**
  **a. Pathophysiology**
    **(1)** The majority of cases are due to an **impacted stone** in the gallbladder neck or the cystic duct. Direct pressure from the stone on the mucosa or unrelieved obstruction causes ischemia, necrosis, ulceration, edema, and impaired venous return. The result can be perforation with consequent bile peritonitis, fistula formation, or pericholecystic abscess.
    **(2)** **Other causes** of acute cholecystitis include sepsis, trauma, or collagen vascular disease.

**b. Clinical findings**
  **(1)** The greatest incidence of acute cholecystitis is in patients aged 30 to 80; women are affected more often than men.
  **(2)** Most patients give a history consistent with chronic cholecystitis: The patient complains of right upper quadrant or epigastric pain, which may radiate to the back or interscapular region.
  **(3)** Fever, nausea and vomiting, and right upper quadrant tenderness with or without rebound tenderness are common. The gallbladder may be palpable.
**c.** The **differential diagnosis** includes:
  **(1)** Perforated or penetrating peptic ulcer
  **(2)** Myocardial infarction
  **(3)** Pancreatitis
  **(4)** Hiatal hernia
  **(5)** Pneumonia
  **(6)** Appendicitis
  **(7)** Hepatitis
  **(8)** Herpes zoster
**d. Diagnostic studies**
  **(1)** A **radionuclide scan** is the diagnostic study of choice.
  **(2)** **Other studies** include a complete blood count; measurements of levels of serum amylase, serum bilirubin, and liver enzymes; an electrocardiogram; and chest x-ray.
  **(3)** Levels of the following substances will be elevated in patients with acute cholecystitis:
    **(a)** Serum alkaline phosphatase in 23%
    **(b)** Serum bilirubin in 45%
    **(c)** SGOT in 40%
    **(d)** Serum amylase in 13%
**e. Treatment**
  **(1)** Cholecystitis should be treated similarly to cholelithiasis, except that:
    **(a)** It more often requires emergency surgery because of complications, including:
      **(i)** Perforation
      **(ii)** Abscess formation
      **(iii)** Fistula formation
    **(b)** It has a higher mortality rate, secondary to sepsis, and so treatment should include antibiotic therapy.
  **(2)** The advantage (if any) of early versus delayed surgical intervention is still debated.
    **(a)** Advocates of **delayed surgical intervention** give the following **reasons**.
      **(i)** Most cases of acute cholecystitis will resolve with medical management.
      **(ii)** Surgery performed during acute inflammation and vascular congestion may cause spreading of the infection.
      **(iii)** Acute inflammation distorts anatomy, leads to technical errors, and may prevent common bile duct exploration.
      **(iv)** Patients often present with associated diseases and thus are not ideal candidates for emergency surgery.
    **(b)** Proponents of **early surgical intervention** cite the following **reasons**.
      **(i)** Some 5% of patients fail to respond to medical management.
      **(ii)** Fully 50% of patients who initially respond will have an exacerbation.
      **(iii)** Early and delayed surgery show no difference in mortality rates.
      **(iv)** Morbidity is lower with early surgical intervention.
  **(3)** We advocate **early surgical intervention** in the treatment of acute cholecystitis with common bile duct exploration. Our **approach** is as follows.
    **(a)** If symptoms began within 72 hours of the time of presentation, cholecystectomy is performed.
      **(i)** If the patient is extremely ill from sepsis or if another medical condition precludes the patient's tolerating cholecystectomy, then cholecystostomy is performed under local anesthesia, and cholecystectomy is performed later, when the patient has recovered from the acute attack.
      **(ii)** If common bile duct exploration is indicated but cannot be performed because of severe inflammation, cholecystostomy is performed.
    **(b)** If symptoms began more than 72 hours before the time of presentation and the patient is responding to medical management (i.e., a nasogastric tube; nothing by mouth; antibiotics), then surgery is delayed for 4 to 6 weeks.
    **(c)** Deterioration or failure to improve on medical management is an indication for surgery.
**3. Emphysematous cholecystitis** is an acute, **usually gangrenous cholecystitis** complicated by secondary invasion by gas-forming organisms.

      **a.** Unlike acute cholecystitis, emphysematous cholecystitis is three times more prevalent in males than in females, and it is often not associated with cholelithiasis.

      **b. Radiologically**, the gallbladder is seen as filled with gas, in the absence of any abnormal communication between the gallbladder and the gastrointestinal tract.

      **c. Treatment** is early cholecystectomy, or cholecystostomy if the patient is too ill to tolerate cholecystectomy. Antibiotics effective against *Clostridia* and coliform organisms are given.

  **4. Chronic cholecystitis**

      **a. Clinical findings.** The patient complains of moderate intermittent pain in the right upper quadrant and epigastric region, nausea, and vomiting. Symptoms are particularly associated with eating fatty foods.

      **b. Diagnosis.** On oral cholecystography, the gallbladder fails to visualize or shows a filling defect. Ultrasonography may show stones.

      **c. Treatment** is cholecystectomy. About 75% of patients operated on for cholecystitis secondary to cholelithiasis are relieved of their symptoms; 25% retain mild symptoms that presumably are unrelated to the biliary tree.

  **5. Acalculous cholecystitis** is acute or chronic **cholecystitis in the absence of stones**. It occurs as a frequent complication of burns, sepsis, trauma, or collagen vascular disease.

      **a. Etiology.** Possible causes include:

        **(1)** Kinking or fibrosis of the gallbladder

        **(2)** Thrombosis of the cystic artery

        **(3)** Sphincter spasm with obstruction of the biliary and pancreatic ducts

        **(4)** Prolonged fasting

        **(5)** Dehydration

        **(6)** Systemic disease, such as the multiorgan failure associated with trauma

        **(7)** Generalized sepsis

      **b. Treatment** is cholecystectomy, or cholecystostomy if the patient is too ill to tolerate cholecystectomy.

**G. Postcholecystectomy syndrome** is the term given to **symptoms that develop after or persist despite cholecystectomy**.

  **1.** In a patient who underwent cholecystectomy for chronic cholecystitis and cholelithiasis, the symptoms are usually **extrabiliary** in origin. Such **causes** include:

      **a.** Hiatal hernia

      **b.** Peptic ulcer

      **c.** Pancreatitis

      **d.** Irritable bowel

      **e.** Food intolerance

  **2.** However, symptoms may be due to a **biliary cause**:

      **a.** A stone in the common bile duct

      **b.** A cystic duct stone

      **c.** Stenosis of the sphincter of Oddi

      **d.** Biliary stricture

  **3.** Although a rare occurrence, the cystic duct stump can undergo inflammation and stone formation.

**H. Bile duct disorders**

  **1. Choledocholithiasis**

      **a. Stones in the common bile duct** can be single or multiple and are found in 10% to 20% of patients who are undergoing cholecystectomy.

      **b.** Most such stones are formed in the gallbladder and pass into the duct. However, primary common duct stones can form.

      **c. Clinical findings.** Some patients are asymptomatic. Others present with right upper quadrant pain that radiates to the right shoulder, or with intermittent obstructive jaundice, acholic stools, and bilirubinuria.

      **d. Diagnosis**

        **(1)** In contrast to findings in neoplastic obstruction of the common bile duct or ampulla of Vater, the gallbladder is not palpable.

        **(2) Diagnostic studies** include ultrasonography, transhepatic cholangiography, or a radionuclide scan.

        **(3) Liver function test results** are consistent with obstructive jaundice, and include elevations in bilirubin and alkaline phosphatase.

**e. Treatment**
  **(1)** This involves cholecystectomy, choledochotomy, common bile duct exploration, stone removal, T-tube placement, and T-tube operative cholangiography.
  **(2) Operative cholangiography and common bile duct exploration**
    **(a)** The use of operative cholangiography has decreased the need for common bile duct exploration while increasing the number of positive explorations.
    **(b)** The only absolute indication for common bile duct exploration is a palpable stone in the common bile duct.
    **(c)** When any of the following are present, operative cholangiography is performed instead, although these were at one time considered to be absolute or relative indications for duct exploration:
      **(i)** Increased size of the common bile duct
      **(ii)** Jaundice
      **(iii)** Small stones in the gallbladder
      **(iv)** A history of cholangitis or pancreatitis
    **(d)** Common bile duct exploration is not necessary if the operative cholangiogram is of good quality and demonstrates both:
      **(i)** No filling defects
      **(ii)** The free flow of contrast medium into the duodenum
    **(e)** Common bile duct exploration is indicated if the operative cholangiogram shows either:
      **(i)** Filling defects within the intra- or extrahepatic biliary tree
      **(ii)** Obstruction of the flow of bile into the duodenum
**f. Retained common bile duct stones**
  **(1)** Stones that remain after surgery complicate up to 10% of common bile duct explorations.
  **(2)** For small stones, no treatment is needed. If stones are larger, treatment options are:
    **(a)** Chemical dissolution by administration of:
      **(i)** Sodium cholate
      **(ii)** Monooctanoin (a medium-chain diglyceride)
      **(iii)** Heparin
    **(b)** Mechanical extraction under radiographic guidance

**2. Cholangitis**, or **inflammation of the bile ducts**, is a potentially life-threatening disease that results from concurrent biliary infection and obstruction. *E. coli* is the most common offending organism.
  **a. Etiology.** Benign postoperative strictures and common bile duct stones account for 60% of the cases. Neoplasms, sclerosing cholangitis, plugged biliary drainage tubes, and biliary contrast studies are other causes.
  **b. Clinical findings. Charcot's triad** of fever, jaundice, and right upper quadrant pain is present in 70% of cases. In severe cases, hypotension may be present.
  **c. Treatment** includes antibiotics, resuscitation with fluids and electrolytes, and relief of the obstruction.
  **d.** The **prognosis** depends on the cause of the obstruction; from best prognosis to worst, the order is stones, benign stricture, sclerosing cholangitis, and neoplasm.

**3. Primary sclerosing cholangitis** is a disease of unknown etiology that affects the biliary tract, resulting in stenosis or obstruction of the ductal system. Progressive obstruction, if not relieved, results in biliary cirrhosis and liver failure.
  **a. Clinical findings**
    **(1) Symptoms and signs** include right upper quadrant pain and painless jaundice, usually without fever or chills. Other symptoms include pruritus, fatigue, nausea, and symptoms of hepatic failure.
    **(2)** Other inflammatory conditions, particularly ulcerative colitis, may be present.
  **b. Histologically**, the bile ducts show edema and areas of inflammation and fibrosis submucosally and subserosally.
  **c. Diagnosis**
    **(1)** The diagnosis is made:
      **(a)** Most commonly by exploratory laparotomy
      **(b)** Nonsurgically by either endoscopic retrograde cholangiography or percutaneous transhepatic cholangiography
    **(2)** The **criteria** needed to fulfill the diagnosis are:
      **(a)** Thickening and stenosis of a major portion of the biliary ductal system
      **(b)** Absence of prior surgery, choledocholithiasis, malignancy, or congenital biliary anomalies
      **(c)** No evidence of primary liver disease, particularly primary biliary cirrhosis

    **d. Operative management** is complex and is strongly determined by the level of bile duct involvement and the amount of fibrosis present.

      **(1)** A careful exploration is performed to determine the presence of disease outside the right upper quadrant.

      **(2)** The region of the gastrohepatic ligament and gallbladder is examined. To confirm the diagnosis, the wall of the common duct is opened and operative cholangiography is performed to determine the extent of luminal narrowing and the absence of stones. The wall of the common duct is biopsied for histologic confirmation and a liver biopsy is performed.

      **(3)** The **goal of operative management** is to restore adequate and, one hopes, permanent biliary drainage.

        **(a) Internal biliary drainage**, via either a hepaticoenteric or choledochoenteric anastomosis, is the preferable method of management. This is most successful when the major area of involvement is the extrahepatic bile ducts.

        **(b) External biliary drainage**, using either a T tube as an internal stent or a percutaneous stent, establishes adequate drainage initially but should only be used as a last resort because of the higher propensity for occlusion and resultant bacterial cholangitis.

        **(c)** Cholecystectomy is performed only when gallbladder disease requires it.

    **e.** The **postoperative course** is strongly dependent upon the presence of preoperative sepsis and the adequacy of drainage. Steroids have not been proven to be of benefit and could potentially complicate the postoperative course.

    **f.** The **prognosis** is poorly defined at present. If the liver parenchyma has been severely damaged, only hepatic transplantation offers a real chance of longevity, and this procedure is only possible when the patient is free of sepsis.

  **4. Fibrosis of the sphincter of Oddi** is a disorder of uncertain etiology that causes colicky right upper quadrant pain, nausea, and vomiting. Treatment is by endoscopic papillotomy, choledochoduodenostomy, and sphincteroplasty.

**I.  Biliary-enteric fistula and gallstone ileus**

  **1. Pathophysiology.** This complication of cholelithiasis usually results from cystic duct obstruction which then progresses to acute cholecystitis, empyema, adhesions to the surrounding viscera, and subsequent perforation and passage of the stone.

  **2.** The **site of communication** with the gallbladder is most commonly the duodenum, but the colon or any other intra-abdominal or intrathoracic viscera may be penetrated.

  **3. Site of obstruction**

    **a.** If the stone travels in the gastrointestinal lumen, the terminal ileum is the most common site of obstruction, as this is the narrowest portion of the small bowel. Stones smaller than 2 cm to 3 cm will usually be passed per rectum.

    **b.** If the stone is passed free into the peritoneal cavity, extraluminal obstruction secondary to inflammation and adhesions can occur anywhere.

  **4. Clinical findings**

    **a.** This is a disease of the elderly, and concomitant multisystem disease is common.

    **b.** The patient presents with symptoms of small-bowel obstruction (nausea, vomiting, obstipation, pain, distention).

    **c.** About 25% of the patients will have symptoms of acute cholecystitis immediately preceding the episode of obstruction. Some 50% to 70% of the patients have a history of cholelithiasis.

  **5. Diagnosis**

    **a.** The correct diagnosis is made preoperatively in fewer than 25% of the cases.

    **b.** The diagnosis is suggested by the history and by plain films of the abdomen. These may show small-bowel obstruction accompanied by air in the biliary tree, or a radiopaque stone in the right lower quadrant. A stone will be visualized in fewer than 15% of cases.

  **6. Treatment**

    **a.** As these patients are often extremely ill, emergency laparotomy may permit only localization of the stone, proximal enterotomy, stone extraction, and closure of the enterotomy.

    **b.** The whole small bowel, common bile duct, and gallbladder must be palpated for stones, as recurrent gallstone ileus will develop in 5% to 9% of the patients.

    **c.** Cholecystectomy and closure of the biliary fistula can be performed either concomitantly, or after an interval, depending on the patient's condition.

**J. Neoplasms**

1. **Benign tumors of the gallbladder** are rare. They include papilloma, adenomyoma, fibroma, lipoma, myoma, myxoma, and carcinoid.

2. **Carcinoma of the gallbladder** accounts for 4% of all carcinomas. It is the most common cancer of the biliary tract and occurs in 1% of all patients undergoing biliary tract surgery.
   a. Although the **etiology** is not known, 90% of the patients have a history of cholelithiasis.
   b. About 80% of the tumors are adenocarcinomas. Metastases occur by lymphatic spread to the pancreatic, duodenal, and choledochal nodes, and by direct extension to the liver.
   c. **Clinical presentation.** The most common complaint is right upper quadrant pain. This is often associated with nausea and vomiting. The **diagnosis** is rarely made preoperatively.
   d. **Treatment.** Cholecystectomy with wedge resection of the liver and regional lymphadenectomy provides the best chance for cure.
   e. **Prognosis** is poor, the 5-year survival rate ranging from 0 to 10%.

3. **Common bile duct malignant tumors** are rare and are difficult to cure.
   a. **Clinical findings**
      (1) The patient usually complains of pruritus, anorexia, weight loss, and an aching right upper quadrant pain. Jaundice is usually severe.
      (2) The following diseases are occasionally associated with this malignancy:
         (a) Chronic ulcerative colitis
         (b) Sclerosing cholangitis
         (c) Chronic parasitic infections of the bile ducts
         (d) Gallstones (present in 18% to 65% of cases)
   b. The **clinical diagnosis** may be made by percutaneous transhepatic cholangiography or ERCP. Both procedures allow the obtaining of biopsy material for pathologic examination.
   c. **Pathologic findings**
      (1) The tumor may be located in the distal common bile duct (one-third of cases), the common hepatic duct or cystic duct (one-third of cases), or the right or left hepatic duct. When the confluence of the hepatic ducts is involved, the tumor is termed a **Klatskin tumor**.
      (2) The tumor initially metastasizes to the regional lymph nodes (16% of cases), spreads by direct extension into the liver (14%), or metastasizes to the liver (10%).
      (3) The gross pathologic finding is a mass involving a portion of the bile ducts. The microscopic appearance is that of adenocarcinoma, although the distinction from sclerosing cholangitis may be difficult.
   d. The **management** of common bile duct tumors is generally surgical, although fewer than 10% are resectable at the time of initial diagnosis.
      (1) Tumors in the distal duct may be resected by pancreaticoduodenectomy, with biliary and gastrointestinal reconstruction. More proximal lesions can sometimes be locally resected, with subsequent biliary reconstruction. The average length of survival after resection is 23 months. Postoperative radiation may improve the life expectancy.
      (2) Unresectable lesions should be bypassed by some form of rigid stent to provide palliative therapy of the biliary obstructive symptoms.
         (a) Laparotomy with no bypass is associated with an average survival time of less than 6 months.
         (b) With T-tube stenting, the average survival time is less than 10 months.
         (c) With transhepatic stenting, the average survival time is 19 months.
            (i) In this procedure, either an internal or external transhepatic stent is placed percutaneously or a U tube is placed surgically.
            (ii) The U tube passes from the skin, through the liver, into the common bile duct and through the tumor, and then back out through the abdominal wall. The U tube can easily be maintained by irrigations and even by percutaneous removal and replacement.
         (d) When a common bile duct tube cannot be placed, an intrahepatic cholangiojejunostomy (**Longmire procedure**) may provide adequate biliary drainage. This is performed by partial hepatic resection followed by suturing a defunctionalized segment of small intestine to the liver edge. This allows bile to leak from the surface of the liver and into the gastrointestinal tract.
   e. **Prognosis**
      (1) Metastatic spread of the tumor is usually slow and is not responsible for death.
      (2) The usual cause of death postoperatively is related to the following problems:
         (a) Progressive biliary cirrhosis due to inadequate biliary drainage
         (b) Persistent intrahepatic infection and abscess formation
         (c) General debility

**K. Anomalies of the biliary tree** are surgically important because the classic anatomic descriptions apply to only one-third of the population. Cystic artery anomalies or hepatic anomalies are seen in one-half of the population

1. **Choledochal cyst**
   a. **Classification.** These **congenital malformations of the pancreaticobiliary tree** are of four types:
      (1) **Type I**: fusiform dilatation of the common bile duct
      (2) **Type II**: diverticula of the common bile duct
      (3) **Type III**: choledochocele involving the intraduodenal portion of the common bile duct
      (4) **Type IV**: cystic involvement of the intrahepatic bile ducts (**Caroli's disease**)
   b. The **pathogenesis** is not known. **Pathologically**, patients show cystic dilatation of the common bile duct, a normal liver parenchyma and (except in Caroli's disease) a normal intrahepatic biliary tree, and partial obstruction of the terminal common bile duct.
   c. **Clinical findings.** The most common presenting symptom is intermittent jaundice. The classic triad of pain, jaundice, and an abdominal mass occurs in only 30% of the cases.
   d. **Diagnosis.** Ultrasonography is the best initial investigative study; next most useful is radionuclide scanning. Transhepatic cholangiography and ERCP can define the extent of the disease but are not necessary.
   e. **Treatment**
      (1) Type I patients are treated with cholecystectomy, cyst excision, and a Roux-en-Y choledochojejunostomy.
      (2) Type II patients are treated by excision of the choledochocele.
      (3) Type III patients are treated by cyst excision and choledochoduodenostomy.
      (4) Type IV patients require liver transplantation; the anomaly is frequently fatal.
   f. **Complications** of choledochal cysts include cholangitis, cirrhosis, and carcinoma.

2. **Congenital biliary atresia** (see Chapter 33, section IX B)

**L. Trauma**

1. **Gallbladder injuries** are uncommon but can be seen after both penetrating and nonpenetrating trauma. Associated visceral injuries are common and most frequently (72%) involve the liver.
   a. **Types of injuries** to the gallbladder include contusions, avulsion, rupture, and traumatic cholecystitis.
   b. **Clinical findings.** Right upper quadrant pain, right chest pain, biliary leakage through a penetrating wound, and shock are the most common presenting symptoms.
   c. **Diagnosis** is most frequently made at laparotomy. A peritoneal tap may be negative.

2. **Extrahepatic bile duct injuries**
   a. **Operative injury.** The majority of extrahepatic bile duct injuries are iatrogenic, occurring after uncomplicated cholecystectomy.
      (1) **Clinical findings.** Only 15% of intraoperative injuries are diagnosed at the time of surgery; 85% present days to years later with progressive jaundice, cholangitis, or cirrhosis and its complications.
      (2) **Diagnosis** is by transhepatic cholangiography.
      (3) In **treatment**, end-to-end (duct-to-duct) anastomosis is always preferable, although a Roux-en-Y choledochojejunostomy is acceptable as well.
      (4) The mortality rate after repair of a chronic biliary stricture is 8% to 10%, and death is usually secondary to liver failure.
   b. **Other extrahepatic bile duct injuries** almost always accompany other visceral injuries and result from trauma such as gunshot wounds. Isolated bile duct injuries are rare.
      (1) **Clinical findings** are the same as those in gallbladder injuries, and **diagnosis** is made at laparotomy.
      (2) **Treatment**, besides administration of antibiotics, involves:
         (a) Meticulous exploration of the ducts
         (b) Mobilizing the duodenum to visualize the retroperitoneum (Kocher maneuver) to rule out retroduodenal perforation of the common bile duct
         (c) Either a primary end-to-end (duct-to-duct) anastomosis or a Roux-en-Y choledochojejunostomy.
   c. **Intraperitoneal extravasation of bile**
      (1) The extravasation of **sterile bile** results in a chemical peritonitis.
         (a) This may be a mild peritonitis, producing ascites, or a localized collection.
         (b) Continuous outpouring of sterile bile may produce an extensive chemical peritonitis and shock.
      (2) **Infected intraperitoneal bile** induces a fulminant and frequently fatal peritonitis.

# 10
# The Pancreas

Bruce E. Jarrell
Jerome J. Vernick
Stephen M. Weiss

## I. ANATOMY

**A.** The pancreas (Fig. 10-1) is a retroperitoneal, pistol-shaped organ. The handle of the pistol lies in the duodenal C-loop, and the barrel extends to the left upper quadrant.

1. The **head of the pancreas** lies over the aorta and under the stomach and transverse colon, posteromedial to the inferior vena cava.
   a. The superior limit of the head is the portal vein. The anterior limit is the gastroduodenal artery.
   b. The common bile duct courses posterior to the head of the pancreas and partially within it.
   c. The head of the pancreas has a common blood supply with the medial wall of the duodenal C-loop. The serosal surface of the duodenum is intimately related to the capsule of the pancreas in that area.

2. The **uncinate process** lies posterior to the superior mesenteric vein and anterior to the inferior vena cava.

3. The splenic artery and vein provide the **blood supply** to the pancreas. The pancreatic body and tail are related to these vessels, which run posterior and superior into the hilus of the spleen.

4. The **tail of the pancreas** is intimately related to the spleen and contains, besides the splenic artery and vein, most accessory spleens (see Chapter II, section VIII C).

5. The **neck of the pancreas** lies at the confluence of the splenic and inferior mesenteric veins. The **posterior aspect of the pancreas** lies over this confluence, at the origin of the portal vein.

6. The superior mesenteric artery and the superior mesenteric vein exit below the pancreas at the junction of the body and head and are surrounded by the uncinate process.

7. The **anterior aspect of the pancreas** lies against the posterior wall of the stomach, forming the posterior border of the lesser omental bursa, or lesser sac.

**B.** The average **weight** of the pancreas is 85 g, and the usual **length** is 12 cm to 15 cm. The normal anteroposterior thickness of the head is less than 2.5 cm; the neck, 1.5 cm; the body, 2 cm; and the tail, 2.5 cm.

**C.** The **pancreatic ducts** drain pancreatic secretions into the duodenum. They comprise two separate systems:

1. The **major system** is the **duct of Wirsung**, which empties into the ampulla of Vater in conjunction with the common bile duct.

2. The **minor system** is the **duct of Santorini**, which empties into a minor papilla approximately 2 cm above and medial to the ampulla of Vater.

## II. PANCREATITIS is an inflammatory process in the pancreas.

**A. Classification**

1. Pancreatitis was classified into four different categories in 1963, in order to clarify the different types of syndromes that are seen and to improve the standardization of treatment and prognosis.

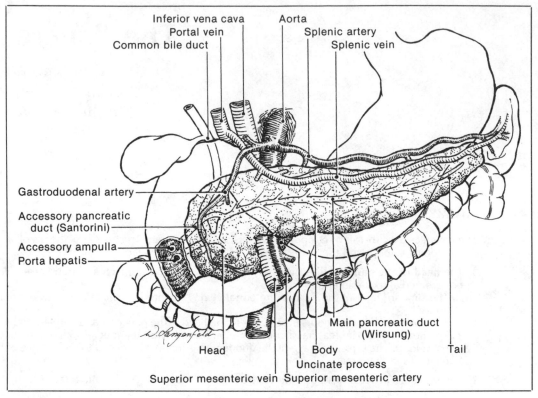

**Figure 10-1.** Anatomy of the pancreas.

**2.** The four **categories of pancreatitis** are as follows:
   **a. Acute pancreatitis** arises in a previously asymptomatic patient and subsides to normalcy after treatment.
   **b. Acute relapsing pancreatitis** is a series of recurrent episodes of acute pancreatitis in an otherwise asymptomatic patient. A quiescent, asymptomatic phase always precedes and follows each attack.
   **c. Chronic relapsing pancreatitis** is a chronic inflammation of the pancreas with chemical evidence of pancreatitis which fluctuates in its intensity and does not return to normal.
   **d. Chronic pancreatitis** shows unrelenting symptoms that are due to inflammation and fibrosis of the pancreas; the pancreatic duct and parenchyma usually show calcification. Chronic pancreatitis is often associated with malabsorption and even with pancreatic endocrine insufficiency.

**B. Etiology.** Approximately 75% of pancreatitis cases can be explained on the basis of biliary tract disease or alcohol abuse, although the exact mechanism for production of pancreatitis in these cases remains theoretical.

   **1. Biliary pancreatitis** is thought to be induced by the inflammation that results from continued passage of stones through a common channel.
      **a.** The pancreatic duct and the bile duct empty into a common papilla, which is subject to trauma in a patient with biliary calculi.
      **b.** The entire common channel can be obstructed if a large calculus becomes impacted in the papilla. This can cause reflux of bile into the pancreatic duct, and experiments have shown that such reflux can induce pancreatitis. However, it is not clear whether this actually occurs in humans.

   **2. Alcohol** is thought to cause pancreatitis by inducing an increase in gastric acidity.
      **a.** The combination of alcohol plus gastric acid causes
         **(1)** Increased pancreatic secretion
         **(2)** Spasm of the sphincter of Oddi
      **b.** The increased intraductal pressure combined with the sphincteric spasm then presumably results in pancreatitis.

C. **Acute pancreatitis**

1. The **clinical presentation** of acute pancreatitis may vary from mild abdominal discomfort to profound shock with hypotension and hypoxemia. Usually the patient presents with epigastric pain that radiates to the back and is associated with nausea and vomiting.

2. There is often a **history** of recent consumption of a heavy meal, many times with generous quantities of alcoholic beverages. The pain typically begins 1 to 4 hours after a meal, and is often less severe when the patient sits slumped forward.

3. **Physical findings** vary with the severity of the inflammatory process.
   a. Most patients have mild to moderate abdominal tenderness.
   b. In severe cases a rigid abdomen with epigastric guarding, rebound tenderness, and marked abdominal pain may be present.
   c. Severe pancreatic inflammation and necrosis may cause **retroperitoneal hemorrhage**.
      (1) This can lead to large third-space fluid losses and hypovolemia, hypotension, and tachycardia.
      (2) It can also allow blood dissection along different tissue planes.
         (a) When this extends to the flank tissues, resulting in flank ecchymoses, it is known as **Grey Turner's sign**.
         (b) When the blood dissects up the falciform ligament and creates a periumbilical ecchymosis, it is known as **Cullen's sign**.

4. The **diagnosis** of acute pancreatitis is aided by the following studies:
   a. **Serum amylase level.** This is elevated in 95% of patients with pancreatitis.
      (1) Approximately 5% of all amylase determinations are falsely positive, and only 75% of patients with abdominal pain and an increased amylase level have pancreatitis.
      (2) The rise in amylase level is not proportional to the severity of the pancreatitis. Some inferences, however, can be made from the degree of elevation.
         (a) An amylase level over 1000 Somogyi units usually indicates biliary tract disease with pancreatitis.
         (b) An amylase level between 200 and 500 units often indicates alcoholic pancreatitis. Some 17% of patients with amylase levels in this range have no other evidence of pancreatitis.
      (3) The pancreas must be intact and functional to synthesize amylase and release it into the circulation. Thus, patients with acute pancreatitis superimposed on chronic pancreatitis may not demonstrate a rise in serum amylase.
      (4) A significant amount of circulating amylase is not of pancreatic origin. The major alternative source is salivary.
   b. **Amylase:creatinine clearance ratio.** Amylase determinations are more sensitive when the amylase clearance rate is compared to the creatinine clearance rate and a ratio is established.
      (1) An amylase:creatinine clearance ratio above 5 is significant and is strongly suggestive of pancreatitis.
      (2) Using this ratio avoids the problem of rapid renal clearance of amylase, which tends to reduce serum levels below the point where a simple serum amylase determination would be positive.
      (3) Impaired renal function affects the creatinine clearance rate sooner than the amylase clearance rate. Even in this situation, however, the amylase:creatinine clearance ratio appears to be more sensitive than the serum amylase level if urine specimens are collected for at least 1 hour.
   c. **Radiographic imaging**
      (1) **Plain films** of the upper abdomen are relatively insensitive with regard to diagnosing pancreatitis. Significant findings include the following:
         (a) Calcification in the area of the lesser sac and pancreas may indicate chronic pancreatitis, which is most often seen in association with alcoholism.
         (b) A gas collection in the lesser sac suggests abscess formation in or around the pancreas.
         (c) Blurred psoas shadows from retroperitoneal pancreatic necrosis may be seen on plain films.
         (d) Soft tissue shadows and gas-containing viscera may be visibly displaced by collections and edema in the lesser sac and structures adjacent to the pancreas.
         (e) An area of colonic spasm adjacent to an inflamed pancreas will cause the gas in the transverse colon to end abruptly (the "cutoff" sign).
         (f) Focal duodenal and jejunal ileus in the area of the pancreas can cause the "reversed 3" or "inverted 3" sign.
      (2) **Barium studies** may demonstrate upper gastrointestinal abnormalities.

        **(a)** The duodenal C-loop may be widened by pancreatic edema.

        **(b)** Hypotonic duodenography may demonstrate the **"pad" sign,** a smoothing out or obliteration of the duodenal mucosal folds by the edematous pancreas and the inflammatory response on the medial aspect of the C-loop.

    **(3)** Angiography is useful for visualization of suspected neoplasms, but is not useful in the diagnosis of pancreatitis.

  **d. Ultrasound imaging** of the pancreas is particularly useful in the diagnosis of pancreatitis.

    **(1)** Changes from the normal anatomy of the pancreas and its vascular landmarks can be delineated.

        **(a)** Acute pancreatitis is suggested by swelling beyond the normal anteroposterior thickness and loss of tissue planes between the pancreas and the splenic vein.

        **(b)** Other anomalies of the pancreas may also be seen. For example, a change in duct size or calcification may be shown.

        **(c)** Chronic pancreatitis is often manifested by the presence of calcification or pseudocysts containing fluid or showing a complex cystic structure.

        **(d)** Ascites, which is easily diagnosed by ultrasound, may or may not be present in chronic pancreatitis.

    **(2)** Various pancreatic disorders can change the ultrasound echogenicity.

        **(a)** Most diseases decrease the echogenicity in the pancreas; this is due to the presence of edema and inflammation. Tumors are also often hypoechogenic.

        **(b)** Increased echogenicity is generally due to gas or calcification.

    **(3)** Fluid densities lying within the pancreas indicate cysts, abscesses, or possibly lymphoma.

    **(4)** Ultrasound may also demonstrate the presence of gallbladder pathology, such as cholecystitis, cholelithiasis, or a dilated common bile duct.

    **(5)** Ultrasound has a major limitation, in that it cannot be performed when excessive bowel gas is present, as occurs with an ileus.

  **e. Computed tomographic (CT) scanning** of the pancreas may also be helpful. It provides higher resolution than ultrasonography does, and it is not limited by blocking of intestinal gas.

    **(1)** The criteria for findings are similar to those described for ultrasound.

    **(2)** Dilute barium ingestion may help to outline the pancreas.

**5.** The **prognosis** in acute pancreatitis is aided by certain signs which are associated with a higher mortality rate and are therefore useful prognostic indicators.

  **a. Signs present when the patient is admitted:**

    **(1)** Patient's age over 55 years

    **(2)** White blood cell count over 16,000/mm³ of blood

    **(3)** Fasting blood sugar level over 200 mg/dl

    **(4)** Lactic dehydrogenase (LDH) over 350 units/ml

    **(5)** Serum glutamic oxaloacetic transaminase (SGOT) over 250 units/ml

  **b. Signs present 48 hours after admission:**

    **(1)** A 10% drop in hematocrit

    **(2)** An increase of 5 mg/dl in blood urea nitrogen (BUN)

    **(3)** Serum calcium levels under 8 mg/dl

    **(4)** Arterial oxygen partial pressure ($Pa_{O_2}$) below 60 mm Hg

    **(5)** Anion base deficit greater than 4 mEq/L

    **(6)** Third-space fluid loss greater than 6 L

  **c. Determining prognosis.** If 0 to 2 of the above signs are present, the mortality rate is 0.9%; if 7 to 8 signs are present, it is 100%.

    **(1)** The poor prognostic signs at 48 hours are generally related to the severe local effects of pancreatitis, which result in massive third-space fluid loss and hemorrhage.

    **(2)** Systemic effects such as shock and hypoxia may also be a consequence of circulating toxins released by the pancreas.

**6.** In the **medical management** of acute pancreatitis certain measures are considered standard. Not all of them are indicated in each case, however, and the patient's symptoms dictate much of the treatment required.

  **a. Nasogastric suction** is used to control nausea and vomiting, decrease pancreatic stimulation, and decrease gastrointestinal distention from an ileus. It also makes the patient more comfortable, although it does not appear to shorten the hospital stay.

  **b. Intravenous fluids** are used to replace the third-space fluid loss from edema and extravasation into the peripancreatic spaces. Crystalloid solutions are usually adequate.

    **(1) Monitoring** similar to that for burn patients should be initiated.

    **(2)** This should include the use of a Foley catheter to measure urine output.

    **(3)** In severe cases with unstable hemodynamics the patient's fluid status should be monitored accurately with a Swan-Ganz catheter.

    **c. Antibiotics** reduce the risk of abscess formation and of lesser sac collections, which often progress to abscess formation.
    **(1)** The early use of antibiotics is thought to promote the maturation of these collections into pseudocysts (see section II F) rather than abscesses.
    **(2)** Antibiotics also act as prophylaxis against cholangitis, which can develop if a swollen pancreatic head obstructs the biliary tract.
    **(3)** If the pancreatitis is due to biliary calculi, the bile is almost certainly contaminated with bacteria, and antibiotics are indicated.
    **d.** In severe pancreatitis, respiratory distress is common, as are **pleural effusions**. These are more often on the left and contain high concentrations of amylase.
    **(1)** The $Pa_{O_2}$ should therefore be monitored closely in patients with severe pancreatitis.
    **(2)** Serial chest x-rays should be obtained to rule out the presence of effusions and parenchymal disease.
    **e.** Oral feedings should be withheld until laboratory test results return to normal and pain is gone for 48 hours. Exacerbations of the pancreatitis are common with premature feedings and removal of the nasogastric tube.

  **7. Surgery in acute pancreatitis**
    **a.** The **indications for surgery** include the following:
    **(1)** To confirm the diagnosis in severe cases that do not respond to the measures just described
      **(a)** The symptoms of severe acute pancreatitis can be mimicked by visceral perforation, mesenteric arterial occlusion, and other intra-abdominal catastrophes.
      **(b)** Surgery may be needed to establish the diagnosis before the situation is irreversible.
    **(2)** To relieve biliary or pancreatic duct obstruction
      **(a)** Early biliary tract surgery has increased the mortality rate in severe pancreatitis. If possible, therefore, surgery should be delayed until the pancreatitis has subsided.
      **(b)** If the patient's status continues to deteriorate, surgical exploration may become necessary.
        **(i)** Cholecystostomy or common bile duct drainage should be considered, with definitive dissection deferred, when there are acute severe inflammatory changes in the duodenum and region of the ampulla.
        **(ii)** Definitive biliary tract surgery to correct the cause of the pancreatitis (e.g., removal of common bile duct stones or gallstones; repair of the sphincter of Oddi) should be done during the same admission as for the treatment of the acute pancreatitis, in order to prevent recurrence.
    **(3)** To drain the lesser sac
      **(a)** Pancreatic or lesser sac drainage increases morbidity if it is done before septic complications have occurred. It is not effective as a prophylactic measure.
      **(b)** Drainage has been shown to improve the prognosis when sepsis has occurred and lesser sac collections are present.
      **(c)** For drainage of established lesser sac abscesses, drains can be inserted after wide opening of the lesser omentum. Irrigation catheters can be used as part of the therapeutic plan.
    **b.** Resection for acute pancreatitis is a dangerous procedure and is not indicated. It has not been shown to decrease morbidity; indeed, in some studies resection increased the mortality rate.
    **c. Peritoneal lavage** may be useful in excluding other severe intra-abdominal processes and may be therapeutic in severe pancreatitis. However, peritoneal lavage appears to improve early mortality rates but not ultimate survival rates in acute severe pancreatitis.
    **(1)** Catheters may be placed percutaneously, and antibiotics may be included in the lavage solution.
    **(2)** Peritoneal lavage can be undertaken as part of a laparotomy performed for diagnosis and lesser sac exploration.
    **(3)** Complications include a deterioration of pulmonary function, which may be compromised by abdominal distention from the dialysis solutions.
    **(4)** A high glucose load in the dialysis solution may induce severe hyperglycemia.

**D. Relapsing pancreatitis** frequently occurs in nonalcoholic patients and results from biliary tract disease—either calculi in the ducts or inflammation and spasm of the sphincter of Oddi.

  **1.** The **diagnosis** of relapsing pancreatitis may be made by demonstrating the presence of biliary stones or biliary sphincter dysfunction.
    **a. Ultrasound** (see section I D 3 d) is useful for diagnosing biliary calculi.
    **b. Microscopic examination of the bile** is useful.

(1) Bile is aspirated through a suction tube placed in the duodenum.
(2) The bile is examined for white blood cells, cholesterol crystals, and microspheroliths.
(3) These are signs of occult biliary disease and are an indication for cholecystectomy.
c. **Provocative testing** (i.e., the **Nardi test**) can be done to determine if narcotic-induced stimulation or spasm will reproduce the abdominal pain and amylase elevation.
 (1) Morphine and neostigmine are given intramuscularly, and baseline levels are obtained for SGOT and serum glutamic pyruvic transaminase (SGPT), γ-glutamyl transpeptidase (GGT), amylase, and lipase.
 (2) Determinations are repeated at hourly intervals for 4 hours, and a final determination is made at 8 hours.
 (3) The test is positive if biliary pain is reproduced within 15 to 20 minutes after the injection and if the enzyme levels increase at least four times over the baseline levels.
 (4) In the presence of sphincteric disease:
  (a) Amylase levels will rise whether or not the gallbladder is present.
  (b) Liver-related enzymes will not rise if the gallbladder is present and can distend to relieve pressure on the hepatic ductal system.
 (5) The test can therefore be used to infer sphincteric disease in any pancreatic or biliary ductal system if the gallbladder is absent.
 (6) Although the test is controversial, in our experience it has been accurate in the diagnosis of perisphincteric disease.
 (7) At the time of surgery, the test results can be confirmed by measuring the pressure and flow in the common bile duct.

2. The **treatment** of relapsing pancreatitis is based on the etiology.
 a. In a patient with biliary calculi, the following procedures may be performed:
  (1) Cholecystectomy
  (2) Common bile duct exploration
  (3) Biliary manometry
  (4) Sphincteroplasty plus pancreaticobiliary septum resection, if indicated
 b. The **treatment of perisphincteric disease** is removal of the gallbladder, if it is present, and a wide sphincteroplasty that includes the pancreaticobiliary septum. The results have been very good in patients with a positive Nardi test.
 c. Many patients have had a cholecystectomy in the past, yet continue to have recurrent pancreatitis, biliary tract disease symptoms, or both.
  (1) These patients often have a positive provocative test and can be treated successfully by sphincteroplasty.
  (2) Patients with a negative provocative test require further workup, including endoscopic retrograde cholangiopancreatography (ERCP; see section III A 3 c). Alcohol abuse should be ruled out.

E. **Chronic pancreatitis** is often progressive.

1. **Pathologic findings** include fibrosis and calcification throughout the gland.
 a. Early pancreatic changes may consist of plugging of the small pancreatic ducts with proteinaceous material containing eosinophils.
 b. With progression of the disease, the calcification becomes prominent and multiple areas of ductal dilatation may result.
 c. The ductal dilatation in its end stages produces a "chain-of-lakes" appearance.
 d. Common bile duct obstruction or duodenal obstruction can occur in advanced cases of chronic pancreatitis as a result of inflammation in surrounding areas.

2. The **etiology** is almost always alcohol-related. There are, however, congenital anomalies that can produce chronic ductal obstruction and chronic pancreatitis.

3. **Clinical findings**
 a. A history of unrelenting pain is usual in advanced cases of chronic pancreatitis. The pain is usually the major indication for surgical intervention.
 b. Pancreatic damage may be severe enough to cause pancreatic endocrine insufficiency with impaired glucose tolerance or true diabetes.
 c. Exocrine pancreatic insufficiency results in malabsorption with consequent weight loss and steatorrhea.
 d. Plain films may show the calcifications in the ductal system or may aid in delineating neighboring areas that are caught in the inflammatory process.

4. **Medical treatment** of chronic pancreatitis consists of:
 a. Analgesia
 b. Endocrine replacement as needed

    **c.** Exocrine replacement with pancreatic enzymes such as pancrelipase (Viokase or Pancrease) or cholecystokinin (pancreozymin)

    **d.** General measures such as avoidance of alcoholic beverages and correction of malnutrition

  **5.** **Surgical treatment** of chronic pancreatitis depends on the condition of the pancreatic ducts, as determined by ERCP. If ERCP is not possible and the patient must be operated upon, operative pancreatograms can be obtained.

    **a.** A dilated, "chain-of-lakes" duct is treated by wide unroofing of the duct and dilated ductules, with drainage of the entire open pancreas into a defunctionalized jejunal loop. A side-to-side procedure may be used, or an invagination in which the pancreas is placed into the jejunal loop (the **Puestow operation**).

    **b.** A distal ductal obstruction is treated by distal pancreatectomy.

    **c.** A proximal ductal obstruction is usually treated by amputating the tail of the pancreas and draining the pancreas retrograde into a defunctionalized jejunal loop (**Duval operation**).

    **d.** For a patient with severe pain and a fibrotic, nondilated duct, possible surgical procedures include:

      **(1)** A 95% pancreatectomy (the **Child operation**)

      **(2)** Either an abdominal or thoracic **splanchnicectomy**

        **(a)** This merely divides the splanchnic nerves and serves only to relieve the pain of pancreatitis with no direct effect on the underlying disorder.

        **(b)** It should be noted that a splanchnicectomy will also eradicate the pain from appendicitis and other intra-abdominal problems, which may lead to the delayed diagnosis of an abdominal emergency.

**F.** A **pseudocyst** is a late complication of pancreatitis.

  **1. Pathogenesis**

    **a.** The pseudocyst begins as a lesser sac collection and forms as a result of fibrosis, thickening, and organization of the organs bordering the collection.

    **b.** The pseudocyst is not lined by epithelium and consists only of the inflammatory response of the neighboring organs.

    **c.** The organs forming the walls are the stomach, duodenum, colon, and transverse mesocolon. The major organ involved is generally the stomach, which forms the anterior surface of the pseudocyst.

    **d.** Maturation of the pseudocyst takes 3 to 5 weeks. It is not truly formed until the walls are sufficiently organized to become firm anatomic structures.

    **e.** The **natural history** of the pseudocyst depends on its size. Small pseudocysts may resolve; large pseudocysts with mature organized walls generally do not resolve.

  **2. Clinical findings**

    **a.** During the maturation phase the patient has recovered from a bout of pancreatitis but has developed a persistent elevation of amylase, a low-grade fever, a minimally elevated white blood cell count, and chronic pain.

    **b.** There is a tendency for continuous minor bleeding into the pseudocyst to cause a gradual decrease in hemoglobin and hematocrit.

    **c.** Pseudocysts are usually **diagnosed** by ultrasound or CT scan.

  **3. Treatment**

    **a. During the maturation phase** the goal is to allow this phase to continue until the walls of the pseudocyst have matured.

      **(1)** The patient is generally treated with total parenteral nutrition or an elemental diet for 3 to 4 weeks, until maturation has occurred. Prematurely starting the patient on a full diet is likely to cause an exacerbation of the pancreatitis.

      **(2)** Maturation-phase treatment sometimes must be cut short due to sepsis or to hemorrhage within the pseudocyst.

    **b.** The **mature pseudocyst** is treated surgically.

      **(1)** This is done by internal drainage, if possible.

        **(a)** The common approach is through the anterior wall of the stomach, to locate the firm connection that usually exists between the posterior stomach and the pseudocyst.

          **(i)** An opening is made between the stomach and the pseudocyst, and the wall of the opening is sutured for hemostasis.

          **(ii)** The pseudocyst then drains into the stomach and generally resolves.

        **(b)** If the pseudocyst is not fixed to an organ that lends itself to internal drainage, a defunctionalized loop of jejunum may be sutured to the pseudocyst wall to establish internal drainage.

      **(2)** External drainage can be used if the pseudocyst is not found to be mature and if suturing of the pseudocyst wall is not safe. The external drainage results in a pancreatic fistula, which usually will heal with continued parenteral nutrition.

(3) Excision of a pseudocyst is rarely done, but this may be indicated if the pseudocyst is small and is located distally in the tail of the pancreas.

## III. PANCREATIC MALIGNANCIES

### A. Pancreatic adenocarcinoma

1. The **incidence** of pancreatic adenocarcinoma is rapidly increasing, especially in males.
   a. It is now the fourth most common cause of cancer death for males in the United States.
   b. It accounts for 25,000 annual fatalities, according to the American Cancer Society estimate for 1983.
   c. The rising incidence may be associated with tobacco and coffee use, diabetes, or asbestos exposure.
   d. The tumor occurs most often between ages 50 and 70.

2. **Clinical findings**
   a. Early symptoms are usually vague, such as epigastric pain, weight loss, backache, and depression.
   b. Thrombophlebitis may be the initial presentation. It is migratory and ultimately develops in as many as 10% of the patients.
   c. The **symptoms at the time of presentation** are related to the **location of the tumor** within the pancreas.
      (1) The head of the pancreas is the most common site. Tumors in this site produce weight loss and obstructive jaundice in three-fourths of the patients.
         (a) The jaundice is painless, although back pain or vague abdominal discomfort may be present in up to one-fourth of patients at this stage.
         (b) Because of the retroperitoneal location of the pancreas, tumors must be very large or metastatic to become evident on physical examination. However, an upper abdominal mass may be palpable.
            (i) It represents the tumor mass in as many as 20% of patients, indicating incurability.
            (ii) If the mass represents an enlarged, nontender gallbladder **(Courvoisier gallbladder)**, the cause is most commonly an obstructing pancreatic neoplasm, but the gallbladder is palpable in fewer than one-half of the patients.
      (2) Carcinomas of the body or tail of the pancreas are less common and generally present at a more advanced stage because only about 10% produce obstructive jaundice.

3. **Diagnosis**
   a. Screening for "early" pancreatic cancer is not likely to be useful because even tumors as small as 2 cm or 3 cm are not usually curable.
   b. **Noninvasive imaging techniques**
      (1) CT scanning and ultrasonography are the most useful tests in diagnosing pancreatic cancer. Tumors 2 cm to 3 cm in size can often be detected by these techniques.
      (2) Upper gastrointestinal radiographs can detect pancreatic tumors after they are large enough to distort the duodenum, a late finding.
   c. **Invasive diagnostic techniques**
      (1) Percutaneous fine-needle aspiration uses ultrasound or CT to direct a small-bore needle to a mass.
         (a) A cytologic specimen is obtained with virtually no risk of complication.
         (b) This technique is highly reliable in diagnosing a malignancy.
      (2) Endoscopic retrograde cholangiopancreatography (ERCP) uses a flexible duodenoscope to cannulate the pancreatic duct. Contrast medium is injected and radiographs are taken.
         (a) Small pancreatic cancers can be demonstrated by this technique, and specimens can be collected from the pancreatic duct for cytologic examination.
         (b) Successful cannulation requires a highly skilled endoscopist.
      (3) Percutaneous transhepatic cholangiography (PTC) is useful in the evaluation of patients with obstructive jaundice.
         (a) A long, small-bore needle is inserted, under local anesthesia, through the liver into a dilated hepatic duct, and contrast medium is injected to identify the site of obstruction.
         (b) Jaundice is relieved preoperatively by passing a catheter through the site of obstruction, because very high bilirubin levels may be associated with an increased risk of postoperative complications.
         (c) Potential complications of the procedure are bleeding from the needle tract in the liver, and sepsis.

**4. Prognosis**

    **a.** The prognosis for patients with pancreatic adenocarcinoma is extremely poor.

        **(1)** Overall, the 5-year survival rate is less than 5%, and cures are extremely rare. Most patients die in less than 1 year.

        **(2)** The median length of survival for patients with unresectable tumors is 6 months.

        **(3)** Even for those few patients with resectable tumors, results of surgery are not good. Only about 10% of patients who undergo resection will live 5 years.

    **b.** The poor prognosis is due in part to the difficulty in making a diagnosis while the tumor is at an early stage: Only about 10% of pancreatic adenocarcinomas are resectable at the time of diagnosis.

**5. Treatment**

    **a. Pancreaticoduodenectomy,** the **Whipple procedure**, is the standard surgical treatment for adenocarcinoma of the head of the pancreas when the lesion is curable by resection.

        **(1) Resectability** is determined at surgery from several criteria:

            **(a)** There are no metastases outside the abdomen.

            **(b)** The tumor has not involved the porta hepatis, the portal vein as it passes behind the body of the pancreas, and the superior mesenteric artery region.

            **(c)** The tumor has not spread to the liver or other peritoneal structures.

        **(2)** Histologic **proof of malignancy** is obtained by needle aspiration, either preoperatively or during surgery.

        **(3)** The **Whipple procedure** (Fig. 10-2) involves removal of the head of the pancreas, duodenum, distal common bile duct, gallbladder, and distal stomach.

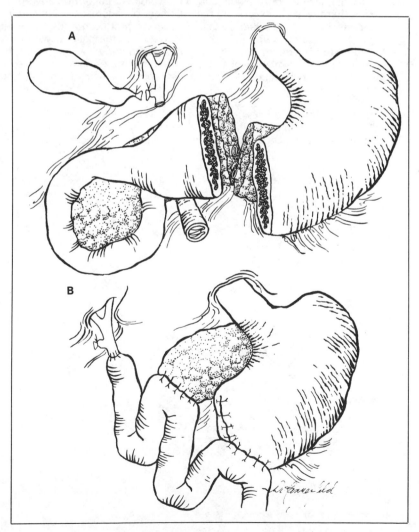

**Figure 10-2.** The Whipple procedure.

        **(a)** The gastrointestinal tract is then reconstructed, with creation of a gastrojejunosto-my, choledochojejunostomy, and pancreaticojejunostomy.

        **(b)** The operative mortality rate with this extensive operation can be as high as 15%.

        **(c)** The complication rate is also considerable, the most common complications being hemorrhage, abscess, and pancreatic ductal leakage.

    **b.** Distal pancreatectomy, usually with splenectomy and lymphadenectomy, is the procedure performed for carcinoma of the midbody and tail of the pancreas.

    **c. Total pancreatectomy** has been proposed for the treatment of pancreatic cancer.

      **(1)** The procedure has two potential advantages:

        **(a)** Removal of a possible multicentric tumor (present in up to 40% of patients)

        **(b)** Avoidance of pancreatic duct anastomotic leaks

      **(2)** However, survival rates are not markedly better, and the operation has not been wide-ly adopted.

      **(3)** In addition, it has resulted in a particularly brittle type of diabetes, making for an un-pleasant postoperative life.

    **d. Palliative procedures** are performed more frequently than curative ones because so many of these tumors are incurable.

      **(1)** Palliative procedures attempt to relieve biliary obstruction by using either the common bile duct or the gallbladder as a conduit for decompression into the intestinal tract.

      **(2)** As many as 20% of patients may require further surgery for gastric outlet obstruction if a gastric bypass procedure is not performed initially. Thus, many centers combine a gastrojejunostomy with choledochojejunostomy as the initial procedure.

      **(3)** Percutaneous transhepatic biliary stents can sometimes be used to provide internal bili-ary drainage for obstructive jaundice, avoiding a major operative procedure.

    **e. Chemotherapy** has been used in the treatment of pancreatic adenocarcinoma. Multidrug regimens that include 5-fluorouracil (5-FU) have produced a response (temporary tumor regression or, rarely, cure) in about 20% to 25% of the patients with metastases.

    **f. Combination treatment** of pancreatic adenocarcinoma has been used experimentally in order to improve local control and to prevent metastases. Intraoperative radiotherapy and the interstitial implantation of radioactive "seeds" are being used, but results are still pre-liminary.

**B. Other pancreatic malignancies** are infrequent. They include cystadenocarcinomas (which typically occur in women), nonfunctional islet cell tumors, and peptide-producing tumors such as insulinomas and Zollinger-Ellison tumors (see Chapter 22, section II).

# Part II
# Study Questions

## QUESTIONS

**Directions:** Each question below contains five suggested answers. Choose the **one best** response to each question.

1. A 60-year-old patient who was known to have colonic diverticular disease was rushed to the hospital because of massive bleeding. Which artery was most likely to be the source of the hemorrhage?

(A) Inferior mesenteric artery, left colic branch
(B) Internal iliac artery, pudendal branch
(C) Internal iliac artery, superior hemorrhoidal branch
(D) Internal iliac artery, inferior hemorrhoidal branch
(E) Left gastroepiploic artery

2. Which of the following statements concerning tumors of the duodenum is true?

(A) Tumors of the duodenum, both benign and malignant, are common disorders
(B) The most common malignant tumor of the duodenum is a malignant lymphoma
(C) Benign duodenal tumors are usually fibromas
(D) Treatment of resectable malignant lesions usually requires pancreaticoduodenectomy (Whipple's procedure)
(E) Benign tumors of the duodenum require vagotomy with antrectomy

3. The carcinoid syndrome can be diagnosed by finding which of the following metabolites in the urine?

(A) 5-Hydroxytryptamine
(B) Serotonin
(C) Metanephrine
(D) 5-Hydroxyindoleacetic acid
(E) Vanillylmandelic acid

4. In which of the following disorders is there an increased risk of adenocarcinoma of the colon?

(A) Granulomatous disease of the colon
(B) Perianal fistula and abscess
(C) Chronic ulcerative colitis
(D) Chronic diverticulitis
(E) Peutz-Jeghers syndrome

5. The most acceptable method of treatment for the first episode of uncomplicated acute colonic diverticulitis is

(A) diverting transverse colostomy
(B) primary resection and reanastomosis
(C) nothing by mouth and intravenous antibiotics
(D) Mikulicz resection
(E) antibiotic enemas

6. All of the following problems commonly occur with the use of balloon tamponade for control of variceal bleeding EXCEPT

(A) pneumonia
(B) aspiration of nasopharyngeal secretions
(C) rebleeding following removal of the tube
(D) gastritis
(E) esophageal ulceration or perforation

7. A 50-year-old man is admitted with massive, bright-red rectal bleeding. He recently had a barium enema that demonstrated no diverticular or space-occupying lesion. Nasogastric suction reveals no blood but does produce yellow bile. The patient continues to bleed. What is the next diagnostic step?

(A) Repeat barium enema
(B) Colonscopy
(C) Upper GI series
(D) Mesenteric angiography
(E) Small bowel follow-through with barium

8. What substance is secreted by the G cells?

(A) Gastrin
(B) Pepsin
(C) Pepsinogen
(D) Gastric acid
(E) Glucagon

9. A patient with Peutz-Jeghers polyps refuses excision. The probability that malignant transformation will occur in the polyps during the next 10 years is

(A) 100%
(B) 75%
(C) 50%
(D) 25%
(E) less than 5%

10. Which of the following tumors of the small intestine have malignant potential?

(A) Adenomatous polyps
(B) Hamartomatous polyps
(C) Juvenile (retention) polyps
(D) Leiomyomas
(E) Fibromas

11. What has been found to be an acceptable screening technique for detecting recurrent colon cancer?

(A) Screening sigmoidoscopy
(B) Screening the stool for occult blood
(C) Stool cytology
(D) Measurement of carcinoembryonic antigen (CEA) levels
(E) Colonoscopy

12. Common duct stones are present in what percentage of patients undergoing cholecystectomy?

(A) 0 to 5%
(B) 10% to 20%
(C) 40% to 50%
(D) 60% to 70%
(E) greater than 70%

13. All of the following findings are useful in determining the prognosis in acute pancreatitis EXCEPT

(A) a white blood cell count over 20,000
(B) a serum calcium level less than 8 mg/dl
(C) hypoxia
(D) a serum amylase level greater than 1000 Somogyi units
(E) patient's age greater than 55 years

14. After absorption, all of the following nutrients are transported across the mucosal cells into the portal venous system EXCEPT

(A) starch
(B) amino acids
(C) vitamin C
(D) triglycerides
(E) tripeptides

15. Sigmoidoscopy will reveal what typical finding in a patient with Crohn's disease involving the rectum?

(A) Normal mucosa
(B) Mucosal ulcers and fissures adjacent to normal-appearing mucosa
(C) Pseudopolyps
(D) Sheets of white blood cells with inflamed mucosa
(E) Edema

16. Which of the following criteria in a patient with alcoholic cirrhosis provides the most acceptable indication for portal-systemic shunting with the best chance of survival?

(A) Proven varices that have never bled but are large
(B) Proven varices that have bled several times in the recent past and have not responded to endoscopic variceal sclerosis
(C) Proven acutely bleeding varices that have not stopped after 10 units of transfused blood
(D) Large esophageal varices and mild encephalopathy
(E) Very high portal pressure discovered during resection of an abdominal aortic aneurysm

17. The most accepted surgical procedure used to treat a chronic pancreatic pseudocyst is

(A) percutaneous drainage
(B) internal drainage to the gastrointestinal tract
(C) pancreatectomy
(D) excision of the pseudocyst
(E) excision of the tail of the pancreas with subsequent pancreatic duct anastomosis to the bowel

18. A 45-year-old man in an executive position is seen because of vomiting bright-red blood. There are no previous symptoms. The man drinks one alcoholic drink per week and has no other significant history. In the hospital, he bleeds 5 units of blood prior to endoscopy. The most likely diagnosis is

(A) gastritis
(B) duodenal ulcer
(C) esophagitis
(D) Mallory-Weiss tear
(E) esophageal varices

19. The usual treatment for massive colonic hemorrhage in a patient with ulcerative colitis is

(A) total proctocolectomy
(B) transverse colostomy to determine which side of the colon is bleeding, followed by hemicolectomy
(C) vasopressin infusion into the inferior mesenteric artery
(D) colonoscopy with coagulation of bleeding sites
(E) high doses of steroids

20. A patient whose job involves world-wide travel presents with a complaint of right upper quadrant pain. Examination reveals hepatomegaly and a positive Casoni test. The most likely diagnosis is

(A) hepatocellular carcinoma
(B) amebic abscess
(C) echinococcal cyst
(D) choledochal cyst
(E) *Candida albicans* abscess of the liver

21. The most common cause of intestinal obstruction in adults is

(A) carcinoma of the colon
(B) carcinoma of the small bowel
(C) adhesive bands
(D) incarcerated inguinal hernia
(E) diverticulitis

22. Massive upper gastrointestinal bleeding occurs in an otherwise asymptomatic, normal man following a violent episode of retching and vomiting without blood. The most likely cause of this man's bleeding is

(A) hiatal hernia
(B) Mallory-Weiss tear
(C) carcinoma of the stomach
(D) duodenal ulcer
(E) gastritis

23. The most common small bowel malignancy is

(A) adenoma
(B) adenocarcinoma
(C) carcinoid tumor
(D) lymphoma
(E) leiomyosarcoma

24. The drug most useful for controlling massive bleeding from erosive gastritis is

(A) epinephrine
(B) dopamine
(C) vasopressin
(D) norepinephrine
(E) propranolol

25. A 50-year-old patient has a 3-cm villous-appearing tumor at 6 cm within the rectum. Biopsy shows that it is a villous adenoma. The most acceptable next step in management is to

(A) observe the lesion for signs of malignancy
(B) reassure the patient that these are not premalignant lesions
(C) fulgurate the lesion
(D) locally irradiate the lesion
(E) surgically excise the lesion

26. Of the factors listed, which most determines long-term survival following a shunting procedure in an alcoholic patient with cirrhosis of the liver?

(A) A low-protein diet
(B) Control of ascites
(C) A low-salt intake
(D) Abstinence from alcohol
(E) Use of lactulose

27. In a 60-year-old patient with jaundice of 2 weeks' duration and with no history of abdominal pain, a markedly distended gallbladder seen on ultrasound is most likely secondary to which of the following diagnoses?

(A) Common duct obstruction from a stone
(B) Common duct obstruction from pancreatitis
(C) Common duct obstruction from a carcinoma of the head of the pancreas
(D) Acute cholecystitis
(E) Alcoholic hepatitis

28. A 15-year-old girl has recurrent abdominal cramping and melena. Physical examination reveals increased pigmentation on her lips and buccal mucosa. Her sister has a similar history and similar physical findings. What is the most likely diagnosis?

(A) Pseudopolyposis
(B) Familial polyposis
(C) Villous adenoma
(D) Juvenile polyposis
(E) Peutz-Jeghers syndrome

29. Which of the following findings in acute pancreatitis is not well visualized with ultrasonography?

(A) Cullen's sign
(B) Biliary obstruction
(C) Pancreatic pseudocyst
(D) Pancreatic abscess
(E) Pancreatic calcification

30. A prophylactic portal-systemic shunt would be indicated in which of the following patients?

(A) A 2-year-old patient with biliary atresia and portal hypertension
(B) An alchoholic cirrhotic with ascites
(C) An alcoholic cirrhotic with mild encephalopathy
(D) A cirrhotic patient with large gastric varices
(E) No patient

31. A 50-year-old chronic alcoholic with known cirrhosis is noted to have a mass in the right lobe of his liver and an elevated α-fetoprotein level. What is the most likely diagnosis?

(A) Hepatocellular adenoma
(B) Hepatocellular carcinoma
(C) Metastatic carcinoma of the colon
(D) Regenerating nodule of cirrhosis
(E) Focal nodular hyperplasia

**Directions:** Each question below contains four suggested answers of which **one or more** is correct. Choose the answer

A  if **1, 2, and 3** are correct
B  if **1 and 3** are correct
C  if **2 and 4** are correct
D  if **4** is correct
E  if **1, 2, 3, and 4** are correct

32. True statements regarding intestinal carcinoma that arises following ulcerative colitis include

(1) it is less malignant than the carcinomas that occur in otherwise normal adults
(2) the incidence of carcinoma increases with the duration of active ulcerative colitis
(3) the carcinoma occurs only in the rectum
(4) the carcinoma is frequently multicentric

33. Characteristics of the short bowel syndrome include which of the following?

(1) Most patients require long-term total parenteral nutrition
(2) It is a commonly occurring syndrome after colectomy
(3) Caloric intake must be reduced significantly
(4) Absorption of water is poor

34. Air within the biliary tree on a plain abdominal roentgenogram usually is associated with which of the following?

(1) Perforated gastric ulcer
(2) Choledochoduodenostomy
(3) Intestinal obstruction
(4) Cholangitis with a gas-forming organism

35. True statements concerning the afferent loop syndrome include which of the following?

(1) The syndrome causes postprandial distention, pain, and nausea that are relieved by vomiting bilious materal not mixed with food.
(2) It occurs frequently in patients with a Billroth I gastrojejunostomy
(3) Treatment consists of providing good drainage of the afferent limb, usually by conversion of a gastrojejunostomy to a Roux-en-Y anastomosis
(4) The syndrome is difficult to correct and recurs frequently after operative revision

36. Morbidity in a patient with a gastrointestinal fistula would likely result from

(1) malnutrition
(2) myocardial infarction
(3) dehydration
(4) pulmonary embolism

37. A hospitalized patient with hepatic failure develops encephalopathy. Which of the following statements can be said about this complication?

(1) In order for a patient to be encephalopathic, the blood ammonia level must be elevated
(2) Encephalopathy may be an early sign of bleeding varices
(3) Encephalopathy decreases after nonselective portal-systemic shunting
(4) Encephalopathy may lead to aspiration of nasopharyngeal or gastric secretions

38. True statements regarding hepatocellular adenoma include

(1) there is a significant risk of spontaneous rupture with hemorrhage
(2) the tumor may present as a palpable liver mass
(3) it may be associated with oral contraceptive use
(4) the tumor is highly malignant

39. A patient with the first episode of acute pancreatitis may manifest

(1) hypotension
(2) Grey-Turner's sign (flank ecchymosis)
(3) "reversed 3" sign on plain roentgenogram of the abdomen
(4) "string" sign on barium study of the colon

40. True statements concerning duodenal ulcers include which of the following?

(1) Most duodenal ulcers are located in the first portion of the duodenum
(2) Most patients present with a history of epigastric pain, which may radiate to the back and which is frequently relieved by food
(3) Most duodenal ulcers can be diagnosed by an upper GI series
(4) The preferred treatment of uncomplicated duodenal ulcer is simple surgical excision

41. Peritoneal-jugular shunting can be described as

(1) the first line of management for newly developed ascites
(2) allowing one-way shunting of ascitic fluid into the circulatory system
(3) raising portal perfusion pressure
(4) stimulating a generalized intravascular coagulopathy, resulting in hemorrhage

42. True statements concerning radiation injury to the small bowel (chronic radiation enteritis) include which of the following?

(1) The 5-year survival rate is less than 50%
(2) The signs and symptoms of chronic radiation injury are similar to those of tumor recurrence
(3) Gastrointestinal bleeding may be caused by a fistula between a major artery and the bowel
(4) The manifestations of chronic injury appear within 1 month of radiation therapy

43. Superior mesenteric artery syndrome has which of the following characteristics?

(1) It occurs in young, thin females
(2) It is an obstruction of the duodenum by the superior mesenteric artery
(3) Typical symptoms are vomiting and postprandial pain
(4) It sometimes can be treated by weight gain

---

SUMMARY OF DIRECTIONS

| A | B | C | D | E |
|---|---|---|---|---|
| 1, 2, 3 only | 1, 3 only | 2, 4 only | 4 only | All are correct |

---

44. Which of the following conditions would be likely to result in generalized portal hypertension?

(1) Hepatic vein thrombosis
(2) Splenic vein thrombosis
(3) Postnecrotic cirrhosis
(4) Hepatocellular carcinoma

45. Common signs and symptoms of Crohn's disease include

(1) abdominal mass
(2) enterovesical fistula
(3) anemia
(4) bloody diarrhea

46. Dehydration is most likely to become a major problem in which of the following types of fistulas?

(1) Pancreatic fistula developing after distal pancreatectomy
(2) Anal fistula
(3) High-output duodenal fistula
(4) Fistula developing after irradiation to the sigmoid colon

47. A patient with obstructive jaundice due to pancreatic carcinoma might have

(1) thrombophlebitis
(2) a mass in the head of the pancreas
(3) a palpable gallbladder
(4) pain early in the course of the disease

48. True statements regarding metastatic hepatic tumors include which of the following?

(1) Solitary, slow-growing hepatic metastasis from colon carcinoma has a 30% to 40% 5-year survival rate after surgical resection
(2) Multiple metastatic liver tumors have not been greatly responsive to chemotherapy
(3) Colorectal cancer metastatic to the liver often is associated with an elevated level of carcinoembryonic antigen (CEA)
(4) Hepatic metastatic tumors are less common than primary hepatic tumors

49. The serum amylase levels of patients with acute pancreatitis can be described as

(1) correlating well with the severity of the pancreatitis
(2) being elevated in 95% of patients
(3) being abnormally low even in the presence of acute pancreatitis in patients with renal failure
(4) being elevated by parotitis

50. True statements regarding the distal splenorenal (Warren) shunt include which of the following?

(1) It selectively decreases the elevated venous pressure in the splenic bed
(2) It maintains good portal venous perfusion to the liver
(3) This procedure is commonly followed by ascites
(4) It may increase the incidence of postoperative encephalopathy

51. A patient with chronic pancreatitis has moderate pain that does not require narcotics. Acceptable methods of treatment would include which of the following?

(1) Puestow procedure
(2) Ninety-five percent pancreatectomy
(3) Distal pancreatectomy with intestinal drainage of the pancreatic duct
(4) Medical management alone

**Directions:** The groups of questions below consist of lettered choices followed by several numbered items. For each numbered item select the **one** lettered choice with which it is **most** closely associated. Each lettered choice may be used once, more than once, or not at all.

**Questions 52–56**

For each type of secretion below, select the cell type that secretes it.

(A) Chief cells
(B) Parietal cells
(C) Brunner's gland cells
(D) G cells
(E) Argentaffin cells

52. Hormone

53. Hydrochloric acid

54. Mucus

55. Intrinsic factor

56. Pepsinogen

**Questions 57–61**

For each characteristic below, select the disorder with which it is most likely to be associated.

(A) Gastric ulcer
(B) Duodenal ulcer
(C) Stress ulceration
(D) Chronic gastritis
(E) Prepyloric ulcer

57. Brought on by ischemia

58. Carries increased risk of cancer

59. Causes gastric outlet obstruction

60. Associated with blood group O

61. Associated with parietal cell antibodies

## ANSWERS AND EXPLANATIONS

**1. The answer is A.** (*Chapter 4 IV C 2 b*) Fully 80% of massive lower gastrointestinal bleeds originate from a mesenteric artery, often the inferior mesenteric artery, if patent, or a branch of the superior mesenteric artery. The hemorrhoidal branches may be responsible for hemorrhage lower in the rectum but account for a minority of lesions.

**2. The answer is D.** (*Chapter 5 VII*) Both malignant and benign duodenal tumors are rare. The most common malignant tumor of the duodenum is adenocarcinoma. These lesions are usually advanced on presentation and if resectable usually require a pancreaticoduodenectomy. Benign tumors found in the duodenum include lipomas, leiomyomas, and adenomas. These usually can be treated by local excision.

**3. The answer is D.** (*Chapter 6 III B 3*) The carcinoid syndrome is caused by the release of serotonin and other vasoactive substances produced by the tumor. Serotonin, or 5-hydroxytryptamine, is broken down in the liver and lungs into 5-hydroxyindoleacetic acid (5-HIAA), which is excreted in the urine. An abnormally high level of 5-HIAA in the urine is diagnostic of the carcinoid syndrome. Metanephrine and vanillylmandelic acid are breakdown products of catecholamines, and elevated urine levels are diagnostic of catecholamine-secreting tumors (e.g., pheochromocytoma).

**4. The answer is C.** (*Chapter 7 XV B 5* e) Chronic ulcerative colitis shows a predictable increase in the incidence of carcinoma of the colon with each additional year of active colitis. The cancers are often multicentric and frequently behave more malignantly than other colonic cancers.

**5. The answer is C.** [*Chapter 7 XVII E 2 c (1)*) Most episodes of acute diverticulitis will resolve with medical management. This includes resting the bowel and administering intravenous fluids and broad-spectrum antibiotics. Surgery is indicated for recurrent episodes as well as for complications such as perforation and abscess formation.

**6. The answer is D.** (*Chapter 9 I E 7 c*) Gastritis is the least common problem following balloon tamponade and is not related to the use of the tube. Gastric ulceration can occasionally occur where the gastric balloon is inflated. Pneumonia, aspiration of nasopharyngeal secretions, rebleeding following removal of the tube, and esophageal ulceration or perforation are common problems with balloon tamponade and can be minimized by keeping the balloon inflated for the briefest amount of time and by careful attention to removing secretions above the tube.

**7. The answer is D.** (*Chapter 4 IV C*) The most likely cause of massive lower gastrointestinal bleeding in the absence of diverticula is an angiodysplastic lesion of the colon, particularly the right colon. An upper GI series and small bowel studies should only be done after an exhaustive colonic workup has failed to demonstrate the source of bleeding. Colonoscopy in the face of massive bleeding is unreliable and difficult, and carries the risk of colonic perforation. In addition, it will not usually demonstrate an angiodysplastic lesion. A repeat barium enema is also unlikely to help. The most helpful study in this patient would be selective mesenteric angiography.

**8. The answer is A.** [*Chapter 5 I B 2 c (2)*] The G cells secrete gastrin, a hormone. Gastrin, in turn, causes the secretion of gastric acid by the parietal (oxyntic) cells and pepsinogen by the zygomatic (chief) cells. Pepsinogen is the precursor of pepsin, an enzyme active in protein digestion. Chief cells are also stimulated by cholinergic impulses and by secretin. Glucagon is a hormone secreted from the wall of the stomach and duodenum and by alpha cells in the pancreas; it has a hyperglycemic effect.

**9. The answer is E.** [*Chapter 7 XI E 3 a (2)*] The polyps of Peutz-Jeghers syndrome are hamartomas with no malignant potential. In this aspect, the disorder contrasts sharply with familial polyposis. Both Peutz-Jeghers syndrome and familial polyposis are autosomal dominant disorders, but carcinoma develops in 100% of untreated patients with familial polyposis by age 50.

**10. The answer is A.** (*Chapter 6 III A 1–2*) The adenomatous polyps found in familial polyposis syndromes are premalignant lesions. The hamartomatous polyps found in patients with Peutz-Jeghers syndrome, leiomyomas, and fibromas have no malignant potential. Juvenile (retention) polyps are benign hamartomas, not true neoplasms, which usually autoamputate.

**11. The answer is D.** (*Chapter 7 XII G 1*) Carcinoembryonic antigen (CEA) levels drop after a successful resection of colorectal cancer, and a later rise in the CEA level signals a recurrence. The measurement of CEA levels is reliable enough to be accepted as a screening test for recurrent colorectal cancer. Examining the stool for occult blood is the technique that is applied to large populations as a screening test for colonic cancer.

**12. The answer is B.** (*Chapter 9 II E 4 c*) Some 10% to 20% of patients with gallstones develop choledocholithiasis. Often the choledocholithiasis is silent and without clinical findings and is discovered only on the operative cholangiogram.

**13. The answer is D.** (*Chapter 10 II C 5*) The serum amylase level is not a prognostic indicator in acute pancreatitis. Any factor that reflects pancreatic necrosis, hemorrhage, infection, or continued third-space loss indicates a poor prognosis.

**14. The answer is D.** (*Chapter 6 II C 3–6*) Monoglycerides and fatty acids are absorbed in the mucosal cells, then synthesized into triglycerides and transported into the intestinal lymphatics as chylomicrons. All other nutrients, including starch, amino acids, vitamin C, and tripeptides, are transported across the mucosal cells into the portal venous system.

**15. The answer is B.** (*Chapter 7 XV C 2*) Crohn's disease of the colon results in serpiginous ulcers of the mucosa and adjacent mucosal edema. One endoscopic finding that helps to differentiate Crohn's colitis from ulcerative colitis is the presence of skip areas of normal mucosa; these are absent in ulcerative colitis. Pseudopolyps are hallmarks of ulcerative colitis, and sheets of white blood cells generally occur in pseudomembranous colitis, which is often caused by *Clostridium difficile*.

**16. The answer is B.** (*Chapter 9 I E 10*) Documented variceal hemorrhage that has recurred in a cirrhotic patient is the most accepted indication for shunting once endoscopic sclerosis has failed. When done electively, the shunting procedure has a mortality rate of 10% or less in low-risk patients. Prophylactic shunts such as those for choices (A) and (E) do not improve survival, and shunt surgery should be withheld in patients with encephalopathy, if at all possible. Shunting a patient who is actively bleeding carries a 50% or greater mortality risk.

**17. The answer is B.** (*Chapter 10 II F 3*) Internal drainage is the preferred method of treatment for a pancreatic pseudocyst. The pseudocyst must be well formed and mature enough to allow sutures to hold within the tissue. Generally a cystogastrostomy is the simplest procedure to perform.

**18. The answer is B.** (*Chapter 4 Table 4-1*) Massive upper gastrointestinal bleeding is usually due to a bleeding source proximal to the ligament of Treitz. The cause is most likely to be a posterior duodenal ulcer that is eroding into the gastroduodenal artery. Gastritis, esophagitis, a Mallory-Weiss tear, and esophageal varices are less likely to occur.

**19. The answer is A.** (*Chapter 7 XV B 6 c*) Total proctocolectomy is the procedure of choice when massive bleeding from a generalized colonic process such as ulcerative colitis is present. Trying to locate the site of bleeding is generally not helpful because multiple sites are often bleeding. Vasopressin may give temporary relief but would have to reach the entire colon, not just the aspect vascularized by the inferior mesenteric artery. Colonoscopy and steroid therapy have little value in the control of massive bleeding.

**20. The answer is C.** (*Chapter 9 I D 4*) An echinococcal parasitic infestation of the liver causes a cyst to form within the parenchyma. Serologic tests and the Casoni skin test are often positive. The major risk of this infestation is either spontaneous rupture, with resultant shock, or leakage at the time of surgery, with the formation of new cysts.

**21. The answer is C.** (*Chapter 4 II A 3 a*) Obstructing adhesive bands following abdominal surgery are the most common cause of intestinal obstruction. Although inguinal hernias were the most common cause in the early 1900s, the policy of repairing hernias electively has greatly reduced this problem. Colonic tumors are the third most common cause. Acute diverticulitis can, on occasion, cause complete obstruction, but it more commonly produces incomplete obstruction.

**22. The answer is B.** (*Chapter 5 IX A*) Massive upper gastrointestinal bleeding in an otherwise normal person following an episode of violent vomiting is a classic history for a patient with a Mallory-Weiss tear of the esophagus. The forceful vomiting tears the esophageal mucosa at the gastroesophageal junction, resulting in bleeding. Hiatal hernia, gastric carcinoma, duodenal ulcer, and gastritis are possible but less likely causes of massive bleeding when the blood appears after a bout of vomiting.

**23. The answer is B.** (*Chapter 6 III B 1–5*) Malignant tumors constitute 75% of symptomatic small bowel tumors, and usually present with bleeding, perforation, or obstruction. Common primary small bowel malignancies in descending order of frequency are: adenocarcinomas (40%), carcinoid tumors (30%), lymphomas (20%), and sarcomas. Adenomas are benign epithelial tumors. Leiomyosarcomas are the most common sarcoma of the small bowel but not the most common malignancy.

**24. The answer is C.** (*Chapter 4 III F 2 d*) The only drug proven to reduce bleeding in this situation is vasopressin. It is contraindicated in the presence of coronary artery disease. It is effective both intravenously and by selective intra-arterial mesenteric infusion, but it often is only a temporary measure.

**25. The answer is E.** (*Chapter 7 XI D 2 e*) Villous adenoma carries about a 35% risk of developing into an adenocarcinoma, and as many as one-third of all specimens are already invaded. Often a biopsy of only one location will not reveal the tumor. Because a tumor may be present, the adenoma should be excised. Local excision is acceptable if no invasion is present, but abdominoperineal resection is necessary if an invasive cancer is present.

**26. The answer is D.** (*Chapter 9 I E 4*) Whether or not a patient with alcoholic cirrhosis continues to abuse alcohol is the most important factor in determining survival. A low-protein diet, control of ascites, a low-salt intake, and the use of lactulose are types of therapy that are indicative of the severity of liver failure.

**27. The answer is C.** [*Chapter 10 III A 2 c (1) (a)*] Painless jaundice in the presence of a distended gallbladder is most likely secondary to a carcinoma of the head of the pancreas. Occasionally a common duct stone will not cause pain but this is unusual. A patient with distal common bile duct obstruction usually has a history of repeated bouts of pancreatitis. Acute cholecystitis is associated with pain. Alcoholic hepatitis usually does not cause a distended gallbladder, and the patient will have an associated history of alcohol abuse.

**28. The answer is E.** (*Chapter 7 XI E*) This patient's history is typical of Peutz-Jeghers syndrome. The association of recurrent bouts of colicky pain with pigmented spots on the lips and oral mucosa is striking. A sibling with similar symptoms is a clue to the hereditary nature of the disorder.

**29. The answer is A.** (*Chapter 10 II C*) Cullen's sign is periumbilical ecchymosis secondary to hemorrhagic pancreatitis with blood dissection up the falciform ligament. Ultrasonography would not be used to identify this sign. However, ultrasonography is a very useful procedure in the diagnosis of pancreatitis as well as its complications.

**30. The answer is E.** (*Chapter 9 I E 10 c*) Prophylactic shunts have not been shown to prolong life and are therefore not recommended for any patient. The presence of large gastric varices is a special type of portal hypertension that may be associated with pancreatitis or another process, resulting in splenic vein thrombosis. Gastric varices alone may be associated with splenic vein thrombosis, resulting in isolated splenic venous hypertension and varices through the short gastric vessel. The usual treatment for this type of portal hypertension is splenectomy.

**31. The answer is B.** [*Chapter 9 I B 2 a (4) (a)*] $\alpha$-Fetoprotein is a protein secreted by embryonal hepatocytes and is present at levels of 400 ng/ml in up to 85% of patients with hepatocellular carcinoma. It has a high sensitivity as a diagnostic "marker" in hepatocellular carcinoma, as it is not often present in other disorders with the exception of hepatoblastoma, a tumor of children.

**32. The answer is C (2, 4).** (*Chapter 7 XV B 5 e*) Carcinoma associated with ulcerative colitis behaves in a very malignant fashion, is often multicentric, and predictably increases in incidence with the duration of active ulcerative colitis. It can occur in the colon or rectum, and colonoscopic monitoring of ulcerative colitis patients is advocated by some authorities.

**33. The answer is D (4).** (*Chapter 6 VII A–D*) With short bowel syndrome, absorption of all nutrients, including water, is poor. While all patients require total parenteral nutrition immediately after the loss of most of their bowel, eventually most patients can be weaned from parenteral nutrition gradually. As a total colectomy leaves the entire small bowel intact (approximately 20 feet in length), it does not cause short-bowel syndrome. Caloric intake must increase because of malabsorption.

**34. The answer is C (2, 4).** (*Chapter 4 I E 3 e*) Any abnormal communication between the bile duct and the gastrointestinal tract may allow air to enter the bile duct. This communication can be secondary to surgery (e.g., choledochoduodenostomy) or can result from an inflammatory process, such as erosion of a gallstone into the duodenum. Cholangitis can also cause air in the bile ducts when the biliary obstruction is complicated by a gas-forming organism. This represents a surgical emergency resulting in death if the biliary tree is not promptly drained.

**35. The answer is B (1, 3).** (*Chapter 5 X B*) The afferent loop syndrome is caused by intermittent mechanical obstruction of the afferent loop of a Billroth II gastrojejunostomy. This obstruction causes discomfort as the afferent loop contracts and becomes distended. As the force of contraction empties the afferent loop, the symptoms are relieved. The symptoms of the afferent loop syndrome can be ameliorated by converting the Billroth II gastrojejunostomy to a Roux-en-Y type of anastomosis. Relief usually is complete after revision, and, if done properly, recurrence of symptoms is very unusual.

**36. The answer is B (1, 3).** (*Chapter 8 III*) Malnutrition and dehydration are common developments in patients with enteric fistulas. Myocardial infarction is not a usual problem. Although patients with fistulas can bleed due to erosion of intra-abdominal blood vessels, myocardial infarction and pulmonary embolism are not complications of fistulas.

**37. The answer is C (2, 4).** [*Chapter 9 I E 5 a (2), g*] Although blood ammonia levels may be elevated with encephalopathy, many times they are normal and fail to correlate with the level of encephalopathy. Encephalopathy makes the patient lethargic and often is followed by pneumonia due to aspiration. Encephalopathy may be induced by excessive protein intake, blood in the gastrointestinal tract, infection, or impaired hepatic perfusion, which occurs after portal-systemic shunting procedures.

**38. The answer is A (1, 2, 3).** (*Chapter 9 I B 1 b*) Hepatocellular adenoma is a benign tumor that occurs in women and is distinctly unusual in men. It may present either as a palpable mass or with spontaneous rupture and is often associated with oral contraceptive use. If oral contraceptives, steroids, and pregnancy are avoided, the tumor often regresses spontaneously. However, the patient who presents with spontaneous rupture requires resuscitation, with surgery once her condition has stabilized.

**39. The answer is A (1, 2, 3).** (*Chapter 10 II C 4 c*) Patients with acute pancreatitis are often critically ill and may even demonstrate blood dissection into the peritoneum, causing flank ecchymosis. The bowel may have an ileus near the pancreas, causing "reversed 3" roentgenographic findings.

**40. The answer is A (1, 2, 3).** (*Chapter 5 III B 1, 4, 5*) Duodenal ulcers commonly are in the first portion of the duodenum. Duodenal ulcer patients frequently are found to have increased acid production. The history is characteristic and consists of epigastric pain radiating to the back, which is frequently relieved by food. Most ulcers are diagnosed by an upper GI series. Endoscopy may be done; however, since the incidence of carcinoma is small in duodenal ulcers, endoscopy is not necessary on a routine basis. The initial treatment of duodenal ulcer is medical management consisting of $H_2$-receptor antagonists, often combined with antacid therapy. Surgical therapy is usually reserved for complications of duodenal ulcer disease.

**41. The answer is C (2, 4).** (*Chapter 9 I F 4*) Peritoneal-jugular shunting allows ascitic fluid to return to the vascular system, but its use is reserved for ascites that fails to resolve despite intensive medical therapy. The shunt usually lowers portal pressure. In some patients there may be factors in the ascitic fluid that result in a disseminated intravascular coagulation.

**42. The answer is A (1, 2, 3).** (*Chapter 6 IV A–C*) Chronic radiation enteritis generally becomes evident months to years after the conclusion of radiation therapy to the small bowel. At that time, the possibility of tumor recurrence must be excluded as the signs and symptoms are similar. Due to the breakdown of tissues that occurs, fistulas may form between the bowel and major arteries (enteroarterial fistula); at times these fistulas cause severe gastrointestinal hemorrhage. The overall prognosis for severe radiation enteritis is poor; the 5-year survival is less than 50%.

**43. The answer is E (all).** (*Chapter 5 VIII C*) The superior mesenteric artery takes a sharp origin from the aorta and courses over the duodenum. In thin patients, this can occasionally cause compression of the duodenum manifested by vomiting and postprandial pain. Patients who are immobile for a long period of time, such as patients in body casts, may also develop the syndrome as retroperitoneal fat is progressively lost. Gaining weight may lift the artery off the duodenum and thus relieve the symptoms. The condition can be treated surgically by releasing the ligament of Treitz, thereby removing the duodenum from beneath the superior mesenteric artery.

**44. The answer is B (1, 3).** (*Chapter 9 I E 3*) Postnecrotic cirrhosis and hepatic vein thrombosis lead to portal hypertension. Splenic vein thrombosis usually results in only localized portal hypertension in the region of the spleen and stomach. Hepatocellular carcinoma does not usually lead to portal hypertension unless the tumor invades the portal vein.

**45. The answer is A (1, 2, 3).** (*Chapter 6 IV B 1–3*) Signs and symptoms of Crohn's disease include an abdominal mass, anemia, diarrhea (usually not bloody), abdominal pain, lethargy, fever, weight loss, and anorectal disease. Complications of the disease include intestinal obstruction, usually due to stricture and inflammation, intra- or retroperitoneal abscesses, and fistulas that form from bowel to skin, bladder, vagina, urethra, or to other loops of bowel.

**46. The answer is B (1, 3).** (*Chapter 8 III B*) Fluid and electrolyte imbalances are frequent complications of fistulas, especially those involving the small bowel, pancreas, or bile ducts. High-output fistulas are fistulas that drain more than 200 ml of fluid per day, which can result in dehydration. The greater the fluid loss associated with a fistula, the greater the likelihood of dehydration. A pancreatic fistula developing after distal pancreatectomy might drain 700 ml of fluid per day, producing dehydration. Patients with colovesical fistulas are likely to develop urinary tract sepsis, but usually not dehydration. Fistulas that develop in an irradiated colon can be very difficult to heal, but sepsis, not dehydration, is more likely to be a serious problem.

**47. The answer is A (1, 2, 3).** (*Chapter 10 III A 2*) Migratory phlebitis is present in about 10% of patients with pancreatic cancer. The most common site of pancreatic cancer is the pancreatic head, which often does not produce symptoms until late in the disease, thus delaying the diagnosis.

**48. The answer is A (1, 2, 3).** (*Chapter 9 I C*) The most common tumor of the liver is a metastatic tumor. Results of treatment for colorectal carcinoma metastatic to the liver have been very disappointing, with fluorouracil (5-FU) as the principal drug being tested. The only bright spot in this disease is the fact that a solitary colon metastasis to the liver can be cured by surgery. Such a lesion should therefore be actively sought, and the patient should be referred to a center specializing in liver resections. Testing for carcinoembryonic antigen (CEA) is often positive in metastatic colon cancer, although CEA is not specific for colon cancer.

**49. The answer is C (2, 4).** (*Chapter 10 II C 4*) The serum amylase levels are elevated in 95% of patients with acute pancreatitis, although the rise in the level is not in proportion to the severity of the pancreatitis. The elevated amylase level does not carry a worse prognosis for patients with acute pancreatitis.

**50. The answer is A (1, 2, 3).** (*Chapter 9 I E 10 f*) The Warren shunt selectively decompresses the splenic venous bed while maintaining excellent hepatic portal perfusion. Maintaining this perfusion generally decreases the incidence of encephalopathy. At the same time, the portal pressure within the mesenteric system is maintained, making ascites a common problem following this procedure.

**51. The answer is D (4).** (*Chapter 10 II E*) Surgical management of chronic pancreatitis should be reserved for the patient who has intractable pain despite intensive efforts at medical management, because the surgical procedure may be difficult, may carry significant risk, and may not resolve the pain.

**52–56. The answers are: 52-D, 53-B, 54-C, 55-B, 56-A.** (*Chapter 5 I B 2, D 2*) The chief or zygomatic cells, found deep in the fundic glands of the gastric mucosa, secrete pepsinogen, the precursor of pepsin, which is the protein-digesting enzyme. The parietal, or oxyntic, cells, located in the gastric fundus and body, produce hydrochloric acid and intrinsic factor. Brunner's glands are located in the proximal duodenum, where they produce an alkaline mucus that presumably protects the mucosa. G cells, in the gastric antrum, secrete the hormone gastrin, which stimulates secretion of hydrochloric acid and pepsinogen. Argentaffin cells are found throughout the stomach; their function is unknown.

**57–61. The answers are: 57-C, 58-D, 59-E, 60-B, 61-D.** (*Chapter 5 III B 3 c, C 3; IV A 2, B 2*) Stress ulcers occur in patients undergoing severe stress—from sepsis, severe trauma, burns, and so forth—which causes ischemia of the gastric mucosa and consequent ulceration. Gastric atrophy occurs in chronic (atrophic) gastritis and increases the risk of gastric cancer. (There is no evidence that persons with simple gastric ulcer have a higher incidence of cancer.) Prepyloric ulcers can obstruct the gastric outlet, causing gastric distention, crampy pain, and nausea. Several factors are known to increase the incidence of duodenal ulcer; these include not only understandable factors such as aspirin or coffee ingestion, but also the blood type O. Parietal cell antibodies are associated with the less common of the two types of chronic gastritis—this type is also associated with vitamin $B_{12}$ malabsorption.

# Part III
# Splenic and Lymphatic Disorders

## I. ANATOMY

**A.** The spleen develops from several masses of mesenchyme in the dorsal mesogastrium. These masses coalesce and move to the left as development progresses. By the end of the third gestational month, the organ is formed. The point where the spleen remains attached to the dorsal mesogastrium becomes the **gastrosplenic ligament**.

**B.** The **adult spleen weighs** between 100 g and 150 g and **measures** 12 cm x 7 cm x 4 cm.

**C.** The spleen is **located** in the left upper quadrant of the abdomen and is protected by the eighth to the eleventh ribs. It is bordered by the left kidney posteriorly, the diaphragm superiorly, and the fundus of the stomach and the splenic flexure of the colon anteriorly.

**D.** The **main blood supply** to the organ is carried by the **splenic artery**, which is a branch of the celiac axis. It travels along the superior border of the pancreas. At the hilus it branches into trabecular arteries, which terminate in small vessels to the splenic pulp. The **splenic vein** crosses behind or at the lower border of the pancreas. It joins the superior mesenteric vein to form the portal vein (Fig. 11-1).

**E.** The **organ itself consists of** an outer capsule and trabeculae, which enclose the pulp. The pulp consists of three zones: the white pulp, the red pulp, and the marginal zone.

**1.** The **white pulp** is essentially a lymph node. It contains lymphocytes, macrophages, and plasma cells in a reticular network.

**2.** The **red pulp** consists of cords of reticular cells with sinuses in between.

**3.** The **marginal zone** is a poorly defined vascular space between the pulps. It contains sequestered foreign material and plasma as well as abnormal cellular elements.

## II. PHYSIOLOGY.
The spleen has multiple functions, some of which remain poorly understood. Its most important functions are its ability to act as a **blood filter** and its role in the **immunologic process** of the body.

**A. Filtering functions**

**1. Splenic blood flow** is approximately 350 L of blood per day. Most blood elements pass through rapidly and uneventfully.

**2.** Under normal circumstances the spleen can **remove old or abnormal red blood cells**.
  **a.** The mechanism is not known exactly, but it is thought that as the cell ages its enzyme activity and metabolic capacity decrease.
  **b.** This leads to biophysical changes in the cell, which are accentuated in the substrate-deprived splenic environment.
  **c.** The spleen removes about 20 ml of aged or abnormal red cells per day.

**3. Abnormal white cells, normal and abnormal platelets, and cellular debris** may also be removed by the spleen. In the splenectomized individual, cells with abnormal **inclusion bodies**, such as Howell-Jolly, Pappenheimer, and Heinz bodies, are seen. This is regarded as evidence that the spleen is capable of removing these abnormal cells or inclusion bodies.

**B. Immunologic functions**

**1.** The spleen is a major site of **production of opsonins**. The entire reticuloendothelial system is

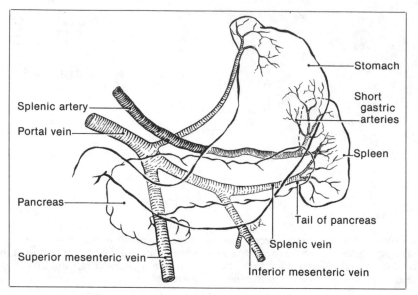

**Figure 11-1.** The spleen: anatomic relationships.

capable of removing bacteria from the circulation, but the spleen, with its highly efficient filtering mechanism, is particularly suited to removing poorly opsonized pathogens.

    **2.** The spleen is also an important site of **antibody synthesis.** This occurs mainly in the white pulp, where soluble antigens stimulate the production of immunoglobulin M (IgM).

    **3.** It is now firmly established that splenectomy leaves some patients more prone to infection.

**C. Storage functions**

    **1.** Approximately one-third of the body's **platelets** are stored in the spleen. In some pathologic states the percentage is increased.

    **2.** The spleen contains approximately 25 ml of **red blood cells** at any one time.

**III. HYPERSPLENISM** is an exaggerated destruction or sequestration of circulating blood elements. This can affect red cells, white cells, and platelets.

    **A. Primary hypersplenism** is essentially a diagnosis of exclusion and is made only after possible causes of secondary hypersplenism have been ruled out.

        **1.** It may, in some cases, actually be an early manifestation of lymphoma or leukemia.

        **2.** It is a rare entity, affecting mainly females. The spleen is almost always enlarged. The hematologic findings may be accompanied by recurring fevers and infections.

        **3.** Primary hypersplenism responds to splenectomy.

    **B. Secondary hypersplenism** is caused by an identifiable underlying disease.

        **1.** The most common cause is **portal hypertension**, which can lead to passive splenic congestion.
            **a.** Although 60% of patients with portal hypertension develop an enlarged spleen, only 15% develop hypersplenism.
            **b.** The hypersplenism is usually mild and clinically insignificant.

        **2. Splenic vein thrombosis** can cause hypersplenism with massive splenomegaly.
            **a.** Pancreatitis is the usual cause of the thrombosis.
            **b.** There may be associated bleeding esophageal varices.
            **c.** The hypersplenism is cured by splenectomy.

        **3. Other causes** of secondary hypersplenism include:
            **a. Inflammatory diseases** including malaria, tuberculosis, brucellosis, mononucleosis, and hepatitis
            **b. Boeck's sarcoid**
            **c. Collagen vascular diseases**

(1) Felty's syndrome (see section V H)
(2) Systemic lupus erythematosus (SLE)
d. **Neoplastic diseases** such as lymphomas and leukemia

## IV. ABSOLUTE INDICATIONS FOR SPLENECTOMY

A. **Splenic tumors**

1. **Primary splenic tumors** are extremely rare.
   a. They include lymphoma, sarcoma, hemangioma, and hamartoma.
   b. Symptoms are caused by the enlarged spleen, and there may be associated hypersplenism.
   c. Splenectomy is indicated.

2. The spleen is a frequent site of **metastasis**, as demonstrated by autopsy studies.
   a. The metastatic tumors are usually not clinically significant.
   b. For this reason and since they are manifestations of advanced disease, splenectomy is not usually indicated unless it is done as part of a staging laparotomy for Hodgkin's disease (see section V I 4).

B. **Splenic abscess** is uncommon, but when present it has a high mortality rate.

1. **Causes** include the following:
   a. **Infection** of a preexisting lesion such as a hematoma
   b. **Direct spread** from adjacent structures such as the pancreas or colon
   c. **Hematogenous seeding** from a remote site (especially in users of intravenous drugs) or during overwhelming bacteremia

2. The **diagnosis** should be suspected if signs of abscess, such as fever and an elevated white blood cell count, occur in association with left upper quadrant fullness or tenderness. It can be confirmed by computed tomography (CT) and scanning with technetium-99m ($^{99m}$Tc).

3. The **treatment** is usually splenectomy and antibiotic therapy. In highly selected cases in which splenectomy is technically hazardous, splenotomy and drainage may be indicated.

C. **Hereditary spherocytosis** is one of a group of hereditary hemolytic anemias and causes the most severe symptoms. It is transmitted as an autosomal dominant trait.

1. It is **characterized** by a **defect of the red cell membrane**.
   a. This results in an increased intracellular concentration of sodium which causes the cell to be spherical (hence the name), small, and more prone to lysis than normal red blood cells.
   b. The cell membrane is thick and rigid, which causes the cells to be held in the splenic pulp.
   c. This leads to cell lysis, due to deprivation of glucose and adenosine triphosphate (ATP). This occurs only in the spleen.

2. The **symptoms** of hereditary spherocytosis include malaise, abdominal discomfort, jaundice, anemia, and splenomegaly.

3. The **diagnosis** is based upon the above clinical findings and the results of laboratory studies, which include:
   a. The demonstration of spherocytes and an elevated reticulocyte count on a Wright-stained blood smear
   b. The demonstration of increased osmotic fragility of the red cells
   c. The demonstration that chromium-51 ($^{51}$Cr) -tagged red blood cells have a greatly shortened half-life and are sequestered in the spleen

4. The disease may be **complicated** by gallstones (rare in patients under the age of 10 years) and by chronic leg ulcers that heal only after splenectomy.

5. The **treatment** is splenectomy.
   a. This cures the anemia and jaundice in all patients. Failure of splenectomy to cure the patient is normally caused by an accessory spleen that has been overlooked during the operation (see section VIII C 2).
   b. The operation should be delayed until the age of 4 years, if possible, to decrease the chance of post-splenectomy sepsis (see section VII B 2).

D. **Massive splenic trauma.** Irreparable splenic injury may necessitate splenectomy. In lesser injuries, splenic repair is preferable (see section VI C).

E. **Bleeding esophageal varices** caused by splenic vein thrombosis (see section III B 2) can be cured by splenectomy if the diagnosis is correct.

## V. RELATIVE INDICATIONS FOR SPLENECTOMY

**A. Congenital hemolytic anemias other than hereditary spherocytosis.** Although splenectomy is not curative, it reduces the need for multiple transfusions in the following conditions:

1. **Enzyme deficiencies** such as glucose-6-phosphate dehydrogenase (G6PD) deficiency and pyruvate kinase deficiency

2. **Hereditary elliptocytosis**

3. **Thalassemia major**, transmitted as a dominant trait and characterized by defective hemoglobin synthesis which causes homozygotes to have severe anemia and hepatosplenomegaly

**B. Sickle cell anemia** may require splenectomy in the rare cases in which excessive splenic sequestration of red cells is documented. Most patients with the disease "autosplenectomize" due to multiple infarcts caused by stagnation and stasis of the abnormal red blood cells.

**C. Idiopathic autoimmune hemolytic anemia** occurs most commonly after the age of 50 years and is found in women twice as often as in men.

1. In this disorder, both warm- and cold-hemolytic antibodies have been described. These presumably shorten the life of the red cells.

2. The anemia is accompanied by reticulocytosis. There is splenomegaly in 50% of the cases. There may be mild jaundice.

3. The direct Coombs' test is positive. $^{51}$Cr-tagged red blood cells demonstrate sequestration in the spleen in 80% of patients.

4. The disease may run a self-limiting course that requires no treatment.

5. In more persistent cases, **medical treatment** consists of administration of steroids and azathioprine. If steroids are ineffective or contraindicated, **splenectomy** is helpful in many patients, especially if they have demonstrated splenic sequestration of $^{51}$Cr-tagged red cells.

**D. Idiopathic thrombocytopenic purpura**

1. This disease is **characterized** by a decreased platelet count accompanied by increased megakaryocytes in the bone marrow. The spleen is usually not enlarged.

2. The **etiology** is unknown but is presumed to be immunologic since most patients with chronic disease have platelet-agglutinating antibodies that rapidly destroy transfused platelets.

3. An **acute form** exists which is more common in children under 16 years of age. Eighty percent of affected individuals recover spontaneously.

4. The **chronic form** is most common in adults, and women predominate in a 3 to 1 ratio.

5. **Steroids** induce remission in 75% of patients, and about 20% of these have a sustained response.

6. **Splenectomy** is indicated in individuals who do not respond to steroids or in those who relapse after steroids are tapered off. It is also mandatory if central nervous system bleeding occurs. It produces a sustained remission in 70% of patients.

**E. Thrombotic thrombocytopenic purpura** is a rapidly progressive and usually fatal disease (approximately two-thirds of patients die within 3 months).

1. The **clinical features** include:
   a. Fever
   b. Thrombocytopenic purpura
   c. Hemolytic anemia
   d. Neurologic disturbances
   e. Renal failure

2. The **diagnosis** is confirmed only by biopsy of the purpuric lesion. This shows a characteristic vascular lesion, which consists of occlusion of arterioles and capillaries by a hyaline membrane.

3. The most efficient **treatment** consists of high-dose corticosteroid therapy combined with dextran administration and prompt splenectomy.

4. The long-term **survival rate** is less than 10% even with optimal therapy.

   **F. Primary hypersplenism** (see section III A).

   **G. Agnogenic myeloid metaplasia** is a mysterious disease that is thought to be related to polycythe-mia vera, myelofibrosis, and myeloid leukemia.

   1. It is **characterized** by connective tissue proliferation in the bone marrow, liver, spleen, and lymph nodes, accompanied by proliferation of the hematopoietic tissue of the liver, spleen, and long bones.

   2. The usual **symptoms** are anemia and splenomegaly, which usually appear in middle-aged or older adults. Secondary hypersplenism may develop, and later in the disease there may be spontaneous bleeding, spontaneous infections, and splenic infarcts.

   3. **Splenectomy** may help to control the hypersplenism. It can reduce the need for transfusions and may also help to control thrombocytopenia. Splenectomy should not be done until the platelet count is less than 100,000 to avoid rebound thrombocytosis.

   **H. Felty's syndrome** is a triad consisting of chronic rheumatoid arthritis, splenomegaly, and granu-locytopenia.

   1. **Spontaneous infections** can occur due to the neutropenia.

   2. Although there are differences of opinion, **splenectomy** is generally regarded as the treatment of choice for this condition.

   **I. Hodgkin's disease**

   1. Advances in therapy have greatly improved chances for the cure or long-term survival of pa-tients with this disease.

   2. Optimal treatment depends upon accurate **staging** of the disease. The **Ann Arbor classifica-tion** is as follows:
   **a. Stage 0:** No detectable disease following excisional biopsy
   **b. Stage I:** Disease limited to a single lymph node region
   **c. Stage II:** Disease limited to two or more lymph node regions on the same side of the diaphragm
   **d. Stage III:** Disease on both sides of the diaphragm but limited to lymph nodes, spleen, or Waldeyer's ring
   **e. Stage IV:** Involvement of bone, bone marrow, lung parenchyma, pleura, liver, skin, gastro-intestinal tract, central nervous system, kidney, or sites other than lymph nodes, spleen, or Waldeyer's ring
   **f.** The stages are **subclassified as A (absence) and B (presence)** of systemic symptoms (i.e., fever, night sweats, and weight loss of greater than 10%).

   3. Patients with clinical stage I or II disease are found to have unsuspected disease in the ab-domen in about 25% of cases.

   4. **Laparotomy** is recommended for stages I, II, and III A. The **staging laparotomy** consists of splenectomy, liver biopsy, and complete abdominal exploration with sampling of lymph nodes from multiple areas.

   5. **Splenectomy** is thought to improve tolerance to chemotherapy. Use of the procedure also avoids the injury to the left kidney and lung that occurs if the spleen is irradiated.

   **J. Non-Hodgkin's lymphoma**

   1. **Staging** for non-Hodgkin's lymphoma uses the same classification as for Hodgkin's disease. Careful evaluation will reveal stage III or stage IV disease in 80% of patients.

   2. **Laparotomy** is useful in stages I, II, and III A disease.
   **a.** Several series have shown an increased incidence of mesenteric nodal or gastric involve-ment by non-Hodgkin's lymphoma.
   **b.** Since these areas are outside the normal field of irradiation, accurate preoperative local-ization is essential in planning therapy.

   3. Laparotomy is not useful in patients in whom chemotherapy is to be the primary mode of treatment.

   4. Non-Hodgkin's lymphoma may present as a gastrointestinal primary malignancy, and in such cases resection may be curative.

**VI. RUPTURE OF THE SPLEEN** may follow either penetrating or nonpenetrating trauma or may oc-cur spontaneously.

**A. Traumatic rupture**

1. **Penetrating trauma.** Knife wounds and gunshot wounds are the most common causes. The resultant wounds are usually obvious. It is very important to realize that the spleen may be injured when the entry wound is in the region of the middle or lower chest as well as when the wounds are in the abdomen.

2. **Nonpenetrating trauma.** The most common cause of nonpenetrating trauma is an automobile accident. When the spleen is injured, there is usually profuse bleeding, but in 5% of blunt injuries, the rupture may be delayed.

3. **Iatrogenic trauma** accounts for 20% of all splenectomies. The trauma results from excessive traction on the splenic attachments or from misplacement of retractors.

4. **Delayed rupture**
   a. Usually the initial injury is a **subcapsular hematoma**. Eventually the red cells lyse, and the osmolality of the hematoma increases, causing it to expand. Rupture may be the eventual outcome.
   b. About 75% of delayed ruptures occur within 2 weeks of the initial injury and present as acute shock from profuse bleeding.

**B. Spontaneous rupture** usually occurs because of splenomegaly due to an associated disease such as mononucleosis or leukemia.

**C. Treatment.** In all cases of isolated splenic injury (with the possible exception of spontaneous rupture), an attempt should be made to salvage the spleen.

1. In minor capsular tears, pressure and application of a topical hemostatic agent will frequently control the bleeding.

2. Deeper lacerations can be treated by splenorrhaphy, using Teflon pledgets, or by partial resection.

3. Massive injuries, especially if there are other injuries that require attention, should be treated by splenectomy.

## VII. COMPLICATIONS FOLLOWING SPLENECTOMY

**A. Postoperative complications**

1. **Atelectasis** of the left lower lung is the most common such complication.

2. **Subphrenic abscess** may develop and is usually accompanied by a left pleural effusion.

3. **Thrombocytosis** postoperatively is common. If the platelet count exceeds 1,000,000, anticoagulation may be required to prevent spontaneous thrombosis.

**B. Postsplenectomy sepsis**

1. Patients are prone to **overwhelming sepsis** following splenectomy.
   a. The syndrome begins with nonspecific, mild, influenza-like symptoms.
   b. These rapidly progress to high fever, shock, and death.

2. In general, the younger the patient and the more serious the disease requiring the splenectomy, the greater the risk for the development of overwhelming sepsis.
   a. The risk is greatest if splenectomy occurs during the first 2 to 4 years of life, particularly if it is done for a disease of the reticuloendothelial system.
   b. In healthy adults who have the spleen removed for trauma, the incidence of overwhelming sepsis is low (0.5% to 0.8%), but it is still higher than that in the normal population (0.01%).

3. About 80% of septic episodes occur within 2 years after splenectomy.

4. **Treatment**
   a. Splenectomized patients should receive **polyvalent pneumococcal vaccine**, which protects them from 80% of pathogenic pneumococci (the most common organisms causing the sepsis).
   b. **Prophylactic penicillin** should probably be given for 2 years following splenectomy, particularly to high-risk patients such as children under the age of 12 years.
   c. Patients should be instructed to seek medical attention immediately if symptoms begin, and penicillin therapy should be started in an attempt to prevent the full-blown syndrome from developing.

## VIII. MISCELLANEOUS LESIONS

**A. Splenosis** is **autotransplantation** of fragments of spleen, which can occur after rupture. It is thought that these fragments can maintain splenic function, including immunocompetence, but this has not been proven.

**B. Aneurysms of the splenic artery**

1. The splenic artery is the second most common site of intra-abdominal aneurysm (the abdominal aorta is most common).

2. The aneurysms occur in older patients as a manifestation of generalized atherosclerosis. They also occur in young women, in whom they are probably congenital. These are important because they are prone to rupture in the last trimester of pregnancy.

3. **Repair** of the aneurysm is indicated if it is enlarging or if it is found in a woman of childbearing age. **Distal aneurysms** require resection and splenectomy. **Proximal aneurysms** may be repaired, allowing the spleen to be preserved.

**C. Ectopic and accessory spleens**

1. An **ectopic spleen** is caused by a long splenic pedicle, which allows the spleen to "wander" about the abdomen.

2. An **accessory spleen** is found in about 10% of autopsies. They are usually located near the hilus or the tail of the pancreas and less frequently in the mesentery. They are only significant if they are overlooked during splenectomy for hematologic disease.

# 12
# The Lymphatic System
R. Anthony Carabasi, III

**I. LYMPHEDEMA** is a condition characterized by swelling of one or more extremities caused by lymphatic insufficiency.

**A.** Lymphedema may be idiopathic (**primary lymphedema**) or may be caused by acquired insufficiency due to infections, obstructions, or surgical destruction of the lymphatics (**secondary lymphedema**).

**1. Primary lymphedema**
   **a.** Primary lymphedema is divided into three **types**, depending on the patient's age at presentation.
   **(1) Congenital lymphedema** is present at birth or occurs early in infancy.
      **(a)** It accounts for fewer than 10% of primary lymphedema cases.
      **(b)** Lymphedema that is both congenital and hereditary is known as **Milroy's disease**.
   **(2) Lymphedema praecox** occurs at any time from puberty until the end of the third decade.
      **(a)** Most cases of primary lymphedema are of this type.
      **(b)** It is three times more common in females than in males.
   **(3) Lymphedema tarda** occurs after age 30.
   **b.** These entities are probably not distinct from one another in any way save the age of onset.
   **(1)** If there are virtually no lymphatics present at birth, the symptoms occur at that time.
   **(2)** If some functioning lymphatics are present at birth, symptoms may be minimal or absent.
   **(3)** However, as growth takes place, and with repeated normal damage from minor infection or trauma, the remaining normal lymphatics are no longer adequate and edema occurs.

**2. Secondary lymphedema.** Secondary lymphedema is due to obstruction from a variety of causes, including infection (see section III), parasites, mechanical injury (including surgery), postphlebitic syndrome, and neoplasms.
   **a.** In developed countries, the most common causes are:
   **(1)** Obstruction by malignancies
   **(2)** Postsurgical lymphedema (e.g., lymphedema following mastectomy)
   **(3)** Lymphatic destruction from therapeutic radiation
   **b.** In less well-developed countries, parasitic obstruction (elephantiasis) is a common cause. *Wuchereria bancrofti* is the most common offending parasite.

**B.** The **diagnosis** of lymphedema is confirmed by lymphangiography, which usually shows hypoplastic and incompetent lymphatics.

**C. Treatment**
   **1.** Simple measures are the first line of treatment.
   **a.** These include elevation of the affected limb, weight reduction, and salt restriction.
   **b.** Compressive stockings may be of benefit if applied properly.
   **c.** It is extremely important to avoid trauma and infection, as these will greatly exacerbate the condition.
   **d.** For severe cases, pulsatile compression devices may help to "squeeze" the edema from the swollen extremity.
   **2.** There are several **surgical approaches** to help uncontrolled lymphedema.
   **a.** The **Thompson procedure** is based on the assumption that dermal lymphatics may be

functional even though the deep lymphatics are incompetent. A dermal flap is buried deep in the swollen extremity, to provide competent lymphatics for drainage.

    **b.** The omentum, which contains an extensive lymphatic network, can also be transposed from the abdomen to the extremity.

    **c.** Microsurgical anastomoses between a lymphatic and a small vein have been tried. Long-term results are not yet available, but this approach may hold promise for the future.

## II. LYMPHATIC TUMORS

  **A. Benign tumors** are most commonly **cystic hygromas**.

    **1.** These are derived from embryonic lymph sacs and are seen during the first year of life.

    **2.** They are most commonly found in the neck, but also occur in the groin, axilla, and mediastinum.

    **3.** Cystic hygromas in the neck may cause respiratory distress and in this case should be excised. Cranial nerves should not be sacrificed, since these are benign tumors.

  **B. Lymphangiosarcoma** is an extremely rare **malignant lymphatic tumor**. It can occur in any extremity affected by chronic lymphedema, but is seen most commonly after a mastectomy that is complicated by lymphedema of the arm (see Chapter 23 section III E 5 c).

  **C. Lymphatic metastases** are seen with many kinds of primary tumor.

## III. LYMPHANGITIS AND LYMPHADENITIS

  **A.** Inflammation in the lymphatic channels (**lymphangitis**) and in the lymph nodes (**lymphadenitis**) is caused by bacterial invasion, usually by staphylococci or by $\beta$-hemolytic streptococci.

  **B.** Usually, an extremity is affected.

    **1.** There is hyperemia around the affected lymphatic, manifested by a red streak, which advances toward the draining lymph nodes.

    **2.** Movement of the affected extremity is painful, and also propels the bacteria along the lymphatic channel, exacerbating the condition.

  **C.** If the process is not arrested by the lymph nodes, septicemia can occur.

  **D. Treatment** consists of immobilizing the limb and giving antibiotics. If a source of bacterial seeding is present (e.g., a paronychia), it should be drained.

  **E.** Uncomplicated cases resolve promptly and usually without sequelae. Repeated insults can result in a chronic secondary lymphedema.

# Part III
# Study Questions

## QUESTIONS

**Directions:** Each question below contains five suggested answers. Choose the **one best** response to each question.

1. Which of the following statements concerning non-Hodgkin's lymphoma is true?

(A) Its staging system is different than that of Hodgkin's disease
(B) It presents as stage III or IV disease in only 10% of patients
(C) Laparotomy is rarely used in staging this disease
(D) It may present as a primary gastrointestinal malignancy
(E) It is found in young patients more commonly than is Hodgkin's disease

2. All of the following statements about primary lymphedema are true EXCEPT

(A) Milroy's disease occurs in women over 30 years of age and tends to run in families
(B) the three types of primary lymphedema differ only in the age of the patient at onset
(C) lymphedema may be exacerbated by repeated damage from minor infections
(D) lymphangiography will confirm the diagnosis
(E) in mild cases, primary lymphedema will respond to compression stockings and elevation

3. Trauma can cause rupture of the spleen or it can occur spontaneously. True statements regarding a ruptured spleen include

(A) the area around small capsular tears should be resected
(B) when massive splenic injury is accompanied by other intra-abdominal injuries there should be an attempt to salvage the spleen
(C) the spleen can be removed with impunity since it has little known immunologic function
(D) delayed rupture of a subcapsular splenic hematoma occurs within 2 weeks of the injury in 10% of cases
(E) none of the above

**Directions:** Each question below contains four suggested answers of which **one or more** is correct. Choose the answer

A   if **1, 2, and 3** are correct
B   if **1 and 3** are correct
C   if **2 and 4** are correct
D   if **4** is correct
E   if **1, 2, 3, and 4** are correct

4.   Postsplenectomy sepsis can be characterized by

(1)  a sudden and catastrophic onset of symptoms
(2)  the greatest risk of development in elderly patients
(3)  a 10% incidence following splenectomy for traumatic injury
(4)  an 80% rate of occurrence within 2 years of splenectomy

5.   Idiopathic thrombocytopenic purpura is characterized by

(1)  an acute form common in children
(2)  a female to male ratio of 3 to 1
(3)  a chronic form common in adults
(4)  decreased peripheral platelets and bone marrow megakaryocytes

**Directions:** The questions below consist of lettered choices followed by two numbered items. For each numbered item select the **one** lettered choice with which it is **most** closely associated. Each lettered choice may be used once, more than once, or not at all.

**Questions 6 and 7**

Match the following.

(A) This is a rare form of malignant lymphatic tumor
(B) This tumor occurs most frequently in the mastectomy patient with lymphedema
(C) Both
(D) Neither

6.   Lymphangiosarcoma

7.   Cystic hygroma

## ANSWERS AND EXPLANATIONS

**1. The answer is D.** (*Chapter 11 V J*) Non-Hodgkin's lymphoma is more commonly found in patients who are over 50 years of age than in a younger age group. The staging of the disease is the same as that for Hodgkin's disease, and stage III or IV disease is present in 80% of patients at the time of diagnosis. Laparotomy is very important since gastric or mesenteric nodal involvement is common and the procedure can guide radiation ports. If the disease presents as a primary gastrointestinal malignancy, resection may be curative.

**2. The answer is A.** (*Chapter 12 I A 1, B, C 1*) The three types of primary lymphedema are congenital lymphedema, lymphedema praecox, and lymphedema tarda; all three types appear to be similar except for the age of the patient at onset. Repeated lymphatic damage from minor infections and trauma reduces the number of normal lymphatics, thereby exacerbating the disorder. Most mild cases are controlled by elevating the affected limb and by using compression stockings; more advanced cases are controlled by pneumatic compression devices. Milroy's disease is a form of congenital lymphedema and thus is present at birth or early in life. It is also hereditary. Lymphedema in a 30-year-old woman would be classified as lymphedema tarda.

**3. The answer is E.** (*Chapter 11 VI A 4, C 1, 3*) In virtually all isolated splenic injuries an attempt should be made to salvage the spleen; however, when other severe intra-abdominal injuries are involved, splenectomy is indicated. Small capsular tears will stop bleeding with pressure and topical application of hemostatic agents and do not require resection. Delayed rupture usually is the result of a subcapsular splenic hematoma that generally ruptures within 2 weeks 75% of the time. The spleen is important as a source of opsonins and immunoglobulins, and postsplenectomy sepsis is now a well-recognized entity.

**4. The answer is D (4).** (*Chapter 11 VII B*) Postsplenectomy sepsis usually begins as a mild influenza-like syndrome. Progression to death after shock develops is usually rapid. Younger patients, especially those who are less than 4 years old, are at greatest risk. Postsplenectomy sepsis following trauma is rare (occurring in 0.5% to 0.8% of cases), but it still has a higher occurrence than in the general population. A polyvalent pneumococcal vaccine should be given to all splenectomized patients; however, it will only protect against 80% of pathogenic pneumococci.

**5. The answer is A (1, 2, 3).** (*Chapter 11 V D*) Idiopathic thrombocytopenic purpura is characterized by a decreased platelet count with increased megakaryocytes in the bone marrow. The acute form, which occurs in children under the age of 16, resolves spontaneously in 80% of cases. The condition occurs three times as often in females as in males. Splenectomy produces a sustained remission in 70% of patients who do not respond to or who relapse after steroid therapy.

**6 and 7. The answers are: 6-C, 7-D.** (*Chapter 12 II A 1–3, B*) Lymphangiosarcoma is a very rare neoplasm of the lymphatic system. Most neoplasms in the lymphatics are metastatic tumors. Lymphangiosarcoma most often occurs after a mastectomy in an arm that has been complicated by lymphedema.

Cystic hygroma is the most commonly occurring benign tumor of the lymphatic system. It occurs during the first year of life, most often in the neck but also in the groin, axilla, and mediastinum. Cystic hygroma in the neck may cause respiratory distress and thus should be excised.

# Part IV
# Vascular Disorders

# 13
# Peripheral Arterial Disease
Bruce E. Jarrell

## I. GENERAL PRINCIPLES OF PERIPHERAL ARTERIAL DISEASE

**A. Atherosclerosis** is a disease process that narrows both large and small arteries of the body. The arteries that are affected vary among individuals and depend upon the involvement of certain risk factors such as lipid disorders, other systemic disease, and hereditary influences. The terminal occlusive stages result in ischemia of the involved tissue followed by necrosis.

1. Pathologically, **arterial occlusion** occurs in three successive **stages**.
    a. In the **early stage**, minimally elevated yellow fatty streaks appear on the arterial intima due to the cholesterol ester lipids that are deposited in both macrophages and smooth muscle cells.
    b. In the **intermediate stage**, the streaks become more organized and fibrous and retain the yellow to yellow-white color.
    c. The **advanced stage** is characterized by thick plaques with calcification, ulceration, and necrosis of the intima.

2. Certain **lipid abnormalities** have a strong association with the development and progression of atherosclerosis. The **five types of hyperlipoproteinemias** may result from hereditary factors or from acquired risk factors such as systemic diseases or dietary habits.
    a. **Type I** is characterized by hypertriglyceridemia and is inherited as a recessive trait. It is not associated with significant atherosclerosis or ischemic heart disease.
    b. **Type II** is associated with greatly accelerated ischemic heart disease. It is divided into two subtypes.
       (1) **Type IIa** has a very strong genetic determination. It is characterized by high levels of cholesterol and responds poorly to dietary manipulation.
       (2) **Type IIb** has elevated levels of cholesterol and triglycerides but responds more readily than type IIa to dietary control of lipids and carbohydrates. It is very common.
    c. **Type III** is very similar to type IIb in that it has elevated levels of triglycerides and cholesterol. It is a rare hereditary disorder of metabolism.
    d. **Type IV** is characterized by hypertriglyceridemia associated with excessive dietary carbohydrates, and dietary manipulation can be beneficial in correcting the disorder. Type IV has a high association with both coronary heart disease and peripheral vascular disease. It is a very common lipid disorder.
    e. **Type V** is a mixed disorder with characteristics of both types I and IV, and it is associated with both hereditary and dietary factors. There is mild elevation of cholesterol levels and marked elevation of triglycerides. There is no known association with atherosclerosis.

**B. Clinical history.** A thorough history and physical examination can lead to the diagnosis of peripheral vascular disease and can suggest the anatomic location of specific occlusive lesions.

1. One of the most characteristic symptoms of peripheral vascular disease is **claudication**—pain in an extremity. It is related to exercise in that the most painful regions are muscle groups that require large amounts of blood during exertion. The pain is relieved by rest. Claudication usually occurs in the calf muscles because of their distal position in the arterial tree and their high metabolic needs during exercise. Occasionally claudication occurs in thigh and buttock muscles when severe aortoiliac disease is present.
    a. **Clinical data**
       (1) Frequently **extremity pulses are diminished** or absent, and occasionally pulses that are palpable at rest disappear with exercise.
       (2) Symptoms stabilize or improve in 80% of patients short-term. They become worse in 20%, of whom one-half develop a more severe form of claudication and one-half develop gangrene.

**b.** Certain **risk factors** are related to claudication.
  **(1)** Eighty-one percent of patients **smoke**.
  **(2)** Forty-three percent of patients have **hypertension**.
  **(3)** **Abnormal lipoproteins** are present in 30%.
  **(4)** Nine percent of patients have **diabetes mellitus**.
**c. Therapy**
  **(1)** **Nonoperative therapy** includes:
    **(a)** Not smoking
    **(b)** Correction of hypertension
    **(c)** Correction of lipid abnormalities
    **(d)** Exercise
  **(2)** **Drug management** of claudication using vasodilators is usually unsuccessful. Frequently, drugs administered for other disorders, especially $\beta$-blocking agents for hypertension or angina, may aggravate claudication by lowering cardiac output and decreasing extremity perfusion.
**d.** The long-term **morbidity** and **mortality** rates of claudication are significant.
  **(1)** There is a 5-year survival rate of 73% and an amputation rate of 7%.
  **(2)** There is a 10-year survival rate of 38% and an amputation rate of 12%.
  **(3)** The 15-year survival rate is 22%.

**2. Ischemic rest pain** is a symptom of peripheral vascular disease and may supplant the intermittent pain of claudication.
  **a.** It is usually a **constant ache**, which is present even when the extremity is under no exertion, and it frequently awakens the patient at night. Occasionally it is associated with numbness. Generally the pain is made worse by elevating the extremity and is relieved temporarily by placing the extremity in a dependent position.
  **b.** In 96% of patients, it **involves the toes or metatarsal heads**. It is not generally associated with calf and thigh pain. Pedal pulses are often absent, especially in the nondiabetic patient.

**3. Gangrene** (tissue necrosis) is further evidence of peripheral vascular disease.
  **a.** It presents as a necrotic toe or as a foot or leg ulcer and results from inadequate arterial inflow and, frequently, from minor trauma to the affected part.
  **b.** Usually some form of amputation is necessary.

**C. Diagnostic procedures**

**1.** Various **noninvasive tests** are useful in the diagnostic assessment of arterial disease.
  **a. Doppler ultrasonic recording of blood flow** permits study of most peripheral arteries.
    **(1)** A triphasic signal indicates normal arterial flow with elastic arterial wall motion.
    **(2)** A biphasic signal is associated with an abnormal artery, which has loss of elasticity and diminished flow.
    **(3)** A monophasic signal indicates a severely diseased artery with diminished flow.
  **b.** Doppler ultrasonography can also be used to determine **systolic arterial pressure**, which is usually slightly higher at the ankle than at the arm. The cuff is placed at the ankle, and the systolic pressure is measured at the dorsalis pedis or the posterior tibial artery location. The ratio of ankle to brachial artery systolic pressure is then evaluated.
    **(1)** Moderate vascular disease with claudication usually results in a ratio of 0.5 to 0.8.
    **(2)** Severe disease with ischemic rest pain usually has a ratio of ankle pressure to brachial pressure of less than 0.5 to 0.8.
    **(3)** Use of the blood pressure cuff when the vessel wall is extremely calcified with loss of compressibility may give spuriously high results. Frequently (generally in diabetics) flow signals are detected above the blood pressure limit of the cuff.
  **c. Plethysmography** measures the change of blood volume in an extremity with each heart beat.

**2. Invasive tests** for assessment of peripheral vascular disease include digital subtraction angiography and percutaneous arterial angiography.
  **a. Digital subtraction angiography** demonstrates arterial anatomy through a single nonselective intravenous injection of radiopaque contrast medium. In terms of injury to arterial structures and renal toxicity, the technique is low-risk; however, risk of allergy to the dye remains. With experience and improved technique, determination of the presence and extent of disease will become more reliable.
  **b. Percutaneous arterial angiography** is the current standard method for evaluating vascular disease. Contrast medium is selectively injected intra-arterially to visualize the vascular anatomy. The **complications** that may arise from use of this technique should be considered.

(1) **Dye-related complications**. Acute renal failure can result from nephrotoxicity of the dye, and acute dehydration can result from brisk diuresis induced by osmotic potency of the dye. Both complications can be minimized by adequate pre- and post-angiographic hydration and by limiting the total amount of dye injected. In addition, allergic reactions to the dye can occur.

(2) **Acute arterial occlusion** occasionally occurs following angiography.

(a) Although **arterial vasospasm** can explain this acute ischemic episode, it is rare, occurring in less than 3% of cases. It is more appropriate to assume that the ischemia occurs secondary to arterial occlusion that is **related to a technical problem**, including:

(i) Simple thrombosis of the artery at the site of needle insertion

(ii) Distal embolization in the lower leg, which is associated with thrombi forming on the angiogram catheter

(iii) Subintimal dissection of an atherosclerotic plaque during catheter manipulation

(b) The **clinical symptoms** of acute arterial occlusion in this setting usually occur immediately following angiography.

(i) There is **absence of pulses** that were present prior to the examination.

(ii) There is **severe constant pain**, **numbness**, and **paresthesia** in the extremity examined.

(iii) There is a **sensation of coolness** progressing up the legs.

(c) The **management** of acute arterial occlusion following angiography should include rapid diagnosis followed by rapid surgical intervention.

(i) In preparation for operation, **anticoagulants** should be administered to prevent progression of the thrombotic process.

(ii) **Preoperative repeat angiography should be avoided** unless a specific need is present. Acute occlusion may proceed to ischemic necrosis rapidly, and repeat angiography will unnecessarily delay surgical exploration and repair of the injury.

(iii) **Surgical exploration** for a thrombus or embolus must be undertaken for good results. Results are excellent if the extremity is revascularized within 2 to 6 hours following the thrombosis.

c. **Brachial artery catheterization** is performed frequently for cardiac catheterization or for angiography when the lower extremity vessels are unsuitable for these techniques. However, there are **complications**.

(1) Thrombosis of the artery may result in **acute hand ischemia**, requiring immediate surgical intervention.

(2) Thrombosis of the radial artery may result in the delayed onset of **hand claudication** in 45% of patients.

d. **Axillary artery catheterization** is performed occasionally when the femoral vessels are not adequate for angiography.

(1) There is a higher risk of causing **cerebral emboli** with this technique than occurs with the catheterization of other vessels.

(2) A **periarterial hematoma** may result following the study. The hematoma may compress the brachial plexus, causing arm paralysis if it is not surgically decompressed.

e. **Translumbar aortography** is performed by catheterizing the suprarenal aorta through use of a long needle, which is inserted posteriorly in the lumbar area. This study is useful when neither femoral nor axillary arteries are sufficient for catheterization. It is also useful when ulcerated plaques are present in the aorta and catheter manipulation could dislodge the plaque. The study may be **complicated**, however, by **retroperitoneal hematomas**.

D. **Arterial dilation** in areas of stenosis by means of a **balloon (Grüntzig) catheter** is a nonoperative technique that fractures atherosclerotic plaques. It may be used in most extremity vessels.

1. The dilation is performed by a radiologist immediately following angiography. An inflatable balloon, which is attached to an angiographic catheter, is fluoroscopically guided to the area of stenosis. The balloon is then inflated with 4 to 8 atm to fracture the plaque.

2. Clinically significant **distal emboli** may follow this procedure in 3% to 5% of the cases.

3. The **patency record** of the technique is 94% at 1 year. The long-term benefits are yet to be determined.

## II. DIABETIC FOOT

### A. Clinical data

1. The toe, foot, and leg of a patient with diabetes mellitus are subject to infection, which can

arise after minor trauma to the affected area. Because of the peripheral neuropathy of diabetes, the trauma can become complicated by trophic ulcers, which, in turn, become easily infected. This infection, which is caused by mixed flora including anaerobic bacteria, results in:
   **a.** Deep plantar space **abscesses**
   **b. Cellulitis** of the dorsum of the foot
   **c. Osteomyelitis** of the metatarsal or phalangeal bones

2. The diabetic has an **increased chance of** developing **atherosclerosis**, which occurs at a younger age and progresses more rapidly than in the nondiabetic.

3. The diabetic can develop **gangrene** with a frequency 40 times that of the nondiabetic; this is due to:
   **a.** Large vessel occlusive disease in which pulses are absent
   **b.** Small vessel disease (microangiopathy) characterized by thickening of the capillary basement membrane

**B. Prevention**

1. Through early care of localized injuries, the patient should be able to control and heal an ulcer before it becomes extensive.

2. Footwear should be properly fitted.

**C. Treatment** includes:

1. Bed rest without elevation of the affected limb

2. Systemic or local administration of antibiotics

3. Debridement of devitalized tissue

4. Immobilization of the affected limb

5. Avoidance of pressure on and weight bearing by the affected area

6. Amputation of necrotic tissue

7. In mild, localized cases, nonoperative treatment of osteomyelitis

**III. AORTOILIAC OCCLUSIVE DISEASE.** Aortoiliac occlusive disease is obstruction of the distal aorta and iliac artery systems (Fig. 13-1) as a consequence of atherosclerosis. It can result in significant buttock or calf claudication and distal extremity gangrene, or it can be totally without symptoms.

**A. Pathology.** In general, there are **three patterns of aortoiliac disease**.

1. Atherosclerosis is limited to the aortic bifurcation and common iliac arteries in 13% of the cases. Over 50% of the patients are female, and frequently they are in a young age-group.

2. Atherosclerosis extends from the aorta to the level of the inguinal ligament, but there is little or no disease more distally. This distribution occurs in 21% of cases.

3. Atherosclerosis extends from the aorta to include femoral and distal vessels. This distribution of disease occurs in 66% of cases, and over 80% of the patients are male and smokers.

**B. Indications for surgery** in aortoiliac occlusive disease are limited to several situations.

1. **Severe claudication or rest pain** is present in 65% of the patients requiring operation.

2. **Tissue necrosis** of the lower extremities or toes necessitates surgery in 35% of patients.

3. Formation of **distal arterial emboli** in the legs occurs rarely in patients with aortoiliac occlusive disease. When it does occur, it usually is evidenced by the presence of a "blue toe" or small petechiae on the foot. The proposed source of these small emboli is an ulcerated plaque located either on the aorta or distal to it (see section V B 1 c).

4. **Impotence in the male** is an indication when it has been shown to be secondary to bilateral internal iliac occlusion.

**C. Operative techniques** for aortoiliac and aortofemoral occlusion include the following.

1. **Aortoiliac endarterectomy** is a technique that removes obstructing atherosclerotic material from the lumen of the vessel, allowing new endothelium to grow over the denuded surface.

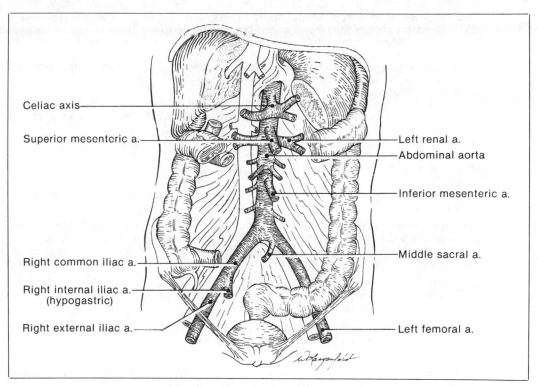

Celiac axis

Superior mesenteric a.

Left renal a.

Abdominal aorta

Inferior mesenteric a.

Middle sacral a.

Right common iliac a.

Right internal iliac a.
(hypogastric)

Right external iliac a.

Left femoral a.

**Figure 13-1.** Arteries of the abdominal region.

The procedure may be used only when the disease is limited to a short segment of vessel. In extensive disease it is very difficult to remove all of the obstructing material that is present.

2. **Aortoiliac** or **aortofemoral grafting** using artificial graft material is the most common way of bypassing severe occlusive disease in the aorta and iliac arteries.
    a. **Operative principles**
        (1) A bilateral leg graft should usually be used because there is a high rate of occurrence of new symptoms in the unoperated leg soon after unilateral grafts are performed.
        (2) The graft should originate from the aorta just below the renal arteries for the most reliable inflow.
    b. The **operative results** of aortoiliac and aortofemoral bypass are very acceptable.
        (1) The technique has a **patency rate** of at least 85% at 5 to 10 years. The patency rate is strongly dependent upon the outflow into the legs that is provided at the distal arterial anastomosis.
        (2) **Improvement of preoperative symptoms** reliably occurs. Good to excellent relief of claudication occurs in 85% of patients in whom it was the initial complaint. Good to excellent results occur in 90% of patients who presented preoperatively with gangrene.
        (3) The **operative mortality rate** varies from 1% to 5%. Most operative deaths occur secondary to acute myocardial infarction.

3. **Femoral-to-femoral artery bypass grafts** are occasionally used in patients with aortoiliac and aortofemoral occlusive disease.
    a. **Indications.** The decision to use this type of graft rather than an aortofemoral graft is based on **three factors**:
        (1) One of the patient's lower extremities is severely ischemic due to poor femoral artery flow.
        (2) The other extremity has excellent femoral artery inflow.
        (3) The patient's risk factors for a major abdominal aortic procedure are prohibitive.
    b. The **operative results** for this procedure are excellent.
        (1) **Graft patency** is 93% at 1 year and 80% long-term.
        (2) The early postoperative mortality rate is about 5%, which is acceptable considering that these patients are at much higher risk than aortoiliac and aortofemoral bypass patients.

**4. Axillofemoral or axillobifemoral artery bypass grafts** are used in patients with severe aortofemoral occlusive disease that affects both femoral arteries. These grafts may be highly effective in healing gangrenous ulcers in patients with an unacceptable operative risk for a more extensive procedure.
 a. **Operative technique.** The arterial inflow of these grafts is based in the axillary artery because neither femoral artery has adequate inflow.
 b. **Complications**
  (1) There is a high rate of thrombosis in these patients, requiring frequent thrombectomy.
  (2) Up to 15% of patients develop infections, requiring the removal of the graft material.

IV. **CHRONIC FEMOROPOPLITEAL DISEASE.** Femoropopliteal occlusive disease is obstruction of the femoral and more distal extremity arteries (Fig. 13-2) as a result of atherosclerosis. It creates a spectrum of symptoms ranging from none to severe claudication and tissue gangrene.

 A. The **pathologic pattern** of femoropopliteal disease includes atherosclerosis of various leg arteries.

  1. The **superficial femoral artery** is the most frequently occluded leg artery. In fact, it is the most frequently occluded of all peripheral arteries. The occlusion is frequently in the distal third of the artery where it traverses the adductor (Hunter's) canal. Occlusion may result in minimal or no symptoms in some patients.

  2. The **profunda femoris artery** supplies blood to the thigh muscles and is frequently affected by atherosclerosis. The artery usually shows high-grade stenosis at its origin, but it is relatively free of disease distally.

  3. At the **trifurcation of the popliteal artery** and its branches, which include the anterior tibial, posterior tibial, and peroneal arteries, there is frequently multiple partial or complete vessel obstruction.

  4. The **pedal arteries** also may have multiple vessel occlusions at the ankle or in the pedal arch network, which generally result in rest pain or gangrene.

 B. **Common physical findings** of femoropopliteal occlusive disease result from impaired, sluggish blood flow to the extremity.

  1. Frequently, an **extremity is pulseless, pale, and cool**.

  2. **Rubor** may be present in the foot, manifested as lobster-red discoloration while standing, which is due to stagnated oxygenated blood in the subdermal plexus.

  3. The **loss of lower extremity hair** and the presence of **nonhealing ulcerations** on the leg frequently indicate arterial insufficiency. It is important to distinguish between venous and arterial causes of the ulcerations.

 C. **Surgery**

  1. There are two principal **indications for surgery** in patients with femoropopliteal occlusive disease.
   a. **Tissue necrosis** of the leg or foot is an urgent reason to proceed with surgery.
   b. **Severe claudication** that interferes with life-style may indicate surgery in some patients. If the pain progresses to rest pain in the foot, then surgery is definitely needed to avoid progression to necrosis.

  2. The **basic operative procedure of a bypass graft** from the femoral artery to the popliteal artery using either the autogenous saphenous vein or artificial graft material shunts blood from the femoral system to the lower leg.
   a. There is an excellent cumulative **patency rate** of up to 80% at 5 years. The **limb salvage rate** is up to 90%.
   b. The graft has a **late failure rate** secondary to occurrence of atherosclerosis within the graft, to occurrence of intimal hyperplasia within the graft, or to progression of atherosclerosis distal to the bypass graft.
   c. This procedure has an **operative mortality rate** of about 3%. The major cause of death is myocardial infarction.

  3. **Alternative surgical procedures** may be necessary if the arterial occlusive disease involves the extremity distally or is diffuse or if the patient is a relatively high surgical risk.
   a. The use of a **femoral-to-tibial artery bypass graft** is indicated when vascular disease is distal to the popliteal artery. The results show a higher failure rate than that of a femoropopliteal bypass graft because there is more extensive vascular disease present.

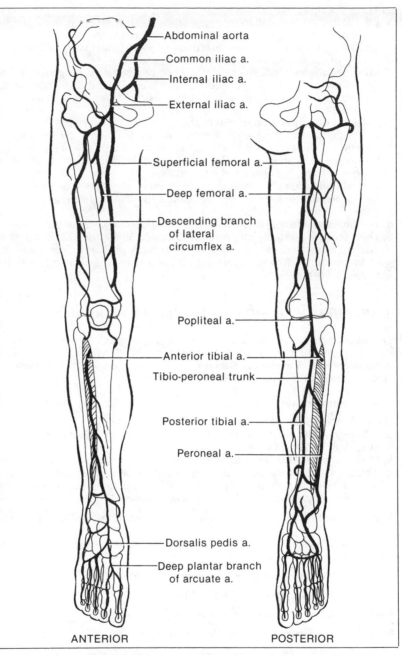

**Figure 13-2.** Arteries of the lower extremity.

  **b. Femoral profundaplasty** is indicated when the distal leg vascular disease is severe and difficult to bypass reliably. Profundaplasty is a technique that relieves the stenosis of the profunda femoris artery, usually by placing a patch over the area of stenosis, resulting in relief of symptoms and, frequently, healing of ulcers.
  **c. Lumbar sympathectomy** is used in patients with severe rest pain or tissue loss, especially in the patient who is not a good candidate for reconstruction. It is a procedure to excise the lumbar sympathetic ganglia of $L_2$, $L_3$, and $L_4$, and results show temporarily increased blood flow to the extremity skin but no change in muscular blood flow. Relief of rest pain occurs temporarily in 50% of cases, and healing of ulcers occurs in 25% of cases.

 **4. Amputation** may not only be lifesaving for some patients but may be expeditious in promoting the total rehabilitation of many patients. Occasionally the result is better than that of an extensive vascular procedure. One-half of all amputations are performed on diabetics.

    **a.** There are **three indications** for amputation.
      **(1)** The presence of **gangrene**, especially when the patient is not a good candidate for reconstruction, is a sign that urgent intervention is required.
      **(2)** The presence of a **serious infection** in the extremity, such as myositis from a gas-forming organism, necessitates prompt amputation.
      **(3)** A **serious medical illness** with a poor rehabilitative prognosis indicates amputation over revascularization. However, there is evidence that the operative mortality rate of amputation may be similar to that of an extremity revascularization procedure for these patients.
    **b.** The **level of amputation** should be the lowest possible position that will heal, to allow the greatest opportunity for rehabilitation. This level is usually chosen on the basis of clinical experience and the presence of a pulse, determined through Doppler ultrasonography, in the proposed location. A prosthesis that is fitted immediately may significantly aid the healing process and the chance of rehabilitation.
    **c.** The **rehabilitation rate** depends on the level of amputation and ranges from 60% to 70% for unilateral below-the-knee amputations to 10% for bilateral above-the-knee amputations.
    **d.** The **healing failure rate** is up to 20% for below-the-knee amputations.
    **e.** The **operative mortality rate** is about 13%, with 50% of deaths occurring secondary to cardiac problems and 25% secondary to respiratory problems. The **long-term mortality rate** of amputation is 50% at 3 years and 70% at 5 years when the amputation is performed for vascular disease.

## V. ACUTE ARTERIAL OCCLUSION OF THE LOWER EXTREMITY

**A.** The **result of acute arterial occlusion** of the lower extremity is sudden cessation of arterial blood flow to the extremity (see Fig. 13-2). Acute ischemia is followed by necrosis if rapid intervention does not take place. The **most common site** of occlusion is the femoral artery, followed by the iliac and popliteal arteries and the aortic bifurcation.

**B.** The **most common cause** of acute occlusion is an embolus or, frequently, multiple emboli.

    **1.** The emboli **originate** from one of several sources.
      **a. Atherosclerotic heart disease** with arterial plaques and thrombi is thought to be the source of emboli in 60% of cases.
      **b. Rheumatic valvular heart disease** is the source of emboli in 21% of cases.
      **c. Abdominal aortic ulcerated plaques** are the source of emboli in 1% to 2% of cases. The small but significant group of patients with these plaques may present with digital emboli, resulting in cyanotic toes (the **"blue toe syndrome"**).

    **2.** A recent onset of arrhythmia, especially atrial fibrillation, may give a clue to the cause.

**C.** The **clinical findings** of a lower extremity embolus result from ischemia of the tissues supplied by the occluded artery. These findings include:

    **1.** Acute onset of **severe pain** and a sensation of **coolness**

    **2.** Acute **loss of motor and sensory function**

    **3.** A **pale, pulseless extremity** without edema

    **4. Ankle blood pressure** that is very low or undetectable

**D.** The **management** of acute arterial occlusion includes **rapid diagnosis** and **expeditious surgical correction** of the occlusion.

    **1.** Patients should be **heparinized** immediately when the clinical diagnosis is made.

    **2.** The **preoperative evaluation** of patients does not generally require an arteriogram because the level of occlusion is usually evident upon physical examination.

    **3.** The patient should be operated on as quickly as possible, preferably within 6 to 8 hours of onset.
      **a.** The surgeon should perform an **embolectomy** using a **Fogarty balloon catheter**. The catheter is passed down the occluded artery past the embolus. It is then inflated and pulled back through the artery, extracting the embolus as it is withdrawn.
      **(1)** The procedure results in good to excellent revascularization in 65% of cases.
      **(2)** The amputation rate is less than 19%.
      **(3)** The mortality rate is 1% to 2%.

    **b. Results of revascularization**
      **(1)** If revascularized within 6 to 8 hours of the onset of symptoms, 80% of patients will have no ischemic sequelae.
      **(2)** If revascularized within 8 to 24 hours, 68% will have no ischemic sequelae.
      **(3)** If revascularized within 1 to 7 days, 57% will have no ischemic sequelae.

  **4. Postoperatively,** patients should be given **anticoagulant therapy**, which lowers the recurrence rate of embolus formation from 38% to 22% long-term.

  **5. Thrombolytic therapy** for emboli using streptokinase is effective for the treatment of acute occlusions. Although the best use of this treatment modality has not been fully defined, it should probably be reserved for very high operative risk patients, such as those with multiple small peripheral emboli. There is a significant hemorrhagic morbidity rate with its use.

  **6.** The **long-term mortality rate** in patients with acute emboli is principally due to death from coronary artery disease.

## VI. MESENTERIC VASCULAR OCCLUSIVE DISEASE. Occlusion of the mesenteric arteries results in ischemia and necrosis of the small bowel, which in turn can result in infarction of part or all of the small bowel and colon, creating an immediate threat to survival.

  **A.** The **usual pathologic findings** are separated into three categories:

    **1. Arterial vascular thrombosis**, secondary to atherosclerosis in 50% of cases, and usually occurring at the origin of the superior mesenteric artery

    **2. Arterial emboli**, usually originating from the heart and frequently causing multiple small occlusions of the branches of the superior mesenteric artery

    **3. Nonocclusive mesenteric insufficiency** secondary to low cardiac output, which is frequently aggravated by superior mesenteric artery stenosis and associated with digitalis therapy

  **B. Clinical findings** depend on the suddenness of the occlusion and the time elapsed since its occurrence.

    **1. Acute occlusion** of the superior mesenteric artery results in moderate abdominal pain, which progresses to hypotension, sepsis, and death. Preexisting heart disease is present in 90% of patients, and patients are frequently receiving digitalis. The usual **symptoms** include:
      **a.** Severe abdominal pain, almost always present early in the course of the disease, with physical findings that are frequently minimal
      **b.** Hypotension, hypovolemia, acidosis, and leukocytosis
      **c.** Heme-positive stools in 25% of cases
      **d.** Frequent diarrhea and vomiting

    **2. Chronic occlusion** of the artery results in a clinical course that is characterized by chronic abdominal complaints; however, it occasionally can result in sudden infarction of the bowel when the stenosis progresses to true occlusion. Involvement of all three mesenteric vessels (i.e., the celiac, superior mesenteric, and inferior mesenteric arteries) by severe occlusive disease is usually necessary before symptoms are present. The usual **symptoms** include the following:
      **a.** Abdominal pain 15 to 60 minutes following a meal
      **b.** Weight loss secondary to food restriction or diarrhea
      **c.** An abdominal bruit, which is present in 78% of cases

  **C.** The **surgical management** of mesenteric occlusion is strongly dependent upon the **stage** at which intestinal ischemia is recognized. The **surgical results** are associated with the acuteness of the occlusion, the extensiveness of the necrosis, and the overall condition of the patient.

    **1. Acute mesenteric ischemia without necrosis** may be diagnosed by angiography and treated in its early stages by hydration, anticoagulation therapy, and intra-arterial vasodilators. The stenosis is then repaired by bypass surgery if indicated.

    **2. Acute ischemia with necrosis** is usually diagnosed when the situation has worsened rapidly. This process is treated by preoperative hydration, laparotomy, and bowel resection. It is repaired by arterial bypass, usually at a later date, if enough of the bowel is present to support life and significant arterial stenosis is present. The rate of mortality is about 85% due to the large area of the bowel that is involved and to delayed diagnosis.

    **3. Chronic ischemia** is diagnosed by a high index of suspicion and through an arteriogram showing a lateral view of the superior mesenteric artery. The stenosis is repaired electively through use of a graft originating on the aorta and bypassing the stenotic segment. The mortality rate in chronic ischemia is low if the disease is recognized before an acute episode occurs. If the stenosis can be repaired, 90% of patients improve.

**VII. RENAL ARTERY STENOSIS.** Stenosis of the renal artery results in ischemia of the renal parenchyma, subsequently stimulating the juxtaglomerular apparatus to release renin. This is followed by systemic vasoconstriction and hypertension.

   **A. Etiology.** The two most common causes of renal artery stenosis are **atherosclerosis** and **fibromuscular dysplasia**. The latter is a disease that produces single or multiple stenoses of the distal main renal arteries, particularly in women.

   **B. The diagnosis** of renal artery stenosis is made through the use of several examination procedures when evaluating patients with hypertension.

   1. A **clinical suspicion** that a hypertensive patient has renal artery stenosis rather than essential hypertension can be diagnostic. The clues are as follows:
      **a.** Recent, rapid onset of hypertension
      **b.** A relatively young age, especially in white females
      **c.** Difficulty controlling blood pressure with antihypertensive medication
      **d.** Flank bruits, which are present in approximately 50% of patients with renal artery stenosis in contrast to only 7% of patients with essential hypertension

   2. **Laboratory tests** are of major assistance in confirming the presence of hypertension caused by renal artery stenosis.
      **a.** Rapid-sequence **intravenous pyelography (IVP)** is used as a screening test to distinguish between renal artery stenosis and essential hypertension, although the test is normal in 20% of patients with proven renal artery stenosis.
         **(1)** The procedure involves the injection of contrast medium and a series of roentgenograms taken immediately following the injection.
         **(2)** Significant findings of rapid-sequence IVP include:
            **(a)** Disparity in kidney size—a difference of about 2 cm is indicative of unilateral renal artery stenosis
            **(b)** Differences in the appearance time of the contrast medium in the calices—a unilateral 1-minute delay is present in only 2% of essential hypertensive patients versus 59% of patients with renal artery stenosis
      **b.** **Selective renal arteriography** is now the definitive diagnostic procedure for demonstrating the presence of renal artery stenosis. The procedure shows anomalous patterns of renal anatomy including multiple renal arteries.
         **(1)** **Pathologic patterns** of renal artery stenosis demonstrated by angiography include:
            **(a)** Atherosclerosis in an older age-group
            **(b)** Fibromuscular dysplastic lesions, especially in young women and children
            **(c)** Inflamed arteries
            **(d)** Associated congenital aortic developmental disorders
         **(2)** The **mortality rate** associated with renal angiography is 0.1%. Major complications (see section I C 2) occur in 1.2% of patients.
      **c.** A selective **renin ratio** compares the renin activity in the individual renal veins and helps to establish the severity of **unilateral** renal artery stenosis.
         **(1)** A renin ratio of 1.5 or greater is considered to be significant and has been predictive of a successful surgical cure of hypertension in 75% to 100% of cases in a number of clinical studies. However, a ratio of less than 1.5 does not necessarily indicate an unsuccessful surgical reconstruction.
         **(2)** Renin ratios are highly sensitive to volume and vasomotor status and should be measured:
            **(a)** After an upright posture has been maintained for several hours
            **(b)** After discontinuance of antihypertensive medication
            **(c)** During volume depletion
            **(d)** Before or long after contrast medium administration because dye stimulates abnormal renin release
      **d.** Renin ratios may be unreliable in establishing the severity of **bilateral** renal artery stenosis. However, urinary findings may be positive for bilateral stenosis.
         **(1)** Significant **urinary findings** include:
            **(a)** A 60% reduction in the urine volume of the stenotic kidney
            **(b)** A 15% reduction in the urine sodium concentration of the stenotic kidney
         **(2)** Technical difficulties can frustrate attempts to measure each kidney's urine output by selective ureteral catheterization.

### C. Surgery

1. The **indications for surgical intervention** in patients with renal artery stenosis include two clinical situations:
   **a. Hypertension**
      **(1)** In a young individual
      **(2)** That is difficult to control
      **(3)** In an individual with significant aortoiliac aneurysmal or occlusive disease requiring an operation for other symptoms
   **b. Impaired renal function**
      **(1)** In the presence of demonstrated high-grade renal artery stenosis (90% occluded)
      **(2)** Especially in a solitary kidney or in the presence of bilateral renal artery stenosis
      **(3)** When angiographic evidence of preservation of functional renal tissue exists, including:
         **(a)** Adequate cortical tissue
         **(b)** Collateral circulation to the kidney
         **(c)** A patent renal artery

2. **Preopertive considerations**
   **a.** Variations in **regional anatomy** must be considered.
      **(1)** The renal artery is usually a solitary branch of the aorta; however, in approximately 30% of patients accessory renal arteries arise from the aorta.
      **(2)** Gonadal and adrenal artery branches frequently supply large amounts of blood to the kidney when renal artery stenosis is present. In addition, many collateral vessels from Gerota's fascia and ureteral vessels become very prominent in the presence of ischemia.
   **b.** It is necessary to screen preoperatively for coronary artery and cerebrovascular disease. Volume depletion also must be corrected preoperatively.

3. The **principles of surgical correction** of renal artery stenosis include:
   **a.** Minimal perirenal dissection so that as few collateral vessels as possible are disrupted
   **b.** Cooling the affected kidney prior to revascularizing it to minimize tubular necrosis and renal dysfunction
   **c.** Total systemic heparinization
   **d.** End-to-end anastomosis using:
      **(1)** Autogenous saphenous vein or the hypogastric artery
      **(2)** A reimplanted or endarterectomized native renal artery
      **(3)** A synthetic Teflon or Dacron graft
      **(4)** The splenic artery when revascularizing the left renal artery
   **e.** Open renal biopsy, when safe, in order to determine the prognosis and curability of hypertension or impaired renal function
   **f.** Nephrectomy only after primary repair has failed or glomerular atrophy is present
   **g.** Staged repair (repair of each artery as a separate surgical procedure) for bilateral arterial lesions
   **h.** Maintenance of adequate volume status, blood pressure, and urine output

4. **Operative results**
   **a.** The cure rates for **hypertension** vary from 30% to 51%, and improvement rates vary from 15% to 50%. The overall success rate is in the range of 60% to 100%.
   **b.** Success rates for **fibromuscular dysplasia** vary from 80% to 100%. Renal artery stenosis that is due to fibromuscular dysplasia is associated with the lowest mortality rates.
   **c.** The success rates for **atherosclerosis** range from 50% to 90%; operations performed for focal atherosclerosis limited to renal arteries are more often successful (87%) than operations performed for generalized atherosclerosis (63%).
   **d.** Improvement in **renal function** may follow revascularization if significant renal artery stenosis (usually with hypertension) exists, if the diminished renal function is not due to intrinsic renal disease, and if angiography demonstrates the patency of intrarenal arteries. In addition, renal function must be demonstrated on a renal scan or by means of a delayed nephrogram.

### D. Medical management

1. For **mild to moderate hypertension** from renal artery stenosis (when the diastolic blood pressure is in the 90 to 100 range), **antihypertensive drugs** can be used to control the blood pressure. However, the risk of medical management is higher when the blood pressure is erratic or difficult to control.

2. Medical therapy with antihypertensive drugs is more reasonable than surgical therapy in pa-

tients with **generalized atherosclerosis**. It is less desirable than surgery in children and in patients with fibromuscular dysplasia.

## VIII. EXTRACRANIAL CEREBROVASCULAR DISEASE

### A. General considerations

1. **Cerebrovascular accident (CVA, stroke)** is ischemic insult of the central nervous system resulting in temporary or permanent neurologic disability. Because of the amount of disability associated with CVA, recognition of significant cerebrovascular disease and prevention of a CVA are critical for optimal patient outcome.

2. **Epidemiology**
   a. CVA is the **third leading cause of death** in the United States and accounts for 10% of all deaths. The **mortality rate** of the first episode is 18%; that of a recurrent stroke is 62%.
   b. It has a higher **incidence** with increasing age (25% of CVAs occur in individuals in the 40- to 55-year-old age-group; 50% occur in the 65- to 79-year-old group). Men are more susceptible than women. In addition, occurrence of CVA is higher when there is evidence of generalized atherosclerosis.
   c. The stroke **recurrence rate** is 10% at 1 year and 20% at 5 years.

3. CVA can occur as a result of disease in either the intracranial or extracranial arteries (Figure 13-3). CVAs due to intracranial causes are discussed in Chapter 31, section XII; those due to extracranial causes are discussed here.

### B. Causes. 
Extracranial causes may be secondary to carotid artery disease or secondary to emboli in the cerebrum that originate from more central sources such as the heart. Most surgically treatable disease occurs at the carotid bifurcation and has one of the following **pathophysiologic characteristics**.

1. **Ulcerated plaques** occur frequently at the carotid bifurcation. These plaques are irregular atherosclerotic areas in the intima of the vessel with local accumulation of platelets, cholesterol, and other debris. They are the probable cause of cerebral infarction in two-thirds of cases originating extracranially.

2. **Stenotic lesions** in the carotid bifurcation are smooth constricted areas in the lumen of the artery with subintimal accumulation of lipid material but an intact intima. Although carotid stenosis is a common angiographic finding, its relationship to CVA is not strong and it is an unlikely cause of cerebral infarction. In general, an arterial stenotic area does not cause a decrease in blood flow until at least a 70% reduction in the cross-sectional area occurs.

3. **Complete occlusion of the carotid arteries** may occur. The occlusion may be silent and therefore completely asymptomatic, or it may be associated with major hemispheric CVA and severe disability or death.

### C. Clinical manifestations. 
CVA may present as many different clinical situations.

1. A **transient ischemic attack (TIA)** is an episode of focal neurologic symptoms. The classic TIA syndrome is characterized by abrupt onset—usually the maximal symptoms occur in less than 5 minutes; rapid resolution within 24 hours—usually within 2 to 15 minutes; neurologic symptoms corresponding to a specific hemispheric arterial distribution; and no residual neurologic deficits.
   a. TIA is **associated with generalized atherosclerosis**. TIA occurs **secondary to a cerebral embolus** originating from an ulcerated carotid plaque, frequently associated with a bruit located high in the neck.
   b. TIA is usually associated with **hemispheric neurologic symptoms**, including:
      (1) A motor deficit contralateral to the involved carotid
      (2) A sensory deficit contralateral to the involved carotid
      (3) Minor or global aphasia
      (4) Homonymous hemianopia
      (5) **Amaurosis fugax**, which is a transient monocular blindness almost always due to an ulcerated carotid plaque. Amaurosis fugax results from an embolus in the ophthalmic artery and is associated with a **Hollenhorst plaque**, a bright spot of cholesterol or platelets seen on retinal examination
   c. TIA is **followed by a CVA** at a rate of 23% in 1 year and 45% in 5 years. (The risk of stroke to the general population is 3% to 7% per year.)
   d. The primary cause of death in patients with TIA is acute myocardial infarction.

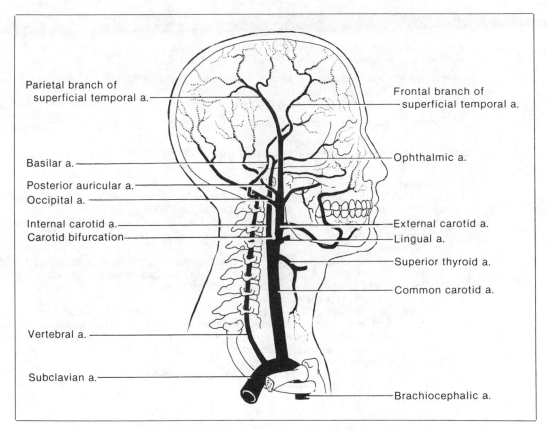

**Figure 13-3.** The arterial supply to the brain.

**2.** A **completed CVA** is a **fixed neurologic deficit**, which does not improve with time.
  **a.** It is the result of:
    **(1)** Cerebral infarction in 79% of cases
    **(2)** Intracerebral hemorrhage in 10% of cases
    **(3)** Subarachnoid hemorrhage in 6% of cases
    **(4)** Other causes in 5% of cases
  **b.** It results in neurologic symptoms that are not necessarily hemispheric. The disability ranges from mild to severe.

**3. Vertebrobasilar artery disease.** A cause-and-effect relationship between the vertebrobasilar system (see Fig. 13-3) and neurologic symptoms can be very difficult to establish because the symptoms are not specific. The following **symptoms** are generally but not exclusively related to the posterior circulation of the central nervous system:
  **a.** A motor deficit, involving any combination of extremities, and including **drop attacks**, which are loss of lower extremity motor function with no loss of consciousness
  **b.** A sensory deficit involving any combination of extremities
  **c.** Loss of vision in both homonymous fields (**homonymous hemianopia**)
  **d.** Ataxia

**4.** An **asymptomatic carotid bruit** occurs high in the neck without an associated history or findings of neurologic disease.
  **a.** It is associated with coronary artery disease (the risk of acute myocardial infarction is doubled in individuals with an asymptomatic bruit).
  **b.** It appears to have a propensity for proceeding to TIA or completed CVA.
    **(1)** Some series show that the risk of CVA with endarterectomy is equivalent to the risk with nonsurgical management in patients with an asymptomatic bruit. These results would support management by simple observation for these patients.
    **(2)** Other series show that the risk of CVA is up to 20% long-term in patients with asymptomatic bruits that are managed by nonsurgical means. These results would support prophylactic carotid endarterectomy.

**D. Medical management** of cerebrovascular disease has been used extensively, but its effectiveness is limited.

**1.** Chronic anticoagulation therapy with warfarin has shown conflicting results in controlling the incidence of recurrent TIA.

**2.** The long-term use of aspirin has been shown to decrease significantly the incidence of both stroke (which drops from 16.5% to 14.3%) and death in men with preceding TIA. However, no effect has been demonstrated in women.

**3.** Long-term therapy with dipyridamole has shown no effect in preventing CVA.

**E. Surgical management** of cerebrovascular disease involves the careful preoperative evaluation of the patient and precise surgical technique.

**1. Preoperative evaluation**
   **a. Laboratory evaluation** of cerebrovascular disease is necessary prior to surgical intervention. There are two types of vascular evaluation currently in use.
      **(1) Angiography** of the carotid, vertebral, and intracranial vessels is the best method available to appraise the nature and extent of disease. The morbidity rates are acceptably low.
      **(2) Noninvasive testing** through the use of ultrasonography devices and ocular pressure measurements is sometimes helpful in following the progression of disease. However, its usefulness in evaluating patients for surgery is unclear.
   **b. Selection of candidates for operation**
      **(1) Candidates for surgery** include patients with TIA associated with an ulcerated carotid plaque and those with a completed hemispheric CVA with a 6-week time lapse since the onset of initial symptoms. The CVA must have resulted in a mild neurologic deficit and must have an associated ulcerated carotid plaque.
      **(2) Surgery is contraindicated** in patients with:
         **(a)** A completely occluded carotid artery corresponding to a neurologic deficit
         **(b)** Severe intracranial disease
         **(c)** Severe evolving CVA
         **(d)** A severe fixed neurologic deficit
         **(e)** Severe medical disability resulting from another disease
      **(3)** Candidates for whom surgical management **may not offer an advantage** over medical management include those with:
         **(a)** Vertebrobasilar TIA
         **(b)** An asymptomatic carotid bruit
      **(4)** In an **emergency carotid event**, surgery is probably more effective than medical management. Such emergencies include:
         **(a)** Crescendo TIAs—multiple daily TIAs uncontrolled by anticoagulants
         **(b)** Mild stroke occurring in the hospital or immediately following cerebral angiography, which can be operated upon within 2 hours
         **(c)** No new neurologic symptoms but more than 95% carotid stenosis in patients with TIA

**2.** The **operative strategy** of cerebrovascular disease includes:
   **a.** Control of operative hypo- and hypertension
   **b.** Monitoring cerebral function during carotid clamping
   **c.** Use of an indwelling carotid shunt while the carotid is clamped in selected patients
   **d.** Use of systemic anticoagulation
   **e.** Removal of embolic debris from the artery
   **f.** Endarterectomy of the carotid bifurcation with careful control of the distal end of the intimal dissection
   **g.** Care not to injure the cranial (i.e., hypoglossal, recurrent laryngeal, and marginal mandibular) nerves

**3.** The **purpose** of endarterectomy is to prevent stroke, and the **postoperative results** vary greatly among surgeons.
   **a.** Preoperative classic TIA **neurologic symptoms are relieved or improved** in 84% to 99% of patients. When the symptoms are nonhemispheric, relief is rare.
   **b.** Postoperative **neurologic deficit** occurs in 1.6% to 6% of TIA patients. The rate of occurrence of postoperative new neurologic deficits in stroke patients is about 5%.
   **c.** The **late stroke rate** following endarterectomy is approximately 13% in a follow-up of 13 years. Late stroke is associated with the recurrence of a bruit, the recurrence of neurologic symptoms, which frequently are identical to previous symptoms, and the recurrence of atherosclerosis or intimal fibrosis.

**4. Mortality rates**. The mortality rates of perioperative TIA range from 0.8% to 1%. Those of perioperative stroke are approximately 4.2%. The **long-term** (5- to 10-year) **mortality rates** range from 9% to 34%: 24% of patients die following acute myocardial infarction; 5% die following a new stroke; and 5% die of other causes. The mortality rates are as high as 42% when patients are operated upon during an acute evolving CVA or following (less than 6 weeks) a recent stroke, in comparison to the 18% to 20% rates of a nonoperated stroke.

## IX. ABDOMINAL AORTIC ANEURYSM

**A. Clinical characteristics.** An abdominal aortic aneurysm is **dilatation of the distal aorta**. It results from a pathologic weakness in the aortic wall and frequently leads to rupture and death if not repaired. Aortic aneurysms are associated with simultaneously occurring aneurysms in other arteries in 20% of cases.

1. **Typical atherosclerotic aneurysm** occurs in the **infrarenal position** in 95% to 98% of cases. Physical examination shows a palpable pulsatile mass, usually in the left upper abdomen; however, the patient is frequently asymptomatic.

2. **Atypical aneurysm**
   a. **Inflammatory aneurysm** comprises 5% of all abdominal aortic aneurysms. It is characterized by a dense fibrotic reaction involving the wall of the aneurysm and the surrounding tissue. Although inflammatory cells and lymphocytes infiltrate the involved tissue, they are culture-negative at the time of surgery. Surgery of an inflammatory aneurysm is usually a difficult procedure.
   b. An **infected abdominal aortic aneurysm** has bacteria in the aneurysm wall. It is usually saccular and is characterized by staphylococci in 41% of cases and by salmonella in 18% of cases.
      (1) The **etiology** of the infected aneurysm varies among patients and includes **bacterial endocarditis** with septic emboli, **direct extension** from an adjacent infection, and **bacteremia** from a distant source with seeding of the mural thrombus and aneurysm wall.
      (2) The usual **clinical findings** are **fever** in one-third of patients, **leukocytosis** in two-thirds of patients, **lumbar vertebral erosion** seen on x-ray in slightly less than one-fifth of patients, and, frequently, **absence of calcification** in the aneurysm wall.
      (3) The **diagnosis** preoperatively may be made by femoral arterial blood culture or by evidence of septic emboli in a distal lower extremity.
      (4) **Management** is similar to that of infected aortic grafts (see section IX C 5).

3. **Laboratory studies**
   a. **Calcification** of part of the abdominal aorta demonstrated by posteroanterior or lateral **abdominal roentgenogram** is present in 60% of patients.
   b. **Ultrasonography** and **computed tomography (CT)** of the abdomen demonstrate the dilated aorta and are the most accurate tests for **aneurysm size**.
   c. **Abdominal angiography** defines the aortic anatomy but may not demonstrate the aneurysm because of a **laminated aortic mural thrombus** filling all but the central lumen of the vessel.

4. **Elective surgical repair.** At surgery, the aneurysm is removed and is replaced by a prosthetic vascular graft.
   a. **Preoperatively,** adequate hydration and optimized cardiac and pulmonary function must be maintained.
   b. **Intraoperative** procedures include:
      (1) Use of a **Swan-Ganz catheter** to monitor fluid status during aortic clamping
      (2) Use of mannitol to minimize the risk of renal failure during aortic clamping
      (3) Use of vasodilators to avoid hypertension and excessive afterload during aortic clamping
      (4) Minimizing the time of aortic clamping
      (5) Careful monitoring for the development of acidosis, hyperkalemia, and hypovolemia when unclamping the aorta
   c. **Postoperative results** of elective repair are excellent. The operative mortality rate is 1% to 5%, with death usually secondary to cardiac complications. Long-term survival is 50% at 5 years, and 10% at 8 years, with most deaths occurring as a result of continued atherosclerosis affecting other major arteries.

**B. Ruptured abdominal aortic aneurysm**

1. The **risk of rupture** is related to the **size** of the aneurysm.
   a. A small aneurysm (4.5 cm to 6 cm in diameter) ruptures in about 20% of patients over a

period of 3 or more years. An aneurysm that is greater than 6 cm in diameter ruptures in about 50% of patients within 2 years. The **mortality rates** of a ruptured aneurysm vary from 50% to 90%.

b. The average **growth rate** of an aneurysm is 0.4 cm in diameter per year. If there is growth greater than 0.5 cm over 3 months, as documented by ultrasonography, rupture is much more likely to occur.

2. The **clinical and laboratory findings** include:

a. Severe central abdominal or back pain, occasionally localizing to the lower abdomen, groin, or testes

b. A pulsatile abdominal mass in over 80% of cases

c. Shock in over 40% of cases (stable blood pressure indicates only that the patient is compensated at the moment and does not indicate the status of the situation)

3. The **surgical repair** of a ruptured aortic aneurysm must be performed as soon as the diagnosis is made. The **operative mortality rates** range between 50% and 67%. Death is usually secondary to massive intraoperative hemorrhage, cardiac complications, or postoperative acute renal failure.

C. **Surgical complications** are not infrequent in either elective or emergency aortic surgery. However, many of these complications can be minimized by careful management and, if recognized early, some can be successfully treated, preventing major morbidity and mortality.

1. **Postoperative renal failure** occurs in 21% of cases of ruptured aneurysms and in 2.5% of aneurysms treated by elective surgery, with mortality rates of up to 90%.

2. **Ischemic colitis** results from ligation of the inferior mesenteric artery in both elective surgery for aneurysms and in surgery for ruptured aneurysms. It occurs to some degree in 7% to 8% of cases, but it results in full-thickness injury with necrosis in 1% to 2% of cases. Ischemic colitis should be suspected in any case of aneurysm with postoperative diarrhea, especially when the stools are heme-positive, and can usually be diagnosed with sigmoidoscopy. The mortality rate can reach 50%.

3. **Acute leg ischemia** occurs postoperatively in up to 7% of cases. It should be suspected if pulses that were present previously are absent.

a. Acute leg ischemia is accompanied frequently by a **compartment syndrome of the calf**, which is characterized by:

(1) Moderate to severe calf pain, which is frequently masked because the postoperative patient is on narcotics

(2) Early loss of fine-touch sensation and two-point discrimination

(3) Tenseness and bulging of the calf muscle compartment

(4) Absence of pulses at and below the muscular compartments, which occurs late in the progression of the ischemia and may result in irreversibility of the damage

(5) Rising tissue pressure within the calf muscle compartment, which causes irreversible muscle necrosis

b. If it is recognized early before muscle necrosis occurs, acute leg ischemia is **treated** successfully by **fasciotomy**. If it occurs secondary to an acute graft or leg thrombosis, **exploration of the femoral vessels** is also indicated.

4. **Spinal cord ischemia** is a **rare complication** (0.25% of cases) and is most common in cases of ruptured aneurysm. It results from **injury to the artery of Adamkiewicz**, which supplies the spinal cord and arises from the left side of the abdominal aorta, usually at $T_8$ to $T_{11}$ but occasionally as low as $L_4$. Spinal cord ischemia produces a **classic anterior spinal artery syndrome**, which is characterized by the following:

a. Paraplegia

b. Rectal and urinary incontinence

c. Loss of pain and temperature sensation but preservation of vibratory and proprioceptive sensation (due to the independent anterior and posterior circulations of the middle and lower spinal cord)

5. **Aortic graft infection** can occur in and around the graft at points of anastomoses. It may **result from bacterial seeding** either at the time of graft implantation or occur at a later date as a result of bacteremia. The most common infecting organism is *Staphylococcus aureus*, but gram-negative bacteria are not infrequently found. The lumina of all currently used grafts are covered with a pseudointima rather than endothelium and have a decreased resistance to infection compared to the native vessel.

a. The **incidence of infection** is between 1% and 4% of all grafts used. It may be decreased significantly by the perioperative use of antibiotics. (There is a 6.8% rate of infection with use of a placebo versus a 0.9% rate with use of antibiotics.)

**b.** The **time of diagnosis** averages 15 months postoperatively but can range from 1 month to many years.

**c.** The **presenting symptoms** of a graft infection vary from fever to inguinal wound infection to proximal aortic pseudoaneurysm formation with disruption of the anastomosis. **Aortoenteric fistula** is occasionally the presenting symptom.

(1) The fistula is a communication between an infected false aneurysm at an anastomosis (usually the proximal one) and a hollow gastrointestinal viscus (usually the distal part of the duodenum).

(2) The diagnosis is likely in any patient with a vascular prosthesis and gastrointestinal bleeding. The fistula is frequently heralded by minor gastrointestinal bleeding several hours to weeks before exsanguination. The mortality rate of a major bleeding episode is 75%. The existence of a fistula may be proven prior to major bleeding by ultrasonography, CT, gallium scanning, or aortography. Upper gastrointestinal endoscopy frequently misses the lesion because of its distal location and minimal duodenal intraluminal involvement.

**d.** The **mortality rate** of graft infection is about 37% to 50%, and the associated leg amputation rate is 20% to 40%. However, the mortality rate may be lowered through:

(1) Early recognition

(2) Removal of all infected prostheses and closure of the aortic stump

(3) Simultaneous revascularization (usually in an extra-anatomic location) through uninfected tissue

(4) Maintenance of an adequate nutritional status

**6. Impotence.** The pudendal nerve branches that mediate erection and ejaculation in the male cross the aortic bifurcation. If this tissue is divided during surgery, impotence may result.

## X. OTHER ARTERIAL ANEURYSMS

**A. Iliac artery aneurysm** usually is an extension of an aortic aneurysm. It may be diagnosed as a pulsatile mass that is palpable on rectal examination; occasionally it ruptures into the sigmoid colon or another part of the gastrointestinal tract and presents as gastrointestinal bleeding. It rarely occurs as an isolated aneurysm.

**B.** An **aneurysm of the splenic artery** is the most common visceral artery aneurysm, representing 60% to 65% of all abdominal aneurysms excluding the abdominal aortic aneurysm. It occurs most commonly (80% of cases) in women, especially in those who have had multiple pregnancies. It is associated with fibromuscular dysplasia or with a local inflammatory process; however, it is not associated with atherosclerosis. Splenic artery aneurysm is **asymptomatic** in 80% of patients.

**1. Diagnosis** is frequently incidental and is made when a plain film of the abdomen shows a left upper quadrant ring-shaped calcification. The diagnosis is confirmed through **angiography**.

**2.** The **rate of rupture** is 9% long-term. It is lower when the aneurysm is not associated with a local inflammatory process. The **mortality rate** related to rupture is 25% in nonpregnant patients, but it rises to 68% in pregnant women.

**3. Indications for surgery** include:

**a.** The presence of symptoms

**b.** Rupture

**c.** An asymptomatic aneurysm in a woman of childbearing age

**d.** A noncalcified aneurysm (which is thought to have a relatively high risk of rupture)

**C. Peripheral arterial aneurysm**

**1. General aspects.** Most (70% to 80%) peripheral aneurysms are multiple, and the most commonly affected arteries are the femoral and popliteal. There is frequent association with an abdominal aortic aneurysm, and 40% of the associated abdominal aortic aneurysms are not palpable. The disease is secondary to atherosclerosis, but occasionally drug abuse is the etiology. Men are predominantly affected.

**2. Popliteal artery aneurysm** is associated with coexisting occlusive peripheral vascular disease in 46% of cases. It is also frequently associated with other arterial aneurysms—78% of those affected have a second aneurysm, and 64% have an abdominal aortic aneurysm.

**a. Clinical findings** include:

(1) An asymptomatic aneurysm in 43% of patients

(2) Pain and paresthesia (10% of patients have posterior tibial nerve compression)

(3) Acute ischemia following thrombosis in 25% of patients

**(4)** Claudication following thrombosis in 20% of patients
**(5)** Occasional foot embolization
**(6)** A palpable posterior knee mass in 60% of patients

  **b.** The aneurysm is **treated surgically** by ligation and total exclusion of the aneurysm. Bypass grafting is performed using either artificial material or an autogenous vein.

  **c.** Long-term follow-up shows associated limb loss in 77% of patients if the aneurysm is untreated.

  **d.** The **mortality rate** with elective repair is 1% to 5%; however, the rate among patients requiring emergency repair is much higher.

**XI. VASOSPASTIC DISEASES** chiefly affect the upper extremities and involve episodic vasoconstriction, usually of the small palmar and digital arteries and arterioles. The common symptoms include pain, numbness, coldness, and, occasionally, skin ulcers. Vasospasm may be associated with systemic diseases, such as collagen vascular disease, or with local processes, such as atherosclerosis, trauma, and embolism.

**A. Disorders**

  **1. Raynaud's phenomenon** is episodic vasoconstriction, most commonly of the fingers but occasionally of the toes, nose, or ears. It is usually initiated by cold exposure or emotional stimuli and occurs mainly in women.

    **a.** The affected digits may go through a classic sequence of color changes, including:
      **(1) Pallor** due to severe vasospasm in the dermal vessels
      **(2) Cyanosis** due to sluggish blood flow and resultant marked blood desaturation from high oxygen extraction
      **(3) Rubor** due to the reactive hyperemia

    **b.** There may be **symptoms** ranging from **numb discomfort,** which is usually localized in the fingers, to **ulceration** or **gangrene.**

    **c.** Raynaud's phenomenon is **frequently associated with a local or systemic disease.** It is the initial symptom of one-third of patients who eventually are found to be sclerodermatous. Eighty percent of patients with **scleroderma** eventually develop Raynaud's phenomenon.

    **d. Management** of Raynaud's phenomenon includes a number of different modalities.
      **(1)** Tobacco should be avoided because it stimulates vasoconstriction, as does contact with the cold.
      **(2)** Use of phenoxybenzamine for $\alpha$-blockade may be therapeutic. Guanethidine, calcium channel blockers such as nifedipine, or intra-arterial reserpine may also be useful.
      **(3)** Emotional problems should be controlled.
      **(4)** Although sympathectomy may help, only 20% to 30% of patients with scleroderma improve.

  **2. Raynaud's disease** is similar to Raynaud's phenomenon; however, the symptoms show no clear association with a systemic disease, and the disease rarely progresses to necrosis. Seventy percent of patients are young women, in whom the occurrence is usually bilateral and symmetrical. **Treatment** is similar to that of Raynaud's phenomenon, and nonoperative management controls 80% of patients. Sympathectomy is reserved for patients with recurrent ulceration, and 50% to 60% of these patients improve.

  **3. Acrocyanosis** is persistent diffuse cyanosis of the hands; although cold may be exacerbating, the symptoms are constant. Ninety percent of patients are women 15 to 35 years of age. There is no skin ulceration, and treatment is similar to that of Raynaud's disease.

  **4. Livedo reticularis** is a continuous vasospastic condition resulting in a mottled or reticulated red-blue discoloration of the extremity. It is more common in the lower extremities, but it also occurs in the arms. The symptoms may increase with cold exposure. It is common in both men and women and rarely results in ulceration. It may be associated with periarteritis nodosa, systemic lupus erythematosus, and cholesterol embolism. The treatment is similar to that of Raynaud's disease.

  **5. Cold hypersensitivity** may occur following frostbite. The affected area is bluish with a burning pain. Medical management and occasionally sympathectomy control the symptoms.

  **B. Associated conditions.** Patients with vasospastic disease should be examined for other disorders, including:

  **1.** Systemic diseases such as collagen vascular disease

  **2.** Cryoglobulinemia or cold hemagglutinins

  **3.** Myxedema

   **4.** Ergotism

   **5.** Thrombocytosis

   **6.** Macroglobulinemia

   **7.** Atherosclerosis involving the larger vessels of the vasospastic region

   **8.** Hazards (generally those related to occupation) in which repetitive vibrations occur

   **9.** Nerve compression syndromes such as the carpal tunnel syndrome

   **10.** Arterial compression syndromes such as the thoracic outlet syndrome

**C. Tests** may be performed to document vasospasm.

   **1. Doppler ultrasonography** examination measures arm and wrist blood pressure.

   **2. Digital plethysmography** determines diminished blood flow.

   **3. Digital temperature recovery time** may measure the digital response to cold temperature. This test is based on a linear correlation between digital temperature and blood flow. The usual rewarming response time after cold exposure is 10 to 15 minutes; in vasospastic disease it ranges from 20 to 25 minutes.

   **4.** The presence of a cervical or an axillary bruit suggests arterial occlusive disease. Arteriography may be necessary to eliminate this possibility totally. During arteriography, tolazoline may be injected intra-arterially and the dye injection repeated. Demonstration of increased blood flow and vasodilation is strong support for the presence of vasospastic disease.

# 14
# Venous Disease and Pulmonary Embolism

Bruce E. Jarrell

## I. VENOUS DISEASE OF THE LOWER EXTREMITIES

**A. Anatomy**. The venous system is divided into four general areas.

1. The **deep venous system** includes the popliteal, femoral, and iliac veins.

2. The **superficial venous system** is made up of subcutaneous veins and the greater and lesser saphenous veins.

3. The **communicating venous system** is a network of veins (**perforating veins**) connecting the superficial and deep systems, with valves that allow flow only from the superficial to the deep system.

4. **Venous valves** are delicate web-like structures in all lower extremity veins that prevent reverse blood flow in the veins. The valves prevent venous hypertension from occurring when the patient is in an erect position. In addition, they assure that blood is pumped from the superficial to the deep system and back towards the heart when the patient is walking.

**B. Etiology**. Venous disease may be caused by either congenital or acquired disorders.

1. **Valvular incompetence** is the congenital or acquired inability of the valves to prevent reflux and gravitational hypertension of the venous system.

2. **Venous thrombosis** is the formation of thrombi in the venous system. The thrombi usually originate at the calf vein level and progress cephalad. They occur as a result of elements of **Virchow's triad**:
   a. **Trauma** to the vein wall (e.g., caused by surgery or physical injury)
   b. **Decreased velocity** of venous blood flow (e.g., due to postoperative immobility or drugs such as estrogen which decrease venous tone)
   c. **Increased coagulability** or a change in the cellular components of blood (e.g., due to surgery or polycythemia vera).

**C. Syndromes**

1. **Superficial thrombophlebitis** is inflammation or thrombosis of the superficial veins.
   a. The **clinical findings** include:
      (1) A tender palpable cord along the course of a vein
      (2) A red, indurated vein
      (3) Varicose (dilated) veins
   b. A pulmonary embolus rarely is present with superficial thrombophlebitis.
   c. **Treatment** includes:
      (1) Bed rest and elevation of the extremity
      (2) Local application of heat for relief of pain
      (3) Support hose worn both during the period of inflammation and for prophylaxis
      (4) Heparin administration (not necessary if only superficial phlebitis is present)

2. **Varicose veins** are dilated networks in the subcutaneous venous system that result from valvular incompetence. Deep venous thrombosis is not often a factor in the development of varicose veins.
   a. **Clinical findings** include:
      (1) Local pain and edema
      (2) Local inflammation

      (3) Local hemorrhage into the surrounding tissue

      (4) Dilated superficial veins

      (5) A positive **Trendelenburg test**, which is a method of proving incompetent valves by occluding the superficial vein and demonstrating filling from the deep system

   **b. Nonoperative management** principally involves the use of support hose, which keep the superficial system collapsed and minimize the effect of venous hypertension on venous dilatation.

   **c. Surgery**

     (1) **Operative indications** include:

      (a) Previous or impending hemorrhage from an ulcerated varicosity (painless exsanguination from these lesions may occur, especially during sleep, if there is bleeding)

      (b) Cosmetic reasons

      (c) Primary incompetence of the greater saphenous vein at the saphenofemoral junction with the development of varicosities along the course of the vein

      (d) Severe recurrent pain over the varicosity

     (2) **Operative strategy** includes:

      (a) Preoperative evaluation of the patency of the deep venous system (ligation of the saphenous vein in the presence of a thrombosed deep system could result in massive venous obstruction and venous gangrene)

      (b) Ligation and removal of the greater saphenous vein when involved

      (c) Ligation of incompetent perforating veins between the superficial and deep systems

**3. Deep venous thrombosis** is thrombosis of part or all of the deep venous system of an extremity. It occurs in 250,000 individuals per year.

   **a. Origin of deep venous thrombosis**

     (1) The condition usually originates in the lower extremity venous system, starting at the calf vein level and progressing proximally to involve the popliteal, femoral, or iliac system. Some 80% to 90% of **pulmonary emboli** originate here.

     (2) Thrombi occasionally develop in other veins, including:

      (a) Pelvic veins, especially in conditions such as pregnancy, pelvic surgery, and gynecologic cancer

      (b) Renal veins, especially when intrinsic renal disease is present

      (c) Inferior vena cava

      (d) Ovarian veins

      (e) Upper extremity and neck veins, particularly in association with athletic activity and use of intravenous cannulas

      (f) The right atrium, in the presence of intrinsic cardiac disorders

   **b.** The **classic clinical syndrome** includes calf or thigh pain, edema, tenderness, and a positive **Homans' sign** (calf pain on dorsiflexion of the foot). However, these findings are nonspecific and are associated with venographically proven deep venous thrombosis in only 50% of patients; 50% of patients with proven venous thrombosis have no associated physical findings in the extremities.

     (1) The presenting symptom in many patients is pulmonary embolism.

     (2) It is very important to ascertain that arterial vascular insufficiency is not present when evaluating venous disease.

   **c.** The **diagnosis** of deep venous thrombosis is made by means of **laboratory tests**.

     (1) **Iodine 125 ($^{125}$I)-labeled fibrinogen scanning** is serial scanning of both lower extremities to detect the uptake of radioactive fibrinogen into a clot. (This method is best for diagnosis of thrombosis of the calf veins.)

     (2) **Doppler ultrasound examination** has an accuracy rate of 80% to 90% for the diagnosis of deep venous thrombosis occurring above the knee. The test determines:

      (a) Variation of flow in the femoral vein occurring with respiration, which indicates the patency of the venous system between the femoral vein and the heart

      (b) Increased femoral venous flow when the blood is rapidly squeezed from the calf veins, indicating patency between the calf veins and the femoral vein

      (c) The presence of normal venous velocity in the femoral, popliteal, and posterior tibial veins

      (d) The presence of a difference in ultrasound findings between the diseased and the normal extremity

     (3) **Impedance plethysmography** measures the variations in the volume of calf blood upon releasing a blood pressure cuff placed so as to cause temporary thigh venous occlusion. This test is accurate for about 90% of cases of deep venous thrombosis occurring above the knee.

     (4) A **venogram** of the ascending venous system is the **most accurate diagnostic method** for deep venous thrombosis. Radiopaque dye is injected into the pedal veins, and a tourniquet is loosely applied at the ankle to direct the flow of dye into the deep venous

system. Inflammation or thrombosis of the veins occurs in 3% of patients who undergo venography unless the vein is flushed with a heparin solution after infusion.

   **d. Treatment of deep venous thrombosis**

      **(1)** Continuous **heparin** infusion is given for 7 to 10 days followed by administration of warfarin or subcutaneous administration of heparin for 3 to 6 months.

      **(2)** Thrombolytic therapy with **streptokinase** or **urokinase** is used if extensive deep venous thrombosis results in impaired perfusion of the extremity.

      **(3) Inferior vena caval interruption** is used only if heparin is contraindicated or if a pulmonary embolus occurs in spite of adequate anticoagulation therapy. However, this treatment prevents only pulmonary embolism and does not treat the deep venous thrombosis.

   **e. Prevention** of deep venous thrombosis

      **(1) Simple preventive measures** include early mobilization after surgery, the use of support hose, which compress superficial veins in the legs and increase flow in the deep veins, and the correction of preoperative risk factors such as polycythemia vera.

      **(2) Intermittent calf compression** by means of a pneumatic cuff increases leg blood flow velocity and helps to prevent stasis.

      **(3)** Venoconstrictive substances such as **dihydroergotamine** may also increase deep venous blood velocity.

      **(4)** Pre- and postoperative administration of prophylactic **heparin** may be effective in preventing deep thrombosis. An intermittent subcutaneous dose of 3000 to 6000 units is given every 8 to 12 hours. At this dose heparin activates antithrombin III, inhibits platelet aggregation, and decreases thrombin availability. In several large series, heparin decreased postoperative phlebitis (there was a 25% incidence in controls versus a 7% incidence in patients treated with heparin) and fatal pulmonary embolism (there was a 7% mortality rate in controls versus a 1% mortality rate in those treated with heparin).

## D. Complications

   **1. Postphlebitic syndrome** occurs in 10% of patients with deep venous thrombosis and is due to permanent obstruction of the deep venous system. (Recanalization of veins occurs late if at all and usually results in incomplete recanalization and valvular incompetence.)

     **a. Physical findings**

      **(1) Chronic venous insufficiency** occurs due to the development of dilated and therefore incompetent venous collaterals around the venous obstruction.

      **(2)** There is minimal to severe **leg edema, pain,** and **nocturnal cramping**.

      **(3)** Venous **claudication** (pain, cramps, and a sensation of heaviness during exercise) occurs.

      **(4)** Abnormal **skin pigmentation** and **dermatitis** usually occur.

      **(5) Stasis ulceration** of the pretibial calf skin due to local superficial venous hypertension (especially during ambulation) causes edema, local thrombosis, and blood extravasation into the subcutaneous tissue followed by necrosis and ulceration. This may occur years after the episode of deep venous thrombosis, but it can result in severe progressive disability.

     **b. Treatment**

      **(1)** Support hose are worn chronically to prevent superficial venous hypertension.

      **(2)** Ligation of local perforating veins is used to lower the venous pressure at the ulcer if it will not heal.

      **(3)** An Unna boot, a medicated pressure bandage, is applied weekly or biweekly until the ulcer heals.

      **(4)** A change of life-style to avoid leg dependency may improve the ulceration.

   **2. Chronic recurrent superficial thrombophlebitis**, in addition to the treatment described in section I C 1 c, is treated with antibiotics because the syndrome often includes a streptococcal lymphangitis, which if untreated will result in additional occlusion of the lymphatics, resulting in more edema, dilatation, inflammation, and so forth, creating a vicious circle.

   **3. Phlegmasia alba dolens** is caused by acute occlusion of the iliac and femoral veins due to deep venous thrombosis. It results in a **pale cool leg** with a diminished arterial pulse due to spasm. Treatment is thrombolytic therapy followed by heparin administration to prevent progression to phlegmasia cerulea dolens.

   **4. Phlegmasia cerulea dolens** is secondary to acute and nearly total venous occlusion of the entire extremity outflow, including the iliac and femoral veins. It is more common in the left leg. Association with another disease is common: 30% of cases occur in postoperative and postpartum patients, and pelvic malignancy is not infrequent.

      **a. Physical findings** include **cyanosis** of the extremity, with massive edema, severe pain, and absent pulses, followed by venous gangrene. Shock may occur as a result of sequestration of a significant amount of blood in the leg.

      **b. Treatment** includes:

        **(1)** Thrombolytic therapy followed by heparin administration

        **(2)** Thrombectomy occasionally if nonoperative therapy is unsuccessful

        **(3)** Bed rest with leg elevation

**II. PULMONARY EMBOLISM** is a mechanical obstruction of the flow of blood in the pulmonary arterial system due to lodgment of a thromboembolus. The resultant effects include decreased cardiac output, pulmonary vasospasm and hypertension, impaired blood oxygenation, and bronchospasm.

**A.** Pulmonary embolism is one of the most common causes of **sudden death in hospitalized patients**.

    **1.** Normal individuals can tolerate a 60% to 70% occlusion of the pulmonary vasculature, but patients with preexisting cardiac or pulmonary disease tolerate much smaller occlusions poorly.

    **2.** Only 10% of all autopsy-proven cases of pulmonary embolism are diagnosed premortem.

    **3.** Frequently pulmonary embolism is sudden and seemingly unheralded, although it is often preceded by the development of small and clinically unrecognized emboli.

    **4.** Ninety percent of deaths occur within 2 hours after the onset of the initial symptoms. Therefore, if the patient lives longer than 2 hours, the chance of survival is very high.

**B.** Pulmonary embolism develops in 10% to 40% of patients with **deep venous thrombosis** (see section I C 3). However, approximately 33% of patients with pulmonary embolism have no antecedent symptoms of deep venous thrombosis.

    **1.** Thrombosis in the venous system is **caused by** situations described in **Virchow's triad** (see section I B 2).

    **2.** Pulmonary embolus formation can be **prevented** through the early diagnosis and prevention of deep venous thrombosis.

**C. Factors that increase the risk** of pulmonary embolism in patients undergoing surgery:

    **1. Pregnant women** and **women in the postpartum period** have an incidence of pulmonary embolism five times greater than the incidence in age-matched controls. Pulmonary embolus formation is a common cause of death after pregnancy.

    **2.** Patients undergoing **estrogen therapy** have an associated risk of pulmonary embolism four to seven times that of controls. The risk is dose-dependent and is eliminated within several weeks after cessation of therapy.

    **3. Heart disease** is associated with a three to four times higher risk of pulmonary embolus formation. This risk is directly related to the severity of the heart disease.

    **4. Obesity** is associated with one and one-half to two times greater risk of pulmonary embolism.

    **5.** Individuals with **carcinoma** have a risk of pulmonary embolism two to three times greater than that of controls.

    **6. Major trauma**, especially spinal cord injury and pelvic or femoral shaft fractures, carries an increased risk of pulmonary embolus formation.

    **7.** Inherent in an episode of pulmonary embolism is an increased risk of later pulmonary embolus formation, especially in cases of surgery.

    **8. Varicose veins** are associated with a two times greater risk of pulmonary embolism.

    **9.** As the **age** of hospitalized patients **increases**, the risk of developing pulmonary emboli increases.

**D. Symptoms** of pulmonary embolism range from none to severe cardiopulmonary dysfunction. In general, the more complicated the symptoms are, the more unreliable the clinical diagnosis is.

    **1.** The **classic signs—hemoptysis, pleural friction rub, cardiac gallop, cyanosis,** and **chest splitting**—are present in only 24% of patients.

    **2.** Common findings include **tachycardia** (in 60% of cases), **tachypnea** (in 85% of cases), and

**dyspnea** (in 85% of cases); however, these findings are nonspecific. **Bronchospasm** and **pleuritic chest pain** also occur frequently.

3. Many changes appear on an electrocardiogram, including **arrhythmias** and evidence of **right ventricular strain**.

4. The plain chest roentgenogram may be totally normal. On occasion, there is a **marked diminution of the pulmonary vasculature**, producing increased radiolucency in the area of the embolus (**Westermark's sign**). A **pleural effusion**, which is usually hemorrhagic, or **pulmonary infiltration** may be present, especially in cases of pulmonary infarction (this occurs in 10% to 25% of cases of pulmonary embolism).

5. **Arterial blood gases frequently show hypoxemia** with a low carbon dioxide partial pressure ($P_{CO_2}$) associated with hyperventilation. Unfortunately, although serial measurements may document a sudden drop in oxygen partial pressure ($P_{O_2}$), a single measurement is unlikely to be accurate in confirming the diagnosis of pulmonary embolism. In addition, a normal $P_{O_2}$ does not eliminate the possibility of pulmonary embolism.

E. **Diagnosis** of pulmonary embolism is based upon the results of several tests.

1. The **pulmonary arteriogram** is the best technique for diagnosing pulmonary embolism. This test is virtually 100% accurate, but it is invasive, as a radiopaque dye is injected directly into the pulmonary artery. The attendant risk of cardiac arrest is small in stable patients, but it can be unacceptably high in hypotensive, unstable patients.

2. **Pulmonary radioisotope scanning** is less invasive than arteriography.
   a. In a **perfusion lung scan**, a radioactive particle, small enough to block a small number of pulmonary capillaries temporarily, is injected. A camera records different views of the uptake in the vasculature.
      (1) A major difficulty with this test is that many acute and chronic pulmonary diseases can result in similar perfusion defects. It is critical to compare the chest roentgenogram with the scan to determine the presence of other abnormalities.
      (2) A normal scan is very reliable in determining the absence of a pulmonary embolus. The presence of segmental or large defects predicts pulmonary embolism in 71% of cases. A subsegmental or small perfusion defect is associated with pulmonary embolism in only 27% of cases.
   b. A **ventilation scan** performed simultaneously with the perfusion lung scan improves the accuracy of the latter. An inert radioactive gas such as xenon is inhaled, and the patency and ventilation of the bronchial tree are assessed.
   c. The situation in which a perfusion defect is present but the ventilation scan is normal is termed a **ventilation perfusion mismatch**. A defect in the same location revealed by both tests is termed a **matched ventilation perfusion defect**.
      (1) A segmental or large perfusion defect mismatched with a normal ventilation scan is associated with pulmonary embolism in 91% of cases.
      (2) Other results lower but do not eliminate the possibility of pulmonary embolism.
         (a) A subsegmental or small perfusion defect mismatched with a normal ventilation scan is associated with pulmonary embolism in only 27% of cases.
         (b) A perfusion defect matched with a ventilation defect is associated with pulmonary embolism in 23% of cases.
   d. When low-probability results are obtained, an additional test should be performed to increase the reliability of those results. A **pulmonary arteriogram** is most reliable. A **leg venogram** is also useful in this situation in documenting the presence of deep venous thrombosis and, therefore, the likelihood of pulmonary embolism.

F. **Treatment** of pulmonary embolism includes supportive measures to maintain circulatory function, and administration of heparin for systemic anticoagulation.

1. **Cardiovascular support** is frequently necessary in patients with significant pulmonary embolism and should be instituted immediately. The supportive measures include oxygen administration, assisted ventilation, correction of cardiac arrhythmias, and treatment of shock by means of adequate hydration and vasopressors. Introduction of a Swan-Ganz catheter is usually necessary for adequate cardiopulmonary monitoring.

2. **Long-term anticoagulation** may be maintained by either oral administration of warfarin or subcutaneous intermittent administration of heparin. The warfarin dosage should be carefully regulated to maintain the prothrombin time at 18 to 21 seconds. However, warfarin interacts with many other drugs, and its effectiveness can be severely altered by these drugs and by hepatic disease.

3. **Thrombolytic therapy** with streptokinase or urokinase may be used in cases of acute life-threatening pulmonary embolism when cardiopulmonary function is severely compromised as evidenced by shock, profound hypoxemia, or elevated pulmonary arterial pressure.
   a. Streptokinase is administered as an initial bolus of 250,000 units followed by a continuous drip of 100,000 units per hour for 1 to 3 days. The dosage is adjusted to maintain the thrombin time at two to five times the control time.
   b. Because thrombolytic therapy results in the lysis of preexisting thrombi, this therapy may be even more dangerous than heparin therapy, and it is **absolutely contraindicated** in patients with recent intracranial hemorrhage, recent surgery, or conditions associated with bleeding, such as peptic ulcer disease, large tumors, or urinary tract diseases.

4. **Heparin as an anticoagulant** should be administered in an initial bolus of 10,000 to 20,000 units to halt the thrombotic process and to stabilize platelets in the embolus to prevent the release of vasoactive and bronchoactive substances. Administration begins with a continuous intravenous drip of heparin at approximately 1000 units per hour; the dosage is then adjusted to maintain the partial thromboplastin time at one and one-half to two times the control time. Heparin is continued for a minimum of 7 days and is followed by long-term anticoagulation therapy for 3 to 6 months.

G. The **complications of anticoagulation therapy** are various.

1. **Major hemorrhage** requiring transfusions occurs in 1% to 2% of patients on anticoagulants; **minor bleeding episodes** are common in over 16%; and fatal hemorrhage occurs in 0.1% to 1%. The risk of hemorrhage is greater if heparin is administered intermittently or is given to elderly or severely hypertensive patients.

2. **Pulmonary embolism recurs** despite anticoagulation therapy in 1% to 8% of patients.

3. **Heparin-induced thrombocytopenia** occurs in up to 5% of patients on heparin and may be related to the development of heparin-induced antibodies directed towards platelets. All heparin infusions must be discontinued if thrombocytopenia occurs, because of the risk of either hemorrhage or heparin-induced necrosis, a form of tissue necrosis that is related to localized intravascular thrombosis.

# 15
# Vascular Grafts
Bruce E. Jarrell

**I. INTRODUCTION.** When arteries and veins develop occlusive lesions, the tissues they supply may need revascularization if an adequate collateral circulation fails to develop and supply enough nutrients to prevent ischemia. Revascularization is frequently performed by bypassing the occlusive lesion with either a biologic or a synthetic vascular prosthesis.

**II. BIOLOGIC PROSTHESES**

  **A.** An **autogenous vein graft** is a vein that is transplanted from one part of the body to another for use in bypassing an occlusion in either an artery or a vein. When use of it is practicable, this graft has a patency rate superior to that of a synthetic graft and is, therefore, the graft of choice.

   **1.** The **saphenous vein** produces a graft that is as long as the lower extremity. Graft diameter is in the range of 2 mm to 8 mm; therefore, the vein can be used only for vessels of that size.

   **2.** **Arterialization** of the saphenous vein results in thickening of the vein wall. Although the majority of these grafts do well, intimal and medial injury and proliferative fibroplasia do occur, resulting in long-term dysplasia with development of stenotic lesions.

   **3.** **Atherosclerotic lesions** appear in 2% to 15% of the arterialized vein with time.

   **4.** Long-term **treatment** with platelet-inhibiting drugs such as aspirin may increase long-term patency.

  **B.** An **autogenous arterial graft** is an artery that is removed from one area of a patient's vascular tree and inserted into another area (e.g., use of a hypogastric artery to bypass renal artery stenosis in a child).

  **C.** A **vascular allograft** is a vessel that is removed from one individual and implanted into another individual.

   **1.** An **arterial allograft** has a high rate of degeneration and is generally not used.

   **2.** A **venous allograft** may be used on occasion if it is modified to decrease the antigenicity by use of techniques such as proteolytic digestion or freezing. If it is unmodified, immune rejection of the graft occurs across both the histocompatibility barrier and the blood group ABO barrier.

   **3.** A **human umbilical vein allograft** is currently used for a bypass graft. The vessel is tanned with glutaraldehyde and is supported externally with a polyester mesh. The graft is rendered nonantigenic by this tanning procedure. Results have shown excellent long-term patency for both lower extremity revascularization and hemodialysis vascular access.

  **D.** A **vascular heterograft** is a vessel that is removed from an animal and rendered nonantigenic by the tanning process. The most commonly used graft is the dialdehyde starch-tanned bovine carotid artery. This graft has been used successfully for both vascular reconstruction and hemodialysis vascular access, but it has a tendency to develop aneurysms (in 3% to 6% of cases) in certain applications.

**III. SYNTHETIC VASCULAR PROSTHESES**

  **A. Types**

   **1. Dacron grafts** are very successful when used for large-vessel replacements, such as in the aorta or iliac vessels. The long-term patency for grafts in the extremities is much less acceptable, however. Dacron may be knitted or woven into a tubular graft.

    **a.** A **woven graft** has a tight structure of low porosity, which allows less ingrowth of tissue into the interstices.

    **b.** A **knitted graft** has a looser structure with resultant higher porosity. The tissue ingrowth into the graft is greater than in a woven graft, allowing a more stable pseudointima to form. The graft requires preclotting with nonheparinized blood to lessen blood loss at the time of implantation.

    **c.** A **velour graft** is a Dacron graft that, in addition to having the characteristics of a knitted Dacron graft, has a loop of yarn occluding some of the pores and projecting onto the surface. This presumably allows the pseudointima to anchor more securely, preventing sloughing of this tissue into the graft lumen.

  **2.** An **expanded polytetrafluoroethylene (PTFE) graft** is a tubular graft extruded from PTFE resin.

    **a.** The porosity is low due to a strongly electronegative charge on the polymer surface caused by the fluoride atoms. Protein aggregates from blood adhere to the surface, and a thin, poorly adherent pseudointima forms on the luminal surface.

    **b.** An outer reinforcing layer is present on some grafts. In addition to increasing the bursting strength of the graft, this layer also prevents the ingrowth of tissue into the graft structure.

    **c.** The PTFE graft gives results superior to those of the Dacron graft when it is used in the lower extremity. The PTFE graft is the second choice to the autogenous saphenous vein graft when use of the vein is not practicable.

**B. Potential problems**

  **1.** All of the currently used synthetic grafts fail to develop a true endothelialized blood lumen.

    **a.** Instead, a **pseudointima** develops, consisting of leukocyte, platelet, and red blood cell debris combined with fibrin and other proteins. This surface is both intrinsically thrombogenic and susceptible to infection from blood-borne organisms.

    **b.** Endothelium covers only 1 cm to 2 cm of graft adjacent to each anastomotic site. This region is called the **pannus.**

  **2.** Whenever a **bacteremia** is anticipated, the patient should be given **prophylactic antibiotics** to prevent seeding of the graft with organisms.

# 16

# Renal Transplantation

Bruce E. Jarrell

## I. INTRODUCTION

**A.** Renal transplantation is a procedure involving the removal of a single kidney from one individual and placing it in another who has markedly impaired renal function. When the operation is successfully performed, most patients return to normal lives, with the ability to be fully employed, physically active, and unencumbered by dialysis. When successful, it is the best treatment for chronic renal failure, and it significantly debilitates patients only in situations of recurrent rejections if excessive steroid therapy is employed.

**B. Classification** of renal and other organ transplants depends on the relationship between the donor and the recipient.

   **1.** An **autograft** is tissue transferred from one area of the body to another in the same individual (e.g., a skin graft).

   **2.** An **isograft** is tissue transferred between genetically identical individuals (e.g., monozygotic twins).

   **3.** An **allograft (homograft)** is tissue transferred between genetically dissimilar individuals of the same species (e.g., cadaver renal transplants).

   **4.** A **xenograft (heterograft)** is tissue transplanted between species (e.g., porcine skin temporarily grafted on human burn victims).

**C. Selection of donors**

   **1. Living related donors** represent approximately one-third of all kidney donors.
      **a.** The genotypes of the related donor and recipient are more compatible (see section I D) than those of an unrelated donor and recipient. There are three potential histocompatibility matches.
         **(1)** A **perfect histocompatibility (two-haplotype) match** is one in which all antigens are matched. Siblings have a 25% chance of having identical antigens.
         **(2)** A **half histocompatibility (one-haplotype) match** is one in which 50% of the antigens are matched. Two siblings have a 50% chance of this occurring; however, this match occurs in essentially all parent/child relationships.
         **(3)** No **histocompatibility match** is present in 25% of siblings. With such a complete mismatch of antigens, the would-be donor is not used.
      **b.** The living related donor must have a normal history and physical examination. The donor must be free of chronic and acute illnesses, especially infections, malignancies, diabetes mellitus, hypertension, psychiatric disorders, and significant cardiac, renal, pulmonary, and hepatic disease. Renal function must be normal.
      **c.** The donor must have an in-hospital evaluation, including intravenous pyelography (IVP) and renal arteriography to demonstrate normal renal and urologic anatomy.
      **d.** The mortality rate among donors is extremely low (0.05%) and is principally a result of general anesthesia problems or postoperative pulmonary embolism.
      **e.** The donor has rapid compensatory hypertrophy of the remaining kidney. Creatinine clearance equals 70% to 80% of the predonation level within 1 year after the donation.

   **2. Cadaver donors** are the source of kidneys for approximately two-thirds of all transplant recipients.
      **a.** The kidneys are from young, previously healthy individuals who sustained irreversible brain injury. The donors must have no evidence of infection, extracranial malignancy,

previous renal disease, hypertension, or diabetes. In addition, renal function must have been normal, with minimal urinary abnormalities, if any.
   **b.** Cadaver donors must fulfill the criteria of brain death as determined clinically by:
   **(1)** Deep coma with no response to painful stimuli
   **(2)** Absence of spontaneous respiration in the presence of a high arterial carbon dioxide tension ($PaCO_2$)
   **(3)** Absence of movement
   **(4)** Absence of all brain stem and higher reflexes
   **(5)** Absence of hypothermia and absence of depressant drugs such as barbiturates in the blood
   **(6)** No change of these findings over a 24-hour period
   **(7)** Optionally, isoelectric electroencephalogram, absence of intracranial blood flow, or visual evidence of gross cerebral tissue destruction
   **c.** The kidneys are surgically removed from heart-beating, brain-dead cadavers and are rapidly flushed and chilled to 4° C. They are preserved for up to 48 hours by cold storage in ice with no perfusion using a concentrated potassium solution (i.e., 115 mEq/L) or with pulsatile perfusion using plasma-type solutions.

   **3. Living unrelated donors** are currently not used in the United States. There is no immunologic advantage to kidneys from these donors over those from cadavers, and there remains the significant risk of the perioperative period.

**D.** For any type of tissue transplant, the **immunologic compatibility of the recipient and the donor** determines the outcome of the transplantation.

   **1. ABO blood group compatibility** must be present. As in blood transfusions, an individual with an O blood type is a universal donor, whereas an individual with an AB blood type may only donate to an AB recipient.

   **2. Crossmatch compatibility** must be present. The recipient's blood is examined for the presence of cytotoxic antibodies specifically directed against antigens on the donor's T lymphocytes. If these antibodies are found, the donor is unacceptable because the recipient's antibodies would immediately attack the new kidney and rapidly destroy it.

   **3. Human leukocyte antigens (HLAs).** Histocompatibility antigen typing is performed. Human beings have HLA-A, -B, -C, and -D loci on the immune regulatory gene area of chromosome 6, which is primarily responsible for humoral and cellular immune responses. Attempts to match these antigens between the donor and recipient are made in order to minimize the genetic dissimilarity between the two.
   **a. HLA-A and -B loci.** Each locus contains subloci characterized by 30 to 40 antigenic specificities. These specificities are characterized by specific antisera directed against T-lymphocyte surface antigens. The microcytotoxicity assay uses complement and requires about 6 hours to perform.
   **(1)** A match between HLA-A and -B indicates an excellent possibility of graft survival when the donor is a living relative.
   **(a)** There is a 90% graft survival rate at 2 years with a perfect HLA-A and -B match.
   **(b)** There is a 65% to 85% graft survival rate at 2 years with a 50% HLA-A and -B match.
   **(c)** There is a 45% to 65% graft survival rate at 2 years with a complete HLA-A and -B mismatch.
   **(2)** The transplantation results are variable when the HLA-A and -B loci of recipients and cadaver donors are matched.
   **(a)** European studies of HLA-A and -B matches show a 70% incidence of functioning grafts at 2 years with a perfect match compared to a 45% incidence at 2 years with HLA-A and -B incompatibility.
   **(b)** American results show a statistical difference between the two groups but to a very small degree.
   **b.** The **HLA-C locus** is not known to affect the outcome of transplantation.
   **c.** The **HLA-D locus** is the locus that determines cellular activity in a mixed lymphocyte reaction.
   **(1)** Blast cells form in a culture of lymphocytes from both donor and recipient, and the degree of histocompatibility between the two is indicated by the number of blast cells.
   **(2)** The mixed lymphocyte reaction correlates in vitro to the host lymphocytic immune reaction towards the donor cellular antigens.
   **(3)** A match of HLA-D loci indicates an excellent possibility of graft survival when the donor is a living relative.
   **(4)** A match of HLA-D loci is untestable with cadaver donors because of the prolonged (5- to 7-day) incubation time required to produce results.

     **d.** The **$D_R$ (D-related) locus** is linked very closely to the HLA-D locus. The $D_R$ antigen is detected serologically in a manner similar to the HLA-A and -B locus microcytotoxicity test and in a similar time frame; however, B lymphocytes rather than T lymphocytes are the target cells because T lymphocytes do not have D-locus antigens upon their surface. A $D_R$-locus perfect match generally results in excellent graft survival (there is an 80% graft survival rate at 2 years compared to a 40% to 60% survival rate when the loci are completely mismatched).

  **4. Pretransplantation transfusion**
     **a. Random third-party-donor blood transfusions,** when given to transplant candidates prior to transplantation, raise the graft survival rate significantly.
       **(1)** There is a correlation between the number of transfusions given and graft survival.
          **(a)** There is a 45% graft survival rate at 1 year for 0 transfusions.
          **(b)** There is a 50% graft survival rate at 1 year for 1 transfusion.
          **(c)** There is a graft survival rate of up to 75% at 1 year for more than 20 transfusions.
       **(2)** There is an immune response in the form of humoral sensitization after transfusion in approximately 10% of patients. These individuals may create antibodies against the antigens of most of the population, which occasionally prevents transplantation.
       **(3)** The risk of transmitting hepatitis or other viral illnesses is present as it is with any transfusion.
       **(4)** The mechanism of graft tolerance after transfusion is unknown. It includes, at least partly, the induction of an active immune blocking phenomenon.
     **b. Donor-specific blood transfusions** are used when a recipient and a living related donor have a half histocompatibility (one-haplotype) match for HLA-A, -B, -C, and -$D_R$ loci in the presence of a reactive mixed lymphocyte reaction. The recipient is transfused with blood from the potential kidney donor on three separate occasions.
       **(1)** Donor-specific transfusions sensitize the recipient to that specific donor in 20% to 30% of cases; thus that individual must be eliminated as a donor.
       **(2)** The transplantation success rate in this group is over 90% at 2 years in comparison to a 65% success rate at 2 years for nontransfused donor/recipient pairs.

  **5. Pretransplantation splenectomy** is performed in transplantation candidates with hypersplenism and pancytopenia. Splenectomy reduces the incidence of leukopenia, so that larger amounts of immunosuppressive drugs may be given. In some centers, pretransplantation splenectomy is associated with an increased rate of graft survival. Although the procedure may not increase the short-term risk of infection, the long-term risk is not known.

## II. SELECTION OF RECIPIENTS AND PRETRANSPLANT MANAGEMENT

  **A.** End-stage renal disease patients on maintenance dialysis are **good candidates for transplantation** when they are between 5 and 60 years of age (although 45- to 60-year-old individuals are considered to be a high-risk group because they are susceptible to infectious complications).

  **B. Acute or chronic infections,** whether bacterial, viral, or fungal, should be absent.

    **1.** A positive purified protein derivative (PPD) tuberculin test is not necessarily a contraindication to transplantation; if it is positive, isoniazid (INH) should be given for at least the first post-transplantation year. If evidence of active turberculosis is present, the transplant should be postponed until no active disease is present.

    **2.** Urine cultures should be negative; if they are positive, a complete urologic examination should be performed. A nephrectomy is performed if the source of infection is renal.

  **C. A normal urinary system is ideal,** and any **urologic problems** should be resolved.

    **1.** Vesicoureteral reflux should be absent; if it is present, a nephrectomy is indicated.

    **2.** Vesical outlet obstruction should be relieved prior to transplantation.

    **3.** A neurogenic bladder may be used as the site for implantation; an ileal loop is rarely necessary.

  **D. The recipient's own kidneys are occasionally removed.** In addition to infection or reflux, indications for removal include the presence of:

    **1.** Severe unmanageable hypertension, especially with elevated renin levels

    **2.** Polycystic kidneys if recurrent cyst hemorrhage or infection occurs. (Polycystic kidneys frequently are associated with a high hematocrit and residual urine output and are best preserved if possible.)

**E.** Autoimmune diseases characterized by glomerular basement membrane antibodies, such as Wegener's granulomatosis, Goodpasture's syndrome, and certain other types of glomerulonephritis (see section VI C 2), should be quiescent prior to transplantation.

**F.** **Secondary hyperparathyroidism** and **severe bone disease** do not constitute a contraindication to transplantation and usually improve postoperatively.

**G.** **Significant gastroenterologic disease** should be identified and resolved prior to transplantation.

　　**1.** Active hepatitis should not be present.

　　**2.** Chronic hepatitis should show minimal activity on biopsy (a positive hepatitis surface antigen is not a contraindication in many centers).

　　**3.** Peptic ulcer disease should be screened for in the older age group; if present, proof of healing should be obtained. Some centers recommend prophylactic acid-reducing operations because the mortality rate from bleeding or perforated ulcer disease post-transplantation varies from 25% to 85%.

　　**4.** Diverticulosis of the colon should also be screened for in the older age group and in patients with polycystic kidneys. If a patient has extensive diverticula or a previous episode of diverticulitis or diverticular bleeding, a prophylactic colectomy should be considered because of the high mortality rate of these colon complications post-transplantation.

**H.** The presence of **malignant disease** either currently or in the recent past is a contraindication to immunosuppression and therefore to transplantation because of the risk of recurrence.

　　**1.** Low-grade malignancies, especially those of the skin and occurring in the distant past, may be an acceptable risk.

　　**2.** A history of Wilms' tumor in infancy may allow transplantation at an older age. This is because the tumor has a very predictable doubling time, which is defined by the age at tumor presentation plus 9 months. If that amount of time has elapsed since surgical removal of the tumor and there is no evidence of recurrence, then it is unlikely to recur.

**I.** **Metabolic diseases** such as oxalosis frequently recur rapidly in transplanted kidneys, and good results of the transplantation may be limited.

## III. RENAL TRANSPLANTATION OPERATION

**A.** **The surgical procedure** in transplantation involves placing the kidney in either iliac fossa retroperitoneally. The vessels are anastomosed to the iliac artery and vein in adults and occasionally to the aorta and inferior vena cava in small children. The ureter is directly implanted into the bladder, usually through use of antireflux anastomosis (Fig. 16-1).

**B.** **Surgical complications** are not uncommon and are usually treatable if they are recognized at an early stage.

　　**1.** **Vascular complications** include renal artery stenosis or thrombosis and renal vein thrombosis. Patients may present with sudden anuria or severe hypertension postoperatively. Rapid diagnosis may be made by means of a renal flow radioisotope scan, arteriography, or reexploration.

　　**2.** **Lymphatic complications** appear as an acute perinephric lymph collection or lymphocele developing as a result of inadequately ligated lymphatics in the operative field. The lymphocele may present as a mass, as wound drainage, or as acute anuria. The best means of confirming the diagnosis is through ultrasound examination. The lymphocele is drained either by surgical exposure or percutaneous needle aspiration.

　　**3.** **Urologic complications** in the transplanted patient include the formation of bladder fistulas as a result of technical problems and ureteric obstruction or infarction due to the interruption of ureteric blood supply, which may occur during donor nephrectomy. Arteries leading to the lower pole of the kidney usually vascularize the upper ureter and must be preserved and revascularized. The diagnosis of urologic complications can be confirmed by means of radioisotope scanning, ultrasound examination, or IVP. Treatment varies according to each diagnosis.

## IV. POSTOPERATIVE MANAGEMENT

**A.** **Immunosuppression** has traditionally included the long-term prophylactic use of azathioprine

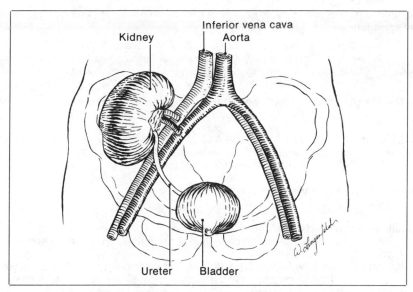

**Figure 16-1.** Placement of the renal transplant.

and prednisone. Antilymphocyte globulin is used short-term for episodes of rejection. However, a new drug, cyclosporine (cyclosporin A), may replace all of these.

1. **Azathioprine** inhibits lymphoid differentiation, especially the differentiation of T lymphocytes. In general, however, it operates as a nonspecific immunosuppressant. It is converted to 6-mercaptopurine by the liver.
   a. Administration of azathioprine is begun prior to the transplant operation at a dose of 1 to 2 mg/kg of body weight and is continued as long as the graft is functional. Up to a 30% dose reduction is necessary if renal function diminishes.
   b. The therapy is monitored by daily white blood cell and platelet counts.
   c. Mild to moderate hepatotoxicity develops in some patients.
   d. If azathioprine is withdrawn, acute graft rejection frequently results, even in cases of long-term graft tolerance.

2. **Prednisone** is a steroid preparation used in combination with azathioprine. It has a nonspecific immunosuppressive action on both cell-mediated and humoral immunity.
   a. High doses (½ to 2 mg/kg body weight per day) are administered early postoperatively, and doses are serially reduced with time.
   b. Prednisone therapy is associated with very significant complications, especially infections and peptic ulcer disease. The likelihood of these complications occurring is partially dose-related.

3. **Antilymphocyte globulin (ALG)** is a serum prepared by immunizing nonhuman animals with human lymphatic cells, allowing an immune response to generate antihuman lymphocyte antibodies, which are then collected and purified for human use. It is a specific immunosuppressive agent directed against T lymphocytes and may be monitored by the absolute T-lymphocyte count in the peripheral blood.
   a. Some centers use ALG prophylactically for 14 days postoperatively, and it is used successfully in many centers for acute rejection episodes.
   b. Therapy is associated with an increase in viral infections, especially from cytomegalovirus (CMV). In addition, there is a low risk of anaphylaxis from the foreign serum.

4. **Cyclophosphamide** blocks the development of immunoblasts and the differentiation of T and B lymphocytes. It is generally used when hepatotoxicity requires the discontinuance of azathioprine.

5. **Cyclosporine (cyclosporin A)** is a new immunosuppressive drug that inhibits antigen recognition and processing by helper T lymphocytes. Early studies have shown excellent graft survival rates with its use. However, it can cause significant renal toxicity and hepatotoxicity, which occasionally require discontinuance of the drug. Cyclosporine does not seem to be associated with as high an increase in opportunistic infections as is azathioprine. Lymphomas may develop in less than 1% of patients.

B. **Postoperative renal function** usually returns rapidly to normal in transplanted kidneys from living related donors and in those from most cadavers, with a brisk diuresis and a rapid drop in serum creatinine.

1. Cadaver donor transplants are occasionally associated with a 1- to 10-day episode of acute tubular necrosis. This is usually a temporary condition resulting from stress during obtaining or preserving the donor kidney and is followed by a diuresis and normal renal function with no ultimate effect on graft success.

2. The transplanted kidney undergoes compensatory hypertrophy with a final creatinine clearance rate of 70% to 80% of normal if rejection does not intervene.

V. **RESULTS OF RENAL TRANSPLANTATION** vary considerably among centers but are still strongly **dependent upon the type of histocompatibility match.** Second and third transplants may be performed safely; the results are generally acceptable and parallel those of earlier transplants.

A. **Living related donor transplants** are the most successful.

1. **Patient survival rates** are 90% to 95% at 5 years.

2. **Kidney survival rates** are also excellent.
   a. Perfect matches (two-haplotype matches) result in a 2-year kidney survival rate of 85% to 95%.
   b. Half matches (one-haplotype) with low donor/recipient mixed lymphocyte cultures (i.e., with good HLA-D matches) have a kidney survival rate of 70% to 85% at 2 years.
   c. Half matches with reactive donor/recipient mixed lymphocyte cultures result in a kidney survival rate of 50% to 70% at 2 years.
   d. Half matches with donor-specific transfusions have a kidney survival rate of 90% at 2 years.

B. **Cadaver donor transplants** show much more variable results; however, the results have improved generally because of blood transfusions, better tissue matching, and administration of cyclosporine.

1. **Patient survival rates** over 5 years are 75% to 85%.

2. **Kidney survival rates** vary.
   a. Four-antigen HLA-A and -B matches result in a 65% 2-year kidney survival rate. With less than a four-antigen match, there is a 40% to 60% 2-year survival rate.
   b. Two HLA-$D_R$ matches show a 65% to 80% 2-year survival rate. However, there is only a 40% to 60% 2-year survival rate with less than two $D_R$ antigens matched.
   c. Not transfusing the recipient before transplantation results in a 25% to 45% 2-year kidney survival rate. On the other hand, giving pretransplantation transfusions results in a 50% to 75% 2-year survival rate.
   d. Early studies of cyclosporine show a 70% to 90% 2-year kidney survival rate with its use.

VI. **COMPLICATIONS**

A. **Renal transplant rejection** is an episode of increased immune activity directed towards destruction of the graft.

1. The **incidence of rejection episodes** varies with the type of donor used.
   a. Perfect-match living related donor transplant recipients experience an episode of rejection in 10% to 20% of cases.
   b. Recipients of transplants from cadavers or from non–perfect-match living related donors experience an episode of rejection in 50% to 90% of cases.

2. There are **four types of rejection**, classified by the time of occurrence in relation to the operation and the type of immune response involved.
   a. **Hyperacute rejection** is associated with preformed antibody and complement deposition on vascular endothelium followed by activation of the coagulation system. It results in a flaccid, cyanotic, anuric, and eventually thrombosed kidney while the patient is still in the operating room. Histologic examination shows polymorphonuclear leukocytes in peritubular and glomerular capillaries, and endothelial necrosis. Hyperacute rejection is treated by nephrectomy, usually at the time of the transplant operation.
   b. **Accelerated acute rejection** is a rapidly evolving rejection that occurs within the first week of transplantation and is associated with sudden anuria. It is probably a second-set, or anamnestic, immune response, mediated by both humoral and cellular elements. Extensive arteriolar necrosis and vasculitis are revealed by histologic examination. Accelerated rejection is treated by high doses of prednisone but with a poor success rate for both immediate and long-term graft survival.
   c. **Acute rejection** usually occurs within the first 3 months post-transplantation and is the

most common type of rejection. It is characterized by a rising serum creatinine level, increasing proteinuria, oliguria, weight gain, fever, and graft tenderness developing over several days. It is usually diagnosed on clinical grounds or by renal biopsy. There is T-lymphocyte–mediated infiltration of vascular and interstitial renal elements. Traditionally, acute rejection has been treated with high doses of methylprednisolone (i.e., 1 g to 6 g over 1 to 2 weeks); however, recently it has been treated by 10 to 21 doses daily of ALG with excellent resolution of the episode in many cases.

    **d. Chronic rejection** is associated with a slow decline in renal function over months or years, usually including a rising serum creatinine level, increasing proteinuria, hypertension, and edema. There is vascular intimal thickening and tubular atrophy. Chronic rejection results from both humoral and cellular destructive events. Although there is no known effective treatment, the process may be slowed by dietary protein restriction.

**B. Infections** are the most dangerous sequelae of immunosuppression and transplantation.

    **1.** The chance of infection is increased by the use of high doses of steroids to treat rejection episodes. Patients over 45 years of age, diabetics, and patients with advanced disease are most susceptible.

    **2.** The most common infection to occur within the first several months post-transplantation is viral, especially CMV. It is not unusual for opportunistic organisms such as *Aspergillus, Cryptococcus*, and *Listeria monocytogenes* to infect the patients.

    **3.** Administration of immunosuppressive drugs should be stopped or markedly reduced in order to allow the immune system to eliminate the organism.

    **4.** There should be aggressive diagnosis so that rapid and appropriate antibiotic treatment can be instituted; when that is accomplished, the patient has an excellent chance of recovery.

**C. Glomerulonephritis** in the transplanted kidney may arise as the recurrence of original disease or de novo.

    **1.** Glomerulonephritis is diagnosed on renal biopsy. Unfortunately, most of these diseases have no specific treatment other than administration of the immunosuppressive drugs used for the transplant or a return to dialysis.

    **2.** Recurrent glomerulonephritis is associated with several types of original disease, including:

        **a. Antiglomerular basement membrane disease** (e.g., Goodpasture's syndrome, Wegener's granulomatosis)

        **b. Acute immune complex disease**

        **c. Membranous glomerulonephritis**

        **d. Focal glomerulosclerosis**

        **e. Membranoproliferative glomerulonephritis**

**D. Long-term complications**

    **1. Cardiovascular disease** continues or worsens post-transplantation in many patients. Any patient with chronic renal failure has a markedly increased risk of death from cardiovascular disease whether he or she is treated by dialysis or transplantation.

        **a. Hypertension** occurs in up to 83% of patients post-transplantion.

        **b. Hyperlipidemia** occurs in up to 78% of patients.

        **c. Coronary heart disease** varies widely in incidence among centers, ranging from 2 times to 25 times the normal risk of death. (Clearly, atherosclerosis continues to progress after the transplantation.)

        **d. Cerebrovascular disease** is reported to be as much as 300 times more common than in control populations.

    **2.** The incidence of **malignant disease** is increased in all transplant patients, warranting careful routine long-term screening.

        **a.** When kidney donors have occult or obvious malignancies at the time of kidney removal, about one-third of recipients develop the same cancer.

        **b.** Primary cancers develop in 5.6% of all transplant recipients. This incidence is 100 times greater than that in age-matched controls. It increases with the increasing duration of immunosuppression.

           **(1)** The etiology is related at least in part to an altered immune status with failure of immune tumor surveillance.

           **(2)** Types of malignancy

               **(a)** Skin cancers represent approximately 40% of all primary post-transplant cancers; in areas in which sunlight exposure is high, the frequency approaches 70%.

               **(b)** Lymphomas represent 25% of all primary post-transplant cancers. This frequency is

350 times the incidence in controls. Most common are reticulum cell sarcomas, frequently involving the central nervous system.

   (c) Other cancers also occur more commonly in transplant patients than in the general population.

3. **Aseptic necrosis of the hip or knee** occurs in up to 10% of transplant patients long-term, probably as a result of steroid therapy. Frequently a prosthetic hip replacement is required for relief of pain. The incidence may be minimized by reducing the use of prednisone therapy.

4. **Obesity and cushingoid features** are common in these patients but frequently become less prominent as the daily dose of prednisone is lowered.

5. **Cataracts** occur more commonly in renal transplant recipients than in age-matched controls.

# 17
# The Heart

R. Anthony Carabasi, III
Scott M. Goldman
Charles J. Lamb

## I. ACQUIRED HEART DISEASE

### A. General considerations

1. **Epidemiology**
   a. Approximately 3 million myocardial infarctions are recorded annually in the United States, with an accompanying mortality rate of 10% to 15%.
   b. Acquired valvular disease is less important than coronary artery disease but still accounts for significant morbidity and mortality.

2. The following are important **signs and symptoms** of acquired heart disease.
   a. **Dyspnea** is usually the result of increased left atrial pressure, which causes pulmonary congestion.
   b. **Peripheral edema** may be the result of significant right-sided congestive heart failure.
   c. **Chest pain** may be caused by angina pectoris, myocardial infarction, pericarditis, aortic dissection, pulmonary infarction, or aortic stenosis.
   d. **Palpitations** may indicate a serious cardiac arrhythmia.
   e. **Hemoptysis** may be associated with mitral stenosis or pulmonary infarction.
   f. **Syncope** may result from mitral stenosis, aortic stenosis, or heart block.
   g. **Fatigue** is the result of decreased cardiac output.

3. **Physical examination** should include:
   a. Measurement of the **blood pressure**
   b. Examination of the **peripheral pulses**
      (1) Pulsus alternans is a sign of left ventricular failure.
      (2) Pulsus parvus et tardus may be seen with aortic stenosis.
      (3) A wide pulse pressure with a "water-hammer pulse" is seen with increased cardiac output or decreased peripheral vascular resistance, as in aortic insufficiency or patent ductus arteriosus.
   c. Examination of the **neck veins**. (Central venous pressure may be indirectly inferred from the height of the internal jugular vein filling.)
   d. Inspection and palpation of the **precordium**
      (1) Normally the apical impulse is appreciated at the midclavicular line, fifth intercostal space. In left ventricular hypertrophy, the apical impulse is increased and displaced laterally.
      (2) With right ventricular hypertrophy, a parasternal heave is appreciated.
      (3) Thrills from valvular disease may be felt.
   e. **Auscultation**, including detection of gallops and murmurs

4. **Preoperative care**
   a. **Laboratory studies** should include the following: complete blood count (CBC), sequential multiple analyzer series 6 (SMA-6), prothrombin time (PT), partial thromboplastin time (PTT), platelet count, serum creatinine, and serum bilirubin.
   b. A **chest x-ray** and **electrocardiogram** are done routinely.
   c. **Cardiac catheterization** is the definitive preoperative study.
   d. **Pulmonary function studies** are important in patients with known pulmonary disease.
   e. **Psychological preparation** of the patient is an important aspect and should include familiarizing the patient with the postoperative procedures in the intensive care unit.
   f. **Perioperative antibiotics** play an important role in the prevention of sepsis.

5. **Postoperative care** is critical in the success of any cardiac operation.

    **a.** An **intensive care unit** especially equipped for this purpose is essential and must be staffed by nursing personnel familiar with the management of cardiac surgery patients.

    **b.** **Drugs** used in the support of the postoperative patient may include drugs administered to improve myocardial contractility, to maintain urine output, or to abolish or control cardiac arrhythmias. In addition, patients may require blood products to increase the hematocrit or to help correct coagulopathies.

**6. Cardiac arrest**

    **a.** Cardiac arrest may be **caused** by any of the following:

      **(1)** Anoxia

      **(2)** Coronary thrombosis

      **(3)** Electrolyte disturbances

      **(4)** Myocardial depressants: anesthetic agents, antiarrhythmic drugs, or digitalis preparations

      **(5)** Conduction disturbances

      **(6)** Vagotonic maneuvers

    **b.** Rapid **evaluation** and **immediate cardiopulmonary resuscitation** are critical, as brain injury will result after 3 to 4 minutes of diminished perfusion.

    **c.** **Treatment** should include:

      **(1)** Establishing an **airway** and giving **ventilatory support**. These are best accomplished by endotracheal intubation and controlled ventilation.

      **(2)** **Cardiac massage.** Closed-chest cardiac massage is usually appropriate. In the patient with cardiac tamponade, acute volume loss, an unstable sternum, or an open pericardium, open-chest cardiac massage may be required.

      **(3)** **Defibrillation**, if cardiac arrest is the result of ventricular fibrillation

      **(4)** Replacement of **blood volume**, if necessary

      **(5)** **Drug therapy.** Commonly used agents include:

        **(a)** Epinephrine, for its cardiotonic effect

        **(b)** Calcium, also for its cardiotonic effect

        **(c)** Sodium bicarbonate, to treat associated acidosis

        **(d)** Vasopressor agents, to support blood pressure

        **(e)** Atropine, to reverse bradycardia

**7. Extracorporeal circulation**

    **a.** The **rationale** for the use of extracorporeal circulation is that it provides the operating team with a bloodless field to work in expeditiously while at the same time perfusing the different organ systems with oxygenated blood.

    **b.** During the procedure, **hypothermia** is employed, which improves the tolerance of the myocardium to ischemia. This is complemented by the use of myocardial perfusion with cardioplegic solutions.

    **c.** **Possible undesirable effects** of extracorporeal circulation include:

      **(1)** Trauma to blood elements, resulting in hemolysis of red cells and destruction of platelets

      **(2)** Mild degrees of renal failure, if the "pump run" is long

      **(3)** Respiratory insufficiency, which is usually self-limited

**8. Prosthetic valves.** These fall into two general categories: tissue valves and metal mechanical valves.

    **a.** **Tissue valves** consist of heterografts of bovine pericardium. Tissue valves do not require anticoagulation postoperatively, which is a strong point in their favor. However, their long-term durability has not been established.

    **b.** **Metal mechanical valves** have proven to be durable for prolonged periods of time but require permanent anticoagulation therapy.

**B. Aortic valvular disease**

**1. Aortic stenosis**

    **a. Etiology**

      **(1)** A history of rheumatic fever is elicited in 30% to 50% of patients, but never in patients with isolated stenosis.

      **(2)** Mitral valve disease may accompany the aortic stenosis in up to 50% of patients, but it is generally thought that acquired aortic stenosis results from degeneration of a calcified aortic valve.

      **(3)** In patients with congenital aortic stenosis, calcific changes usually become apparent by the fourth decade, and symptomatic by age 63.

    **b. Pathology**

      **(1)** Calcification of the leaflets occurs in a congenitally malformed valve.

**(2)** This results in a decreased cross-sectional area of the valve, which may be as narrow as 0.5 cm² to 0.7 cm² in severe aortic stenosis (the normal aortic valve is 2.5 cm² to 3.5 cm²).

**(3)** Severe stenosis increases left ventricular work, resulting in concentric left ventricular hypertrophy (without associated dilation). Eventually, myocardial decompensation will occur.

**c. Clinical presentation**
  **(1)** The **classic symptoms** are angina, syncope, and dyspnea.
  **(2)** Symptoms usually occur late in the course of the disease and represent myocardial decompensation. Sudden death is a frequent occurrence in untreated patients at this stage.
  **(3)** Life expectancy averages 4 years after the onset of symptoms, and 2 years after the onset of dyspnea.

**d. Diagnosis**
  **(1)** **Physical examination** reveals the classic systolic crescendo-decrescendo murmur, heard best in the second right intercostal space.
    **(a)** Often, in loud murmurs, an associated thrill is appreciated. Radiation of the murmur to the carotids is common.
    **(b)** A narrowed pulse pressure is frequently found.
  **(2)** The **chest x-ray** usually shows a heart of normal size. Calcification of the aortic valve may be seen.
  **(3)** The **electrocardiogram** demonstrates left ventricular hypertrophy.
  **(4)** **Cardiac catheterization** is important, to measure the gradient across the aortic valve and to calculate the cross-sectional area. In addition, it should identify any associated coronary artery disease (which exists in 25% of the patients) or mitral valvular disease.

**e. Treatment**
  **(1)** Surgical correction of aortic stenosis is recommended for patients with a valve area smaller than 0.7 cm².
  **(2)** The appearance of syncope, angina, or dyspnea is an indication for prompt surgical intervention.
  **(3)** Surgical correction consists of resection of the diseased valve and replacement with one of the prosthetic valves.

**2. Aortic insufficiency**
  **a. Etiology**
    **(1)** Myxomatous degeneration accounts for most cases of aortic insufficiency.
    **(2)** Other causes include syphilitic aortitis, aortic dissection, Marfan's syndrome, bacterial endocarditis, rheumatic fever, and annuloaortic ectasia.
  **b. Pathology**
    **(1)** The underlying pathologic process may be a fibrosis and shortening of the valve leaflets (as occurs in rheumatic fever) or a dilatation of the aortic annulus (as occurs in Marfan's syndrome).
    **(2)** Left ventricular dilatation is seen. If uncorrected, this may lead to left ventricular failure with pulmonary congestion. Secondary mitral insufficiency may occur at this stage.
  **c. Clinical presentation**
    **(1)** There is a greater variability in time between the onset of aortic insufficiency and the appearance of symptoms than occurs with aortic stenosis.
    **(2)** Early **symptoms** include palpitations secondary to ventricular arrhythmias, and dyspnea on exertion.
    **(3)** Later, severe congestive heart failure is seen. Death results from progressive cardiac failure.
  **d. Diagnosis**
    **(1)** **Physical examination**
      **(a)** The characteristic decrescendo murmur is heard along the left sternal border. The duration of the murmur during diastole often correlates with the severity of the aortic insufficiency. The murmur radiates to the left axilla.
      **(b)** The pulse pressure is often increased. Short, intense peripheral pulses (**"water-hammer pulses"**) are characteristic.
    **(2)** The left ventricular enlargement can be seen on the **chest x-ray**.
    **(3)** **Cardiac catheterization with aortography** is used to quantitate the degree of aortic insufficiency.
  **e. Treatment**
    **(1)** Surgery is recommended whenever any ventricular decompensation is demonstrated. Patients at this stage may or may not have significant symptoms.
    **(2)** Valve replacement with a prosthesis is the indicated therapy.

**C. Mitral valve disease**

**1. Mitral stenosis**

   **a. Etiology.** Although only 50% of patients report a history of rheumatic fever, this is thought to be the cause of mitral stenosis in virtually all cases. Congenital defects causing mitral stenosis are very rare.

   **b. Pathology**

      **(1)** The time interval between the episode of rheumatic fever and the manifestation of mitral stenosis averages between 10 and 25 years.

      **(2)** The underlying pathologic change is a fusion of the commissures, with or without shortening of the chordae tendineae. The severity of the stenosis and the choice of operative approach depend on the extent of these changes.

      **(3)** The normal **cross-sectional area** of the mitral valve is 4 cm² to 6 cm². In mild mitral stenosis, the area is reduced to 2 cm² to 2.5 cm²; in moderately severe stenosis to 1.5 cm² to 2 cm²; and in severe stenosis to 1 cm² to 1.5 cm².

      **(4) Pathophysiologic changes** include:

         **(a)** Increased left atrial pressure

         **(b)** Decreased cardiac output

         **(c)** Increased pulmonary vascular resistance

         **(d)** Atrial fibrillation

   **c. Clinical presentation**

      **(1)** Dyspnea is the most significant symptom. It indicates pulmonary congestion secondary to increased left atrial pressure.

      **(2)** Other manifestations include:

         **(a)** Paroxysmal nocturnal dyspnea and orthopnea

         **(b)** Chronic cough and hemoptysis

         **(c)** Systemic arterial embolization

         **(d)** Pulmonary edema

      **(3)** Long-standing pulmonary hypertension may result in right ventricular failure and secondary tricuspid regurgitation.

   **d. Diagnosis**

      **(1) Physical examination.** The typical patient is thin and cachectic. Auscultation reveals the **classic triad** of a diastolic rumble, opening snap, and loud first heart sound.

      **(2)** The **chest x-ray** typically shows a prominent pulmonary vasculature in the upper lung fields. The cardiac silhouette may be normal or may show a double density of the right heart border. A lateral chest x-ray with a "barium swallow" may detect left atrial enlargement.

      **(3)** The **electrocardiogram** may be normal or may show P-wave abnormalities, signs of right ventricular hypertrophy, and right axis deviation.

      **(4) Cardiac catheterization** is used to detect any associated valvular disease or coronary artery disease and to calculate the mitral cross-sectional area.

      **(5)** M-mode and 2-D **echocardiography** may complement cardiac catheterization in the diagnosis of mitral stenosis.

   **e. Treatment.** Surgery is recommended for all patients with symptomatic mitral stenosis.

      **(1)** Mitral valve commissurotomy should be attempted for a patient with simple fusion of the commissures, although a later prosthetic valve replacement may be necessary.

      **(2)** Mitral valve replacement is required for patients with severe disease of the chordae tendineae and papillary muscles.

      **(3)** Permanent anticoagulant therapy is especially important for nontissue prosthetic valves in the mitral position, to prevent thromboembolization.

**2. Mitral insufficiency**

   **a. Etiology.** Mitral insufficiency is not usually due to rheumatic fever. Other causes include:

      **(1)** Myxomatous degeneration

      **(2)** Papillary muscle dysfunction or rupture secondary to coronary artery disease

      **(3)** Bacterial endocarditis

   **b. Pathology**

      **(1)** The pathogenesis in mitral insufficiency secondary to rheumatic fever is similar to that in mitral stenosis. Why insufficiency predominates in some patients and stenosis in others is not understood.

      **(2)** Pathophysiologic changes include:

         **(a)** Increased left atrial pressure during systole

         **(b)** Late-appearing pulmonary vascular changes, including increased pulmonary vascular resistance

   **c. Clinical presentation**

      **(1)** Many years may elapse between the first evidence of mitral insufficiency and the patient's complaints of symptoms.

**(2)** In general, symptoms occur late in the course of cardiac decompensation, and include dyspnea on exertion, fatigue, and palpitations.
   **d. Diagnosis**
      **(1) Physical examination** reveals a systolic murmur at the apex that radiates to the axilla, accompanied by an accentuated apical impulse. The duration of the murmur in systole correlates with the severity of the disease. Atrial fibrillation may also occur.
      **(2)** The **chest x-ray** demonstrates an enlarged left ventricle and atrium.
      **(3)** The **electrocardiogram** shows evidence of left ventricular hypertrophy in 50% of cases.
      **(4) Cardiac catheterization** helps to estimate the degree of insufficiency by demonstrating the degree of reflux of dye into the left atrium.
   **e. Treatment**
      **(1) Medical therapy** with digitalis, diuretics, and vasodilator agents, has a significant place in the treatment of stable mitral insufficiency and in preparation for surgery.
      **(2) Indications for surgery** include:
         **(a)** Progressive congestive heart failure
         **(b)** Progressive cardiac enlargement
         **(c)** Mitral insufficiency of acute onset, as from ruptured chordae tendineae secondary to bacterial endocarditis
         **(d)** Disease in more than one valve
      **(3)** Mitral valve repair with annuloplasty has gained popularity recently, but mitral valve replacement remains the preferred treatment of mitral insufficiency.

**D. Tricuspid valve, pulmonic valve, and multiple valvular disease**

   **1. Tricuspid stenosis and insufficiency**
      **a. Etiology**
         **(1)** Disease of the tricuspid valve is almost always due to rheumatic fever, and is most commonly found in association with mitral valve disease. Isolated tricuspid disease is rare.
         **(2)** Tricuspid insufficiency, which is more common than tricuspid stenosis, is sometimes seen in the carcinoid syndrome, secondary to blunt trauma, or secondary to bacterial endocarditis in drug addicts.
         **(3)** Functional tricuspid insufficiency is the result of right ventricular dilation secondary to pulmonary hypertension and right ventricular failure. Functional insufficiency is more common than organic tricuspid valve disease.
      **b. Pathology**
         **(1)** The pathogenesis in tricuspid valve disease secondary to rheumatic fever is similar to that in mitral valve disease.
         **(2)** Elevation of right atrial pressure secondary to tricuspid stenosis leads to edema, hepatomegaly, and ascites.
      **c. Clinical presentation**
         **(1)** Moderate isolated tricuspid insufficiency is usually well tolerated.
         **(2)** When right-sided heart failure occurs, symptoms (edema, hepatomegaly, ascites) develop.
      **d. Diagnosis**
         **(1) Physical examination**
            **(a) Tricuspid insufficiency** produces a systolic murmur at the lower end of the sternum.
            **(b) Tricuspid stenosis** produces a diastolic murmur in the same region.
            **(c)** A prominent jugular venous pulse may be observed.
            **(d)** The liver may be pulsatile.
         **(2)** The **chest x-ray** shows enlargement of the right heart, which may also be reflected on the electrocardiogram.
         **(3) Cardiac catheterization** is the most accurate guide to diagnosing tricuspid disease. It should include evaluation of any associated aortic or mitral valve lesions.
      **e. Treatment**
         **(1)** Isolated tricuspid disease, especially tricuspid insufficiency, may be well tolerated without surgical intervention.
         **(2)** In mild to moderate tricuspid insufficiency associated with mitral valve disease, opinion varies concerning the need for tricuspid surgery.
         **(3)** In the case of extensive tricuspid insufficiency associated with mitral valve disease, the consensus is that either tricuspid repair or tricuspid valve replacement is appropriate.
         **(4)** Tricuspid stenosis, when significant, is remedied by commissurotomy or valve replacement.

   **2. Pulmonic valve disease**
      **a.** Acquired lesions of the pulmonic valve are uncommon. The carcinoid syndrome, however, may produce pulmonic stenosis.

    **b.** Surgical repair or replacement of the valve is carried out when warranted by the degree of dysfunction.

  **3. Multiple valvular disease**
    **a.** More than one valve may be involved in rheumatic fever, as indicated in the foregoing discussions.
    **b.** Abnormal physiologic responses to multivalvular disease may be additive but usually reflect the most severely affected valve.
    **c. Treatment** involves repair or replacement of all valves with significant dysfunction.

**E. Coronary artery disease**

  **1. Etiology and epidemiology**
    **a. Atherosclerosis** is the predominant pathogenetic mechanism underlying obstructive disease of the coronary arteries. Uncommon causes of coronary artery disease include vasculitis (occurring with collagen vascular disorders), radiation injury, and trauma.
    **b.** Atherosclerotic heart disease represents the most common cause of death in the United States and most other developed nations.
    **c.** Coronary artery disease is four times more prevalent in males than in females.
    **d.** Epidemiologic studies have identified the following **risk factors for coronary artery disease:**
      **(1)** Hypertension
      **(2)** Smoking
      **(3)** Hypercholesterolemia
      **(4)** A family history of heart disease

  **2.** The **pathophysiologic effects** of coronary artery disease on the myocardium include:
    **a.** Decreased ventricular compliance
    **b.** Decreased cardiac contractility
    **c.** Myocardial necrosis

  **3. Clinical presentation.** Coronary artery disease may take the form of:
    **a. Angina pectoris**
      **(1)** Angina pectoris typically presents as substernal chest pain lasting 5 to 10 minutes. The pain may be precipitated by emotional stress, exertion, or cold weather and is relieved by rest.
      **(2)** Angina may be characterized by its patterns of occurrence:
        **(a)** Stable angina: angina that is unchanged for a prolonged period
        **(b)** Unstable angina (new-onset angina): angina that shows a recent change from a previously stable pattern
        **(c)** Angina at rest
        **(d)** Postinfarction angina
    **b. Myocardial infarction**
    **c. Sudden death**
    **d. Congestive heart failure**

  **4. Diagnosis**
    **a.** The diagnosis of angina pectoris due to coronary artery disease is most often made from the patient's history.
    **b. Electrocardiogram**
      **(1)** The electrocardiogram is normal in up to 78% of patients when they are at rest without pain.
      **(2)** ST-segment changes and T-wave changes may be seen.
      **(3)** Evidence of a previous infarction may be apparent.
    **c.** Exercise stress testing will induce angina in approximately 80% of patients.
    **d.** A radiothallium scan of the heart may be helpful.
    **e. Cardiac catheterization and coronary angiography** provide the most accurate means of determining the extent of coronary artery disease. In addition, left ventricular function may be assessed by the ventriculogram and hemodynamic measurements.

  **5. Treatment**
    **a.** Management of coronary artery disease is initiated with **medical therapy** in patients with stable angina and with no evidence of congestive heart failure.
      **(1)** Drugs used include nitrates, $\beta$-blockers, digitalis derivatives, and calcium channel blockers.
      **(2)** In addition, the patient is encouraged to adopt a low-fat diet and to stop smoking.
    **b. Surgical treatment**
      **(1)** Coronary artery obstructive disease is treated surgically by providing a **bypass** around

physiologically significant lesions, using a reversed autogenous saphenous vein or internal mammary artery or percutaneous transluminal coronary angioplasty (PTCA)

(2) Obstruction is considered physiologically significant when the diameter of the vessel on angiography is narrowed by 50%.

(3) Coronary artery bypass is generally indicated for:

(a) Intractable or unstable angina pectoris

(b) Angina pectoris with any of the following:

(i) Left main coronary artery obstruction

(ii) Obstruction of the three main coronary arteries (**"triple-vessel disease"**) with depressed ventricular function

(iii) Proximal obstruction of the left anterior descending artery

(4) Stable angina pectoris with single-vessel right coronary artery or circumflex coronary artery disease is not usually considered an indication for surgery.

(5) Severe congestive heart failure without angina is a definite contraindication to bypass surgery.

(6) Acute myocardial infarction that presents in less than 4 hours in some centers is an indication for immediate bypass surgery or PTCA.

c. **Prognosis after bypass surgery**

(1) The results of coronary artery revascularization depend on the patient's preoperative left ventricular function. A left ventricular systolic ejection fraction of less than 0.3 constitutes an increased but acceptable operative risk.

(2) In patients with stable angina, the accepted operative mortality rate is around 1%.

(a) About 85% to 95% of patients are helped significantly, with 85% having complete freedom from angina.

(b) Angina may be expected to recur in 50% of patients after 8 to 10 years.

(3) Surgery increases survival in patients with "left main disease," and in those with triple-vessel disease and depressed ventricular function.

6. **Surgical treatment of myocardial infarction complications**. Myocardial infarction and many of its complications are treated medically, but some complications warrant surgery. These include the following:

a. **Ventricular aneurysms.** The scarred myocardium may produce either akinesia or dyskinesia of ventricular wall motion, decreasing the ejection fraction.

(1) This may result in congestive heart failure, ventricular arrhythmias, or systemic thromboembolization.

(2) Surgical correction of the aneurysm is undertaken when these problems occur.

(3) Coronary revascularization may also be warranted at the same time.

b. **Ruptured ventricle** is less common than aneurysm formation. If possible, surgical repair should be undertaken without delay, because the mortality rate is 100% without surgery.

c. **Rupture of the interventricular septum** also carries a high mortality rate. Again, early operative repair is important.

d. **Papillary muscle dysfunction or rupture**

(1) Usually the posterior papillary muscle is involved.

(2) Treatment is by mitral valve replacement.

(3) Long-term survival is independent of the extent of preexisting myocardial damage.

F. **Cardiac tumors**

1. **Types of tumors**

a. **Benign tumors**

(1) **Myxomas**, which account for 75% to 80% of benign cardiac tumors, may be either pedunculated or sessile. The vast majority are pedunculated and are found in the left atrium, attached to the septum.

(2) Other benign tumors include rhabdomyomas (most common in childhood), fibromas, and lipomas.

b. **Malignant tumors.** Overall, primary malignant tumors account for 20% to 25% of all primary cardiac tumors. Most common are the various types of sarcomas.

c. **Metastatic tumors**

(1) Autopsy studies show cardiac involvement by metastatic disease in about 10% of patients who have died of malignancy.

(2) Melanoma, lymphoma, and leukemia are the tumors which most often metastasize to the heart.

2. **Clinical presentation.** Cardiac neoplasms may be manifested by pericardial effusion, resulting in cardiac tamponade; or by congestive heart failure, arrhythmias, peripheral embolization (especially with myxomas), or other constitutional signs and symptoms.

**3. Treatment** is by surgical excision if possible.

**G. Cardiac trauma.** As with other forms of trauma, injuries to the heart may be divided into several categories.

**1. Penetrating injury** may involve any part of the heart.
   **a.** Penetrating wounds may result from gunshots, knives, and so forth. In addition, penetrating injury may be iatrogenic, as results from catheters or pacing wires.
   **b.** Bleeding into the pericardium is a common consequence. **Pericardial tamponade** may result, manifested by:
      **(1)** Distended neck veins
      **(2)** Hypotension
      **(3)** Pulsus paradoxus
      **(4)** Decreased heart sounds
   **c.** Open thoracotomy may be required.

**2. Blunt trauma** may be more extensive than is usually appreciated.
   **a.** A **history** of a significant blow to the chest, with or without fractured ribs or sternum, should create a high index of suspicion.
   **b.** A patient with such a history should be observed and monitored in a similar manner to a patient suffering from myocardial infarction, because the trauma is likely to cause a similar myocardial ischemia.
      **(1)** Serial electrocardiograms and cardiac enzyme studies should be obtained.
      **(2)** Echocardiography may be helpful in determining myocardial injury.
      **(3)** The appearance of new murmurs should be investigated and may call for cardiac catheterization.
   **c.** Blunt trauma may cause rupture of a tricuspid, mitral, or aortic valve, requiring treatment by valve replacement.

**H. Pericardial disorders**

**1. Pericardial effusion**
   **a.** The pericardium responds to noxious stimuli by an increased production of fluid.
   **b.** A pericardial effusion volume as small as 100 ml may produce symptomatic tamponade if the fluid accumulates rapidly, while larger amounts may be accommodated if they accumulate slowly.
   **c.** Pericardial effusion is treated by tube pericardiostomy.
   **d.** Chronically occurring effusions, such as those that occur with malignant involvement of the pericardium, may require pericardiectomy.

**2. Pericarditis** may be acute or chronic.
   **a. Acute pericarditis**
      **(1) Causes** of acute pericarditis include:
         **(a)** Bacterial infection, as from staphylococci or streptococci. Acute pyogenic pericarditis is uncommon and is usually associated with a systemic illness.
         **(b)** Viral infection
         **(c)** Uremia
         **(d)** Trauma causing hemopericardium
         **(e)** Malignant disease
         **(f)** Connective tissue disorders
      **(2) Management** consists of treating the underlying cause. Open pericardial drainage may be required.
      **(3)** Most cases of acute pericarditis resolve without serious sequelae.
   **b. Chronic pericarditis**
      **(1)** Chronic pericarditis may represent recurrent episodes of an acute process or undiagnosed long-standing viral pericarditis. The etiology is often impossible to establish.
      **(2)** Chronic pericarditis may go unnoticed until it results in the chronic constrictive form, causing chronic tamponade.
      **(3) Chronic constrictive pericarditis**, which is often seen in patients aged 10 to 30 years, may be related to tuberculosis. It may present with ascites, peripheral edema, dyspnea on exertion, and easy fatigability.
         **(a)** Cardiac catheterization may be needed to make the diagnosis.
         **(b)** Once the diagnosis has been established in the symptomatic patient, pericardiectomy should be undertaken.

## II. CONGENITAL HEART DISEASE

**A. General considerations**

1. The **incidence** of congenital heart disease is approximately 3 per 1000 births. The incidence is ten times greater in members of the same family.

2. In most cases the **etiology** is unknown.
   a. Rubella occurring in the first trimester of pregnancy is known to cause congenital heart disease (e.g., patent ductus arteriosus).
   b. Down's syndrome is associated with septal defects.

3. The **most common forms** of congenital heart disease are:
   a. Ventricular septal defect (20%)
   b. Atrial septal defect (10% to 15%)
   c. Pulmonic valvular stenosis (10%)
   d. Aortic valvular stenosis (10%)
   e. Patent ductus arteriosus (10%)
   f. Coarctation of the aorta (10% to 15%)
   g. Transposition of the great vessels (10%)
   h. Atrioventricular septal defects (< 5%)

4. **History**
   a. The mother should be questioned about difficulties during the pregnancy, especially in the first trimester.
   b. The mother often states that the patient shows the following:
      (1) Easy fatigability and decreased exercise tolerance
      (2) Poor feeding habits and poor weight gain
      (3) Frequent pulmonary infections
   c. A history of cyanosis should be sought, as this indicates a right-to-left shunt.

5. **Physical examination**
   a. Abnormalities in growth and development should be identified.
   b. Cyanosis and clubbing of the fingers may be noted.
   c. Examination of the heart should proceed in the same manner as in the adult.
      (1) Systolic murmurs are frequently found in infants and small children, and may not be of clinical significance.
      (2) A gallop rhythm is of great clinical importance.
      (3) Congestive heart failure in children is frequently manifested by hepatic enlargement.

**B. Patent ductus arteriosus**

1. **Pathophysiology**
   a. In the normal infant born at term, the ductus arteriosus closes within the first few days of life.
   b. Hypoxia and certain prostaglandins may act to keep the ductus open.
   c. The natural history in patent ductus arteriosus is variable.
      (1) A small percentage of patients will experience heart failure within the first year of life, while others will suffer from pulmonary vascular disease.
      (2) Many patients will remain asymptomatic and will be diagnosed later upon routine examination.
      (3) Patent ductus arteriosus may be seen in combination with other defects, such as ventricular septal defect and coarctation of the aorta.

2. **Clinical presentation**
   a. Common presenting complaints are dyspnea, fatigue, and palpitations, signifying congestive heart failure.
   b. On **physical examination** the classic "machinery-like" murmur is usually heard, but it may be absent until age 1 year.
   c. Other signs include a widened pulse pressure and bounding peripheral pulses.
   d. Cyanosis may be seen in patent ductus arteriosus that is associated with other anomalies or in right-to-left shunt from pulmonary vascular disease.

3. **Diagnosis** is based primarily on the physical findings. Cardiac catheterization is useful in determining the existence of other associated lesions.

4. **Treatment**
   a. Surgical management consists of ligation of the ductus. This is reserved for:
      (1) Premature infants with pulmonary dysfunction
      (2) Infants who suffer from congestive heart failure within the first year of life
      (3) Asymptomatic children with a patent ductus that persists until the age of 2 or 3 years
   b. Indomethacin, a prostaglandin inhibitor, has been used in attempts to close the ductus in premature infants with symptomatic simple patent ductus arteriosus.

### C. Coarctation of the aorta

   **1.** Coarctation is found twice as often in males as in females.
   **a.** It is **classified** as either juxtaductal, arch, or abdominal.
   **b.** Coarctation may be fatal in the first few months of life if left untreated.
   **c.** Associated intracardiac defects, present in up to 60% of patients, include patent ductus arteriosus and ventricular septal defect.

   **2.** The **clinical presentation** varies.
   **a.** Some children are asymptomatic for varying periods of time.
   **b.** In others, symptoms suggesting congestive heart failure are present shortly after birth.
   **c.** Headaches, epistaxis, lower extremity weakness, and dizziness may be seen in the child with symptomatic coarctation.

   **3. Diagnosis**
   **a. Physical findings** include:
      **(1)** Upper extremity hypertension
      **(2)** Absent or diminished pulses in the lower extremity
      **(3)** A systolic murmur
   **b. Chest x-ray** may reveal "rib-notching" in older children, representing collateral pathways.
   **c. Cardiac catheterization** is required to define the location of the coarctation and any associated cardiac defects.

   **4. Treatment**
   **a.** Surgical correction of the coarctation is indicated for all patients, and is delayed until age 5 or 6 years in asymptomatic patients.
   **b.** Operative treatment involves:
      **(1)** End-to-end anastomosis
      **(2)** Insertion of a prosthetic patch graft
      **(3)** A subclavian flap procedure
   **c.** Any associated defects must also be corrected.

   **5. Complications**
   **a.** Residual hypertension may be a problem postoperatively.
   **b.** Spinal cord injury due to ischemia during surgery may manifest itself postoperatively.
   **c.** Postoperative mesenteric ischemia is seen in a small but significant number of cases and is related to postoperative hypertension.

### D. Atrial septal defects

   **1. Classification.** Atrial septal defects occur twice as frequently in females as in males. Three types are commonly seen:
   **a. Ostium secundum defects**, which account for the majority of atrial septal defects, are found in the midportion of the atrial septum. The association of a secundum defect with mitral stenosis is known as **Lutembacher's syndrome**.
   **b. Sinus venosus defects** are located high up on the atrial septum and are often associated with anomalies of pulmonary venous drainage.
   **c. Ostium primum defects** are components of atrioventricular septal defects and are located on the atrial side of the mitral and tricuspid valves.
   **d.** A **patent foramen ovale** is **not** considered an atrial septal defect.

   **2. Pathophysiology**
   **a.** An increased pulmonary blood flow in association with a decreased systemic flow results in mild retardation of growth and development (gracile habitus).
   **b.** Pulmonary hypertension is rare but can occur.
   **c.** Cardiac failure may occur at any tme but occurs most often in the fourth decade.

   **3. Clinical presentation**
   **a.** Mild dyspnea and easy fatigability are seen in infancy and early childhood. Such **symptoms** increase in severity with age and are manifested frequently in early adulthood as congestive heart failure, often brought on by the onset of atrial fibrillation.
   **b. Physical examination** reveals a systolic murmur in the left second or third intercostal space and a fixed split second heart sound.
   **c.** The **chest x-ray** reveals moderate enlargement of the right ventricle and prominence of the pulmonary vasculature.
   **d.** The electrocardiogram reveals right ventricular hypertrophy.

   **4. Diagnosis** can be made on **cardiac catheterization** from the "step-up" in oxygen saturation in the right atrium. The amount of left-to-right shunt may be calculated.

5. **Treatment** is based on the size of the left-to-right shunt.
   a. Surgical closure of the defect is indicated if the pulmonary blood flow is one and one half to two times greater than the systemic blood flow.
   b. Surgery carries a mortality risk of less than 1%.

E. **Ventricular septal defects**

1. Ventricular septal defects are the most common congenital heart defects. Associated anomalies are common, usually coarctation of the aorta.

2. **Classification.** Ventricular septal defects may be classified according to their location in the ventricular septum:
   a. Infracristal (membranous), the most common type
   b. Supracristal
   c. In the atrioventricular canal
   d. Muscular

3. **Pathophysiology.** The size of the left-to-right shunt depends on the size of the defect.
   a. Defects greater than 1 cm in diameter cause significant shunts.
   b. With large shunts—greater than a 2 to 1 pulmonary-to-systemic flow—cardiac failure and pulmonary hypertension usually result.
   c. Progressive sclerotic changes in the pulmonary vascular bed may result in reversal of the shunt, causing cyanosis, clubbing, and polycythemia; this is known as **Eisenmenger's syndrome.**
      (1) At this point, operative intervention is not possible.
      (2) Eisenmenger's syndrome may also be caused by patent ductus arteriosus, atrial septal defects, and other malformations.

4. **Clinical presentation**
   a. Small ventricular septal defects rarely cause significant symptoms in infancy or early childhood, and may undergo spontaneous closure before they are recognized.
   b. **Symptoms** are usually seen with ventricular septal defects greater than 1 cm in diameter.
      (1) Children with larger defects usually have dyspnea on exertion, easy fatigability, and an increased incidence of pulmonary infections.
      (2) Severe cardiac failure may be seen in infants, but is less common in children.
      (3) Physical examination reveals a harsh pansystolic murmur.

5. **Diagnosis**
   a. This is aided by the chest x-ray and electrocardiogram, especially in large ventricular septal defects, which show evidence of biventricular hypertrophy.
   b. **Cardiac catheterization** is essential for delineating the severity of the left-to-right shunt and pulmonary vascular resistance. In addition, catheterization demonstrates the location of the defect and identifies any associated defects.

6. **Treatment**
   a. Surgical closure of the defect should be performed in the following situations:
      (1) In an infant with significant cardiac failure or increased pulmonary vascular resistance
      (2) In an asymptomatic child with a significant shunt who has not had spontaneous closure by age 2 years
      (3) In any patient with pulmonary blood flow one and one-half to two times greater than systemic flow
   b. The operative mortality risk, which is generally less than 5%, is related to the degree of preoperative pulmonary vascular disease.

F. **Tetralogy of Fallot**

1. **Pathophysiology**
   a. The tetralogy of Fallot, one of the most common **cyanotic congenital heart disorders**, consists of:
      (1) Obstruction to right ventricular outflow
      (2) A ventricular septal defect
      (3) Hypertrophy of the right ventricle
      (4) An overriding aorta
   b. The addition of an atrial septal defect (which is of little further physiologic significance) turns the condition into the **pentalogy of Fallot.**
   c. The four defects result in a right-to-left shunt, resulting in desaturation of the blood and cyanosis.
   d. Exercise tolerance is limited because of the inability to increase pulmonary blood flow.

**2. Clinical presentation**
  **a.** Cyanosis and dyspnea on exertion are routinely seen in patients with tetralogy of Fallot.
    **(1)** Children soon learn that by squatting they can temporarily alleviate these symptoms. Though the mechanism is obscure, it may have to do with increasing pulmonary blood flow by increasing peripheral vascular resistance.
    **(2)** The cyanosis is seen at birth in 30% of the cases, by the first year in 30%, and later in childhood in the remainder. Polycythemia and clubbing accompany the cyanosis.
  **b.** Cerebrovascular accidents and brain sepsis constitute the major threats to life, as cardiac failure is rare.

**3. Diagnosis**
  **a. Physical examination** reveals clubbing of the digits and cyanosis. A systolic murmur is often heard.
  **b. Cardiac catheterization** is important for determining the level of pulmonic outflow obstruction and the size of the main and branch pulmonary arteries.

**4.** The choice of **treatment** depends on many variables, including the anatomy of the defect and the age of the child.
  **a.** Total correction is undertaken after the age of 2 years.
  **b.** Controversy exists over whether the defect should be corrected before this age. Many feel that a palliative systemic-to-pulmonary (Blalock-Taussig) shunt should be done initially, followed by definitive correction at a later date.
  **c.** The risk of surgery depends on the age of the patient and the degree of cyanosis.
  **d.** After correction, a dramatic improvement is usually seen.

# Part IV
# Study Questions

## QUESTIONS

**Directions:** Each question below contains five suggested answers. Choose the **one best** response to each question.

1. The arterial replacement prosthesis of choice for a femoropopliteal bypass graft in a young man is

(A) a Dacron tube graft
(B) an umbilical vein allograft
(C) an autogenous arterial graft
(D) an autogenous saphenous vein graft
(E) an arterial allograft

2. All of the following patients are at increased risk of developing deep venous thrombosis or pulmonary embolism EXCEPT

(A) an obese woman who needs a gastric bypass
(B) a 36-year-old man who has experienced spinal cord injury
(C) a woman with a history of congestive heart failure who needs an appendectomy
(D) a 32-year-old woman who is scheduled for a left colectomy for carcinoma
(E) a 25-year-old man who is scheduled for inguinal herniorrhaphy

3. All of the following complications of myocardial infarction are indications for surgical correction EXCEPT

(A) ventricular premature beats
(B) a ventricular aneurysm
(C) a ruptured ventricle
(D) a ruptured intraventricular septum
(E) papillary muscle dysfunction

4. All of the following statements concerning angiography are true EXCEPT

(A) angiographic dye is hypertonic and may cause renal failure
(B) digital subtraction arteriography visualizes arteries using an intravenous injection of radiopaque contrast medium
(C) hand claudication is a complication of brachial artery angiography
(D) limb ischemia after angiography is most likely due to vasospasm
(E) retroperitoneal hematomas may occur following translumbar aortography

5. Which of the following donor types offers the greatest chance for successful renal transplantation?

(A) One-haplotype match, living related donor
(B) Two-haplotype match, living related donor
(C) Cadaver allograft donor
(D) Isograft donor
(E) Xenograft donor

6. Clinical findings associated with varicose veins include all of the following EXCEPT

(A) deep venous thrombosis
(B) a positive Trendelenburg test
(C) valvular incompetence
(D) local hemorrhage
(E) pain relief with support hose

7. Coarctation of the aorta is best characterized by which of the following statements?

(A) It is found twice as often in females as in males
(B) Physical findings include decreased pulsations in the upper and lower extremities
(C) Surgical correction is indicated in all patients, ideally when the child is 1 to 2 years old
(D) Hypotension is a frequent postoperative problem
(E) Headaches, lower extremity weakness, and dizziness are seen in the child with symptomatic coarctation

8. Foot ulcers secondary to arterial insufficiency are successfully treated by all of the following techniques EXCEPT

(A) debridement of devitalized tissue
(B) elevation of the affected extremity
(C) antibiotic administration
(D) bed rest
(E) amputation of necrotic tissue

9. All of the following immunologic criteria are routinely examined prior to transplantation from a cadaver donor EXCEPT

(A) HLA-A and -B locus typing
(B) crossmatch compatibility
(C) mixed lymphocyte reaction
(D) ABO blood group compatibility
(E) HLA-$D_R$ locus typing

**Directions:** Each question below contains four suggested answers of which **one or more** is correct. Choose the answer

A  if **1, 2, and 3** are correct
B  if **1 and 3** are correct
C  if **2 and 4** are correct
D  if **4** is correct
E  if **1, 2, 3, and 4** are correct

10. Postphlebitic syndrome is associated with which of the following conditions?

(1) Chronic stasis ulceration
(2) Venous valvular incompetence
(3) Venous claudication
(4) Recurrent pulmonary embolism

11. True statements concerning vascular grafts include which of the following?

(1) Atherosclerotic lesions may appear in arterialized saphenous vein bypass grafts
(2) Synthetic vascular grafts spontaneously develop a lining of endothelial cells
(3) Vascular heterografts, such as the tanned bovine carotid artery, have been used successfully
(4) Arterial allografts from human cadaver donors have a high rate of success when used for aortic bypass

12. The management of stable angina pectoris should include

(1) coronary angiography
(2) medical therapy with nitrates, $\beta$-blockers, and antihypertensive medications
(3) a low-fat diet
(4) coronary artery bypass

13. Contraindications to renal transplantation in a potential recipient include

(1) positive tuberculin test, but no other evidence of active tuberculosis
(2) an unhealed duodenal ulcer
(3) polycystic kidneys
(4) antiglomerular basement membrane disease

14. True statements concerning diagnostic procedures for pulmonary embolism include which of the following?

(1) A ventilation-perfusion scan is more accurate than a perfusion scan alone for detecting pulmonary embolism
(2) Pulmonary arteriography is only 75% accurate in detecting clinically significant pulmonary emboli
(3) A normal lung scan essentially rules out a pulmonary embolus
(4) A perfusion lung scan is helpful in differentiating pulmonary embolism from chronic pulmonary disease

15. Diabetic patients are at risk for developing which of the following foot complications?

(1) Gangrene
(2) Severe infection
(3) Plantar space abscess
(4) Peripheral neuropathy

16. True statements concerning the etiology and epidemiology of coronary artery disease include which of the following?

(1) Atherosclerosis is the predominant pathogenetic mechanism underlying obstruction of the coronary arteries
(2) Atherosclerotic heart disease is the most common cause of death in the United States
(3) Coronary artery disease is four times more prevalent in males than in females
(4) Hypertension and smoking are important risk factors associated with coronary artery disease

17. True statements concerning deep venous thrombosis include which of the following?

(1) Most of the time it originates in the lower extremity venous system
(2) Heparin infusion is the treatment of choice
(3) It is most accurately diagnosed by venography
(4) About 50% of patients have no physical findings in the extremities

18. Long-term complications of renal transplantation include

(1) skin cancers
(2) coronary artery disease
(3) lymphoma
(4) hyperlipidemia

19. Conditions associated with renal artery stenosis include

(1) fibromuscular dysplasia
(2) uncontrollable hypertension
(3) hypovolemia
(4) disparity in kidney size

20. The management of cardiac arrest should include which of the following protocols?

(1) Immediate resuscitation, as irreversible brain damage will result after 3 to 4 minutes of diminished perfusion
(2) Establishment of an airway and ventilatory support
(3) Closed-chest cardiac massage
(4) Defibrillation, if cardiac arrest is due to ventricular fibrillation

21. Immunosuppressive drug therapy can be complicated by

(1) cushingoid facies
(2) cytomegalovirus (CMV) infection
(3) hypertension
(4) cerebrovascular disease

22. True statements concerning femoropopliteal occlusive disease include which of the following?

(1) Femoropopliteal grafts are more likely to remain patent over time than are femoral-tibial bypass grafts
(2) Dependent rubor is a common problem
(3) The saphenous vein is the preferred vessel for a bypass graft
(4) The most commonly occluded vessel in the leg is the distal profunda femoris artery

23. True statements concerning cardiac tumors include which of the following?

(1) Myxomas account for approximately 75% to 80% of benign cardiac tumors
(2) Primary malignant tumors are responsible for only 20% of all primary cardiac tumors
(3) Approximately 10% of patients dying of malignant tumors will have cardiac involvement at the time of autopsy
(4) Tumors most often metastasizing to the heart include melanoma, lymphoma, and leukemia

24. True statements concerning acute arterial occlusion include which of the following?

(1) It may be caused by emboli that originate from a cardiac source
(2) It results in severe pain
(3) It requires immediate heparinization
(4) It should be treated by balloon catheter embolectomy

25. True statements concerning pericardial effusions include which of the following?

(1) The pericardium responds to noxious stimuli by an increased production of fluid
(2) A rapidly accumulating pericardial effusion must have a volume of at least 200 ml before symptoms will occur
(3) Pericardial effusion is treated by tube pericardiostomy
(4) Chronically occurring effusions (e.g., from malignant involvement of the pericardium) are best treated by repeated pericardiocentesis

26. True statements concerning reconstructive techniques for aortoiliac disease include which of the following?

(1) Death is most commonly caused by stroke
(2) Long-term patency for aortoiliac bypass grafts is excellent
(3) Axillofemoral grafts are associated with a low rate of infection (< 2%)
(4) Reconstruction relieves claudication and other ischemic leg symptoms in most patients

**Directions:** The questions below consist of lettered choices followed by two numbered items. For each numbered item select the **one** lettered choice with which it is **most** closely associated. Each lettered choice may be used once, more than once, or not at all.

### Questions 27 and 28

Match the phrase describing valvular disease with the appropriate lesion.

(A) Aortic stenosis
(B) Mitral stenosis
(C) Both
(D) Neither

27. A history of rheumatic fever can be documented in approximately one-half of patients

28. Dyspnea is a significant symptom

## ANSWERS AND EXPLANATIONS

**1. The answer is D.** (*Chapter 15 II A 1–4, B, C 1, 3; III A 1*) The graft of choice for a femoropopliteal by-pass is an autogenous saphenous vein graft. This type of graft is a vein that is transplanted from one part of the body to another for use in bypassing an occlusion in either an artery or vein. An autogenous arterial graft is an artery that is removed from one area of the vascular tree and inserted into another area. Of the vascular allografts—that is, vessels removed from one individual and implanted into another individual—arterial allografts are not used because of a high rate of degeneration, while umbilical vein allografts have shown excellent long-term patency for both lower extremity revascularization and hemodialysis vascular access. Dacron grafts are very successful when used for large-vessel replacements, such as in the aorta or iliac vessels.

**2. The answer is E.** (*Chapter 14 I C 3 a; II C 1–9*) Patients who are undergoing uncomplicated surgery (e.g., inguinal herniorrhaphy) and who are otherwise young and healthy are not at risk for developing pulmonary embolism. Obesity, a history of congestive heart failure, spinal cord injury, and carcinoma do place the surgical patient at increased risk for pulmonary embolism and deep venous thrombosis.

**3. The answer is A.** (*Chapter 17 I E 6*) Myocardial infarction and many of its complications are treated medically, including a variety of arrhythmias that can occur. However, some complications require surgery. The scarred myocardium of a ventricular aneurysm may produce akinesia or dyskinesia of the ventricular wall which will decrease the ejection fraction. In addition, thrombosis can form in this area, and distal thromboembolization may result. Aneurysms should be corrected if either of these two complications are present. Rupture of the ventricle and rupture of the intraventricular septum carry extremely high mortality rates and require surgical correction as early as possible. Severe papillary muscle dysfunction or papillary muscle rupture results in valvular incompetence. This should be corrected promptly with surgical replacement of the valve.

**4. The answer is D.** [*Chapter 13 I C 2 a, b (1), (2) (a), c (1), e*] Invasive tests for the assessment of peripheral vascular disease include digital subtraction angiography and percutaneous arterial angiography. Digital subtraction angiography demonstrates arterial anatomy through a single nonselective intravenous injection of radiopaque contrast medium. This technique is of low risk in terms of injury to arterial structures and renal toxicity, but risk of allergy to the dye remains. Percutaneous arterial angiography demonstrates the vascular anatomy by the selective injection of contrast medium intra-arterially. Acute renal failure may result from the nephrotoxicity of the dye. Brachial artery catheterization is frequently performed for cardiac catheterization or for angiography when the lower extremity vessels are unsuitable; however, acute hand ischemia or hand claudication may result. Translumbar aortography is performed by catheterizing the suprarenal aorta by a long needle. This study is used when neither the femoral nor the axillary arteries are suitable; however, retroperitoneal hematomas may complicate this procedure. Although ischemia after angiography may be caused by vasospasm, this is a rare occurrence; the occlusion is more often the result of technical problems, such as simple thrombosis at the needle insertion site, thrombi formed on the angiogram catheter, or release of an atherosclerotic plaque during catheter manipulation.

**5. The answer is B.** (*Chapter 16 I C*) The genotypes of a related donor and recipient are more compatible than those of an unrelated donor and recipient. In a two-haplotype match all antigens are matched; in a one-haplotype match only 50% of the antigens are matched.

**6. The answer is A.** (*Chapter 14 I C 2 a, b*) Varicose veins are dilatated networks in the subcutaneous venous system that result from valvular incompetence. Clinical findings include edema, pain, inflammation, dilatated superficial veins, local hemorrhage into the surrounding tissue, and a positive Trendelenburg test, which indicates incompetent valves. Nonoperative management involves the use of support hose to keep the superficial vessels collapsed, thereby minimizing the effect of venous hypertension on venous dilatation. Deep venous thrombosis is not often a factor in the development of varicose veins.

**7. The answer is E.** (*Chapter 17 II C*) Coarctation is found twice as often in males as in females. Associated intracardiac defects are commonly seen with this condition. Physical findings include upper extremity hypertension with absent or diminished pulses in the lower extremity. Surgical correction is the treatment of choice, ideally when the child is between 5 and 6 years old, although symptoms may mandate earlier repair. Residual hypertension may be a problem postoperatively. Spinal cord injury due to ischemia and postoperative mesenteric ischemia may also be seen in a small number of cases.

**8. The answer is B.** (*Chapter 13 II C 1–7*) Foot ulcers can develop secondary to arterial insufficiency; however, with early care, ulcers can be controlled and healed before they become extensive. Ulcers can be successfully treated by debridement of devitalized tissue, immobilization of the affected limb, systemic or local administration of antibiotics, amputation of necrotic tissue, avoidance of weight bearing on an affected limb, and bed rest without elevation of the affected limb; elevation of an ischemic limb will decrease arterial perfusion, thereby impeding the healing process.

**9. The answer is C.** *(Chapter 16 I D)* Although the mixed lymphocyte reaction may be used to predict success in kidney transplantation from a cadaver donor, the test is not usually performed because it requires 5 to 7 days. Cadaver kidneys must be transplanted within 1 to 2 days following removal.

**10. The answer is A (1, 2, 3).** *(Chapter 14 I D 1 a)* The postphlebitic syndrome generally presents as a lower leg complication due to a permanent obstruction of the deep venous system. It occurs in 10% of patients with deep venous thrombosis. Physical findings include chronic venous insufficiency, venous valvular incompetence, leg edema, pain, nocturnal cramping, venous claudication, abnormal skin pigmentation, and dermatitis. Stasis ulceration may occur years after the episode of deep venous thrombosis, but it can result in severe progressive disability. Pulmonary embolism is not likely to occur as part of this syndrome, although it can occur after any episode of deep venous thrombosis.

**11. The answer is B (1, 3).** *(Chapter 15 II A 2, 3, C 1, D; III B 1)* Arterialization of the saphenous vein grafts results in thickening of the vein wall. Although most of these grafts do well, atherosclerotic lesions appear in 2% to 15% of arterialized veins with time. Vascular heterografts, vessels removed from animals and rendered nonantigenic by the tanning process, have been used successfully for both vascular reconstruction and hemodialysis vascular access; however, they have a tendency to develop aneurysms (in 3% to 6% of cases) in certain applications. Arterial allografts have a high rate of degeneration and are generally not used. All of the currently used synthetic grafts fail to develop a true endothelialized blood lumen; instead a pseudointima develops that is thrombogenic and susceptible to infection.

**12. The answer is A (1, 2, 3).** *(Chapter 17 I E 4, 5)* Initially, angina pectoris is managed with medical therapy. Nitrates, $\beta$-blockers, and antihypertensive medicines are frequently effective in ameliorating the symptoms. In addition, the patient is encouraged to modify his or her life-style in order to eliminate all risk factors. Cardiac catheterization and coronary angiography provide the most accurate means of determining the extent of coronary artery disease. Surgical treatment is indicated if the angina is intractable or unstable. In selected lesions, such as left main coronary artery obstruction or three-vessel coronary artery disease, surgery is the preferred treatment.

**13. The answer is C (2, 4).** *(Chapter 16 II B 1, D 2, E, G 3; VI C 2)* Unhealed duodenal ulcers may become worse, with bleeding or perforation, if steroids are given after renal transplantation. Circulating antiglomerular basement membrane antibodies will attack the new kidney as well as the original kidneys, resulting in rapid destruction of the graft. Therefore, both duodenal ulcer disease and autoimmune diseases characterized by glomerular basement membrane antibodies should be inactive before proceeding with transplantation.

**14. The answer is B (1, 3).** *(Chapter 14 II E)* Pulmonary ventilation is assessed with an inert radioactive gas, such as xenon, which is inhaled; the technique improves the accuracy of the perfusion scan. Pulmonary arteriography is diagnostic in about 100% of cases, but it is an invasive procedure with a risk of causing cardiac arrest. A perfusion lung scan can show similar results with pulmonary embolism or chronic pulmonary disease; however, a normal scan rules out an embolus.

**15. The answer is E (all).** *(Chapter 13 II A 1–3)* The toe, foot, and leg of a patient with diabetes mellitus are subject to infection, even after minor trauma, because of the peripheral neuropathy of diabetes. Infections, in turn, can result in deep plantar space abscesses, cellulitis of the dorsum of the foot, osteomyelitis, and gangrene. The diabetic patient is 40 times more likely to develop gangrene than the nondiabetic patient due to large vessel occlusive disease, in which the pulses are absent, and small vessel disease (microangiopathy), which is characterized by thickening of the capillary basement membrane.

**16. The answer is E (all).** *(Chapter 17 I E 1)* Atherosclerosis is the predominant mechanism of injury to coronary arteries. The most common lesion is obstruction. Uncommon causes of coronary artery injury include vasculitis, radiation injury, and trauma. Hypertension and smoking are important risk factors as are hypercholesterolemia and a family history of heart disease.

**17. The answer is E (all).** *[Chapter 14 I C 3 a (1), b, c (4), d (1)]* The origin of deep venous thrombosis is most often in the lower extremity venous system. The classic clinical picture includes calf or thigh pain, edema, tenderness, and a positive Homans' sign; however, 50% of patients with proven venous thrombosis have no physical findings in the extremities. While venography is the most accurate diagnostic technique, Doppler ultrasonography and impedance plethysmography are also highly accurate, provided that the thrombosis occurs above the knee. The treatment of choice for uncomplicated deep venous thrombosis is continuous heparin infusion for 7 to 10 days, followed by administration of warfarin or subcutaneous administration of heparin for 3 to 6 months.

**18. The answer is E (all).** (*Chapter 16 VI D*) Malignancy is more likely to occur following transplantation because of the immunosuppressive therapy administered. The incidence of primary cancers is 100 times greater than in controls. Vascular complications, including hypertension, hyperlipidemia, coronary artery disease, and cerebral vascular disease, are common after both dialysis and transplantation.

**19. The answer is E (all).** (*Chapter 13 VII A, B 1, 2*) A common cause of renal artery stenosis is fibromuscular dysplasia, particularly in young women. The hypertension inherent in renal artery stenosis must be differentiated from essential hypertension: Suspicion is confirmed by a history of recent, rapid onset of the hypertension, by difficulty in controlling blood pressure with antihypertensive medication, and by the presence of flank bruits. Renal artery stenosis can be diagnosed in most cases by rapid-sequence intravenous pyelography (IVP)), selective renal arteriography, and renin ratios. A signifcant finding on IVP is a disparity in kidney size—a difference of about 2 cm is indicative of unilateral renal artery stenosis. Renin ratios are highly sensitive to volume and vasomotor status. Volume depletion must be corrected preoperatively.

**20. The answer is E (all).** (*Chapter 17 I A 6*) Immediate resuscitation, establishment of an airway, ventilatory support, closed chest cardiac massage, and defibrillation are all appropriate protocols for the management of cardiac arrest. In addition, drug therapy may also be appropriate. Agents that may be useful include epinephrine and calcium for their cardiotonic effects, sodium bicarbonate to treat the associated acidosis, and vasopressors to support blood pressure. If bradycardia is present, atropine may reverse this and should be given promptly.

**21. The answer is E (all).** (*Chapter 16 VI B 2, D 1 a, d, 4*) Infections are the most dangerous sequelae of transplantation and subsequent immunosuppression. Cerebrovascular disease is 300 times more common than in control populations. Other long-term complications include malignancy, aseptic necrosis of the hip or knee as a result of steroid therapy, and cataracts. Cyclosporine has been reported to cause hypertension, especially in children.

**22. The answer is A (1, 2, 3).** (*Chapter 13 IV A 1, B 2, C 2 a, 3 a*) Femoropopliteal occlusive disease is obstruction of the femoral and more distal extremity arteries as a result of atherosclerosis. The most frequently occluded leg artery is the superficial femoral artery, particularly where it enters the adductor canal. The distal profunda femoris artery is usually spared from significant occlusive disease. Physical findings, which result from impaired, sluggish blood flow to the extremity, include an extremity that is pulseless, pale, and cool; rubor in the affected foot, manifested as lobster-red discoloration while standing; loss of lower extremity hair; and the presence of nonhealing ulcerations. There is an excellent cumulative patency rate of up to 80% at 5 years after the basic operative procedure of a bypass graft from the femoral artery to the popliteal artery. Femoral-tibial bypass grafts, which are used for vascular disease distal to the popliteal artery, result in a higher failure rate than the femoropopliteal bypass graft because of the more extensive vascular disease present.

**23. The answer is E (all).** (*Chapter 17 I F 1*) Myxomas are the most common benign cardiac tumor. Most are pedunculated and are found in the left atrium. Myxomas may embolize and present as isolated distal embolic events. Primary malignant tumors of the heart are rare, and the most common types are sarcomas. Cardiac involvement by metastatic disease is somewhat more common, especially in patients with melanoma, lymphoma, or leukemia.

**24. The answer is E (all).** (*Chapter 13 V A, B 1, C 1–4, D 1, 3 a*) Acute arterial occlusion is the sudden cessation of arterial blood flow to the extremities, which results in ischemia that may be followed by necrosis if rapid intervention does not occur. The most frequent cause of the occlusion is the lodgment of emboli that originate from atherosclerotic heart disease (60%), rheumatic heart disease (21%), and abdominal aortic ulcerated plaques (1%–2%). Clinical findings include severe pain; a pale, cool, pulseless extremity; acute loss of motor and sensory function; and low or undetectable ankle blood pressure. Patients should be heparinized immediately (i.e., when the clinical diagnosis is made) and operated on within 6 to 8 hours of the onset of symptoms. The surgeon should perform an embolectomy using a Fogarty balloon catheter.

**25. The answer is B (1, 3).** (*Chapter 17 I H 1*) A pericardial effusion volume as small as 100 ml may produce symptomatic tamponade if the fluid accumulates rapidly. Larger amounts may be tolerated if the accumulation is gradual. Chronically occurring effusions, such as those that occur with malignant involvement of the pericardium, may require creation of a pericardial window to allow drainage of fluid into the chest or peritoneum.

**26. The answer is C (2, 4).** (*Chapter 13 III C 1–4*) Operative techniques for aortoiliac and aortofemoral occlusion include aortoiliac endarterectomy, aortoiliac or aortofemoral grafting, femoral-to-femoral artery bypass grafts, and axillofemoral artery bypass grafts. Aortoiliac grafting using artificial graft material is the most common way of bypassing severe occlusive disease in the aorta and iliac arteries. The technique has a patency rate of 85% at 5 to 10 years. Good to excellent relief of claudication and ischemic leg symptoms results postoperatively. Axillofemoral grafts, on the other hand, are associated with a high rate of thrombosis and infection. The most common cause of death following vascular reconstruction is myocardial infarction.

**27 and 28. The answers are: 27-C, 28-C.** (*Chapter 17 I B 1 a, b, C 1 a, b*) A history of rheumatic fever is elicited from 30% to 50% of patients with aortic stenosis. The classic symptoms are angina, syncope, and dyspnea. Calcification of the leaflets occurs in a congenitally malformed valve, resulting in a decreased cross-sectional area of the valve, which may be as narrow as 0.5 cm² to 0.7 cm² in severe aortic stenosis (an indication for surgery). Severe stenosis increases left ventricular hypertrophy, and eventually myocardial decompensation occurs. Surgical correction consists of repair of the diseased valve or removal of the valve and replacement with a prosthetic device.

Although rheumatic fever is thought to be the cause of mitral stenosis, in the majority of medical centers only 50% of the patients with mitral stenosis have a documented history of rheumatic fever. The normal mitral valve has a cross-sectional area that is between 4 cm² and 6 cm². In severe cases of mitral stenosis, this area is reduced to between 1 cm² and 1.5 cm². The pathophysiologic changes in mitral stenosis include increased left atrial pressure and decreased cardiac output. Dyspnea is the most significant presenting symptom and indicates pulmonary congestion secondary to increased left atrial pressure. Surgery is the recommended treatment for virtually all patients with symptomatic mitral stenosis.

# Part V
# Endocrine Disorders

# 18
# The Thyroid Gland

Herbert E. Cohn

## I. INTRODUCTION

**A.** The indications for operations on the thyroid gland have varied since excision was first described by Kocher in the late 1800s.

**B.** In early years, operations on the thyroid were done primarily to relieve the pressure symptoms of large iodine-deficiency goiter, to control hyperthyroidism, or to remove thyroid neoplasms.

**C.** With the advent of iodized salt, iodine-deficiency goiters have almost been eliminated, and hyperthyroidism is now controlled mainly by nonoperative means.

**D.** However, surgery remains the mainstay of treatment for thyroid neoplasms, and in many instances is important in their diagnosis.

## II. ANATOMY

**A.** The thyroid is an H-shaped gland consisting of two lobes and an interconnecting isthmus. A pyramidal lobe located in the midline and extending above the isthmus is present in a small percentage of cases.

**B. Arterial supply**

  **1.** The superior thyroid artery, which is the first branch of the external carotid, supplies the superior pole of the thyroid.

  **2.** The inferior thyroid artery, which arises from the thyrocervical trunk as a branch of the subclavian artery, supplies the lower pole of the gland.

  **3.** Occasionally, a thyroidea ima artery arises from the aortic arch and connects to the thyroid isthmus on its inferior aspect.

**C. Venous drainage** of the thyroid is an interconnecting system of veins without valves.

  **1.** The superior thyroid veins drain along the course of the superior thyroid arteries into the internal jugular vein.

  **2.** The middle thyroid vein drains directly into the internal jugular vein.

  **3.** The inferior thyroid veins drain from the lower pole and isthmus either directly into the internal jugular vein or into the innominate vein.

**D. Lymphatic drainage**

  **1.** The thyroid gland always drains to the ipsilateral lymph nodes in either the anterior or posterior triangle of the neck, along the course of the internal jugular vein to the nodes in the tracheoesophageal groove or to the antero- or paratracheal nodes in the mediastinum.

  **2.** The **nodes in the tracheoesophageal groove** are most important in the spread of thyroid malignancies, since involvement of these nodes may cause tumor extension into the underlying recurrent nerve, trachea, or esophagus.

**E. Important anatomic relationships**

  **1. Recurrent (inferior) laryngeal nerve**

    **a.** The recurrent laryngeal nerve runs in the tracheoesophageal groove in intimate relationship to the posteromedial aspect of the thyroid gland.

        **(1)** On the right the nerve recurs around the subclavian artery and runs an oblique course from lateral to medial, crossing the inferior thyroid artery before entering the tracheoesophageal groove.

        **(2)** On the left the nerve recurs around the ligamentum arteriosum in the mediastinum and runs a course parallel to the tracheoesophageal groove throughout its course in the neck.

    **b.** The nerve divides into an external branch which is sensory to the larynx and an internal branch which supplies the intrinsic muscles of the larynx.

    **c. Injury to the recurrent laryngeal nerve** (see section IV B 8 d) most commonly occurs where the nerve crosses the inferior thyroid artery or where it penetrates the cricothyroid membrane, but can occur anywhere along its course. Injury can be avoided by visualizing the nerve throughout its course during operations requiring complete thyroid lobectomy.

**2. Superior laryngeal nerve**

    **a.** The superior laryngeal nerve has an external branch which is sensory to the larynx and an internal branch which is motor to the cricothyroid muscle.

    **b.** The nerve is intimately intertwined with the branches of the superior thyroid artery.

    **c.** It can be injured during mobilization of the upper pole of the thyroid, especially when the lobe is enlarged.

        **(1) Injury** results in voice weakness, which is especially noticeable in singers or orators.

        **(2)** Injury can be avoided by ligation of the branches of the superior thyroid artery at their junction with the gland rather than along the course of the artery in the neck.

**3. Parathyroid glands** (see also Chapter 20)

    **a.** The superior parathyroids are located at the junction of the upper and middle third of the thyroid on the posteromedial aspect.

    **b.** The inferior parathyroids are located in relationship to the lower pole of the thyroid, either on the surface of the gland or within a 3-cm circle the center of which is formed by the junction of the inferior thyroid artery and the recurrent laryngeal nerve.

    **c. Injury to the parathyroids** during thyroid surgery usually occurs during total lobectomy or total thyroidectomy.

        **(1)** The injury usually results from disruption of the blood supply to the parathyroids.

        **(2)** If this occurs, the consequence is either temporary or permanent hypoparathyroidism, unless the parathyroids can be successfully reimplanted (see Chapter 20, section I A).

## III. ABNORMALITIES OF THYROID DESCENT (see also Chapter 24, section III B)

**A. Route of descent**

    **1.** The thyroid migrates downward from its point of origin at the foramen cecum at the base of the tongue.

    **2.** It descends to assume its normal position on either side of the trachea at the level of the thyroid and cricoid cartilages.

    **3.** Abnormalities of descent of the thyroid may result in ectopic placement of thyroid tissue in the tongue, in the midline of the neck, or in the mediastinum.

**B. Glottic (lingual) thyroid** occurs when the thyroid fails to descend into the neck and remains at the base of the tongue. It may be the only functioning thyroid tissue in the individual.

    **1.** Symptoms of obstruction or difficulty with speech are usually related to goiter formation in the lingual mass.

    **2.** Diagnosis is by inspection or indirect laryngoscopy. A radioiodine thyroid scan should be done to identify the mass as thyroid tissue.

    **3.** Suppression of thyroid-stimulating hormone (TSH) with thyroxine should be the first step in management, since glottic thyroid tissue is usually hypofunctioning.

    **4.** Surgical removal should be considered when a patient has obstructive symptoms, especially if hormonal therapy is ineffective.

**C. Ectopic midline thyroid tissue**

    **1.** This diagnosis should be considered when a midline mass is encountered below the hyoid bone.

**2.** If there is no thyroid gland in the neck, the ectopic thyroid should be confirmed by radioiodine scan, since removal of the ectopic tissue would leave the patient without functioning thyroid tissue.

### D. Mediastinal thyroid

**1.** Most aberrant thyroids in the mediastinum are located in the anterior superior mediastinum. They may represent:
  **a.** Substernal extensions from an enlarged thyroid
  **b.** Normal thyroid tissue resulting from aberrant embryologic descent of the thyroid into the mediastinum

**2.** Normal functioning thyroid tissue will take up radioiodine and can thus be confirmed by a radioiodine scan of the mediastinum.

**3.** However, many substernal extensions of the thyroid (i.e., **substernal goiters**) result from adenomatous hyperplasia and as a result do not take up radioiodine.

**4.** Substernal goiters usually occur in older age-groups.
  **a.** They usually result in tracheoesophageal compression.
  **b.** They do not respond to nonoperative attempts to relieve pressure symptoms by suppressing TSH with thyroxine.

**5.** Operation is usually advised to relieve pressure symptoms or to diagnose an otherwise undiagnosed mediastinal mass.

**6.** Substernal goiters can almost invariably be removed through a cervical incision without the need for sternotomy, since their blood supply is derived from the neck.

### E. Thyroglossal duct cysts and sinuses

**1.** Thyroglossal duct cysts usually present as midline masses located between the hyoid bone and the thyroid isthmus. They are always connected to the base of the tongue, traversing the center of the hyoid bone.

**2.** They may be solid or cystic and may communicate with the skin, forming a sinus.

**3.** These lesions may present at any age, but most are seen in children.

**4.** A history of redness and inflammation from infection in the cyst is present in one-third of the cases.

**5.** Treatment involves radical excision, including a portion of the hyoid bone and the proximal duct extending to the base of the tongue (Sistrunk procedure).

## IV. THYROID DYSFUNCTION REQUIRING SURGERY

### A. Normal thyroid function

**1.** The **follicular cells** of the thyroid are derived primarily from the floor of the foregut. These cells produce the thyroid hormones **triiodothyronine** ($T_3$) and **thyroxine** ($T_4$; tetraiodothyronine).
  **a. Hormone synthesis and release**
    **(1)** Iodine and tyrosine combine to form $T_3$ and $T_4$.
    **(2)** Both of these hormones bind with thyroglobulin, and are stored in the gland until released into the blood stream.
    **(3)** Release is under the control of TSH from the pituitary and thyrotropin-releasing hormone (TRH) from the hypothalamus.
    **(4)** A feedback mechanism regulating $T_3$ and $T_4$ release is related to the level of circulating $T_3$ and $T_4$.
  **b. Hormonal action**
    **(1)** The thyroid hormones activate energy-producing respiratory processes, resulting in an increase in the metabolic rate and an increase in oxygen consumption.
    **(2)** Increased glycogenolysis results in a rise in blood sugar.
    **(3)** The thyroid hormones also enhance metabolic, circulatory, and somatic neuromuscular actions of catecholamines.
      **(a)** The result is an increase in the pulse rate, cardiac output, and blood flow.
      **(b)** Nervousness, irritability, muscular tremors, and muscle wasting can also occur.
      **(c)** These effects can be blocked by the use of $\beta$-blockers such as propranolol.

**2.** The **parafollicular** or **C cells** are derived from the ultimobranchial body. These cells are part of the APUD (amine precursor uptake and decarboxylation) cell system (see Chapter 22, section II) and produce **thyrocalcitonin**.

**B. Graves' disease** (diffuse toxic non-nodular goiter)

**1. Pathogenesis.** Graves' disease is thought to be an autoimmune disease resulting from a defect in cell-mediated immunity.

**a.** A substance known as **long-acting thyroid stimulator (LATS)** is produced which increases the size of the thyroid and its production of thyroid hormone.

**b.** This results in a clinical syndrome of hypermetabolism with associated abnormal eye signs and an unusual form of pretibial edema.

**2. Symptoms and signs due to the hypermetabolic state**

**a.** Symptoms include palpitations, sweating and intolerance to heat, irritability, insomnia and nervousness, weight loss, and fatigue.

**b.** Signs include an audible bruit over the gland, tremors of the hands and tongue, cardiac arrhythmias, and a widening of the palpebral fissure of the eye.

**3. Signs due to the abnormal deposition of mucopolysaccharide and round-cell infiltration** in the tissues include exophthalmos, edema of the eyelids, chemosis, and pretibial edema.

**4. Diagnosis**

**a.** This is confirmed by the presence of an elevated total serum $T_4$, an increase in the $T_3$ resin uptake ($T_3RU$), and an increase in $T_3$ by radioimmunoassay.

**b.** An elevation of the free thyroxine index (the $T_3RU$ value times the total serum $T_4$) and an increase in radioiodine uptake distinguish this form of thyrotoxicosis from thyrotoxicosis without hyperthyroidism (caused by thyroiditis, factitious thyrotoxicosis, or struma ovarii).

**c.** A thyroid scan shows an enlarged thyroid with uniform uptake throughout.

**d.** The serum cholesterol level is decreased, and the blood sugar and alkaline phosphatase are increased.

**5. Medical treatment.** The preferred method of treatment is medical, since the disease has a tendency to remit spontaneously after 1 or 2 years in adults or after 3 to 6 months in children.

**a. Radioiodine ($^{131}I$)** administered orally is simple, safe, and inexpensive.

(1) It avoids the need for surgery, and apparently does not increase the risk of carcinoma.

(2) It has, however, several disadvantages.

(a) It may produce chromosomal abnormalities in the fetus if administered during pregnancy.

(b) It may cause an increase in germ cell chromosomal abnormalities in later life if administered during childhood or early adulthood.

(c) Because of its slow onset of effectiveness, concomitant use of antithyroid drugs may be necessary if the patient is severely symptomatic.

**b. Antithyroid drugs** are effective in about 50% of patients, especially those with symptoms of short duration and with a small gland.

(1) These drugs act by altering various stages of iodine metabolism.

(a) Propylthiouracil and methimazole act through competitive inhibition of peroxidase, blocking the oxidation of iodine to elemental iodine. Propylthiouracil also interferes with the peripheral conversion of $T_4$ to $T_3$.

(b) Iodine in high concentrations blocks the release of thyroid hormones by inhibiting proteolysis. However, glands treated with iodine suppression escape this therapeutic effect after 10 to 14 days of therapy.

(c) Propranolol, a $\beta$-adrenergic blocker, reduces the secondary effects of hypermetabolism, such as tachycardia, without affecting the production of $T_3$ or $T_4$.

(2) Antithyroid drugs are rapidly effective and can reverse symptoms in a short period of time.

(3) Their main disadvantage is that the incidence of recurrence is high if the drugs are stopped, so that prolonged therapy is required.

(4) Their use must be stopped if drug toxicity occurs, manifested by fever, rash, arthralgia, a lupus-like syndrome, and agranulocytosis.

**6. Surgical treatment**

**a.** The preferred operation is bilateral subtotal thyroidectomy.

**b.** This is **indicated** for Graves' disease:

(1) When medical therapy has failed because

(a) Remission has not occurred after treatment for 1 year in adults or for 3 months in children

(b) The patient refuses to take the medication

(c) The patient develops an allergic reaction to antithyroid drugs

**(2)** When radioiodine therapy is not advisable because

    **(a)** The patient is a woman in her childbearing years, for whom radioiodine is contraindicated because of its possible carcinogenic or teratogenic effects

        **(i)** On the patient's own germ cells

        **(ii)** On the fetus if the woman should be pregnant

    **(b)** The patient is a child, for whom radioiodine is contraindicated because of its unknown late carcinogenic or teratogenic effects

  **c.** The **objectives of surgery** are:

    **(1)** To remove enough thyroid tissue to correct the hyperthyroidism, while leaving enough tissue to prevent hypothyroidism (usually 10 g to 20 g)

    **(2)** To do this with a minimum of perioperative complications

  **d.** Despite this, the incidence of postoperative hypothyroidism may be as high as 40%.

**7. Preoperative preparation of the patient.** To minimize the risk of thyroid storm (see section IV 8 a) the patient should be euthyroid prior to operation.

  **a.** Usually, antithyroid drugs are given until the patient is euthyroid, and then Lugol's solution or saturated potassium iodide is given for 7 to 10 days before surgery.

    **(1)** This reduces the risk of thyroid storm both during and after surgery. It also reduces the size and vascularity of the thyroid gland, which increases the technical ease of surgery.

    **(2)** However, it takes several weeks or longer to achieve the euthyroid state. Moreover, in a pregnant woman thyroid drugs can cross the placenta and can cause fetal goiter.

  **b.** Alternatively, especially if patients have had adverse reactions to antithyroid drugs, propranolol can be given in conjunction with Lugol's solution.

    **(1)** This is rapidly effective in restoring the euthyroid state and in reducing thyroid size and vascularity. Moreover, it is not known to cause any fetal abnormalities should the patient be pregnant.

    **(2)** The propranolol must be given for 4 or 5 days postoperatively to prevent thyroid storm, since the half-life of circulating thyroid hormone is 5 to 10 days.

**8. Complications of thyroidectomy**

  **a. Thyroid storm** is a severe hypermetabolic state that causes hyperpyrexia and tachyarrhythmias due to uncontrolled hyperthyroidism.

    **(1)** Thyroid storm is rarely seen when the patient is adequately prepared preoperatively.

    **(2)** It occurs most often when a patient has undiagnosed hyperthyroidism and is operated on for some unrelated emergency.

    **(3)** Treatment is with large doses of antithyroid drugs, iodine, and propranolol.

  **b. Hemorrhage** is a possible complication due to the increased vascularity of the hyperactive thyroid.

    **(1)** Postoperative hemorrhage can cause airway obstruction due to tracheal compression and laryngeal edema.

    **(2)** Treatment is by opening the wounds, evacuating the clot, and controlling the bleeding.

  **c. Hypoparathyroidism** usually develops within the first 24 hours following surgery and results in a subnormal serum calcium concentration.

    **(1)** Symptoms of hypocalcemia include numbness and tingling circumorally or in the fingers and toes, nervousness, and anxiety.

    **(2)** Increased neuromuscular transmission is evidenced by positive Chvostek's and Trousseau's signs.

    **(3)** Treatment is with intravenous calcium gluconate, followed by oral calcium therapy after several days if hypocalcemia persists.

    **(4)** Serum calcium levels should be checked daily for at least 3 days after thyroidectomy, to alert one to the possibility of this complication.

  **d. Recurrent laryngeal nerve injury** produces vocal cord paralysis.

    **(1)** Unilateral injury is usually manifested by hoarseness. If the nerve is intact, the patient will usually recover a normal voice in 3 weeks to 3 months postoperatively.

    **(2)** If the injury is bilateral, airway obstruction results, due to paralysis of the vocal cords in the midline adducted position.

        **(a)** This requires emergency intubation or tracheostomy.

        **(b)** If the nerve is intact and the injury is temporary, recovery usually occurs in 3 to 6 months.

        **(c)** If the injury is permanent, it will require either a permanent tracheostomy or lateral fixation of the arytenoid cartilages with Teflon injections into the cord.

**C. Plummer's disease (toxic nodular goiter)** is a hyperthyroid state caused by either an autonomously hyperfunctioning nodule in an otherwise normal gland, or several hyperfunctioning nodules in a multinodular gland.

1. The disorder is most commonly seen in women beyond the age of 50 years and is usually associated with a history of preexisting multinodular goiter.

2. **Clinical presentation**
   a. Symptoms are not those of the classic hyperthyroidism seen with Graves' disease but are usually related to cardiac arrhythmias, such as palpitations.
      (1) Muscle weakness may be seen, but is rarely profound.
      (2) Hypermetabolic symptoms are infrequent.
   b. Signs suggesting Plummer's disease are arrhythmias, occasional muscle wasting, and the presence of a multinodular goiter.

3. **Laboratory studies**
   a. $T_3$ and $T_4$ are elevated.
   b. Radioiodine uptake is increased in the hyperfunctioning nodules.
   c. The nodules will not be suppressed by exogenously administered $T_4$ (thyroxine).

4. **Treatment**
   a. Since the hyperthyroidism of Plummer's disease results from an abnormality within the thyroid gland itself, thyroidectomy is the preferred form of treatment.
   b. Preoperative preparation and perioperative management are the same as for Graves' disease.

## V. ENLARGEMENTS OF THE THYROID (GOITERS)

A. Enlargements in the thyroid gland have been collectively referred to as **goiters**.

1. Goiters may be diffuse or focal, and may be either smooth or nodular.

2. They may be associated with normal thyroid function or with thyroid hyperfunction or hypofunction.

3. In general,
   a. Diffuse non-nodular goiters with normal or decreased function are due to benign causes
   b. Focal or nodular goiters with normal function may be due to thyroid neoplasms

B. **Diffuse thyroid enlargements**

1. **Colloid and iodine-deficiency goiters**
   a. These are large, bulky, soft enlargements of the thyroid which may grow to sizable proportions.
   b. They occur infrequently in the United States.
   c. They occasionally produce compressive symptoms requiring surgery, but more often than not are removed for cosmetic reasons.
   d. Other treatment is medical and depends on the cause of the goiter.

2. **Thyroiditis.** Inflammations of the thyroid can be acute, subacute, or chronic.
   a. **Acute thyroiditis** is an uncommon disorder caused by the hematogenous spread of microorganisms into the thyroid gland.
      (1) Staphylococci and streptococci have been incriminated, but any organism can be causative.
      (2) The condition may occur in an immunocompromised patient.
      (3) The clinical picture is that of acute inflammation, with pain and tenderness, swelling, and redness over one or both lobes.
      (4) The diagnosis is established by needle aspiration with appropriate bacteriologic studies.
      (5) Treatment is by open drainage or localized resection, with administration of appropriate antibiotics.
   b. **Subacute thyroiditis (giant cell, granulomatous, or de Quervain's thyroiditis)** is thought to be viral in origin and is often preceded by an upper respiratory infection.
      (1) It is characterized by sore throat, enlargement of the gland (which may be asymmetrical), and tenderness and induration over the gland.
      (2) Patients may have symptoms of hyperthyroidism due to the release of thyroid hormone from the gland secondary to the inflammation, but the radioiodine uptake is always decreased, distinguishing it from Graves' disease.
      (3) The disorder is self-limiting, usually lasting from 2 to 6 months.
      (4) Symptoms are controlled with either aspirin or corticosteroids.
         (a) Beta-adrenergic blockade may be used to relieve the symptoms of hyperthyroidism.

      **(b)** Antithyroid drugs are ineffective, since the hyperthyroidism is not caused by increased thyroid hormone synthesis.

    **(5)** Occasionally, subacute thyroiditis is painless, causing hyperthyroidism without symptoms of inflammation in the gland, so that it may resemble Graves' disease clinically.

      **(a)** This form is also distinguished from Graves' disease by the low radioiodine uptake.

      **(b)** Painless thyroiditis not infrequently occurs during the postpartum period.

  **c. Chronic thyroiditis** occurs in two major forms, Hashimoto's and Riedel's.

    **(1) Hashimoto's thyroiditis (struma lymphomatosa)** is a relatively common autoimmune disorder that occurs predominantly in women.

      **(a)** This disease is considered to be autoimmune in nature since it coexists with other autoimmune conditions and is associated with the presence of antithyroid antibodies in the serum.

      **(b)** Because it is a rather common form of thyroid enlargement today, it should be considered in any woman who has a goiter and hypothyroidism. It is usually unassociated with any other symptoms.

      **(c)** The enlargement in the thyroid is most commonly diffuse and less commonly nodular or asymmetrical.

      **(d)** Thyroid function studies are usually normal. Radioiodine uptake and scans show decreased uptake with patchy distribution.

      **(e)** This form of thyroiditis is usually treated with long-term thyroxine therapy. The gland will usually regress in size unless there is considerable fibrosis.

      **(f)** There does not appear to be a predilection for thyroid cancer, but thyroid cancer should be suspected when the thyroiditis is associated with one or more nodules. Needle biopsy is helpful in confirming the diagnosis.

      **(g)** Surgery for thyroiditis is indicated:

        **(i)** When a dominant mass is not suppressed by thyroxine therapy

        **(ii)** When the gland continues to enlarge despite thyroxine therapy

        **(iii)** When the history and physical findings or the needle biopsy is suggestive of thyroid malignancy

    **(2) Riedel's (fibrous) thyroiditis** is a relatively rare form of thyroiditis in which the thyroid parenchyma is almost completely replaced with dense fibrous tissue.

      **(a)** Because the gland is usually stony hard, the condition is difficult to distinguish from thyroid malignancy.

      **(b)** Riedel's thyroiditis usually occurs in middle age and may cause pressure symptoms such as cough, dyspnea, or dysphagia.

      **(c)** Surgery, namely resection of the isthmus, is needed both to confirm the diagnosis and to relieve the symptoms.

## C. Nodular thyroid enlargements

  **1. Diffuse multinodular goiter** is the most common form of thyroid enlargement. It is the cause of a palpable nodule in the thyroid in as many as 10% of the adult population.

  **2.** It is **caused** by adenomatous hyperplasia of the thyroid gland.

    **a.** The thyroid enlargement is thought to be due to long-standing stimulation of the thyroid by TSH during a period of suboptimal thyroid hormone production.

    **b.** The progression to multinodularity occurs through a process of cyclic changes of hyperplasia and colloid formation.

  **3.** The nodules in the glands show a wide variety of **pathologic findings**.

    **a.** Some are filled with colloid, while others show evidence of cystic degeneration.

    **b.** There may be focal calcification, hemorrhage, or scarring.

  **4.** Most patients are asymptomatic, and the nodularity is detected on routine physical examination.

  **5.** Occasionally, attention may be drawn to the nodules because of pain, difficulty in swallowing, or dyspnea if the nodules enlarge either spontaneously or due to hemorrhage.

  **6.** Thyroid function studies are normal, as are thyroid antibodies. Radioiodine uptake is normal but scanning shows variegated uptake of the radioiodine in the areas of multinodularity.

  **7.** Despite the relatively high incidence of adenomatous hyperplasia, the presence of biologically active thyroid cancer in multinodular goiters without clinical evidence of malignancy occurs in fewer than 1% of cases.

  **8. Treatment**

    **a.** If there are no clinical signs of malignancy and the gland is not symptomatic, no treatment is necessary and simple observation is appropriate.

**b.** If the gland is cosmetically objectionable or if pressure symptoms develop, then exogenous thyroid hormone should be given.
   **(1)** The purpose of thyroxine therapy is to suppress endogenous TSH stimulation of the gland and allow the gland to shrink.
   **(2)** Lifelong suppressive therapy with thyroxine should be given to minimize recurrence.
**c.** Subtotal thyroidectomy is advisable if the glands are large enough to produce compressive symptoms and do not regress with thyroxine therapy.
**d.** If patients develop clinical signs of malignancy, this should be confirmed by needle aspiration biopsy, and appropriate surgery should be performed.

## VI. THYROID NEOPLASMS

**A.** The most common reason for thyroid surgery today is to diagnose or treat a suspected thyroid neoplasm that cannot be diagnosed by conventional means.

   **1.** Not infrequently, a solitary or prominent thyroid nodule is detected on physical examination in an asymptomatic patient.

   **2.** The concern is that the nodule will be malignant, although the majority of solitary thyroid nodules are benign.

**B.** The **clinical pathologic classification** of primary thyroid malignancies is shown in Table 18-1.

**C.** **Factors to consider in assessing thyroid nodules**

   **1. The patient's age**
   **a.** In children, 50% of thyroid nodules are malignant.
   **b.** During the childbearing years the vast majority of nodules are benign.
   **c.** The incidence of cancer in nodules increases by about 10% per decade after age 40 years.

   **2. The patient's sex**
   **a.** Thyroid cancer is more common in women than in men.
   **b.** Benign thyroid nodules are also more common in women.
   **c.** Therefore, the likelihood that a nodule will prove to be malignant is greater in men than in women.

   **3. A family history of thyroid malignancy.** Medullary carcinoma of the thyroid may be transmitted as a mendelian dominant trait, but other thyroid cancers are not transmitted genetically.

   **4. A history of radiation exposure**
   **a.** Exposure of the head or neck region to therapeutic x-rays has been found to increase the incidence of thyroid cancer 5- to 10-fold.
   **(1)** The radiation exposure has been as low as 50 rads and as high as 6000 rads.
   **(2)** The radiation has been given for a variety of disorders, such as an enlarged thymus in infancy, enlarged tonsils and adenoids during childhood, congenital hemangiomas of the head or neck region, acne vulgaris, and Hodgkin's disease.
   **b.** The resulting thyroid cancers are no different from those that occur without a prior history of radiation, but the latent interval from the time of radiation exposure until the development of thyroid cancer varies with the age at which the radiation exposure occurred.
   **(1)** When the thyroid is irradiated during infancy, the mean interval until development of thyroid cancer is 10 to 12 years.
   **(2)** When the thyroid is irradiated during adolescence, the mean interval until development of thyroid cancer is 20 to 25 years.
   **(3)** When the thyroid is irradiated during adulthood, the mean interval until development of thyroid cancer is 30 years.

   **5. The characteristics of the nodule**
   **a. Consistency**
   **(1)** Nodules that are firm in consistency suggest malignancy.
   **(2)** Soft nodules are likely to be benign.
   **(3)** However, long-standing adenomatous hyperplasia may be associated with calcification in the nodule, and malignant nodules may undergo cystic degeneration so that they may be somewhat soft to palpation.
   **b. Infiltration** of the nodule into the surrounding thyroid or overlying structures such as the strap muscles or trachea suggests malignancy. However, malignant nodules may have no sign of infiltration and may mimic benign nodules.
   **c.** If the nodule is solitary, it has a 20% chance of being malignant. **Multiple nodules** are present in as many as 40% of proven cases of thyroid malignancy.

**Table 18-1.** Clinical Pathologic Classification of Primary Thyroid Malignant Lesions

| Pathologic Variety | Local Invasion by Primary Lesion | Multicentricity Thyroid | Regional Lymph Node Metastases | Distant Metastases |
|---|---|---|---|---|
| Carcinoma | | | | |
| Well-differentiated | | | | |
| Papillary* | Uncommon | Common | Common | Uncommon |
| Follicular* | | | | |
|   Low-grade, encapsulated | Rare | Rare | Uncommon | Occasional |
|   High-grade, angioinvasive | Common | Occasional | Common | Common |
| Hürthle cell tumors | Uncommon | Common | Common | Occasional |
| Sclerosing ("occult" or minimal) | Uncommon | Rare | Occasional | Rare |
| Medullary (parafollicular C-cell origin) | Common | Constant in familial / Occasional in sporadic | Common | Common |
| Anaplastic | Always | Common | Common | Common |
| Lymphoma | Involves entire gland | Involves entire gland | Systemic disease usual but not constant | |

Note.—Reprinted with permission from Block MA and Cerny JC: Endocrine system. In *General Surgery—Therapy Update Service.* Edited by Beahrs OH and Beart RW Jr. Media, PA, Harwal Publishing Co, 1984, p 2-7.

*Associated foci of anaplastic carcinoma convert this to virulence of anaplastic variety.

d. Nodules that **suddenly appear** or **suddenly increase in size** should be suspected of being thyroid neoplasms. Hemorrhage into a preexisting nodule such as adenomatous hyperplasia can cause a sudden increase in the size of the nodule, but this is frequently associated with pain.

6. **Ipsilateral lymph node enlargement** suggests thyroid malignancy. In children, as many as 50% of thyroid cancers are first detected because of cervical lymph node enlargement.

7. **The mobility of the vocal cords.** This should be assessed preoperatively in all patients undergoing thyroid operations.
   a. Ipsilateral vocal cord paralysis in a patient with a thyroid nodule is almost diagnostic of a thyroid malignancy that has infiltrated the recurrent laryngeal nerve.
   b. The paralysis may not be associated with noticeable voice changes, and therefore the cords should be examined by either indirect or direct laryngoscopy, or by nasal pharyngoscopy.
   c. Examination should be repeated postoperatively if voice abnormalities occur.

D. **Diagnostic studies.** Although it is the mainstay in distinguishing benign from malignant thyroid nodules, clinical evaluation alone may be insufficient, and therefore other diagnostic studies may be needed.

1. **Thyroid function tests** are of little value in diagnosing thyroid cancer.
   a. Nearly all thyroid cancers are nonfunctioning, as are the nodules of adenomatous hyperplasia.
   b. Therefore, fewer than 1% of all thyroid malignancies will be associated with hyperfunction.

2. **Antithyroid antibodies** may be elevated in patients with Hashimoto's thyroiditis, but thyroid cancer may coexist with thyroiditis, and therefore a positive antibody test does not preclude the diagnosis of thyroid cancer.

3. A **thyrocalcitonin assay** will be elevated in patients with medullary carcinoma of the thyroid.

4. **Radioisotope scanning** of the thyroid may be done with radioiodine or with technetium-99m ($^{99m}$Tc) pertechnetate.
   a. These isotope tracers are taken up by normally functioning thyroid tissue, which appears as a "hot" area on a thyroid scan.
   b. Nodules that do not take up the tracers appear as "cold" areas.
   c. Approximately 20% of cold nodules will be malignant, and approximately 40% of thyroid cancers will take up the radioisotope tracer to some degree.
   d. Thus, radioisotope scanning may exclude nodules which are not malignant if they appear "hot," but does not discriminate benign "cold" nodules from malignant ones.
   e. Iodine-123 ($^{123}$I) and -125 ($^{125}$I) give less radiation exposure than iodine-131 ($^{131}$I) because they have shorter half-lives than $^{131}$I. They do not provide any better discrimination than $^{131}$I between benign and malignant thyroid nodules.
   f. $^{99m}$Tc pertechnetate is trapped but, in contrast to radioiodine, is not organified by the thyroid gland.
      (1) Nodules that are "cold" to radioiodine will also be "cold" to $^{99m}$Tc.
      (2) However, tumors of the thyroid may take up $^{99m}$Tc and appear "hot" on the scan due to the vascularity of the tumor.
      (3) Therefore, all nodules that are "hot" on a $^{99m}$Tc scan should be scanned with radioiodine to determine their function.
      (4) $^{99m}$Tc delivers only a fraction of the radiation that is delivered by $^{131}$I. It does not discriminate any better than does $^{131}$I between benign and malignant thyroid nodules.

5. **Ultrasonography**
   a. Using an ultrasound probe, one is able to map an image of the size and shape of the thyroid gland and the nodules that it contains.
   b. Thyroid nodules thus can be identified as either cystic, solid, or complex (that is, a mixture of solid and cystic components).
   c. While ultrasonography is able to distinguish pure cysts of the thyroid, which are rarely malignant, from complex or solid masses, it cannot distinguish benign from malignant complex or solid masses.
   d. Ultrasonography is helpful in identifying thyroid nodules that are not clinically palpable and in directing a needle to a nonpalpable nodule for biopsy.

6. **Needle biopsy** of the thyroid is designed to obtain cells for histopathologic or cytopathologic examination as an aid in the diagnosis of thyroid nodules and the planning of therapy.

**a.** Needle biopsy is considered to be the most useful diagnostic tool for distinguishing benign from malignant thyroid nodules, short of surgery itself.

**b. Types of needle biopsy**

   **(1) Core biopsy**

   **(a)** Using a 14-gauge, specially designed needle (Vim-Silverman or Tru-Cut), this biopsy technique obtains from the thyroid nodule a cylinder of tissue that is then fixed and stained for histopathologic analysis.

   **(b)** It is the most accurate method of assessing the histologic nature of a thyroid nodule.

   **(c)** However, because of the large size of the needle, it is unsuitable for biopsying small nodules.

   **(d)** The incidence of complications is relatively high.

   **(2) Large-needle biopsy**

   **(a)** A plug of tissue is aspirated from the nodule by applying suction to a syringe attached to an 18- or 20-gauge needle that is inserted into the nodule. Fragments of tissue are obtained in this way for histopathologic preparation, as well as cells for cytopathologic preparation.

   **(b)** This technique has the same advantages as core biopsy, and has a lower rate of complications.

   **(3) Fine-needle aspiration**

   **(a)** This technique obtains a specimen for cytopathologic examination.

   **(b)** In contrast to the other techniques, which provide a core of tissue, fine-needle aspiration allows individual cells and clusters of cells to be examined.

   **(c)** The technique requires interpretation by a well-trained thyroid cytopathologist.

   **(d)** It has a good degree of accuracy and specificity in diagnosing thyroid malignant lesions and, due to the small size of the needle, is associated with virtually no complications.

   **(e)** Its main disadvantage is that it obtains only cells for evaluation.

**c.** Combining either core or large-needle biopsy with fine-needle aspiration is considered to be the best method for diagnosing or excluding malignancy in a thyroid nodule. However, none of these biopsy techniques can be relied upon to distinguish benign from malignant follicular neoplasms.

## E. Operative approach to the thyroid nodule

**1. General considerations**

**a.** Operative removal is the mainstay of treatment for thyroid carcinoma.

**b.** The extent of the operation will depend upon:

   **(1)** The type of thyroid cancer found

   **(2)** The extent of the tumor, as determined from the preoperative assessment and the operative findings

   **(3)** The biologic aggressiveness of the tumor (see section VI E 2)

**c.** For a solitary nodule confined to one lobe, the minimal operation is total removal of that lobe and the isthmus, and removal of the anterior portion of the opposite lobe.

**d.** A frozen section of the resected tissue must always be obtained in order to determine whether the nodule is benign or malignant.

   **(1)** If the lesion is grossly benign in appearance and the frozen section reports a benign lesion, but the permanent sections reveal it to be papillary or follicular carcinoma, the extent of further surgery will be determined by the biologic aggressiveness of the lesion.

   **(2)** If the lesion grossly appears to be malignant and is confined to one lobe without invasion of surrounding tissues, then total removal of that lobe and the isthmus, and near-total removal of the opposite lobe is appropriate therapy.

   **(3)** If the lesion grossly appears malignant and extends beyond the thyroid or involves both lobes, then total thyroidectomy is indicated.

**e.** Lymph node resection is indicated when nodes appear to be grossly involved.

   **(1)** The resection should generally concentrate on nodes in the interjugular location.

   **(2)** Prophylactic removal of uninvolved lymph nodes is of no proven benefit.

**f.** The parathyroid glands and the recurrent laryngeal nerve should be identified in all operations. The parathyroid glands should be reimplanted in an appropriate skeletal muscle site if their blood supply is compromised during thyroidectomy.

**g.** The complication rate following total thyroidectomy, and especially the incidence of permanent hypoparathyroidism, is significantly greater than the rate following near-total thyroidectomy. Therefore, total thyroidectomy should not be done unless it is of proven clinical benefit.

2. **Biologic aggressiveness of thyroid cancers.** Three risk groups have been defined for patients with well-differentiated thyroid cancer, based on an analysis by the Lahey Clinic.
   a. The **low-risk group** consists of women under age 50 years and men under age 40 years with papillary thyroid carcinoma.
      (1) Unless both lobes are grossly involved with tumor, patients in this group do as well with near-total thyroidectomy as with total thyroidectomy.
      (2) The remaining thyroid remnant is ablated postoperatively with $^{131}$I.
      (3) After surgery, patients should receive exogenous thyroid hormone for life, in doses sufficient to suppress endogenous TSH production.
      (4) With comparable treatment, the recurrence rate and death rate in this group were found to be significantly lower than in the high-risk group.
   b. The **medium-risk group** consists of women under age 50 and men under age 40 with follicular carcinoma.
      (1) In this group, there is a higher incidence of recurrence after near-total thyroidectomy than in the low-risk group. Therefore, total thyroidectomy is indicated as the primary treatment.
      (2) Radioiodine is administered postoperatively if there is any uptake in the neck on a scan after surgery.
      (3) Patients should receive exogenous thyroid hormone for life, to suppress endogenous TSH production.
   c. The **high-risk group** consists of women over age 50 and men over age 40 with **either** papillary or follicular carcinoma.
      (1) In this age-group, the tumors are much more aggressive and require a more aggressive initial approach, since local recurrences are more difficult to treat and the mortality rate is significantly greater.
      (2) Total thyroidectomy is indicated in these patients.
      (3) Lymph node dissection of palpable nodes should be more extensive than in the lower-risk groups.
      (4) As in the medium-risk group, radioiodine ablation of any tissue demonstrating radioiodine uptake postoperatively should be carried out, and exogenous thyroid hormone should be administered to suppress TSH production.

F. **Types of thyroid malignancy**

   1. **Papillary carcinoma**
      a. **Incidence**
         (1) Papillary carcinoma accounts for 80% of all thyroid cancers in children, and 60% in adults.
         (2) It affects women twice as often as men, and is the most common histologic type seen in patients with a prior history of radiation exposure.
      b. The tumor is characterized by a slow rate of growth, with spread to regional lymphatics in 50% of the cases. It spreads by way of the bloodstream in fewer than 5% of cases.
      c. Tumors range in size from occult (less than 0.5 cm in diameter) to tumors which involve an entire lobe or both lobes.
      d. In 40% of cases, the tumor is multicentric in origin.
         (1) Microscopic multicentric lesions rarely develop into clinical carcinoma.
         (2) Macroscopic multicentric lesions will usually behave biologically like papillary cancer.
      e. Some tumors are well encapsulated, with minimal invasion of adjacent normal thyroid. Others are poorly encapsulated, with invasion to perithyroidal structures.
      f. **Prognosis**
         (1) This is excellent with occult or well-encapsulated intrathyroidal carcinoma. Patients with these tumors have a 20-year survival rate of better than 90%.
         (2) Prognosis is poor when the tumor is poorly encapsulated and extends by extrathyroidal invasion. The 20-year survival rate is less than 50%.
         (3) Prognosis is also poorer as the patient's age increases beyond 40 years.
         (4) Survival does not appear to be adversely affected by lymphatic spread.

   2. **Follicular carcinoma**
      a. **Incidence**
         (1) Follicular carcinoma accounts for approximately 20% of all thyroid malignancies. It is more common in areas of the world where iodine-deficiency goiter is in evidence.
         (2) It also affects women twice as often as men.
         (3) Its relative frequency increases after age 40.
      b. Follicular carcinoma spreads primarily through the bloodstream by way of angioinvasion. It rarely spreads to regional lymph nodes except for locally invasive nodules that extend into the perithyroidal tissue.

   **c.** The tumor is slow-growing and usually unifocal.

   **d.** When found cytologically to be combined with papillary elements, its biologic behavior is similar to that of papillary carcinoma.

   **e. Prognosis**

      **(1)** Prognosis is good when there is minimal vascular invasion, with a better than 80% 20-year survival rate.

      **(2)** Prognosis is poor when there is gross invasion, with a less than 20% 20-year survival rate.

**3. Medullary carcinoma**

   **a. Incidence**

      **(1)** Medullary carcinoma of the thyroid accounts for fewer than 10% of all thyroid cancers.

      **(2)** It occurs at all ages, without predilection for either sex.

      **(3)** It most commonly occurs sporadically, but also can be genetically transmitted.

         **(a)** When it occurs sporadically, it usually appears as a solitary lesion.

         **(b)** When transmitted genetically, it may occur as a solitary lesion or may be a part of multiple endocrine adenomatosis (MEA) syndrome type II (Sipple's syndrome; see Chapter 22, sections I B 2, I C 2, and I D 2).

   **b.** Early spread to the lymphatics is characteristic, and spread by way of the bloodstream is also common.

   **c.** There are two types of medullary carcinoma, which are indistinguishable histologically:

      **(1)** Those characterized by aggressive, rapid growth, rapid spread, and early metastasis

      **(2)** Those characterized by slow growth and a prolonged course despite metastasis

   **d.** Since these tumors arise from the C cells of the thyroid, they produce thyrocalcitonin.

      **(1)** This hormone can be detected by radioimmunoassay in early stages of tumor development.

      **(2)** In patients with hereditary MEA type II, the disease can be detected in this way prior to the development of clinically evident malignancy.

   **e. Prognosis** is poorer than for papillary or follicular carcinoma, and is related to the stage of the tumor at the time of its initial treatment.

      **(1)** Stage I medullary carcinoma has a 50% 20-year survival rate.

      **(2)** Stage II has a less than 10% 20-year survival rate.

      **(3)** Death results from generalized metastasis.

      **(4)** Hereditary MEA syndrome is totally curable by total thyroidectomy if detected and treated prior to the development of clinically evident malignancy.

**4. Anaplastic carcinoma of the thyroid**

   **a. Incidence**

      **(1)** This tumor accounts for fewer than 10% of all thyroid cancers.

      **(2)** It is most common between ages 50 and 70, and shows no predilection for either sex.

   **b.** Anaplastic carcinomas are characterized by either small cells, giant cells, or spindle cells.

   **c.** They usually arise from a preexisting, well-differentiated thyroid neoplasm such as a follicular lesion.

   **d.** They grow rapidly into local structures such as the trachea and esophagus, and metastasize early by way of the lymphatics and the bloodstream, so that they are usually incurable at the time of initial presentation.

   **e. Prognosis**

      **(1)** This is poor, with a fatal outcome in almost all instances, regardless of the type of treatment.

      **(2)** When treatment appears successful, the lesion may well have been a lymphoma instead of a small-cell anaplastic carcinoma, and the histologic nature of the neoplasm should be confirmed by electron microscopy.

**5. Lymphosarcoma (lymphoma) of the thyroid**

   **a.** This tumor accounts for fewer than 1% of all thyroid malignancies and affects mostly women aged 50 to 70.

   **b.** Pathologically, these are usually small-cell tumors and may be difficult to distinguish from small-cell anaplastic carcinoma except by electron microscopy.

   **c.** The lesion may occur primarily in the thyroid gland as an extranodal growth, or it may be part of a generalized lymphomatous process.

   **d.** The focal type is best treated by radiation therapy, whereas the diffuse type will probably require systemic multidrug chemotherapy.

   **e.** Prognosis is variable and depends on the cell type and whether the tumor is focal or diffused.

# 19
# The Adrenal Gland

Herbert E. Cohn
John S. Radomski

## I. GENERAL CONSIDERATIONS

**A.** The adrenal glands are of importance to the surgeon primarily because they are the source of several tumors, benign and malignant, and of hyperplasias, primary and secondary.

**B.** Some of these lesions produce syndromes due to the overproduction of normal adrenal hormones. These include Cushing's syndrome, Conn's syndrome, and pheochromocytomas.

**C.** The diagnosis and treatment of these disease states require a thorough knowledge of the production, action, and metabolism of the adrenal hormones.

## II. EMBRYOLOGY. The adrenal gland consists of two distinct parts, the **cortex** and the **medulla**, each of which has a different embryologic origin.

**A.** The **adrenal medulla** originates from ectodermal cells of neural crest origin.

  **1.** These cells migrate from the sympathetic ganglion and combine to form the medulla, which is surrounded by mesodermal cortex.

  **2.** Additional **collections of adrenal medullary tissue** can form. These are most frequently found in the paraganglia, in the organ of Zuckerkandl just below the origin of the inferior mesenteric artery, and in the mediastinum.

**B.** The **adrenal cortex** is derived from mesodermal cells near the genital ridge.

  **1.** These cells coalesce to form a complete layer around the ectodermal cells that will form the adrenal medulla.

  **2.** Occasionally these cells become separated from the main cortex and form **adrenocortical rests**. These are most commonly found in the ovary or testis, and near the adrenal glands and kidneys.

## III. ANATOMY

**A.** There are two adrenal glands, each one lying on the medial aspect of the superior pole of a kidney. The normal combined weight of the two glands is about 10 g.

**B.** **Histologically**, three areas can be recognized in the cortex:

  **1.** The **zona glomerulosa** is the outer zone where the production of **aldosterone** takes place.

  **2.** The **zona fasciculata** is the intermediate zone where cortisol and the other **glucocorticoids** are produced.

  **3.** The **zona reticularis** is the inner zone where **androgens and estrogens** are made.

**C.** **Vasculature**

  **1.** The **arterial supply** to the adrenals varies, but arises from three primary sources:
    **a.** The phrenic artery
    **b.** The aorta
    **c.** The renal artery

  **2.** The **venous drainage** is more constant.

**a.** There is usually a large single vein on each side of the body. The right adrenal vein drains into the vena cava, and the left adrenal vein empties into the left renal vein.
**b.** Small accessory veins can occur.

**3. The adrenal portal system.** Venous blood from the cortex, containing high levels of glucocorticoids, drains into the medulla, helping to induce the enzyme phenylethanolamine-N-methyltransferase. This enzyme methylates norepinephrine to form epinephrine.

## IV. ADRENAL HORMONES AND CATECHOLAMINES

**A.** The **adrenal cortex** produces three main classes of **steroid hormones:** the glucocorticoids, the mineralocorticoids, and the sex steroids—androgens and estrogens.

**1. Glucocorticoids.** The most important physiologically is cortisol.
   **a.** Production of cortisol takes place primarily in the zona fasciculata. There is a diurnal variation, with the highest levels occurring around 6:00 A.M.
   **b. Regulation**
      **(1) Adrenocorticotropic hormone (ACTH; corticotropin)** is produced by the anterior pituitary gland. ACTH stimulates the production of cortisol by the adrenal. **Cortisol,** in turn, exerts a negative feedback on ACTH production at the hypothalamic-pituitary level.
      **(2) Corticotropin-releasing factor (CRF)** is produced by the hypothalamus and stimulates the release of ACTH from the pituitary.
   **c. Free cortisol** is the active hormone. Normally, most circulating cortisol is bound to corticosteroid-binding globulin (CBG). When large amounts of cortisol are produced, the binding sites become saturated and the levels of free hormone will rise.
   **d.** Cortisol is **metabolized** in the liver by conjugation with glucuronide. This renders it water-soluble for urinary excretion. The level of urinary 17-hydroxycorticosteroids reflects glucocorticoid production and metabolism. However, in states of hypercortisolism the urinary free cortisol is more accurate.

**2. Mineralocorticoids. Aldosterone** is the major mineralocorticoid produced by the adrenal gland.
   **a.** Aldosterone is produced in the zona glomerulosa of the adrenal cortex.
   **b. Regulation**
      **(1)** Aldosterone production is regulated chiefly by the **renin-angiotensin system**.
         **(a)** Renin is released by the juxtaglomerular cells of the kidney in response to a fall in blood pressure.
         **(b)** Renin converts angiotensinogen (made in the liver) to angiotensin I.
         **(c)** Angiotensin I is converted to angiotensin II by angiotensin-converting enzyme, which is produced by endothelial cells.
         **(d)** Angiotensin II stimulates the adrenal cortex to release aldosterone.
      **(2)** Aldosterone production is minimally controlled by ACTH.
      **(3)** The sympathetic nervous system can also stimulate the release of aldosterone.
   **c.** Aldosterone is **metabolized** in a similar manner to cortisol. It is excreted in the urine in small quantities and can be measured by radioimmunoassay.

**3. Androgens and estrogens** are produced in the zona reticularis of the adrenal cortex. The urinary level of 17-ketosteroids reflects the androgen production. Estrogens can also be measured in the urine.

**B.** The **adrenal medulla** is the site of **catecholamine** production.

**1.** Figure 19-1 summarizes the pathways of catecholamine production and metabolism in the adrenal medulla.

**2.** Dopamine can be metabolized by an alternate pathway to homovanillic acid.

**3.** The levels of metanephrine, normetanephrine, vanillylmandelic acid (VMA), and the individual catecholamines can be measured in the urine to detect neoplasms (see section IX D).

## V. CONGENITAL VIRILIZING ADRENAL HYPERPLASIA

**A. Pathogenesis**

**1.** If an adrenocortical hormone or an enzyme is missing from the pathway of cortisol production, the consequent shortage of cortisol will cause an increase in ACTH activity, and adrenal hyperplasia will result. The cortisol precursors will then be shunted into the production of androgens.

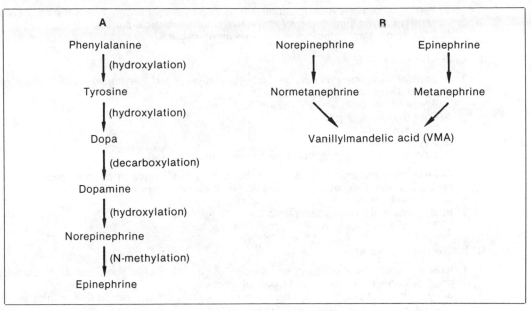

**Figure 19-1.** Pathways of (A) catecholamine production and (B) metabolism.

**2.** Although several different enzymes can be congenitally absent, the most common defect is a block in hydroxylation at C-21 of the cortisol molecule.

**B. Clinical presentation**

   **1.** Virilization results from the hormonal defect. In the female, this produces pseudohermaphroditism, and in the male, macrogenitosomia precox.

   **2.** In a minority of cases, the block is more complete, and a severe salt-losing state with vascular collapse results from the aldosterone deficiency.

**C.** The **diagnosis** can be suspected from the characteristic virilization and the excess levels of 17-ketosteroids in the urine.

**D. Treatment**

   **1.** The metabolic deficiency is treated with steroid replacement.

   **2.** In females, plastic surgical procedures are often necessary to correct the genital deformities.

   **3.** An accurate sex assignment must be made in female pseudohermaphrodites by means of karyotyping and Barr body analysis.

**VI. ADRENOCORTICAL INSUFFICIENCY (ADDISON'S DISEASE).** This condition is important to the practicing surgeon because patients with Addison's disease are not capable of undergoing the stress of surgery without receiving corticosteroid support.

**A. Types.** Addison's disease may be primary or secondary.

   **1.** In **primary adrenocortical insufficiency**, the function of the adrenal cortex is diminished or absent because of adrenal pathology. Some **causes** are:
   **a.** An autoimmune attack on the adrenal gland
   **b.** Bilateral adrenal tuberculosis
   **c.** Adrenal fungal infections
   **d.** Bilateral adrenal hemorrhage. This can occur:
      **(1)** Secondary to meningococcal septicemia
      **(2)** Postpartum
      **(3)** In patients on anticoagulant therapy

   **2. Secondary adrenocortical insufficiency** is due to atrophy of the adrenal cortex secondary to a decreased pituitary production of ACTH.

**a.** The usual **cause** is ACTH suppression by corticosteroid drugs. This is the most common cause of adrenal insufficiency encountered in the surgical patient.
**b.** Primary pituitary pathology is a less common cause.

**B. Clinical presentation**

1. A **cortisol deficiency** occurs in both the primary and secondary forms. Some of the **manifestations** are:
   **a.** Anorexia, malaise, and weight loss
   **b.** Poor tolerance of stress
   **c.** Hypoglycemia
   **d.** Hypotension
   **e.** Occasionally, hyperpigmentation of the skin

2. **Aldosterone deficiency** occurs only in the primary form, since aldosterone production is not primarily under feedback control via ACTH. It causes a tendency for:
   **a.** Volume depletion
   **b.** Hyponatremia and hyperkalemia
   **c.** Azotemia and acidosis

**C. Preparation for surgery**

1. After a patient discontinues steroid therapy, it can take up to a year for the hypothalamic-pituitary-adrenal axis to return to normal function.
   **a.** Usually, a patient who has taken steroids regularly for any period during the past year is assumed to have inadequate adrenal reserve.
   **b.** If there is time, an ACTH stimulation test may be performed to assess the patient's adrenocortical reserve.

2. **Perioperative steroid replacement** is handled on an individual basis, and depends on how long the patient was taking steroids, the dose that was taken, and the magnitude of the planned procedure. The following is a general **guideline** for a patient undergoing a major operation who is a **chronic steroid user:**
   **a.** Hydrocortisone (300 mg) is given on the day of surgery (100 mg before surgery, 100 mg during, and 100 mg after).
   **b.** The steroid dose is tapered off over the next 3 to 5 days, until the patient is back on his or her preoperative oral dose.

# VII. HYPERADRENOCORTICALISM (CUSHING'S SYNDROME)

**A.** Cushing's syndrome results from the effects of chronically elevated cortisol levels.

**B.** At least three different **mechanisms** can cause Cushing's syndrome:

1. **Adrenal Cushing's syndrome** accounts for about 15% of the cases.
   **a.** It is caused by an excess of cortisol that is produced autonomously by the adrenal cortex. This can be due to an adenoma, a carcinoma, or bilateral nodular dysplasia.
   **b.** The remaining adrenocortical tissue atrophies, and ACTH levels are low because of suppression by the excess cortisol.

2. **Ectopic Cushing's syndrome** also represents about 15% of the cases.
   **a.** In this form, ACTH is produced by an extra-adrenal, extrapituitary neoplasm. The result is a hyperplasia of the adrenocortical tissue, with consequent hypercortisolism.
   **b.** The cause is most commonly an oat cell carcinoma of the lung, but the syndrome can also occur with bronchial carcinoids, thymomas, and pancreatic and liver tumors.

3. **Pituitary Cushing's syndrome**, or **Cushing's disease**, accounts for about 70% of the cases of Cushing's syndrome.
   **a.** It results from an overproduction of ACTH by the pituitary, which results in bilateral adrenal hyperplasia.
   **b.** The source of the excess ACTH has been debated.
   **(1)** Pituitary tumors, either chromophobic or basophilic adenomas, probably account for the majority of cases. Some autopsy series have shown pituitary tumors in at least 60% of patients with Cushing's disease.
   **(2)** However, in the remaining patients no tumor was found. This raises the possibility of an abnormality in the hypothalamic-pituitary axis resulting in increased ACTH secretion.

### C. Clinical presentation

1. The presentation of Cushing's syndrome is extremely variable and consists of any combination of various features.

2. Some of the more common manifestations are listed in Table 19-1.

**Table 19-1.** Common manifestations of Cushing's syndrome

| | |
|---|---|
| Hypertension | Peripheral muscle wasting |
| Diabetes | Striae |
| Hypokalemic alkalosis | Easy bruisability |
| Osteoporosis | Hirsutism |
| Buffalo hump | Acne |
| Truncal obesity | Menstrual irregularities |
| Muscle weakness | Emotional lability |

### D. Diagnosis.
No one test is conclusive for Cushing's syndrome. The laboratory test results and the clinical situation must all be considered together in order to make an accurate diagnosis.

1. **Plasma total cortisol** is the most direct measurement, since Cushing's syndrome is a state of hypercortisolism.
   a. The accuracy of this determination is increased by measuring morning and afternoon samples, as well as a morning sample after a suppressing dose of dexamethasone the night before.
   b. Plasma cortisol levels are suggestive of Cushing's syndrome if they exceed 30 μg/dl at 8:00 A.M. and 15 μg/dl at 5:00 P.M., or 10 μg/dl at 8:00 A.M. following a midnight dose of 1 mg dexamethasone, especially if these results are reproducible on several different days.
   c. The overnight dexamethasone suppression test is not fully reliable, as both false-positives and false-negatives occur. Adjusting the dose of dexamethasone on the basis of the patient's weight may reduce the number of false-positive and false-negative results.

2. If further confirmation is needed, the level of **urinary free cortisol** is the most reliable urinary index of hypercortisolism, due to the increased renal clearance of unmetabolized cortisol.

3. The normal **diurnal rhythm** of cortisol secretion is usually lost in Cushing's syndrome.

### E.
Once the diagnosis of Cushing's syndrome has been made, the underlying pathophysiologic mechanism (see section VII B) must be identified.

1. The **plasma ACTH level** gives a good indication of the type of Cushing's syndrome.
   a. Extremely low values are seen with adrenal Cushing's syndrome, due to the suppressive effects of cortisol.
   b. Very high levels occur with ectopic Cushing's syndrome, due to the autonomous ACTH production.
   c. In pituitary Cushing's syndrome, the values remain in the normal range in about 50% of the cases, but are elevated in the other 50%.

2. The problem occurs in **differentiating ectopic from pituitary Cushing's syndrome** when the ACTH level is in the intermediate range. Three methods are helpful in making this distinction:
   a. **High-dose dexamethasone suppression test**
      (1) After the diagnosis of Cushing's syndrome has been made, the patient is given dexamethasone 8 mg/day for 2 days and the urine is collected for measurement of 17-hydroxycorticosteroids.
      (2) In pituitary Cushing's syndrome the 17-hydroxycorticosteroid levels will usually decrease below 50% of normal, whereas they will show no suppression in the ectopic syndrome.
      (3) However, there have been enough recorded exceptions in both cases to make this test of questionable value.
   b. **Jugular versus peripheral ACTH levels**
      (1) Samples of venous blood are drawn from a peripheral site and, by catheterization, from the inferior petrosal sinus.
      (2) Ratios of petrosal to peripheral ACTH greater than 2.0 have correlated with a pituitary source for the Cushing's syndrome, and ratios less than 1.5 with an ectopic source.
   c. **Plasma lipotropic hormone (LPH, lipotropin) concentration.** This tends to be higher than the ACTH concentration with ectopic Cushing's syndrome, while the opposite holds true for pituitary Cushing's syndrome.

**F. Localization of the tumor**

1. In **pituitary Cushing's syndrome**, polytomography of the sella turcica has localized some pituitary tumors, but computed tomography (CT) is more sensitive and is specific for detecting small adenomas.

2. In **ectopic Cushing's syndrome** a chest film will usually show the offending neoplasm. However, a technique such as CT may be needed to detect pancreatic or hepatic tumors.

3. For **adrenal Cushing's syndrome**, several techniques are available.
   a. **CT** can correctly identify over 90% of adrenal lesions, including adenomas larger than 1 cm in diameter, carcinomas, and bilateral hyperplasia.
   b. **Radioisotope scanning**
      (1) Radioiodine-labeled 19-iodocholesterol can successfully localize functioning adrenocortical tumors, but the radiation dose is in the millicurie range and several days are needed before enough of the isotopic label accumulates to provide an image.
      (2) A new radiocholesterol analog, NP-59, may offer quicker images with less radiation.
   c. **Arteriography** will localize adrenal tumors and is helpful in assessing the arterial supply of a neoplasm before its surgical removal.
   d. **Retrograde adrenal venography** can also localize adrenal tumors and allows for bilateral cortisol measurements. However, there is a 5% risk of adrenal hemorrhage and possible infarction.
   e. **Venacavography** is helpful, if a malignancy is suspected, to assess the intravenous extension of the tumor.

**G. Treatment**

1. **Curative therapy**
   a. In **ectopic Cushing's syndrome**, treatment is directed toward the underlying neoplasm secreting ACTH. Removal of the tumor is curative. However, because of the diffuse nature of oat cell lung cancers, often only palliative therapy can be offered.
   b. In **adrenal Cushing's syndrome**, treatment involves total adrenalectomy of the gland affected by adenoma or carcinoma. Even if all of the malignant tissue cannot be removed, palliative therapy will be easier if as much tumor as possible is resected.
   c. In **pituitary Cushing's syndrome**, treatment depends on the cause.
      (1) If a pituitary adenoma is localized, then the procedure of choice is a trans-sphenoidal resection of the tumor.
      (2) **Pituitary irradiation** from an external source has provided effective treatment in up to 80% of children. However, for adults the cure rate is only about 15% to 20%.
         (a) Implantation of yttrium-90 may improve results but this requires a separate operation for implantation and may cause progressive hypopituitarism.
         (b) Another disadvantage of radiation therapy is the lag period of up to 18 months before effects are seen.
      (3) **Bilateral total adrenalectomy**
         (a) With the advent of effective trans-sphenoidal removal of pituitary adenomas, bilateral adrenalectomy is now reserved for cases where no pituitary adenoma is found, where radiation has failed, or where the patient is too sick to tolerate the prolonged radiation process or to await its ultimate effect.
         (b) The advantage of bilateral adrenalectomy is its immediate and complete control of the cushingoid state.
         (c) The disadvantages are the increased morbidity and mortality secondary to the operative procedure.
            (i) It produces a permanent addisonian state.
            (ii) In at least 15% of the cases an ACTH-secreting pituitary tumor develops (**Nelson's syndrome**). Therefore, all patients treated for Cushing's disease with bilateral total adrenalectomy must be monitored yearly with visual field examination and sellar tomography.

2. **Palliative chemotherapy** can be offered to those patients with unresectable or incompletely resected malignancies, and also during the lag phase to those undergoing radiation treatment.
   a. Remissions can be obtained in about 60% of the cases but relapse is rapid after drug cessation.
   b. Two groups of drugs exist with differing sites of action.
      (1) Drugs acting on the adrenal cortex, inhibiting steroid synthesis, include mitotane (formerly called o,p'-DDD), metyrapone, trilostane, and aminoglutethimide.
      (2) Centrally acting drugs appear to be less toxic and faster-acting. They apparently act by affecting the hypothalamic release of CRF, and therefore pituitary ACTH production.

These drugs include cyproheptadine (a serotonin antagonist) and bromocriptine (a dopamine agonist).

## VIII. PRIMARY HYPERALDOSTERONISM (CONN'S SYNDROME)

**A.** Conn's syndrome is due to the excess secretion of aldosterone by the adrenal cortex.

   **1.** It is due to a unilateral adenoma of the adrenal in 85% of the cases, and to bilateral adenomas in fewer than 5%.

   **2.** Bilateral hyperplasia causes about 10% of the cases.

   **3.** Rarely, the syndrome is due to an adrenocortical carcinoma.

**B.** It is important to **distinguish primary from secondary hyperaldosteronism**.

   **1.** In the **secondary form** there is an increase in plasma renin and subsequently in aldosterone. This results from a decrease in pressure on the juxtaglomerular cells of the kidney. Common causes include renal artery stenosis, malignant hypertension, and edematous states such as congestive heart failure, cirrhosis, and the nephrotic syndrome.

   **2.** In the **primary form** plasma renin levels are normal or low.

**C.** It is also important to distinguish hyperaldosteronism due to an adenoma from that due to hyperplasia, since surgical excision is curative for most cases of adenoma, but the response is not as good in hyperplasia.

**D. Signs and symptoms.** The increased secretion of aldosterone leads to hypertension, muscle weakness and fatigue, polyuria and polydipsia, and headaches.

**E. Diagnostic laboratory tests.** Most of the laboratory abnormalities follow from the hypersecretion of aldosterone.

   **1. Plasma electrolytes.** Frequently the potassium level is low and the sodium level is high-normal. The carbon dioxide content may be elevated due to alkalosis.

   **2. Sodium loading.** Hypokalemia and a significant increase in urinary potassium may be induced (or will persist if already present) by giving the patient a high-sodium diet (200 mEq/day).

   **3. Plasma and urinary aldosterone levels**
      **a.** One of the commonest causes of a missed diagnosis is the measurement of aldosterone before potassium repletion.
      **b.** After potassium repletion, the serum and urinary aldosterone levels are markedly elevated in most patients with Conn's syndrome.

   **4. Plasma renin activity.** This helps to distinguish primary from secondary hyperaldosteronism. The activity is very high in the secondary form, but low, even undetectable, in the primary disease.

   **5. Postural response of aldosterone.** The response of aldosterone production to 4 hours of upright posture is helpful in distinguishing hyperaldosteronism due to an adenoma from that due to hyperplasia. In patients with an adenoma there is no change or a decrease in aldosterone production. With hyperplasia there is an increase in aldosterone levels.

**F. Localization of adenomas**

   **1.** Selective sampling of the adrenal venous blood to determine aldosterone concentration is the most accurate means of identifying an adenoma.

   **2.** CT has been shown to be at least 80% accurate in detecting adrenal adenomas and is much less invasive than adrenal venous sampling. The latter can be performed should CT fail to reveal a lesion.

   **3.** Iodocholesterol scanning (see section VII F 3 b) can be used to localize aldosterone-producing adenomas.

**G. Treatment**

   **1. Surgical treatment**
      **a.** For patients with primary hyperaldosteronism due to an adrenocortical adenoma, the treatment of choice is total adrenalectomy of the involved gland.

**b.** It is important to restore the potassium levels to normal prior to surgery.

**2. Medical management. Spironolactone** is a direct antagonist to aldosterone at the kidney tubule.

    **a.** It will gradually lead to a reduction in blood pressure and a return of serum potassium levels to normal.

    **b.** It is used in patients with primary hyperaldosteronism caused by adrenal hyperplasia, since the results of surgery have been disappointing in these patients.

    **c.** Spironolactone is also used in the preoperative restoration of normal serum potassium levels.

## IX. PHEOCHROMOCYTOMA

**A.** Pheochromocytomas are functionally active tumors, which arise from the neural crest–derived chromaffin tissue.

    **1.** Pheochromocytomas produce excess amounts of catecholamines, particularly norepinephrine and epinephrine.

    **2.** The majority of these tumors (about 90%) are benign, but some (10%) are found to be malignant. There is a higher incidence of malignancy with extra-adrenal tumors.

        **a.** Histologic examination is not an accurate means of determining the malignancy of a pheochromocytoma.

        **b.** Malignancy is determined by the presence of metastases or direct invasion by the tumor.

    **3.** Pheochromocytomas can occur as part of the syndrome of multiple endocrine adenomatosis type II (Sipple's syndrome—see Chapter 22, section I B 2). The adrenal medullary abnormality is bilateral in up to 80% of these cases.

**B. Location**

    **1.** About 90% of all pheochromocytomas are found in the adrenal medulla. Approximately 10% of these are bilateral.

    **2.** Of the extra-adrenal 10%, most are found in the organs of Zuckerkandl, the extra-adrenal paraganglia, the urinary bladder, and the mediastinum.

**C. Signs and symptoms**

    **1.** Hypertension results from the excessive production of catecholamines.

        **a.** The hypertension is sustained in about half the patients and intermittent in the others.

        **b.** However, patients with the sustained variety can have paroxysms of more severe hypertension superimposed.

    **2.** Other findings include attacks of headaches, sweating, palpitations, tremor, nervousness, weight loss, fatigue, abdominal or chest pains, polydipsia and polyuria, and convulsions.

**D. Laboratory diagnosis**

    **1.** The most reliable diagnostic **screening test** has been urinary levels of metanephrine and VMA. These are elevated in 90% to 95% of the cases.

    **2.** The accuracy increases to virtually 100% if fractionated plasma and urinary catecholamines are measured as well.

    **3.** Thus, the need for potentially hazardous provocative tests using histamine, tyramine, and glucagon has been greatly reduced. These tests are used only in the rare patient with equivocal biochemical findings.

**E. Tumor localization**

    **1. CT** has emerged as the most accurate, minimally invasive means of localizing pheochromocytomas. It has an accuracy above 95%.

    **2. Arteriography** should be used only after adequate $\alpha$-adrenergic blockade, since it can precipitate a hypertensive crisis.

    **3. Scintigraphy** with radioiodine-labeled m-iodobenzylguanidine (MIBG), which structurally resembles norepinephrine, has been helpful in cases where CT has failed to localize the tumor, especially with small extra-adrenal tumors.

    **4. Vena cava sampling.** If the pheochromocytoma still has not been localized, samples of blood can be taken by catheter from different parts of the vena cava and other veins for hormonal analysis.

**F. Surgical therapy**

**1. Preparation** for surgery should include **adrenergic blockade** with both α- and β-blockers.
  **a.** Adrenergic blockade is helpful for three reasons:
    **(1)** It provides preoperative control of hypertension.
    **(2)** It reduces the risk of dramatic swings in blood pressure during surgery.
    **(3)** It provides vasodilation, allowing restoration of a normal blood volume (blood volume can be about 15% below normal in patients with pheochromocytomas).
  **b. Alpha-blockade** is achieved first. Phenoxybenzamine therapy is begun 2 weeks prior to surgery, starting with 40 mg/day and adjusting the dose until hypertension and associated symptoms are controlled.
  **c. Beta-blockade** is then obtained with propranolol, starting about 3 days before surgery, to control tachycardia. A starting dose of 40 mg/day may need adjustment if tachycardia persists.

**2. Operation**
  **a.** For **monitoring**, the patient should have at least an arterial and a central venous pressure line, because of the potential for wide blood pressure changes and the large fluid requirements. A Swan-Ganz catheter should be used in elderly patients and in those with cardiac disease.
  **b.** The **approach** should be transabdominal in all cases because of the high incidence of multiple and extra-adrenal tumors.
  **c. Procedure.** Total adrenalectomy is carried out for pheochromocytomas.

**3. Special situations**
  **a. Malignant pheochromocytomas** are treated by surgical excision of the tumor. If this cannot be accomplished, then as much tumor as possible is resected and pharmacologic control of the catecholamine excess is started. Chemotherapy can be used for extensive metastatic disease.
  **b.** When pheochromocytoma is a component of **multiple endocrine adenomatosis**, a bilateral total adrenalectomy should be performed. If only one gland is removed, there is a high incidence of recurrence on the other side.

# X. ADRENAL CYSTS

**A.** Adrenal cysts occur infrequently, showing up in fewer than 0.1% of autopsies.

**B.** Most adrenal cysts are either endothelial cysts (lymphangiomatous or angiomatous) or pseudocysts resulting from hemorrhage into normal adrenal tissue or into an adrenal neoplasm. Rarely, they are retention cysts or cystic adenomas.

**C.** A large cyst can present as a palpable mass, and can cause dull aching or gastrointestinal symptoms due to pressure. With cystic neoplasms, symptoms are those of the underlying process.

**D.** CT is the best method available for diagnosing adrenal cysts.

**E.** Since a neoplasm cannot be excluded, these cysts should be surgically excised.

# XI. OTHER ADRENAL TUMORS

**A. Virilizing tumors of the adrenal cortex**

**1.** These are either adenomas or carcinomas of the adrenal cortex.

**2. Symptoms**
  **a. In females**, hirsutism, amenorrhea, and an enlarged clitoris are characteristic. In female patients, it is important to exclude other causes of virilization, particularly congenital virilizing hyperplasia in the young and an arrhenoblastoma of the ovary in older patients.
  **b. In males**, pseudoprecocious puberty occurs.
  **c.** In all patients, some of the features of Cushing's syndrome may be evident. The urinary 17-ketosteroids are increased.

**3.** CT provides the best localization of the tumor.

**4.** Treatment consists of complete surgical excision. Mitotane is used for metastatic disease.

B. **Feminizing tumors of the adrenal cortex**

   1. These also are either adenomas or carcinomas of the adrenal cortex.

   2. In females, the tumor causes rapid premature sexual development. In males, there will be gynecomastia, decreased libido, and testicular atrophy.

   3. Localization is by CT.

   4. Complete surgical excision offers the only hope for cure. Mitotane is used for metastatic disease.

C. **Nonfunctioning adrenal masses**

   1. Autopsy series have uncovered small, nonfunctioning adrenal adenomas in up to 9% of patients. With the growing use of CT scanning, an increasing number of these are being discovered during life.

   2. Although adenomas cannot be distinguished from carcinomas except by excision and inspection, carcinomas are rare when lesions are nonfunctional and smaller than 3 cm in diameter.

   3. These patients should probably be followed up with a repeat CT in 3 months. However, if a nonfunctioning mass is larger than 3 cm or is enlarging, surgical excision is the safest course to take.

   4. A CT-directed biopsy of nonfunctional tumors less than 3 cm in diameter may help to distinguish benign cortical adenomas from early cortical carcinomas.

# 20

# The Parathyroid Gland

Herbert E. Cohn

**I. GENERAL CONSIDERATIONS.** The parathyroid glands are important to the surgeon for two reasons:

  **A.** It is imperative that the integrity of the parathyroids be preserved during operations in the neck, in order to avoid injury to the parathyroids.

    **1.** The consequence of injury to the parathyroids can be permanent hypoparathyroidism.

    **2.** There is no satisfactory replacement for endogenously produced parathyroid hormone, and the patient with hypoparathyroidism is doomed to a lifelong process of episodic symptomatic hypocalcemia despite lifelong calcium and vitamin D therapy.

  **B.** The surgeon is called upon to treat patients with symptomatic hyperparathyroidism, and therefore must have a thorough knowledge of the cause and management of various hyperparathyroid conditions.

**II. EMBRYOLOGY.** In most persons, there are two superior and two inferior parathyroid glands, which differ in their embryologic origin.

  **A. Superior parathyroids**

    **1.** The superior parathyroid glands arise from the fourth branchial arch, in close proximity to the origin of the thyroid (the floor of the foregut), and descend into the neck.

    **2.** Because of the embryologic origin, abnormal parathyroid locations may be either:
      **a.** Intrathyroidal
      **b.** Within the posterior mediastinum, in relationship to the tracheoesophageal groove or the esophagus

  **B.** The **inferior parathyroids** arise from the third branchial arch in relationship to the thymic anlage.

    **1.** They cross the superior glands in their descent into the neck.

    **2.** Not infrequently, they are associated with the thymus gland in the anterior superior mediastinum.

**III. ANATOMY**

  **A.** Some 85% to 95% of individuals have four parathyroid glands but as few as three glands and as many as five have been identified in 10% to 15% of the population. The average parathyroid gland varies from 40 mg to 70 mg in weight.

  **B. Location**

    **1.** The two **superior parathyroid glands** usually lie at the junction of the upper and middle third of the thyroid gland, on its posteromedial surface and in the tracheoesophageal groove.
      **a.** They usually lie posterior to the recurrent laryngeal nerve and are in close proximity to the thyroid gland.
      **b.** Occasionally they may even be intrathyroidal.

    **2.** The **inferior parathyroid glands** lie within a circle with a 3-cm diameter the center of which is the point where the recurrent laryngeal nerve crosses the inferior thyroid artery.

**a.** The inferior parathyroids usually lie in a plane anterior to the recurrent laryngeal nerve.
**b.** They frequently are in close proximity to or within the cervical limb of the thymus gland.

C. **Blood supply**

1. The **arterial supply** to the parathyroid is derived mainly from the inferior thyroid artery arising from the thyrocervical trunk.

2. Since in 10% of autopsies the superior parathyroids are found to receive their blood supply from the superior thyroid artery, this artery should always be left intact when the superior parathyroid glands are exposed, for fear of disrupting their blood supply.

3. The **venous drainage** from the parathyroids is into the superior, middle, and inferior thyroid veins. These veins can be cannulated to provide blood specimens for parathyroid hormone analysis as a means of localizing sources of increased parathyroid hormone production.

D. **Histopathology**

1. The normal parathyroid gland has a significant amount of fat interspersed with chief and oxyphil cells.

2. Hypercellular glands, seen in hyperparathyroid states, have a paucity of fat. The hypercellularity is mostly oxyphil-cell hyperplasia but occasionally chief-cell hyperplasia may also be noted.

3. Histologically, one cannot distinguish the hypercellularity of a hyperplastic gland from that of a gland harboring an adenoma.

## IV. PARATHYROID HORMONE (PARATHORMONE, PTH)

A. Parathormone is a major **regulator of calcium metabolism**.

1. It acts in conjunction with calcitonin and activated vitamin $D_3$ to regulate the plasma concentration of the ionized form of calcium.

2. There is normally a reciprocal relationship between the serum calcium concentration and parathormone secretion.
   **a.** As serum calcium falls, the secretion of parathormone increases.
   **b.** As serum calcium rises, the secretion of parathormone decreases.

3. Parathormone exerts its biologic effect on bone, intestine, and kidney.
   **a.** Parathormone increases the mobilization of calcium and phosphate from bone by stimulating osteoclastic and osteolytic activity.
   **b.** It acts synergistically with 1,25-dihydroxyvitamin $D_3$ to increase the absorption of calcium and phosphorus from the gut.
   **c. Renal effects**
      **(1)** Parathormone raises the renal threshold for calcium by promoting the active reabsorption of calcium in the distal nephron.
      **(2)** It also lowers the renal threshold for phosphate by inhibiting phosphate reabsorption in the proximal tubule.
      **(3)** Parathormone secretion and phosphate depletion stimulate the activation of 1,25-dihydroxyvitamin $D_3$ via the activation of $1\alpha$-hydroxylase.

B. The net effect of increased, unopposed parathormone secretion on bone, intestine, and kidney is to produce:

1. Hypercalcemia

2. Altered calcium excretion
   **a.** Initially, hypocalciuria occurs, due to increased calcium reabsorption.
   **b.** This reverts to hypercalciuria in chronic hyperparathyroid states when the hypercalcemia exceeds the renal threshold for calcium.

3. Hypophosphatemia

4. Hyperphosphaturia

C. Serum parathormone levels can be measured by radioimmunoassay. Normal values vary from laboratory to laboratory, depending in part upon whether the C or N terminal of the parathormone molecule is used in the assay.

## V. HYPERPARATHYROIDISM

### A. Primary hyperparathyroidism

1. **Incidence.** Primary hyperparathyroidism is a relatively common disorder, accounting for 1 in every 800 hospital admissions. It most commonly occurs sporadically, but may occur as:
   a. Part of a multiple endocrine adenomatosis syndrome (see Chapter 22, section I)
   b. Familial hyperparathyroidism
   c. Ectopic or pseudohyperparathyroidism due to the production of a parathormone-like substance from a tumor of extraparathyroidal origin.

2. **Etiology and pathology**
   a. Fully 90% of primary hyperparathyroidism cases are due to a solitary adenoma of one of the four glands.
   b. About 8% to 10% are due to four-gland hyperplasia.
      (1) The hyperplasia may occasionally be asymmetrical, with one or two glands grossly enlarged.
      (2) Microscopically, however, all glands will show hypercellularity.
   c. Parathyroid carcinoma accounts for 1% of primary hyperparathyroidism cases.
   d. About 0.4% are due to multiple adenomas involving more than one gland.
   e. Microscopically, the glands have a paucity of fat and appear hypercellular (see section III D).

3. **Clinical presentation**
   a. The majority of patients with primary hyperparathyroidism are asymptomatic, and the altered state is discovered only because an elevated serum calcium level is noted on routine multichannel biochemical screening.
   b. When patients are symptomatic, the symptoms follow the mnemonic "stones, bones, moans, and abdominal groans."
      (1) **Stones.** Renal lithiasis occurs in 50% of patients with symptomatic primary hyperparathyroidism (although primary hyperparathyroidism occurs in fewer than 10% of all patients who have renal lithiasis).
      (2) **Bones.** Osteitis fibrosa cystica (von Recklinghausen's disease of bone) is seen mostly in patients with secondary or tertiary hyperparathyroidism, which are due to chronic renal disease (see section V B, C).
      (3) **Moans.** Psychiatric manifestations—personality disorders or frank psychoses—may accompany primary hyperparathyroidism, but are relatively uncommon.
      (4) **Abdominal groans**
         (a) The incidence of peptic ulcer disease is increased in primary hyperparathyroidism, usually associated with hypergastrinemia that results from the hypercalcemia.
         (b) Cholelithiasis or pancreatitis may also occur, accounting for abdominal symptoms.
   c. The majority of patients will have nonspecific symptoms such as weakness, easy fatigability, lethargy, constipation, and arthralgia.

4. **Laboratory studies**
   a. An elevated serum calcium level is the cornerstone of diagnosis.
      (1) This should be demonstrated on at least three blood specimens, drawn on three different occasions.
      (2) While primary hyperparathyroidism is a relatively common cause of hypercalcemia, other causes must be excluded, such as metastatic bone disease, myeloma, sarcoidosis, the use of thiazide diuretics, milk-alkali syndrome, hypervitaminosis, thyrotoxicosis, and Addison's disease.
   b. A serum parathormone level that is disproportionately high for the serum calcium level (measured concomitantly) is diagnostic for primary hyperparathyroidism (see Fig. 20-1).
      (1) In patients with metastatic bone disease, hypercalcemia occurs without a disproportionate elevation of parathormone.
      (2) In patients with secondary hyperparathyroidism, the serum parathormone level is elevated and the serum calcium is low.
      (3) In patients with hypoparathyroidism, the serum calcium and serum parathormone are both low.
      (4) The serum parathormone level can also be elevated in patients with **pseudohyperparathyroidism**.
         (a) This disorder is characterized by an extraparathyroidal source of parathormone.
         (b) Tumors arising from the APUD (amine precursor uptake and decarboxylation) cell system (see Chapter 22, section II A 3) may produce a parathormone-like substance that is indistinguishable from parathormone by normal laboratory means.

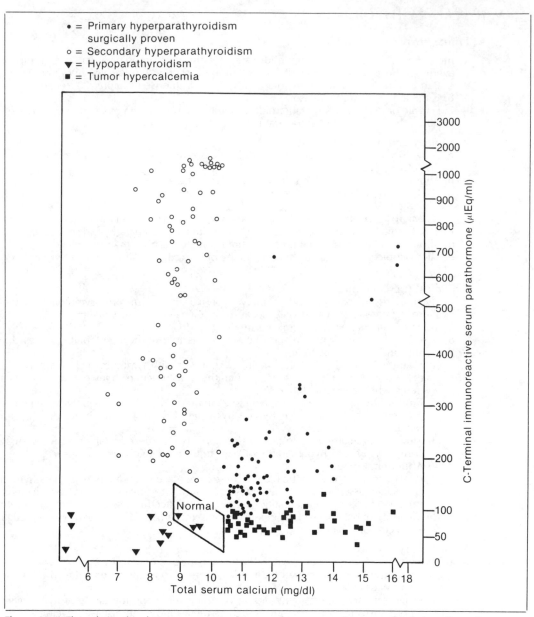

**Figure 20-1.** The relationship between serum calcium and serum parathormone levels in primary hyperparathyroidism (•), secondary hyperparathyroidism (○), hypoparathyroidism (▼), and hypercalcemia due to metastatic bone disease (▪).

   **c. Other laboratory tests**
      **(1)** The serum phosphorus level is decreased and the serum chloride:phosphorus ratio usually exceeds 33:1.
      **(2)** The tubular reabsorption of phosphorus is less than 80%, so that hyperphosphaturia is present.
      **(3)** Measurement of urinary cyclic AMP demonstrates it to be elevated.
      **(4)** Urinary calcium excretion is increased when the patient is on a calcium-restricted diet.

**5. Radiographic studies**
   **a.** X-rays of the skull may show a "ground-glass" appearance in the outer two-thirds of the skull. Skull x-rays are also obtained to search for enlargement of the sella turcica due to a pituitary tumor, which may connote multiple endocrine adenomatosis.

   **b.** X-rays of the proximal ends of the long bones may demonstrate bony reabsorption or brown tumors of the bone.

   **c.** X-rays of the fingers may demonstrate subperiosteal absorption on the radial side of the middle phalanges and in the tufts of the terminal phalanges. Abnormal calcification in the digital vessels may also be seen.

**6. Indications for surgery.** Once the diagnosis of primary hyperparathyroidism is confirmed biochemically, patients should be selected for operation.

   **a.** All symptomatic patients with biochemically proven hyperparathyroidism should be considered for surgery.

   **b.** Operation is also advised for an asymptomatic patient whose serum calcium levels exceed 11 mg/dl, especially if the patient has a decrease in bone density, hypercalciuria, or a decrease in renal function due to other diseases such as hypertension or diabetes mellitus.

**7. Preoperative localization of the parathyroid glands**

   **a.** In general, localization techniques should be reserved for patients who are being considered for reexploration because of persistent or recurrent hyperparathyroidism following unsuccessful parathyroid surgery.

   **b.** Localizing the abnormal parathyroids preoperatively is helpful for several reasons.

   **(1)** It helps to reduce the operating time.

   **(2)** It helps to define the anatomy of the neck in patients who have had prior surgery, in whom the normal anatomy may be distorted.

   **(3)** It helps to define the pathology in patients who have had prior unsuccessful surgery for primary hyperparathyroidism and who still have either persistent or recurrent hypercalcemia.

   **c. Methods of preoperative localization**

   **(1) Ultrasonography** will define an enlarged parathyroid in 70% to 80% of the cases. The ultrasound criteria for an enlarged parathyroid gland are both:

   **(a)** A hypoechoic area in close proximity to either pole of the thyroid gland

   **(b)** The presence of internal echoes that exclude a pure cyst or vascular structure

   **(2) Dual-tracer imaging**, using technetium-99m ($^{99m}$Tc) and thallium-201 ($^{201}$Tl), is helpful in localizing 70% to 80% of enlarged parathyroids due either to adenoma or to hyperplasia.

   **(a)** $^{201}$Tl is taken up by both the thyroid and the parathyroid, whereas $^{99m}$Tc is trapped only in the thyroid.

   **(b)** An enlarged parathyroid gland can therefore be localized by scanning the neck after administering $^{201}$Tl, then rescanning the neck with $^{99m}$Tc, followed by computer subtraction of the $^{99m}$Tc from the $^{201}$Tl image.

   **(3) Thyrocervical angiography** by the Seldinger technique

   **(a)** If the thyrocervical trunk is selectively cannulated, and angiograms of the thyroid and parathyroid are obtained, enlarged glands in the neck can be seen.

   **(b)** If the internal mammary artery is selectively cannulated, enlarged parathyroids in the mediastinum can be seen.

   **(c)** Stroke has been reported as a complication of thyrocervical angiography and therefore this technique should not be used indiscriminately.

   **(d)** It is reserved primarily for patients who have previously been operated upon unsuccessfully, or who develop recurrent hyperparathyroidism after operation, and in whom other techniques of localization are unsuccessful.

   **(4) Selective venous sampling and parathormone assay**

   **(a)** The Seldinger technique can be used in the venous system to obtain blood samples from different venous sites for parathormone assay.

   **(i)** Retrograde injection of the thyroid veins is performed, and each of the draining thyroid veins is selectively cannulated.

   **(ii)** A disproportionately high parathormone level in one or more of the venous samples helps to localize the lesion to one side of the neck or the other.

   **(iii)** Significant elevation in samples obtained from veins on both sides of the neck suggests four-gland hyperplasia.

   **(b)** Because the study is costly and time-consuming, it too is reserved only for patients in whom initial surgery was unsuccessful, or who had a recurrence of hyperparathyroidism after initial successful treatment.

   **(5) Computed tomography (CT) and magnetic resonance imaging**

   **(a)** Using these techniques with and without contrast is allowing parathyroid localization with increasing frequency. CT is particularly successful in localizing enlarged parathyroids in the mediastinum.

   **(b)** However, at the present time these studies are not nearly as successful as the previously described techniques.

**8. Operative management**
  **a. General considerations**
    **(1)** Successful surgery requires a thorough knowledge of the anatomy of the normal parathyroids and their abnormal locations.
    **(2)** When possible, all four parathyroid glands should be identified at surgery.
  **b.** When a solitary adenoma is present, it should be removed and at least one other parathyroid gland should be biopsied. Biopsy of the gland will demonstrate its normal cellularity and exclude the possibility of asymmetrical hyperplasia.
  **c. Management of four-gland hyperplasia**
    **(1)** Two options are currently available:
      **(a)** Subtotal parathyroidectomy, leaving a well-vascularized remnant (100 mg of parathyroid tissue in the adult and 150 mg in the child) to provide for normal parathyroid function
      **(b)** Total removal of all parathyroids, with autotransplantation of minced parathyroid tissue into a well-vascularized, accessible forearm muscle so that recurrence can be treated without reoperation on the neck
    **(2)** There is a 5% recurrence rate after subtotal parathyroidectomy, but a real danger of permanent hypoparathyroidism after total parathyroidectomy and reimplantation if the autotransplant does not survive.

**9. Postoperative management. Postoperative hypocalcemia** usually develops after successful therapy.
  **a.** If asymptomatic, postoperative hypocalcemia requires no treatment.
  **b.** Symptomatic hypocalcemia always requires treatment.
    **(1)** In severely symptomatic patients, treatment should begin with intravenous calcium gluconate.
    **(2)** Mildly symptomatic patients may be given oral calcium in the form of calcium lactate, calcium carbonate, or calcium glubionate. Doses ranging from 4 g to 20 g per day may be required.
  **c.** If hypocalcemia remains symptomatic despite calcium supplementation, additional therapy with vitamin D may be needed. Supplemental calcium and vitamin D therapy should be continued until serum calcium levels return to normal.
  **d.** Patients with significant bone disease will require prolonged calcium therapy to permit remineralization of the calcium-depleted skeleton.

**B. Secondary hyperparathyroidism**

  **1.** Secondary hyperparathyroidism is characteristically seen in patients with chronic renal failure.
    **a.** These patients are unable to synthesize the active form of vitamin D.
    **b.** Therefore, they develop chronic hypocalcemia, hyperphosphatemia, and impaired calcium absorption.

  **2.** If untreated, secondary hyperparathyroidism may result in symptomatic bone demineralization, metastatic calcification in soft tissues, and accelerated vascular calcification. It occasionally can cause severe pruritus and painful skin ulcerations.

  **3.** Initial treatment is with:
    **a.** Dialysis with a high-calcium bath
    **b.** The use of phosphate-binding antacids
    **c.** Administration of calcium supplements plus the active form of vitamin D

  **4.** In patients who are refractory to medical therapy, subtotal parathyroidectomy is indicated, since this form of hyperparathyroidism is always associated with four-gland hyperplasia.

**C. Tertiary hyperparathyroidism**

  **1.** This term refers to the hyperparathyroidism which persists in patients with chronic renal disease despite a successful renal transplant.
    **a.** Apparently, the parathyroid hyperplasia of long-standing renal disease becomes autonomous despite the return of serum calcium levels to normal.
    **b.** Patients are often hypercalcemic, hypophosphatemic, and hypercalciuric.
    **c.** Tertiary hyperparathyroidism may produce the same symptoms as those seen in secondary hyperparathyroidism.

  **2.** When persistent, the condition is treated by subtotal parathyroidectomy.

# 21
# The Thymus
Herbert E. Cohn

**I. GENERAL CONSIDERATIONS.** The thymus assumes importance to the surgeon for several reasons.

    **A.** The thymus gland serves as a source of origin for a variety of tumors.

    **B.** It is significantly involved in the development of cellular immunity and as such has been implicated in a variety of disease states.

**II. ANATOMY AND EMBRYOLOGY**

    **A.** The thymus gland is a multilobulated structure with many fibrous septa.

    **B.** It arises from the third branchial pouch and descends into the anterosuperior mediastinum.

        **1.** Because of its bilateral origin, the thymus develops two lobes and a roughly H-shaped configuration.

        **2.** Two limbs of the thymus extend into the neck and are often associated with the inferior parathyroid glands.

        **3.** The inferior limbs extend along the surface of the pericardium and abut the pleura.

    **C.** Each lobule in the thymus has a cortex and a medulla.

        **1.** The **cortex** consists primarily of lymphocytes which appear to migrate to the medulla and then emigrate from the thymus.

        **2.** The **medulla** also contains Hassall's corpuscles.
            **a.** These are composed of concentric layers of epithelial cells.
            **b.** Their function is not known.

    **D.** The thymus reaches maximal size shortly after birth and then begins to involute during adolescence and early adult life.

    **E. Blood supply**

        **1.** The **arterial supply** to the thymus is derived from small branches of the internal mammary or pericardiacophrenic arteries.

        **2. Venous drainage** is primarily to a single thymic vein that drains into the left innominate vein.

**III. THYMIC FUNCTION**

    **A.** The thymus is essential for the development of **cellular immunity**, which controls such processes as delayed hypersensitivity reactions and transplant rejection.

        **1.** The thymic-dependent portion of the immune system consists principally of the thymus and a circulating pool of small lymphocytes that produce cell-mediated immune reactions.
            **a.** While removal of the neonatal thymus in certain strains of mice leads to significant impairment in immunologic capacity, it has no such effect in the human newborn.
            **b.** However, impaired thymic development may be associated with immunologic deficiency disorders.

   **2.** The thymus is the first organ to begin the manufacture of lymphocytes during fetal life, but the vast majority of cells produced in the thymus die there.

**B. Association of thymic lesions with clinical syndromes**

   **1.** Histologic abnormalities in the thymus, such as lymphoid hyperplasia or thymic tumors, are frequently seen in association with certain autoimmune diseases, such as:
   **a.** Myasthenia gravis (see section V)
   **b.** Systemic (disseminated) lupus erythematosus
   **c.** Erythroid agenesis
   **d.** Hypogammaglobulinemia
   **e.** Rheumatoid arthritis
   **f.** Dermatomyositis

   **2.** This suggests a possible relationship between thymic function and disorders of the immune system.

## IV. THYMIC TUMORS

**A.** Thymic tumors (**thymomas**) are among the most common tumors of the anterosuperior mediastinum in the adult.

   **1.** While thymic tumors can occur at any age, they are most common in the fifth and sixth decades of life.

   **2.** Males and females are equally affected.

   **3.** Some 40% to 50% of patients with thymomas have associated myasthenia gravis.

**B.** Two-thirds of thymic tumors are considered to be benign, and of these, 10% are simple cysts (see Chapter 24, section III A 1).

**C. Pathology**

   **1.** While thymic tumors have been described according to their cell of origin as lymphoid, epithelial, spindle cell, or mixed, it is almost impossible to distinguish benign from malignant thymic tumors microscopically.

   **2.** The best index of the benign or malignant nature of the tumor is its tendency to invade contiguous structures.
   **a.** Benign tumors are well encapsulated.
   **b.** Malignant tumors are invasive.
      **(1)** Malignant thymomas spread by direct invasion of contiguous structures and onto adjacent pleural surfaces.
      **(2)** Distant spread is extremely rare.

**D. Diagnosis**

   **1.** The majority of patients with thymomas are asymptomatic and the tumor is discovered incidentally on a routine chest x-ray.

   **2.** Symptoms, when present, are related to invasion by malignant thymomas and consist of chest pain, dyspnea, or superior vena cava syndrome.

   **3.** The existence of a thymoma is suggested by either:
   **a.** An abnormality on chest x-ray or computed tomography (CT) scan (Fig. 21-1).
   **b.** The presence of myasthenia gravis
      **(1)** This condition should prompt a search of the mediastinum for a thymic tumor.
      **(2)** A lateral chest x-ray is most helpful, since small tumors may be obscured by the great vessels in standard posterior–anterior chest x-rays.

   **4.** Recently, CT has been helpful in identifying the degree of invasion of thymic tumors.

**E. Treatment**

   **1.** Most thymic tumors are removed through a sternal-splitting median sternotomy.

   **2.** Tumors that are not associated with myasthenia gravis or another clinical syndrome require mediastinal exploration and total removal of the tumor.
   **a. Benign tumors** can be removed by local excision.

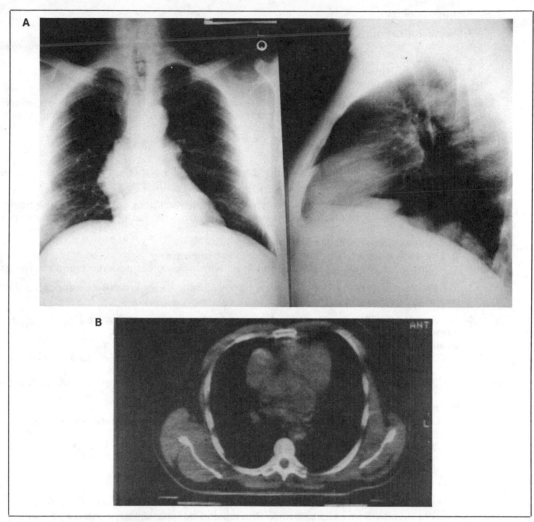

**Figure 21-1.** (A) Posterior–anterior and lateral chest x-ray showing an anterior mediastinal mass in the right hemithorax in a patient with a thymoma. (B) CT scan from the same patient showing an anterior mediastinal mass without fixation to the underlying pericardium.

  **b. Malignant tumors**
    **(1)** If possible, all areas of invasion should be removed.
    **(2)** When invasive thymic tumors are nonresectable or cannot be removed completely, postoperative radiation may be of value.

  **3.** When thymic tumors occur in association with myasthenia gravis or other clinical syndromes, both the tumor and the entire remaining thymus gland should be removed.

  **4.** Epithelial thymomas appear to have a poor prognosis. Spindle cell thymomas appear to have a better prognosis.

## V. MYASTHENIA GRAVIS

### A. General considerations

  **1.** Myasthenia gravis is a disease of neuromuscular transmission that causes skeletal muscle weakness. It is thought to be an autoimmune disease.

  **2.** The disease is characterized by spontaneous remissions and by exacerbations that are often precipitated by upper respiratory infection.

  **3.** The most common symptoms are ptosis, double vision, dysarthria, dysphagia, nasal speech, and weakness of the arms and legs.

**B. Pathophysiology**

    **1. Normal neuromuscular transmission**

        **a.** The neurotransmitter acetylcholine is produced at the nerve terminal of the myoneural junction.

        **b.** The acetylcholine binds to receptor sites on the muscle end plates.

        **c.** This action triggers muscle contraction.

    **2.** In myasthenia gravis, it appears that antibodies to acetylcholine receptors develop, which decrease the available number of receptor sites on the muscle end plates, resulting in reduced muscle contraction.

**C. Treatment**

    **1.** Patients with myasthenia gravis respond to drugs that stimulate the neuromuscular junction, such as neostigmine and pyridostigmine.

    **2.** However, even in patients without thymic tumors, thymectomy appears to be the treatment of choice for all forms of myasthenia except purely ocular myasthenia. Thymectomy appears to:

        **a.** Increase the percentage of permanent remissions

        **b.** Decrease the morbidity and mortality of the disease

        **c.** Improve the response to medication in patients who do not undergo complete remission

    **3.** In patients with thymic tumors, surgical removal of the tumor is advised, although the effect on the myasthenia is unpredictable.

    **4.** Appropriate pre- and postoperative management has significantly reduced the morbidity and mortality rates of surgery.

        **a.** Surgery in patients with myasthenia gravis creates several problems.

            **(1)** The sternal-splitting incision reduces the ability of patients with impaired muscle strength to ventilate properly and to mobilize secretions.

            **(2)** The use of parasympathomimetic drugs improves muscle strength but also increases pharyngeal and tracheobronchial secretions.

        **b.** Preoperative plasmapheresis has been used to good effect.

            **(1)** It eliminates the need for parasympathomimetic drugs and eliminates circulating acetylcholine receptor antibodies.

            **(2)** This produces significant improvement in perioperative muscle strength and virtually eliminates the need for prolonged ventilatory support.

**D. Results of operative therapy in myasthenia gravis**

    **1.** Without surgery, spontaneous remissions occur in 18% of patients with myasthenia gravis, whereas thymectomy induces complete remission in approximately 38% of patients.

    **2.** Sustained improvement is achieved with medication in only 33% of patients without surgery, and in 85% of patients following thymectomy.

    **3.** Best results from thymectomy are usually seen in young patients with myasthenia of relatively short duration who are becoming increasingly refractory to medication.

# 22
# Multiple Endocrine Adenomatosis and Tumors of the Endocrine Pancreas

Herbert E. Cohn
Bruce E. Jarrell

## I. MULTIPLE ENDOCRINE ADENOMATOSIS

**A. Multiple endocrine adenomatosis (MEA)** syndromes, or **multiple endocrine neoplasia (MEN)** syndromes, are characteristic patterns of endocrine hyperfunction inherited as autosomal dominant traits.

1. Many of the endocrine cell types involved originate from the neuroectoderm and have the ability to secrete peptide hormones, amines, or both, but no unifying molecular defect is currently known.

2. Certain features are present in all MEN syndromes.
  a. All are autosomal dominant traits with significant phenotypic variability.
  b. The involved endocrine glands develop either hyperplasia, adenoma, or carcinoma.
  c. The neoplasias in the involved glands can develop simultaneously or at different times.
  d. Ectopic hormone production is common.

**B.** Three **types** have been identified:

1. **Type I (Wermer's syndrome)** involves principally the parathyroid glands, pancreatic islets, and pituitary gland.
  a. **Hyperparathyroidism** (see Chapter 20, section V) is present in 90% or more of the patients, with over one-half having hyperplasia of multiple parathyroid glands.
  b. **Pancreatic tumors** are present in 80%.
    (1) These are usually non-beta islet cell tumors, and usually cause the Zollinger-Ellison syndrome (see section II C).
    (2) However, other syndromes can occur (see section II and Chapter 10, section III).
  c. **Pituitary tumors** are present in 65% of the cases. These are usually chromophobe adenomas, producing acromegaly, galactorrhea, amenorrhea, or Cushing's syndrome.
  d. Approximately 90% of patients present with hypercalcemia, hypoglycemia, peptic ulcer, or complaints secondary to a pituitary mass.

2. **Type II (Sipple's syndrome)** comprises medullary carcinoma of the thyroid, pheochromocytoma, and parathyroid hyperplasia.
  a. **Medullary thyroid carcinoma** (see Chapter 18, section VI F 3) occurs in all patients.
    (1) It is usually multifocal and is often preceded by nonmalignant hyperplasia of the parafollicular C cells.
    (2) Serum calcitonin levels are elevated, although in the premalignant state stimulation with calcium pentagastrin may be necessary to identify this.
  b. **Pheochromocytomas** (see Chapter 19, section IX) occur in approximately 40% of patients.
    (1) They are usually bilateral and occasionally are malignant.
    (2) They often present later than the medullary thyroid cancer.
  c. **Parathyroid hyperplasia**, with consequent hyperparathyroidism, develops in 60% of patients and resembles that of type I.

3. **Type III (mucosal neuroma syndrome)** is considered a variant of type II and is sometimes labelled **type IIb**; Sipple's syndrome then becomes **type IIa**.
  a. As in type II, patients develop medullary thyroid carcinoma and pheochromocytoma.
  b. However, the features most characteristic of type III are a distorted body habitus and the development of multiple neuromatous mucosal nodules.
  c. In addition, type III presents at a much earlier age, usually in the first or second decade of life, and assumes a much more aggressive course.

**C. Diagnosis**

**1. MEA type I (Wermer's syndrome)**

**a.** Most patients with MEA type I present with symptoms of peptic ulceration related to the pancreatic gastrinoma (see section II C) or with symptoms related to the pituitary tumor (see section I B 1 c).

**b.** The hyperparathyroidism is usually asymptomatic and is usually detected only by an elevated serum calcium level.

**2. MEA type II (Sipple's syndrome)**

**a.** The diagnosis is suspected in all kindred of any patient with **medullary carcinoma of the thyroid**.

(1) The inherited trait can be diagnosed in the premalignant stage, when **C cell hyperplasia** is present before the medullary carcinoma develops.

(2) Finding an elevated serum thyrocalcitonin level leads to the diagnosis. Infusion of calcium and pentagastrin helps to stimulate an abnormal thyrocalcitonemia in those with C-cell hyperplasia or occult medullary carcinoma before either is clinically detectable.

**b.** The **hyperparathyroidism** is usually detected by elevations in the serum calcium and parathyroid hormone levels.

**c. Pheochromocytomas** or **adrenal medullary hyperplasia** may be asymptomatic, but should be detectable by biochemical screening for elevated serum and urine catecholamines.

**3. MEA type III (mucosal neuroma syndrome)**

**a.** Because MEA type III assumes so aggressive a course, early diagnosis is important so that effective treatment can begin promptly.

**b.** The diagnosis is similar to that for type II. The early appearance of mucosal neuromas and the body habitus should help in making the diagnosis.

**D. Treatment**

**1. MEA type I**

**a.** If only the pancreatic and parathyroid components of this syndrome are present, the **hyperparathyroidism** is treated first.

(1) This may reduce the production of gastrin and relieve the peptic ulceration.

(2) Subtotal parathyroidectomy is required, since the parathyroid disorder is usually four-gland hyperplasia.

(3) If the hypergastrinemia and peptic ulceration persist, treatment is directed towards the **Zollinger-Ellison syndrome** (see also section II C 4). This involves:

(a) Removal of the gastrin-producing tumor, if possible

(b) Removal of the end-organ (i.e., total gastrectomy) if the tumor cannot be removed and if the use of histamine$_2$- (H$_2$-) receptor antagonists does not control the ulceration.

**b.** The **pituitary tumors** are usually treated by stereotactic transsphenoidal hypophysectomy, using an operating microscope to minimize the risk of injury to the posterior pituitary.

**2. MEA type II**

**a.** If **medullary carcinoma** is treated during the premalignant stage, when only C-cell hyperplasia is present, total thyroidectomy is curative.

**b.** If a **pheochromocytoma** or **adrenal medullary hyperplasia** is detected, it should be treated prior to thyroidectomy, since otherwise these hormone-producing disorders can lead to hypertensive crises during thyroidectomy.

**c. Hyperparathyroidism** can be treated at the time of total thyroidectomy by the protocol described in Chapter 20, section V A 9.

**3. MEA type III** is treated similarly to type II. Because type III assumes so aggressive a course, prompt and effective treatment is important.

## II. TUMORS OF THE ENDOCRINE PANCREAS

**A. Pathophysiology**

**1.** The pancreatic islet cells and the endocrine cells of the gut originate from embryonic cells that have certain cytochemical properties in common.

**a.** They have a high amine content.

**b.** They have the ability for amine precursor uptake.

**c.** They produce the enzyme amino acid decarboxylase.

**2.** These cells have been labeled **APUD cells** (standing for **a**mine **p**recursor **u**ptake and **d**ecarboxylation).

**3.** Tumors that arise from these cells are termed **apudomas**. The various kinds of apudomas arising in the pancreas include:
  **a. Insulinomas**
  **b. Gastrinomas (Zollinger-Ellison syndrome)**
  **c. Glucagonomas**
  **d. Vipomas** (for vasoactive intestinal peptide, or **VIP**)
  **e. Somatostatinomas**

**B. Insulinomas**

**1.** An insulinoma is a tumor originating in the beta cells of the pancreatic islets that releases abnormally high amounts of insulin.
  **a.** Approximately 80% to 90% of insulinomas are solitary, benign adenomas.
  **b.** About 10% are malignant, with the potential to metastasize.
  **c.** The remainder are islet cell hyperplasia (termed **nesidioblastosis** in children).

**2.** The abnormally elevated insulin levels and the resultant hypoglycemia produce various **symptoms:**
  **a.** Bizarre behavior; unconscious episodes
  **b.** Palpitations, nervousness, and other symptoms of sympathetic discharge
  **c. Whipple's triad:**
    **(1)** Episodes of illness precipitated by fasting
    **(2)** Hypoglycemia during the episodes, usually with blood glucose levels below 60 mg/dl
    **(3)** Relief of hypoglycemic symptoms by oral or intravenous administration of glucose

**3.** The **diagnosis**, once suspected, must be confirmed by documenting the abnormal circulating insulin levels.
  **a.** An effective screening test is to have the patient fast for 72 hours or until symptoms of hypoglycemia appear, and then to test the insulin and glucose levels. An elevated insulin level in the presence of a low glucose level (insulin to glucose ratio greater than 0.25) effectively confirms an insulinoma.
    **(1)** Essentially all patients with insulinomas will become hypoglycemic within 72 hours.
    **(2)** As many as 40% will develop symptoms within 2 hours of beginning the fast.
  **b.** Comparing insulin and proinsulin levels can be helpful.
    **(1) Proinsulin** is the single-chain intracellular precursor that is cleaved, prior to secretion, into insulin and C peptide.
    **(2)** Normally, less than 20% of the total circulating immunoreactive insulin is proinsulin.
    **(3)** In patients with insulinoma, proinsulin levels frequently represent more than 20% of the total circulating insulin.
  **c. Provocative tests** may be necessary to prove the diagnosis.
    **(1)** Tolbutamide or glucagon may be infused intravenously: an elevated insulin level is diagnostic of insulinoma.
    **(2)** Fish insulin may be infused: endogenous insulin levels will be suppressed in the normal individual but not in the insulinoma patient. (Fish insulin is not immunoreactive with human insulin.)
    **(3)** Calcium may be infused: this will cause the release of insulin and proinsulin in insulinoma patients, resulting in symptoms of hypoglycemia.

**4. Surgical management**
  **a.** This is based on preoperative localization of the tumor.
    **(1)** Over 75% of all insulinomas are smaller than 1.5 cm, so that both arteriography and computed tomography (CT) are less sensitive for detecting insulinomas than for larger tumors.
    **(2)** Selective arteriography may discover 50% of these tumors.
  **b.** Exploration of the entire pancreas, examining for a palpable mass, is first undertaken.
    **(1)** If the tumor is palpable or is visible as a reddish-brown discoloration, it should be either enucleated or removed as part of a distal pancreatectomy.
    **(2)** If lymph nodes adjacent to the tumor are firm and enlarged, suggesting carcinoma, or if the tumor feels malignant (i.e., firm and infiltrative), then a standard form of resectional therapy should be performed, such as pancreaticoduodenectomy or total pancreatectomy with lymphadenectomy.
  **c.** If no lesion is palpable (as occurs about 10% to 20% of the time), and if preoperative tests have clearly documented hyperinsulinism but not the tumor location, then the management is debatable.
    **(1)** The classic procedure is to resect the tail of the pancreas and examine the specimen pathologically. If a tumor is still not found, all of the pancreas but the head and the uncinate process is removed and the operation terminated.

**(2)** The surgeon may proceed to total pancreatectomy if the tumor is not found in the tail of the pancreas.
**(3)** The surgeon may resect only 80% to 90% of the pancreas and then observe the patient for hyperinsulinism postoperatively. If medical measures then fail to control the patient's symptoms, a total pancreatectomy may be necessary.
    **d.** When islet cell hyperplasia is present, an 80% to 90% subtotal pancreatectomy will usually control the symptoms.
    **e.** Blood glucose levels should be monitored in the operating room to prevent hypoglycemia.

**5. Medical management** is limited to patients who are incurable operatively or who have malignant disease.

**6. Prognosis**
    **a.** Approximately 65% of patients are cured by surgery.
    **b.** The operative mortality rate is 10%.
    **c.** Patients with malignant insulinomas have a 60% 2-year survival rate.

**C. Zollinger-Ellison syndrome (gastrinoma)**

**1. Pathogenesis**
    **a.** Symptoms in this disorder result from oversecretion of gastrin.
    **b.** The consequence is peptic ulceration because of high gastric acid secretion.
    **c.** The cause is usually a non-beta islet cell tumor of the pancreas (that is, a D-cell or A-cell tumor).
    **d.** Zollinger-Ellison syndrome may be a component of MEA type I.

**2. Clinical presentation**
    **a.** Abdominal pain secondary to the peptic ulceration is present in more than 90% of the patients.
    **b.** Diarrhea is common. It results from:
        **(1)** Gastric hypersecretion, which
            **(a)** Creates a low duodenal pH
            **(b)** Inactivates pancreatic enzymes, resulting in steatorrhea
        **(2)** Gastrin-stimulated intestinal motility, which impairs fluid and electrolyte absorption
    **c.** Gastrointestinal hemorrhage from the peptic ulceration occurs in up to 40% of patients.
    **d.** Other gastrointestinal complications such as ulcer perforation and gastric outlet obstruction also occur.
    **e.** Profound dehydration and malnutrition may be present.

**3. Diagnosis**
    **a.** The following conditions should alert the physician to the possibility of Zollinger-Ellison syndrome:
        **(1)** Recurrent ulcer symptoms
        **(2)** Recurrent ulcer following a standard surgical procedure for peptic ulcer disease
        **(3)** An ulcer that is refractory to intensive treatment with antacids or $H_2$-receptor blockers
    **b.** Laboratory findings provide the diagnosis.
        **(1)** Gastric acid hypersecretion is present in 70% to 80% of patients. It is manifested by:
            **(a)** A 12-hour overnight basal acid output (BAO) of more than 100 mmol of hydrochloric acid
            **(b)** A 1-hour BAO of more than 15 mmol
            **(c)** Little or no increase in gastric acid secretion after stimulation by pentagastrin or betazole
                **(i)** This test demonstrates that the parietal cells are under maximal stimulation.
                **(ii)** Results are expressed as the ratio of basal to maximal acid output (BAO to MAO), which usually exceeds 0.6 in patients with Zollinger-Ellison syndrome.
        **(2)** Elevated levels of serum gastrin are the key to the diagnosis.
            **(a)** Gastrin levels are determined by radioimmunoassay, which measures both the heptadecapeptide itself and its precursor form, G-34 or "big gastrin."
            **(b)** Most patients with Zollinger-Ellison syndrome have a fasting serum gastrin level of 500 pg/ml or more (the normal level is 20 to 150 pg/ml).
            **(c)** Some patients have an intermediate serum gastrin level of 200 to 500 pg/ml. A gastrin stimulation test may then aid in the diagnosis.
                **(i)** In Zollinger-Ellison syndrome, an infusion of calcium will raise the gastrin level by more than 300 pg/ml and an infusion of secretin will raise it by 100 pg/ml or more.
                **(ii)** Peptic ulcer patients and normal persons will not show this response.
            **(d)** Extremely high gastrin levels (over 5000 pg/ml) or the presence of $\alpha$-chain human chorionic gonadotropin in the serum strongly suggests a malignant gastrinoma.

(3) Serum gastrin levels may also be elevated by pathologic processes other than non-beta islet cell carcinoma of the pancreas, including:
   (a) Non-beta islet cell adenomas
   (b) Antral G-cell hyperplasia
   (c) Gastric outlet obstruction
   (d) A retained gastric antrum following incomplete antrectomy for peptic ulcer disease
   (e) Conditions that cause gastric hypoacidity (which is a stimulus for gastrin production). These include:
      (i) Pernicious anemia
      (ii) Atrophic gastritis
      (iii) Gastric carcinoma
c. X-ray films will usually show upper gastrointestinal ulceration.
   (1) Frequently, multiple ulcers are seen.
   (2) Ulcers are sometimes seen in the distal duodenum and jejunum.

4. **Treatment** of Zollinger-Ellison syndrome is centered around removal of the causative tumor plus control of the end-organ (gastric mucosal) response.
   a. The tumor should be removed if possible because approximately 60% are malignant.
      (1) Unfortunately, the tumor is frequently multifocal or difficult to identify at laparotomy.
      (2) Only about 20% are resectable.
      (3) Lesions in the wall of the duodenum (present in fewer than 5% of cases) and lesions in the tail of the pancreas are the most common types of resectable tumors.
   b. The end-organ response, namely gastric hypersecretion, and the complications it causes may be treated either by surgical means or by the use of $H_2$-receptor blockers.
      (1) Total gastrectomy is the classic treatment of choice.
         (a) It should be done even in the presence of metastasis because of the slow-growing nature of the tumor.
         (b) It results in control of the severe gastrointestinal hypersecretion and ulceration, and it is well tolerated by most patients.
      (2) Prolonged $H_2$-receptor blockade with cimetidine may control the gastrointestinal manifestations of Zollinger-Ellison syndrome, but the failure rate is as high as 15%.

5. The **prognosis** of Zollinger-Ellison syndrome is good if the gastrointestinal hyperacidity can be controlled by surgical or medical measures. Although two-thirds of the causative tumors are malignant, they are very slow-growing and patients may live a long time.

D. **Pancreatic cholera** is a syndrome of severe diarrhea associated with hypersecretion of a pancreatic non-beta islet cell tumor.

   1. The **symptoms** are:
      a. Watery diarrhea
      b. Hypokalemia and a resultant profound muscular weakness due to the high potassium content in the stool
      c. Achlorhydria

   2. The syndrome has therefore been called **WDHA syndrome**.

   3. The probable **cause** is an increase in the secretion of VIP due to a pancreatic tumor.
      a. The tumor is solitary in 80% of the cases and is usually localized to the body or tail of the pancreas.
      b. One-half of the tumors are malignant and frequently have metastasized by the time of surgery.

   4. The **treatment** is surgical excision when possible. If not, "debulking" the tumor may improve the diarrhea.

   5. **Prognosis** is poor. The average length of survival after surgery is 1 year.

E. **Glucagonomas** are tumors of the pancreatic $alpha_2$ islet cells that cause hypersecretion of glucagon.

   1. The patient is usually diabetic and has weight loss, dermatitis, anemia, and stomatitis.

   2. The tumor is usually benign and is cured by resection.

## QUESTIONS

**Directions:** Each question below contains five suggested answers. Choose the **one best** response to each question.

1. Which of the following factors is helpful in differentiating ectopic Cushing's syndrome from Cushing's syndrome of pituitary origin?

(A) Absence of diurnal variation in cortisol secretion
(B) Results of a low-dose dexamethasone suppression test
(C) Determination of urinary free cortisol
(D) Determination of plasma adrenocorticotropic homone (ACTH) levels
(E) Differential ACTH levels in jugular versus peripheral blood samples

2. All of the following statements about substernal goiters are correct EXCEPT

(A) they are usually seen in older age-groups
(B) they may result in tracheoesophageal compression
(C) they infrequently take up radioiodine
(D) they frequently respond to thyroid suppressive therapy, eliminating the need for operative removal
(E) they frequently result from adenomatous hyperplasia

3. Tumors primary to the thymus gland may be associated with which of the following disorders?

(A) Lupus erythematosus
(B) Scleroderma
(C) Myasthenia gravis
(D) Stricture of the esophagus
(E) Pericarditis

**Directions:** The group of questions below consists of lettered choices followed by several numbered items. For each numbered item select the **one** lettered choice with which it is **most** closely associated. Each lettered choice may be used once, more than once, or not at all.

**Questions 4–7**

For each of the characteristics listed below, select the disorder with which it is most commonly associated.

(A) Graves' disease

(B) Plummer's disease

(C) Medullary carcinoma of the thyroid

(D) Follicular carcinoma of the thyroid

(E) Hashimoto's thyroiditis

4.  Frequently associated with goiter and hypothyroidism

5.  Usually associated with cardiac arrhythmias and a history of preexisting multinodular goiter

6.  Frequently associated with pretibial edema, eyelid edema, and chemosis

7.  Usually causes elevation of serum thyrocalcitonin

## ANSWERS AND EXPLANATIONS

**1. The answer is E.** (*Chapter 19 VII E*) Both the ectopic and the pituitary type of Cushing's syndrome result in a loss of the normal diurnal variation in plasma cortisol levels. Both types also cause elevations of both urinary free cortisol and plasma adrenocorticotropic hormone (ACTH) levels. Although high-dose dexamethasone usually suppresses urinary secretion of 17-hydroxycorticosteroids in pituitary Cushing's syndrome but not in ectopic Cushing's syndrome, a low-dose dexamethasone suppression test is not helpful in differentiation. However, plasma ACTH levels are higher in jugular venous blood samples than in peripheral venous samples in patients with pituitary Cushing's syndrome, whereas the levels are not different in patients with ectopic Cushing's syndrome.

**2. The answer is D.** (*Chapter 18 III D 3, 4*) Substernal goiters usually enlarge as a result of adenomatous hyperplasia and thus do not take up radioiodine. They usually occur in older age-groups, and usually result in tracheoesophageal compression. They rarely respond to thyroid stimulating hormone suppression, and almost always require operative removal both for diagnosis and for the relief of pressure symptoms.

**3. The answer is C.** (*Chapter 21 III B 1*) Thymic tumors are associated with myasthenia gravis and with immune disorders such as hypogammaglobulinemia. Thymic tumors secrete a chemical that becomes associated with acetylcholine receptors, stimulating an immune response followed by myasthenia gravis. Many patients with generalized myasthenia gravis improve after a complete thymectomy.

**4–7. The answers are: 4-E, 5-B, 6-A, 7-C.** [*Chapter 18 IV B 1 b, C 1; V B 2 c (1), F 3 d*] Graves' disease is thought to be an autoimmune disease resulting from a defect in cell-mediated immunity. An abnormal deposition of mucopolysaccharides and round-cell infiltration in tissues result in a clinical syndrome of exophthalmos, edema of the eyelids, chemosis, and pretibial edema. Plummer's disease is also a hyperthyroid state, like Graves' disease, but presents with a clinical syndrome of cardiac arrhythmias, muscle wasting, and the presence of a multinodular goiter. Hashimoto's thyroiditis is a relatively common form of thyroid enlargement that should be considered in any woman who has a goiter and hypothyroidism. Medullary carcinoma of the thyroid arises from the C cells of the thyroid, which have the potential to produce thyrocalcitonin.

# Part VI
# Breast Disorders

# 23
# The Breast

Bruce E. Jarrell
Francis E. Rosato

## I. GENERAL CONSIDERATIONS

**A. The anatomy of the breast** and its **lymphatic drainage** are described in Figure 23-1.

1. It is clinically significant that the lymphatic vessels drain principally to the axillary lymph node chain.

2. More medial areas of the breast tend to drain to the internal mammary node chain but do not cross the midline.

3. Some lymphatic vessels also drain across the diaphragm where they may communicate with the liver.

**B. Examination of the breast** should be done systematically.

1. **Visual inspection** can reveal visible abnormalities that may not be palpable. Breast and nipple asymmetry, dimpling, ulcerations, nodules, and edema are abnormal and may be visible only in one position of the patient or with the patient's arms at the sides or elevated.

2. **Palpation** for masses, which may not be visible, in the breast tissue, tail of Spence, axilla, and supraclavicular area should be done with the patient in several positions.

## II. BENIGN CONDITIONS of the breast may present with pain, nipple complaints, or lumps. Although there are many diagnoses in this group of disorders, several are more common and of greater importance.

**A. Fibroadenoma** occurs in young women who are usually under 35 years of age, and it may be multiple in 10% to 15% of patients. It is usually a discrete mass 1 cm to 4 cm in size and is unattached to surrounding tissue. Treatment is by excisional biopsy.

**B. Cystosarcoma phylloides** is a giant fibroadenoma containing many more cellular components than the usual fibroadenoma. Very rarely does the tumor undergo transformation into a malignant sarcoma. The treatment is wide local excision. If inadequately excised, the tumor has a tendency to recur locally.

**C. Chronic cystic mastitis**, or **fibrocystic disease of the breast**, is a very common entity characterized by painful multiple bilateral cystic masses that change during the menstrual cycle.

1. The diagnosis is made by breast cyst aspiration and cytology of the aspirated fluid.
   **a.** If the mass completely disappears, **observation** is indicated.
   **b.** If the mass recurs or does not disappear completely, **excisional biopsy** is indicated.

2. The risk of carcinoma is two times higher in individuals with this disorder (when there is atypicality of cells) than in the general population, and, therefore, frequent examination should be performed.

3. If multiple biopsies have been performed or dense fibrous disease is present, a prophylactic subcutaneous mastectomy may be justified.

**D. Intraductal papilloma** is a benign lesion that produces a serosanguineous nipple discharge, which may or may not be associated with a subareolar mass. Excision of the involved mammary duct is necessary to determine if the lesion is a malignant papillary adenocarcinoma.

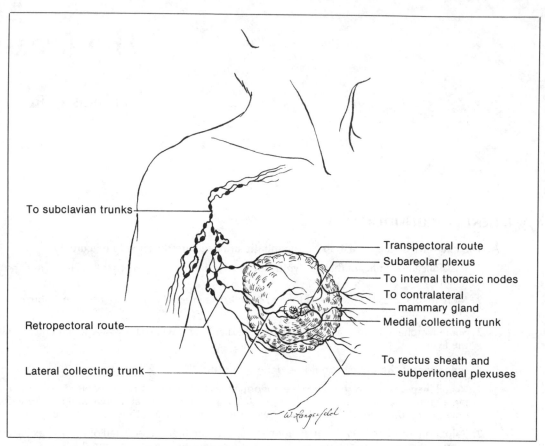

To subclavian trunks

Transpectoral route
Subareolar plexus
To internal thoracic nodes
To contralateral
mammary gland
Medial collecting trunk

Retropectoral route

Lateral collecting trunk

To rectus sheath and
subperitoneal plexuses

*W. Langerfeld*

**Figure 23-1.** Right breast showing lymphatic drainage.

## III. CARCINOMA OF THE FEMALE BREAST

### A. Epidemiology

1. **Frequency.** By the age of 70 years, 9% of all women in the United States will have contracted carcinoma of the breast.
   a. It is the principal cause of cancer deaths in women, with an incidence of 75 cases in 100,000 population.
   b. The age-adjusted mortality rate and incidence have shown no appreciable change since 1930, which indicates that not only does breast cancer remain a major threat to human life but also that therapy has not been improved since that time.

2. **Geographically**, carcinoma of the breast has an **increased incidence** in the north central part of the United States, in the area of the Great Lakes. The incidence is somewhat decreased in the Sun Belt.

3. There are multiple **factors that increase the risk** of developing carcinoma of the breast.
   a. A **family history** positive for breast carcinoma produces a twofold to threefold increased risk. This applies only to first-degree relatives, such as a patient's mother, maternal grandmother, maternal aunts, and sisters.
      (1) A first-degree relative of a patient with premenopausal breast carcinoma has a threefold increase in risk.
      (2) A first-degree relative of a patient with bilateral breast carcinoma has a fivefold increase in risk.
      (3) A first-degree relative of a patient with bilateral premenopausal breast carcinoma has an eightfold increase in risk.
   b. A **history of chronic cystic mastitis** results in a one- and one-half–fold to twofold increased risk of breast carcinoma.
   c. A **previous incidence of contralateral breast cancer** carries a relatively high risk of breast carcinoma occurring in the unaffected breast. If an adenocarcinoma was present previous-

ly, the risk is increased twofold; if the preceding tumor was a lobular carcinoma, there is a 25% to 50% likelihood of developing carcinoma in the other breast.
  d. A **higher socioeconomic status** carries a higher risk of developing breast carcinoma.
  e. Individuals of **Western Hemisphere extraction** have a greater risk of developing breast carcinoma than do those of Eastern Hemisphere extraction; however, the relative "immunity" enjoyed by Easterners is lost after one generation in the Western Hemisphere. The difference in risk is not related to the mass of breast tissue.
  f. **Nulliparous women** have a twofold to threefold increased risk of breast carcinoma when compared to parous women. The risk is lowest in women who become pregnant prior to the age of 23 years.
  g. Women with **wet cerumen** have a higher risk of breast cancer than do those with dry cerumen.
  h. **Estrogen compounds** have a variable effect in animals on the development of breast carcinoma. Although estradiols and ketones do not produce carcinoma, estratriols do.
    (1) There is no current evidence that breast cancer is caused in humans by exogenous estrogens.
    (2) There is an association, however, with endometrial carcinoma. It is probably prudent to withhold exogenous estrogen from patients who previously have had breast cancer and from those in high-risk groups since estrogens can support the growth of an already established carcinoma.
  i. A **mammography pattern** of dense breasts, which is known as **Wolfe's DY pattern**, has been shown to have a high association with carcinoma of the breast. This pattern is characterized by sheet-like areas of increased density in the breast which demonstrate predominately fatty or ductular tissue.

**B. Clinical evaluation** determines if carcinoma of the breast is present and if the lesion is operable.

  1. **Excisional biopsy** is the preferred method of diagnosing a breast lesion; however, it is not always possible to perform on large masses or on those deeply placed. The biopsy may be done as an outpatient procedure, and although mastectomy may be delayed by weeks, there is no indication that this delay is detrimental to the patient.

  2. **Common presenting symptoms** include the following.
    a. **Breast lumps** are the presenting symptoms in 85% to 90% of patients with carcinoma. Approximately one-half are discovered by patients on self-examination, and one-half are discovered on routine surveillance.
      (1) A breast mass may be evaluated by **aspiration alone** only if the following criteria are met.
        (a) It should not be a solitary mass.
        (b) There should be no evidence of axillary nodal involvement.
        (c) There should be associated cystic findings.
        (d) The mass should be entirely collapsible on aspiration.
        (e) The mass should not reappear prior to 3 months.
        (f) Cytology performed on the aspirate must not be suspicious for tumor cells.
      (2) Lumps that show obvious signs of malignancy should be **biopsied** without delay. These signs include the following.
        (a) The mass is large or hard.
        (b) There is marked unilateral breast enlargement.
        (c) There is skin dimpling, redness, or edema.
        (d) There is a spontaneous **nipple discharge**.
          (i) Although most nipple discharges are benign and present as serosanguineous drainage from an intraductal papilloma, 10% are malignant. In addition, although most nipple discharges associated with breast carcinoma are bloody, one-third of bloody discharges are not associated with malignancy.
          (ii) Nipple discharge should be evaluated through mammograms and cytology of the discharged fluid. When a mass is present in association with the discharge, excision of the mass is indicated.
          (iii) When a mass is not present but the quadrant of the breast from which the discharge originated can be localized by local compression, a breast quadrantectomy is indicated.
          (iv) When the source of nipple discharge cannot be localized to a specific area of the breast, correct **treatment** is controversial. Generally, if the patient is over 40 years of age, a mastectomy or central duct excision is performed. In younger patients, frequent observation may be warranted.
      (3) Lesions that are most likely benign but are **solid on aspiration** should probably be biopsied, although they may be safely watched through one or two menstrual cycles.

Most are fibroadenomas in younger women, but well-defined papillary or medullary carcinomas can also be present.

  **b. Breast pain** may be a presenting symptom of carcinoma and should be completely evaluated to eliminate the possibility of malignancy.

  **c.** Evidence of **metastatic disease** may also be the initial symptom.

**3. Patients may have no symptoms** or signs of breast cancer but may be in a **high-risk category**. They may be evaluated by the following methods.

  **a.** Frequent **physical examinations** of the breast by both the physician and patient can reveal symptoms.

  **b.** Mammograms reveal the breast architecture using low-dose radiation.

   **(1)** The suspicious signs for malignancy are asymmetry, skin thickening, and an irregular mass or distorted architecture. Speckled calcification is the most ominous finding, although other patterns of dense breasts are associated with carcinoma.

   **(2)** Mammograms are useful in certain situations:

    **(a)** Supporting a clinical diagnosis of absence of malignancy when no palpable lesion is present

    **(b)** Following patients who have had previous breast carcinoma for signs of contralateral breast carcinoma

    **(c)** Screening high-risk patients for subclinical tumors

  **c.** Regardless of mammographic findings, all dominant masses that are present in more than one examination should be biopsied. Fifteen percent of proven breast carcinomas have negative mammograms.

**4. Patients may present with axillary node enlargement** but no palpable primary breast tumor. This situation represents an occult breast carcinoma in one-third to one-half of cases after other likely diagnoses, such as Hodgkin's disease, lung or pancreatic cancer, and squamous cell carcinoma of the skin, have been ruled out. In this situation, a blind mastectomy (i.e., removal of a breast without evidence of malignancy) is indicated.

**C. Preoperative evaluation** of the patient with proven carcinoma of the breast should determine whether spread outside the axilla has occurred, thus indicating inoperability.

**1. Criteria for inoperability** as defined by Haagensen:

  **a.** Extensive edema of the breast

  **b.** Satellite nodules of carcinoma

  **c.** Inflammatory carcinoma

  **d.** A parasternal tumor, indicating spread to the internal mammary nodes

  **e.** Supraclavicular metastasis

  **f.** Arm edema

  **g.** Distant metastasis

**2. Determination of distant metastasis**

  **a. Extensive examination** for distant spread of disease is a preoperative requirement.

   **(1)** A bone scan should be performed if nodes are clinically positive or if nodes are clinically negative but the patient has symptoms of bone pain.

   **(2)** Of the liver function tests, the alkaline phosphatase is the most sensitive in detecting hepatic metastasis. A liver scan is performed only if the alkaline phosphatase is abnormal or there is other evidence of distant metastasis.

   **(3)** A chest roentgenogram detects pulmonary parenchymal or bone metastasis.

   **(4)** A radioisotope or computed tomography (CT) scan of the brain should be done if neurologic signs or symptoms are present.

   **(5)** A mammogram is useful not only to determine additional foci in the involved breast but to determine the presence of metastatic or synchronous disease.

   **(6)** Although the adrenal glands and ovaries are often involved by metastatic disease, there are no good screening tests for these areas. If warranted, a more extensive evaluation may be performed with an abdominal CT scan.

  **b.** If the presence of metastatic disease seems likely, based on one or more of the screening tests, a **pathologic sample** of the suspected metastasis must be obtained to prove the diagnosis.

  **c.** Even if no evidence of metastatic disease is found, there are patients with apparently early disease who later prove to have had **occult dissemination** at the time of initial diagnosis. This figure may approach 25% in some series and represents a very disappointing group to treat.

**3. Pregnancy** at the time of diagnosis of carcinoma of the breast is not a contraindication to mastectomy. It is associated with an increased incidence (75%) of positive axillary nodal involvement and, therefore a worse prognosis. Chemotherapy obviously presents a danger to the fetus and should be avoided.

**D.** The **prognosis** of patients with carcinoma of the breast is strongly dependent upon a number of clinical and histologic factors at the time of diagnosis.

  **1.** The **histologic type** of carcinoma strongly influences the prognosis. The carcinomas may be categorized by the ability of a cell type to metastasize.

    **a. Nonmetastasizing carcinoma** is noninvasive and represents 5% of all breast carcinomas. The 5-year survival rate of affected patients is 95%.

      **(1)** In situ intraductal papillary carcinoma is nonmetastasizing but may develop into invasive ductal carcinoma in up to 50% of cases within 5 years. Treatment therefore should be the same as for invasive ductal carcinoma.

      **(2)** Noninvasive lobular carcinoma is an in situ carcinoma that has a 15% to 20% chance of developing into frank adenocarcinoma within 20 years. The opposite breast is involved by adenocarcinoma as often as the breast containing the noninvasive lobular carcinoma. Either prophylactic bilateral mastectomy or close long-term observation is appropriate treatment.

    **b. Paget's disease of the breast** is carcinoma involving the nipple. It may be either invasive or in situ breast carcinoma which originates from the underlying ducts. Paget's cells infiltrate the epidermis of the nipple, resulting in an eczematous dermatitis. Generally, treatment is similar to that for invasive carcinoma.

    **c. Metastasizing carcinoma**

      **(1) Carcinoma that rarely metastasizes** is invasive and represents 15% of all cases of breast carcinoma. The 5-year survival rate for patients with this type of carcinoma is 80%. Examples include:

        **(a)** Colloid carcinoma, which contains a preponderance of mucin-producing cells

        **(b)** Medullary carcinoma, which shows lymphocytic infiltration in a sheet-like pattern and has a well-circumscribed margin

        **(c)** Well-differentiated adenocarcinoma

        **(d)** Tubular carcinoma, which has a low incidence of nodular metastasis and has a good prognosis, even if axillary nodes are involved

        **(e)** Invasive lobular carcinoma, which is characterized by small cells infiltrating the lobules, is usually multifocal and frequently bilateral, often presents with pain, is slow growing, and metastasizes late

      **(2) Moderately metastasizing carcinoma** is highly invasive and spreads early to regional lymph nodes. It represents 65% of all breast carcinomas. The 5-year survival rate for individuals with this type of carcinoma is 60%. Examples include:

        **(a)** Infiltrating adenocarcinoma of ductal origin, which is the **most common carcinoma of the breast**

        **(b)** Intraductal carcinoma with stromal invasion

        **(c)** Infiltrating lobular carcinoma

      **(3) Highly metastasizing carcinoma** represents fewer than 15% of carcinomas of the breast. It includes any of the previously mentioned tumors that show vascular invasion or are undifferentiated, with cells growing in a nonductal or nontubular arrangement. The 5-year survival rate is 55%.

    **d. Inflammatory carcinoma** is any breast carcinoma with local inflammatory signs, including redness, localized warmth, swelling, and pain. Histologically, tumor-plugged subdermal lymphatic vessels are found almost universally. Individuals with inflammatory carcinoma have a very poor prognosis; fewer than 3% survive 5 years.

  **2. Size of the primary tumor**, as well as **size, number, and location of the involved lymph nodes**, influences patient survival. Most classification systems (see section D 5) are based on these variables. Classification of breast carcinoma into stages I and II generally indicates operability and therefore better prognosis, whereas classification into stages III and IV indicates inoperability and a worse prognosis.

    **a. Primary tumor size**

      **(1)** Patients with tumors less than 1 cm in diameter have a 10-year survival rate of 80%.

      **(2)** Patients with tumors 3 cm to 4 cm in diameter have a 10-year survival rate of 55%.

      **(3)** Patients with tumors 5 cm to 7.5 cm in diameter have a 10-year survival rate of 45%.

    **b. Size and structure of lymph nodes** involved by metastases based on clinical examination

      **(1)** If no palpable lymph nodes are present, the 10-year survival rate for patients is 60%.

      **(2)** If palpable, freely movable lymph nodes are present, the 10-year survival rate for patients is 50%.

      **(3)** If the lymph nodes are fixed to surrounding structures, the 10-year survival rate for patients is 20%.

    **c.** The **number** of lymph nodes involved by metastases may be assigned erroneously if based on clinical evaluation of the axilla. In 25% of the patients whose axillary nodes are not palpable, a tumor is seen microscopically in the nodes. In 25% of patients with palpable nodes, no tumor is found on pathologic examination of the axillary contents. There is a linear relationship between the number of axillary nodes found on pathologic examination and the incidence of recurrence and patient survival.

      **(1)** Patients with negative axillary nodes have a 10-year survival rate of 65%.

      **(2)** Patients with one to three positive axillary nodes have a 10-year survival rate of 38%.

      **(3)** Patients with more than four positive axillary nodes have a 10-year survival rate of 13%.

    **d. Location** of lymph nodes involved by metastases

      **(1) Level I axillary nodes** are located low in the axilla and extend between the lateral border of the pectoralis minor muscle and medial border latissimus dorsi muscle. The 5-year survival rate for patients with involvement of this level of lymph nodes is 65%.

      **(2) Level II axillary nodes** are located posterior to the pectoralis minor muscle insertion. The 5-year survival rate of patients with involvement of nodes up to this level is 45%.

      **(3) Level III axillary nodes** are located medial to the superior border of the pectoralis minor muscle. The 5-year survival rate of patients with involvement of nodes at this level is 28%.

**3. Other clinical characteristics** of breast carcinoma significantly **worsen the prognosis** and lower the survival rate of patients. These include:

    **a.** Edema or ulceration of the surrounding skin

    **b.** Tumor fixation to the chest wall or overlying skin

    **c.** Satellite skin nodules

    **d.** Inflammatory carcinoma

    **e.** Peau d'orange, which is an orange-peel consistency of breast skin due to dermal lymphatic invasion

    **f.** Skin retraction or dimpling of the breast skin due to shortening of tumor-involved Cooper's ligaments

    **g.** Involvement of the medial portion of the inner lower quadrant of the breast, which is the least favorable anatomic location for a carcinoma

    **h.** Arm edema

    **i.** Evidence of distant metastasis

**4. Estrogen receptor status** of tumors (see section G 2 a) also affects the overall patient survival; that is, if there are hormone receptors in cancer cells, breast cancer may respond to hormonal therapy. Receptor-positive tumors respond more often to hormonal therapy and have a better prognosis than those that are receptor-negative.

**5. Staging categories** are attempts to summate all of the prognostic indicators and relate them to patient survival. Stage I, with no nodal involvement, has the best patient prognosis; stages II and III have an intermediate patient survival rate; and stage IV is characterized by metastatic disease and poor patient prognosis. Below is the staging system of the American Committee on Cancer Staging and End Results Reporting.

    **a. Tumor, nodes, and metastasis (TNM) classification**

      **(1) Primary tumor (T)**

        **(a) TIS**: carcinoma in situ

        **(b)** $T_0$: no primary tumor found

        **(c)** $T_1$: primary tumor, less than 2 cm in diameter

        **(d)** $T_2$: primary tumor, 2 cm to 5 cm in diameter

        **(e)** $T_3$: primary tumor, greater than 5 cm in diameter

        **(f)** $T_4$: extension to chest wall

      **(2) Nodal involvement (N)**

        **(a)** $N_1$: mobile axillary nodes with or without tumor

        **(b)** $N_2$: fixed axillary nodes

      **(3) Distant metastasis (M)**: metastatic disease outside of the breast and axilla

    **b. Clinical staging** is performed with consideration of the TNM classification.

      **(1) Stage I** is characterized by an 85% 5-year survival rate; the tumor is less than 2 cm in diameter. There is no nodal involvement and no distant metastasis.

      **(2) Stage II** is characterized by 66% 5-year survival rate; the tumor is 2 cm to 5 cm in diameter. The axillary nodes are palpable and movable. There is no distant metastasis.

      **(3) Stage III** patients have a 41% 5-year survival rate; the tumor is greater than 5 cm in diameter or is characterized by local invasion. Nodes are palpable outside of the axilla. There is no distant metastasis.

      **(4) Stage IV** is characterized by a 10% 5-year survival rate. There is distant metastasis.

**6. Cure rates** in breast carcinoma cannot be determined until the occurrence of at least 10 disease-free years. The stage of tumor at diagnosis is the most important factor determining cure rate. The best way to improve the cure rate is early detection of cancer, which is accomplished through self-examination and screening programs.

    **a. Self-examination** by the patient and education of the patient to report any abnormality are largely responsible for detection of carcinoma at an earlier stage.

    **b. Screening programs** using physical and mammographic examination of asymptomatic women have detected early cancers.

        **(1)** Six cases of cancer out of one thousand are detected and at an early stage of disease. In 80% of screened women there is no axillary node involvement; of the usual presenting cases, only 45% are without axillary node involvement.

        **(2)** Early breast carcinoma cannot be detected reliably by mammography or physical examination alone, but combined-modality screening detects 80% of cases.

        **(3)** The current recommendation is to screen women over 50 years of age, women over 40 years of age who are in a high-risk category, and women with a history of breast carcinoma.

**E. SURGERY**

    **1. Essential components of surgical therapy** include the following:

        **a. Removal of all breast tissue** in the affected breast is necessary because of the high occurrence of multicentricity of breast lesions. Some 30% to 35% of patients have premalignant or malignant lesions in the affected breast in a quadrant other than that in which the tumor has been discovered.

        **b. Removal of axillary nodes** to ascertain accurate staging is necessary because of the possible erroneous classification of axillary metastasis based on clinical examination alone. Many surgical procedures differ primarily in their treatment of the axillary contents.

    **2. Principally used surgical procedures** may be curative or palliative. The choice of procedure is based on the clinical staging, on the pathologic cell type and its invasive characteristics, and on factors relating to the operative risk of the patient, such as age and a history of other serious disease.

        **a.** Limited procedures include **segmental and simple mastectomy**, which is removal of part or all of the affected breast tissue.

            **(1)** Its use is best limited to small primary lesions, especially those that are less aggressive, or in high-risk patients.

            **(2)** It is most commonly used to treat fibrocystic breast disease, in situ carcinomas, and intraductal papillomas.

        **b.** Simple mastectomy may also be combined with a **partial or level I axillary lymph node dissection**.

            **(1)** A level I axillary dissection is 97% accurate in predicting metastatic disease if the nodes at this level are not involved. This allows more accurate staging of a breast lesion on which to base later treatment decisions.

            **(2)** Whether or not this is adequate treatment for a metastasizing breast carcinoma is controversial.

        **c. Radical mastectomy** is the current standard surgical procedure for the treatment of carcinoma of the breast.

            **(1)** The **Halsted radical mastectomy** removes a generous amount of skin, the entire breast, the pectoralis major and minor muscles, and the axillary contents inferior to the axillary vein.

                **(a)** This procedure adequately removes all axillary lymph nodes, the interpectoral fascia nodes (Rotter's nodes), and the primary tumor. Also sacrificed sometimes is the thoracodorsal nerve innervating the latissimus dorsi muscle.

                **(b)** The long thoracic nerve should be carefully preserved to prevent denervation of the serratus anterior muscle, which results in a "winged scapula."

                **(c)** The Halsted procedure is extremely effective in preventing the local recurrence of disease but has the disadvantage of causing an obvious deformity.

            **(2)** The **modified radical mastectomy** (Patey procedure) is similar to the Halsted procedure with the exception that part or all of the pectoralis major muscle is left intact.

                **(a)** It has the advantages of a better cosmetic outcome and a stronger possibility of breast reconstruction by subpectoral placement of a prosthesis.

                **(b)** Critics of this procedure fear inadequate removal of interpectoral or level III axillary nodes, resulting in a lower cure rate. However, several major studies have shown results comparable to those of the Halsted procedure in long-term survival rates and patterns of recurrence.

        **d. Extended radical mastectomy**, which includes removal of the mediastinal lymph nodes, has been advocated for large or medially placed primary tumors or when there is evidence of internal mammary metastasis. Currently, it is rarely used because of increased surgical morbidity and unimproved rates of survival when compared to radiation therapy and other modalities of therapy.

   **3. Reconstruction of the breast** following mastectomy (see Chapter 30, section I F) may be performed safely. It is not ideal to reconstruct the breast immediately, but it is best to wait at least 6 months until wound healing is complete.

   **4. Adjuvant therapy** is designed to eradicate occult distant metastasis or local residual tumor in patients with stage II or stage III disease with positive axillary nodal involvement but no other evidence of metastasis.

   **a. Chemotherapy** with a triple-drug regimen is the most common form of adjuvant treatment and involves the use of cyclophosphamide, methotrexate, and fluorouracil in monthly cycles for 1 year.

   **(1)** The results show improvement in both the disease-free interval and the overall survival of premenopausal women. The results in postmenopausal women are unclear but are probably improved.

   **(2)** The side effects include the following:

   **(a) Myelosuppression**, requiring monitoring of bone marrow function

   **(b) Immunosuppression** with impaired defense mechanisms, particularly against infection

   **(c) Carcinogenesis**, particularly related to cyclophosphamide, which has been associated with bladder carcinoma and possibly with the late onset of leukemia

   **b. Radiation therapy** as adjuvant therapy was examined in the National Surgical Adjuvant Breast Project (NSABP), no. 4. The results showed no advantage of adjuvant radiation therapy whether patients demonstrated positive or negative nodal involvement.

   **c. Oophorectomy** was shown in the NSABP, no. 3, to have no effect on long-term survival rates, although it possibly prolonged the disease-free interval prior to recurrence.

   **5. Postoperative care** of the mastectomy patient involves total rehabilitation and observation for tumor recurrence and complications.

   **a. Immediate care** includes both mobilization of the arm to prevent limitation of motion and psychological support for the return to normal living. A breast prosthesis should also be supplied.

   **b. Follow-up care** should be done for life to detect local and distant recurrences and new primary tumors in the contralateral breast (see section G).

   **c. Edema of the arm occurs** in 10% to 30% of women following radical mastectomy and interruption of axillary lymphatic vessels. This may occur acutely or chronically and may be aggravated by radiation therapy to the region. All causes of minor trauma (including needle puncture) to the affected arm must be avoided.

   **(1) Treatment**

   **(a)** Because each infection increases lymphatic obstruction by obliterating remaining open channels with fibrosis in reaction to the bacteria, even minor skin infections should be treated early with antibiotics.

   **(b)** Chronic edema may be treated with a firm, fitted elastic sleeve.

   **(2) Complications.** Chronic edema of 10 years or longer may lead (although rarely) to the development of lymphangiosarcoma in the affected arm.

**F. Other forms of treatment.** Radiation therapy may be used for the treatment of both the primary tumor and metastatic lesions.

   **1.** Wide removal of the tumor (quadrantectomy) and a level I axillary dissection are performed first, followed by radiation therapy of the breast with a booster dose directly to the tumor site.

   **a.** In the World Health Organization study using this technique for tumors less than 2 cm in diameter without clinically positive nodes, the results were comparable to radical mastectomy in patients followed for 8 years.

   **b.** The technique is generally reserved for older women with stage I carcinoma or for women who elect not to have a radical mastectomy. However, the applicability of this treatment has definitely been increasing in the last several years.

   **2.** Radiation therapy may be an extremely effective form of palliative therapy in patients with bone or central nervous system metastasis, resulting in relief of pain and control of local disease.

**G. Recurrent disease**

   **1. Types**

   **a. Local recurrence** is defined as recurrence of the carcinoma within the operative field. It occurs in up to 15% of patients after radical mastectomy and in more patients with axillary metastasis. A recurrence usually presents within 2 years of surgery and is treated by either local excision or radiation therapy.

   **b. Second breast carcinoma** should be closely examined to determine whether the second lesion is a primary or metastatic lesion. New primary lesions should be treated similarly to any other primary lesion. Metastatic lesions should be treated by lumpectomy only, followed by hormonal therapy or chemotherapy (see section G 2). Determination of the type of lesion is based on several criteria.

     **(1)** Wide histologic disparity favors a second primary tumor.

     **(2)** If nuclear differentiation is greater in the second breast, a second primary tumor is most likely.

     **(3)** If the interposed time between occurrence of the two lesions is greater than 5 years, the tumor is probably a second primary. If the interposed time is less than 5 years, it is more likely to be a metastatic lesion.

     **(4)** Location of the new tumor fully in the breast favors a new primary. Location of the new lesion in the fatty area of the tail of Spence or near the sternum favors a metastatic lesion.

     **(5)** If the lesion is single, a new primary lesion is favored. If it is multiple, it is probably metastatic.

     **(6)** Contiguous in situ changes are usually only seen in a new primary lesion.

**2. Treatment.** Recurrent disease should be proven on biopsy with determination of the estrogen receptor status of the tumor. Treatment should follow by means of either hormonal therapy or chemotherapy.

   **a. Hormonal therapy** is based on the estrogen receptor status of the tumor. Breast tissue normally develops with specific binding sites for control of hormones, including estrogen and progesterone. Fifty percent of tumors have hormone receptors that are sensitive to inhibition by endocrine manipulation, whereas only ten percent of tumors without these receptors respond to similar manipulation.

     **(1)** Sixty-four percent of estrogen receptor–positive tumors respond to hormonal therapy, whereas only four percent of estrogen receptor–negative tumors respond.

     **(2)** In estrogen receptor–positive patients with recurrent disease, a change in the hormonal environment usually affects the tumor size. In premenopausal patients this change may be accomplished by adrenalectomy or oophorectomy; in postmenopausal patients estrogen therapy is used.

     **(3) Tamoxifen** is an antiestrogen drug and is used in both pre- and postmenopausal patients to treat recurrent disease.

     **(4) Male hormone therapy** may also be useful in the treatment of both pre- and postmenopausal patients.

     **(5)** Patients who respond to one modality of treatment generally continue to respond to sequential hormonal therapy, whereas nonresponders do not. Few patients are cured once metastasis occurs, but hormonal therapy is very effective in prolonging survival and in reducing tumor size.

   **b. Chemotherapy** is used in patients with recurrent disease who are estrogen receptor–negative or who do not respond to hormonal therapy. Combinations of cyclophosphamide, methotrexate, fluorouracil, and doxorubicin are usually used in these cases. Temporary favorable responses, as determined by a measurable decrease in tumor size or the relief of pain, are obtained in 60% to 80% of patients with stage IV disease with the initiation of this therapy.

**IV. CARCINOMA OF THE MALE BREAST** is uncommon, but it has a worse **prognosis** than carcinoma of the female breast.

   **A.** Broken down by stage, not only is the survival rate worse than in women, but the usual case presents at a much later stage. The survival rates are as follows:

     **1. Stage I** disease results in 38% 10-year survival rate.

     **2. Stage II** disease results in 10% 10-year survival rate.

     **3. Stages III and IV** disease are uniformly lethal.

   **B. Treatment** is similar to that for carcinoma of the female breast; castration is the principal means of endocrine control.

# Part VI
# Study Questions

## QUESTIONS

**Directions:** The question below contains five suggested answers. Choose the **one best** response.

1. All of the following statements concerning fibrocystic disease of the breast are true EXCEPT

(A) painful bilateral cystic masses change during the menstrual cycle
(B) excisional biopsy may be indicated
(C) the chance of developing cancer is enhanced five to seven times
(D) usual onset is in the third or fourth decade of life
(E) needle aspiration may be helpful in diagnosis

**Directions:** The question below contains four suggested answers of which **one or more** is correct. Choose the answer

A  if **1, 2, and 3** are correct
B  if **1 and 3** are correct
C  if **2 and 4** are correct
D  if **4** is correct
E  if **1, 2, 3, and 4** are correct

2. True statements concerning hormone receptors in breast cancer include

(1) elevated hormone receptors indicate a better prognosis
(2) as hormonal receptor status may change over time, treatment should depend on the most recent determination of receptor status
(3) therapy with male hormones is useful in treating premenopausal patients
(4) if a patient does not respond to one form of hormonal therapy, a different hormone should be tried

**Directions:** The group of questions below consists of lettered choices followed by several numbered items. For each numbered item select the **one** lettered choice with which it is **most** closely associated. Each lettered choice may be used once, more than once, or not at all.

## Questions 3–5

For each condition associated with breast cancer, select the therapy that is most appropriate.

(A) Radical mastectomy
(B) Adjuvant chemotherapy
(C) Primary radiation therapy
(D) Oophorectomy
(E) No treatment required

3. Noninvasive lobular carcinoma in situ

4. Myelosuppression

5. Level I axillary dissection

## ANSWERS AND EXPLANATIONS

**1. The answer is C.** (*Chapter 23 II C*) At most, the risk of cancer in individuals with fibrocystic breast disease is twice that of unaffected women, and may be even lower. It is important to remember that benign cysts do not progress to cancer; it arises de novo. In patients with cystic breasts, any malignant lesions must be detected before they become untreatable.

**2. The answer is A (1, 2, 3).** (*Chapter 23 III D 4, G 2 a*) The estrogen receptor status is a predictor of responsiveness to hormonal therapy, and estrogen-positive tumors often have a better prognosis than estrogen-negative tumors, all other things being equal. Patients who do not respond to one form of hormonal therapy generally will not respond to another form. Male hormones are useful in treating both premenopausal and postmenopausal patients.

**3–5. The answers are: 3-E, 4-B, 5-C.** [*Chapter 23 III D 1 a (2), E 2 c, 4 a (2), c, F 1, 2*] The choice of surgical procedure for the treatment of breast cancer is based on the clinical staging, on the pathologic cell type and its invasive characteristics, and on factors relating to the operative risk of the patient. Radical mastectomy, the current standard surgical procedure for the treatment of breast cancer, removes a generous amount of skin, the entire breast, the pectoralis major and minor muscles, and the axillary contents inferior to the axillary vein. This procedure is very effective in preventing local recurrence of disease but has the disadvantage of causing an obvious deformity.

Adjuvant therapy is treatment designed to eradicate occult distant metastasis or local residual tumor in patients with positive axillary nodal involvement. Chemotherapy is the most common form of adjuvant therapy, resulting in improvement in both the disease-free interval and the overall survival of premenopausal women. Side effects, however, include myelosuppression, which requires monitoring of bone marrow function, and immunosuppression, particularly against infection. Oophorectomy as adjuvant therapy has been shown to have no effect on long-term survival rates, although it perhaps prolongs the disease-free interval prior to recurrence.

Radiation therapy for primary tumors involves wide removal of the tumor and a level I axillary dissection. This is followed by radiation of the breast and a booster dose directly to the tumor site.

Noninvasive lobular carcinoma is an in situ carcinoma that has a 15% to 20% chance of developing into frank adenocarcinoma within 20 years. The opposite breast is involved by adenocarcinoma as often as the breast containing the noninvasive lobular carcinoma. Either prophylactic bilateral mastectomy or close long-term observation is appropriate therapy.

# Part VII
# Head and Neck Disorders

# 24
# Benign Lesions of the Head and Neck

Robert T. Sataloff
Joseph R. Spiegel
David A. Zwillenberg

## I. GENERAL CONSIDERATIONS

**A.** Familiarity with the benign conditions reviewed in this chapter is essential to the physician, who must distinguish life-threatening illnesses from those of little consequence, choose appropriate therapy, and avoid injudicious surgery.

**B. General points to remember**

**1.** The most common neck mass is a reactive node, and these are most often secondary to bacterial or viral infections of the ear, nose, paranasal sinuses, teeth, tonsils, or skin and soft tissues of the head and neck.

**2.** Most neck masses in children are benign.

**3.** Most neck masses in adults are malignant.

**4.** The **"rule of sevens"** is a useful guide:
  **a.** A mass that has been present for 7 days is inflammatory.
  **b.** One present for 7 months is malignant.
  **c.** One present for 7 years is congenital.

**C. Workup for lesions that do not appear to be congenital** (see section III)

**1.** The **history** should be detailed, especially regarding:
  **a.** Any **family history** of malignancy
  **b.** Any **past malignancy** in the patient
  **c. Risk factors** associated with malignancy, such as:
    **(1)** Smoking
    **(2)** Alcohol consumption
    **(3)** Exposure to radiation, certain fumes, sawdust, or other potential carcinogens
  **d.** Any **recent relevant illness**, such as:
    **(1)** Upper respiratory infection, sinusitis, or tonsillitis
    **(2)** Otitis or conjunctivitis
    **(3)** Dental problems

**2.** The **physical examination** should include careful inspection of the scalp, eyes, ears, nose, mouth (including the teeth and tonsils), hypopharynx, and nasopharynx for signs of infection, ulceration, or unsuspected additional abnormalities.

**3.** Appropriate **laboratory tests** should be performed; these may include:
  **a.** Complete blood count and differential
  **b.** Chest x-ray
  **c.** Tuberculin test for tuberculosis
  **d.** A heterophil titer ("mono spot" test) for mononucleosis
  **e.** Thyroid function tests or thyroid scan
  **f.** Serologic tests for syphilis
  **g.** Viral titers, especially for Epstein-Barr virus, which is associated with nasopharyngeal carcinoma and Burkitt's lymphoma

**4. Radiologic studies** will probably be in order. These may include soft-tissue x-rays of the neck, xeroradiograms, a "GI series" and "barium swallow," or scanning procedures such as computed tomography (CT), magnetic resonance imaging (MRI scan), bone scan, or other radioisotope scans.

5. If a primary neoplasm is suspected, endoscopy is indicated to search for the tumor. Endoscopic biopsy and radiologic studies should precede any incision in the neck (see Chapter 25, section I B).

D. Appropriate **treatment** depends on the findings during the workup.

1. Antibiotics should be administered if a bacterial infection is present.

2. Antituberculosis drugs may be needed.

3. Consultation with a specialist in another field may be helpful.
   a. A dental consultation may be useful if the teeth seem to be the source of a problem.
   b. If dandruff, scabies, or another dermatologic condition is noted, a dermatology consultation is indicated.

4. Should a mass not shrink significantly or disappear within a reasonable period of time, usually 6 weeks, then surgical treatment or biopsy may be indicated.
   a. If cervical adenopathy persists, then
      (1) The presence of enlarged or cryptic tonsils is believed by many to be an indication for tonsillectomy.
      (2) Equivocal dental findings are an indication for dental treatment.
   b. If neither tonsils nor teeth are implicated, then persistent cervical adenopathy is an indication for excisional biopsy after a complete evaluation for malignancy.
   c. A neck mass biopsy is the last step in a proper workup.

## II. NECK ABSCESSES

A. A patient presenting with fever and a fluctuant neck mass most probably has an abscess.

1. The source of infection should be identified and drainage should be carried out.

2. Due to the danger to the carotid artery, airway, and cranial nerves, deep neck abscesses should be treated only by those knowledgeable in the standard techniques and anatomy of the area, and they should be treated on an emergency basis.

B. **Types of abscesses**

1. **Bezold's abscesses** are neck abscesses arising from the ear.

2. **Ludwig's angina** is an abscess occupying sublingual space.
   a. It generally arises from a dental source.
   b. It can cause death from airway obstruction.

3. **Parapharyngeal abscesses** arise from the posterior teeth or tonsils and involve the carotid sheath. They can cause mediastinitis and carotid "blowout" (erosion of the artery wall leading to massive hemorrhage).

4. **Retropharyngeal abscesses** can cause mediastinitis.

5. **Peritonsillar abscesses (quinsy)** arise as a complication of acute tonsillitis.
   a. They present with ipsilateral palatal edema, contralateral deviation of the uvula, "hot potato" voice, and trismus.
   b. They are the most common source of abscesses in the parapharyngeal space.
   c. They are usually treated with intraoral incision and drainage or aspiration. Tonsillectomy is sometimes required.

## III. CONGENITAL MASSES

A. **Parenchymal cysts**

1. **Thymic cysts**
   a. The thymus arises from the third pharyngeal pouch and migrates caudally and medially to descend into the superior mediastinum.
      (1) During this descent an attachment may be left in the neck.
      (2) Thymic tissues may present in the neck as separate nodules of mature thymus or may occur in association with ciliated or columnar epithelial remnants of the pharyngeal outpouching.
   b. **Characteristics**
      (1) Some 95% of thymic cysts are unilateral, and 90% of thymic ectopias are cystic.
      (2) Thymic cysts may occur anywhere on a line from the mandibular angle to the suprasternal notch and are generally found in children. There is a male predominance.

**(3)** They may be uni- or multilocular.

**(4)** Loculated cysts generally contain amber to brown fluid which may be clear or turbid.

  **c. Complications**

    **(1)** The cysts are often asymptomatic but may be painful if infected or if they grow suddenly.

    **(2)** Midline cysts may cause dysphagia.

    **(3)** Both benign and malignant hyperplasia have been reported in these cysts.

    **(4)** Myasthenia gravis is not found in association with cervical thymic cysts.

  **d. Differential diagnosis**

    **(1)** Branchial cleft cysts seldom extend to the clavicle and often present with signs of acute inflammation.

    **(2)** Cystic hygromas are lateral, spongy, and more diffuse. They are generally seen in infants.

  **e.** Surgery is the **treatment** of choice.

**2. Parathyroid cysts**

  **a.** These unusual cysts generally present as a solitary mass at either inferior pole of the thyroid gland.

  **b.** They are seen in adults, usually between ages 30 and 50.

  **c. Symptoms**

    **(1)** Tracheal deviation is usual and causes a variable degree of respiratory obstruction.

    **(2)** Hoarseness may occur due to pressure on the recurrent laryngeal nerve.

  **d. Treatment** consists of surgical excision.

**B. Lesions of thyroid origin**

**1.** The thyroid gland originates at the foramen cecum and descends central to the thyroid and cricoid cartilages.

  **a.** The thyroglossal duct may pass in front of, through, or behind the hyoid bone.

  **b.** It is generally obliterated but may persist.

  **c.** Elements of thyroidal primordium may remain at any site in its passage.

    **(1)** These may give rise not only to cysts and fistulas but also to accessory thyroid tissue and neoplasms.

    **(2)** Most cystic remnants occur in the midline around the hyoid bone.

    **(3)** Solid tumors of thyroglossal duct origin occur almost exclusively within the tongue and above the hyoid bone.

**2. Thyroid rests**

  **a.** Thyroid rests may be lingual or may occur in the neck.

  **b.** Endotracheal ectopias may occur.

  **c.** Palpation of the normal position of the thyroid will often reveal easily palpable tracheal rings in patients with these rests.

  **d. Therapy** is dictated by:

    **(1)** The degree of obstruction present

    **(2)** The presence of other thyroid tissue

      **(a)** A thyroid scan should be performed prior to the removal of lesions suspected of being thyroid rests, in order to ensure that there is functional thyroid tissue in the usual location.

      **(b)** Some 70% to 80% of patients have no other functional thyroid.

**3. Thyroglossal cysts, sinuses, and fistulas**

  **a.** These occur in the midline unless previous surgery has produced distortion.

  **b.** About 20% are suprahyoid, 15% occur at the hyoid, and 65% are infrahyoid.

  **c. Fistulas** are almost always the result of infection with spontaneous or surgical drainage. Fistulas can drain internally, externally, or both (**complete fistulas**).

  **d. Thyroglossal duct cysts** present by age 10 in half of the cases.

    **(1)** There is no sexual predominance, but there is a racial predominance; the cysts occur more often in whites.

    **(2)** Cysts usually measure 2 to 4 cm in diameter and gradually increase in size, although the size may fluctuate.

    **(3)** They rise and fall with the larynx during swallowing.

  **e. Treatment** is total surgical excision, including:

    **(1)** The cyst and sinus to the base of the tongue

    **(2)** The whole fistula if one is present

    **(3)** The middle third of the hyoid bone

**C. Cutaneous branchiogenic cysts** are extremely rare asymptomatic nodules which are noted soon after birth and gradually increase in size. They are located in the suprasternal notch. Treatment is by local surgical excision.

D. **Teratomas** are growths composed of multiple tissues foreign to the part of the body in which they arise.

1. **Types**
   a. **Epidermoid cysts**, the most common type, are lined by squamous epithelium and are without adnexa.
   b. **Dermoid cysts** are epithelium-lined cavities containing skin appendages (e.g., hair, glandular tissue, and follicles).
   c. **Teratoid cysts** are lined with simple stratified squamous epithelium or respiratory epithelium, and contain cheesy keratinous material. They are rare in the head and neck.

2. **Cervical teratomas**
   a. These masses are most commonly present at birth. Appearance after age 1 year is rare.
      (1) The lesions are usually 5 to 12 cm in their long axis and are semicystic, although they may be solid.
      (2) They are usually unilateral.
   b. Infants with cervical dermoids usually have stridor, apnea, or cyanosis due to tracheal compression or deviation.
      (1) Dysphagia may also be present.
      (2) Some infants are asymptomatic at birth but become symptomatic within weeks or months.
   c. There is an increased incidence of maternal hydramnios, but affected infants show no increase in associated anomalies.
   d. Early excision in infants is mandatory.

3. **Malignant teratomas** of the neck are rare and occur exclusively in adults. Prognosis is very poor.

4. **Nasal dermoids** are often apparent shortly after birth.
   a. They show a male predominance of 2 to 1.
   b. The nasal dorsum is the most common site but they may occur in the tip of the nose or the columella.
   c. They must be differentiated from encephaloceles and gliomas.
   d. Early removal is important.
   e. Recurrences secondary to incomplete removal are common.

E. **Vascular tumors** (see also Chapter 30, section II B 3)

1. **Hemangiomas** constitute the most common tumors of the head and neck in children. Females are more often affected than males, and the lesions are usually solitary.
   a. **Types**
      (1) **Nevus flammeus (port-wine stain)** and **strawberry nevus** are **capillary hemangiomas** characteristically found in the dermis.
         (a) They rarely appear in adults.
         (b) They have an early period of evolution, then may develop suddenly and get quite large, after which they often regress.
      (2) **Cavernous hemangiomas** are more permanent. Spontaneous regression is more likely in those present at birth than in those appearing afterwards.
      (3) **Arteriovenous hemangiomas** occur almost exclusively in adults and have a predilection for the lips and perioral skin.
      (4) **Invasive hemangiomas** occur in the deep subcutaneous tissues, deep fascial layers, and muscles.
         (a) These hemangiomas present as neck masses, predominantly in children.
         (b) They tend to recur long after excision but do not metastasize.
         (c) The masseter and trapezius are the muscles most commonly involved in the head and neck.
         (d) **Intramuscular hemangiomas** most commonly present in young adults as palpable, mobile, noncompressible masses.
            (i) They generally are without thrills, pulsations, or bruits.
            (ii) Pain secondary to compression of other structures is usually present.
      (5) **Subglottic hemangiomas** are usually capillary in type. Due to their location they often present, at birth or soon thereafter, with stridor and usually with cutaneous involvement as well.
   b. **Treatment**
      (1) Congenital **cutaneous hemangiomas** are generally treated expectantly, at least initially.

   **(a)** When patients reach school age, cosmetically deforming lesions may be excised.
   **(b)** Steroids may be used to help slow a rapid growth phase if necessary.
   **(2) Subglottic lesions** may require tracheotomy, steroids, and, in some cases, laser excision.
   **(3)** Surgery may be needed for extensive lesions.
   **(4)** Radiation therapy has been used to suppress tumor growth. However, radiation alone will not effect a cure, and its use in these lesions is controversial.

2. **Cystic hygromas** are found predominantly in the neck and are usually noted at birth or soon thereafter.
   a. They are more common in the posterior triangle.
      (1) They may reach up into the cheek or parotid region and down into the mediastinum or axilla.
      (2) Larger masses will extend past the sternocleidomastoid muscle into the anterior compartment and may cross the midline.
      (3) They may involve the floor of the mouth and the base of the tongue.
   b. There is no predilection for either sex or for either side of the body.
   c. The hygromas can be progressive, static, or regressive.
   d. **Symptoms and signs** may include:
      (1) Difficulty in nursing
      (2) Facial or neck distortion
      (3) Respiratory distress
      (4) Brachial plexus compression with pain or hyperesthesia
      (5) A sudden increase in size secondary to spontaneous hemorrhage, which can be fatal.
   e. **Physical examination**
      (1) Small lesions are unilocular and firm.
      (2) Large tumors are loculated, shiftable, and compressible.
      (3) The hygromas generally display transillumination.
   f. The cyst walls are usually tense and since the loculi tend to communicate, rupture of one locule can cause a partial collapse of all of them.
   g. **Surgery** is the mainstay of **treatment**.
      (1) Recurrences are common because the cysts insinuate themselves into adjacent structures, so that resection is often incomplete.
      (2) The greater the lymphangiomatous component of a hygroma, the more likely it is to recur.

3. **Oral and perioral lymphangiomas** are relatively common lesions that are usually found at birth or soon thereafter. They behave very much like cystic hygromas.

F. **Branchial cleft anomalies**

   1. **Embryology**
      a. In the fourth week of gestation, five ridges appear on the ventrolateral surface of the embryonic head, with a groove between each. These form the branchial arches and clefts, respectively.
      b. The pharyngeal pouches develop internally at the same level as the external grooves.

   2. Branchial cleft anomalies occur as one of several **types:**
      a. A **sinus**, or **incomplete fistula**, has either an internal or an external opening.
      b. A **complete fistula** has both an internal and an external opening.
      c. A **cyst** has neither an internal nor an external opening.
      d. **Combinations** of any of the above types can occur.

   3. **Anatomy.** Branchial cleft anomalies are located along the anterior border of the sternocleidomastoid muscle or deep to it. They can occur anywhere between the external auditory canal and the clavicle.
      a. **First branchial cleft anomalies** are always superior to the hyoid bone.
         (1) If a fistula is present it will course superiorly to end near the external auditory canal.
         (2) The cyst and tract may lie in the parotid gland, with a variable relationship to the facial nerve.
      b. **Second cleft anomalies** are the most common type.
         (1) An external opening, when present, will be about two-thirds of the way down the sternocleidomastoid anteriorly.
         (2) The fistula, if present, will ascend with the carotid sheath and cross over the hypoglossal and glossopharyngeal nerves and between the external and internal carotid arteries to end at the tonsillar fossa. This is the **most common branchial anomaly**.
      c. **Third cleft anomalies** are rare.
         (1) The external opening will occur in the same position as in a second cleft fistula.

**(2)** The tract ascends along the carotid sheath posterior to the internal carotid artery, over the hypoglossal nerve, under the glossopharyngeal nerve, and over the vagus nerve to open in the pyriform sinus.

**d. Fourth branchial cleft anomalies** have never been seen in their entirety.

**(1)** Theoretically, they would have an external opening anterior to the sternocleidomastoid muscle in the lower neck.

**(2)** They would descend along the carotid sheath into the chest, passing under the subclavian artery on the right and the aortic arch on the left, ascend into the neck to cross the hypoglossal nerve, then descend to open into the esophagus.

**4. Clinical presentation**

**a.** Branchial cleft cysts are generally smooth, round, nontender masses.

**b.** An increase in size during upper respiratory infections is common.

**c.** An infected branchial cleft cyst may abscess or rupture spontaneously to form a sinus.

**d.** The size and the location of a branchial cleft anomaly determine the symptoms.

**(1)** Large cysts may cause dysphagia, stridor, and dyspnea.

**(2)** Small cysts are often not discovered until adulthood because of their slow rate of growth and minimal symptoms.

**5. Treatment**

**a.** Complete excision without damage to the surrounding vital structures is the definitive treatment. Antibiotics are given if the lesion is infected.

**b.** Incision and drainage are avoided, if possible, since these will make subsequent excision more difficult.

**G. Encephaloceles** are congenital brain herniations.

**1.** They are usually discovered early in life. About 75% are occipital, 15% are sincipital, and 10% enter the nose or nasopharynx.

**2.** These lesions may or may not communicate centrally. **Communicating** lesions will increase in size and tension when the infant cries; **noncommunicating** ones generally do not.

**3.** Meningitis or cerebrospinal fluid leaks are not uncommon, particularly with manipulation.

**4.** Encephaloceles may be confused with nasal dermoids or polyps.

**5. Treatment** should include total removal. The lesions need not be treated as emergencies if the threat of meningitis is not deemed serious.

# IV. NONCONGENITAL LESIONS

**A. Leukoplakia** and **keratosis** are white lesions occurring on the mucosa of the mouth, pharynx, or larynx. **Erythroplakia** is a similar red patch.

**1.** These lesions are associated with repeated trauma (from poorly fitting dentures, decayed teeth, and so forth) in patients who smoke or use alcohol.

**2.** There is little correlation between the clinical appearance of the lesions and their histology, although erythroplakia is somewhat more likely to be carcinoma.

**3. Biopsy**, to rule out squamous cell carcinoma, should be performed:
**a.** In high-risk patients (smokers and drinkers)
**b.** If the lesion persists after the removal of an irritative focus

**4.** Benign leukoplakic lesions require no treatment but do require continued observation.

**B. Squamous papillomas** of the oral cavity usually occur singly but may be multiple.

**1.** They are usually pedunculated and cauliflower-like in appearance.

**2.** Recurrence is rare after excision.

**C. Nasal vestibular papillomas** are **warts** that are similar in appearance and behavior to cutaneous warts elsewhere on the body.

**D. Inverted papillomas**

**1.** These lesions occur mainly in men aged 30 to 50.
**a.** The lesions typically arise from the lateral nasal wall, and can invade the sinuses and orbits.
**b.** Grossly, the lesions appear bulky and deep red to grey in color; they vary in consistency.

    **c.** Unlike nasal polyps of allergic origin (see section IV F), they are unilateral.

  **2.** Patients generally present with nasal obstruction, a postnasal drip, and headaches. A few have epistaxis.

  **3.** The incidence of malignant transformation ranges from 2% to 15%.

  **4.** The treatment of choice is complete excision. Recurrence is common because excision is often incomplete.

**E. Laryngeal papillomas** are the most common laryngeal tumors of childhood and the **most common benign laryngeal lesions** found at any age.

  **1.** The **juvenile type** occurs predominantly in childhood and tends to involute at puberty.
    **a.** Multiple papillomas are most common and may involve the airway from the epiglottis to the bronchi.
    **b.** The etiology is believed to be viral.
    **c.** Hoarseness is an early sign and obstruction is a later one.
    **d.** Recurrence and spread are common.
    **e. Treatment**
      **(1)** A tracheotomy may be necessary but should be avoided if possible because it predisposes to tracheal seeding of the papillomas.
      **(2)** Laryngoscopic removal, often by the use of a carbon dioxide laser, is the mainstay of therapy.
      **(3)** Interferon therapy appears helpful but the lesions tend to recur when it is stopped.

  **2.** In the **adult type** the papilloma is generally single.
    **a.** As in the juvenile form, the papilloma tends to recur following excision.
    **b.** Recurrent lesions can undergo malignant transformation, particularly in patients exposed to radiation.

**F. Nasal polyps** are very rare before age 5 and occur predominantly in men.

  **1.** Nasal polyps are believed to be an allergic response, but this is not clearly established.
    **a.** They may be associated with asthma and an idiosyncratic reaction to aspirin.
    **b.** In children, the presence of nasal polyps should prompt a sweat test to rule out cystic fibrosis.

  **2.** Polyps may recur frequently.

  **3.** Involvement of the paranasal sinuses is common, and ethmoid or maxillary sinus surgery may be necessary to afford the patient an adequate nasal airway and relief of symptoms.

**G. Fibrous lesions**

  **1. Nodular (proliferative) fasciitis** presents as a rapidly growing, discrete soft-tissue mass.
    **a.** Most probably a reactive, non-neoplastic response to injury, it may occur at any time from childhood to age 70.
    **b.** The lesions may be mistaken for sarcoma.
    **c.** Fascia is the primary tissue involved.
    **d.** The lesions generally do not recur after excision.

  **2. Proliferative myositis** occurs in adults and appears to be post-traumatic in origin.
    **a.** Like nodular fasciitis, it can be confused with sarcoma.
    **b.** The lesion involves muscle diffusely.
    **c.** Occasionally, spontaneous regression occurs.
    **d.** Lesions do not recur after excision.

  **3. Traumatic myositis ossificans**, bony deposits in muscle due to trauma, generally presents as a painful mass in the muscle 1 to 4 weeks after a single severe trauma.
    **a.** In the head and neck, the masseter or sternocleidomastoid is generally involved.
    **b.** X-ray reveals feathery opacities or irregular radiodensities.
    **c.** The condition must be differentiated from **myositis ossificans progressiva**, which is a progressive, systemic illness.
    **d.** Persistent painful masses are excised. Local recurrence is common.

  **4. Desmoid tumors** are benign, locally invasive, encapsulated tumors.
    **a.** They arise from the muscular fasciae and are often associated with prior trauma.
    **b.** These tumors are uncommon in the head and neck but, when found, usually arise from the sternocleidomastoid.
    **c.** Complete surgical excision is the treatment of choice.

**H. Tumors of skeletal muscle**

1. Extracardiac **rhabdomyomas** have a predilection for the head and neck.

2. They show a slight male predominance.

3. Signs and symptoms depend on the site and size of the tumor.

4. Rhabdomyomas tend to recur if incompletely excised.

**I. Tumors of peripheral nerves** (see also Chapter 30, section II B 5)

1. **Schwannomas** are solitary, encapsulated tumors attached to or surrounded by a nerve.
   a. They are not associated with von Recklinghausen's disease or with malignant change, in contrast to neurofibromas.
   b. They are primarily located centrifugally and are often painful and tender.

2. **Acoustic neuromas** are a type of schwannoma.
   a. They arise from the eighth cranial nerve, usually start within the internal auditory canal, and can involve the cerebellopontine angle.
   b. Signs and symptoms may include hearing loss, tinnitus, imbalance, and vertigo.
   c. Early discovery is important, as it will result in earlier resection with a consequent decrease in morbidity and mortality.

3. **Neurofibromas** are usually multiple and unencapsulated.
   a. Neurites (axons) pass through the tumor.
   b. In 8% of patients neurofibromas undergo malignant changes.
   c. Usually these lesions are located centripetally and are characteristically asymptomatic.
   d. The lesions generally occur as a component of von Recklinghausen's disease but may occur as solitary lesions or, rarely, as multiple lesions that are not a part of von Recklinghausen's disease.
   e. Café-au-lait spots, vitiligo, gliomas, osseous changes, meningitis, spina bifida, syndactyly, hemangiomas, or retinal and visceral manifestations may be present.

4. **Traumatic neuromas** are reactive hyperplasias due to a nerve's attempts at regeneration following injury.
   a. They are generally oval or oblong, gray, firm, and unencapsulated.
   b. Persistent hyperesthesia and tenderness are the usual signs.

5. Most neurogenous tumors of the head and neck can be excised safely without sacrificing nerves. If an important nerve must be cut, it should be reanastomosed or a nerve graft interposited.

**J. Granular cell tumors**

1. **Congenital epulis** occurs on the gum pads of newborns in the region of the future incisors.
   a. The female to male ratio is 8 to 1.
   b. The lesion can be quite large, does not recur after excision, and may spontaneously regress.

2. The **nonepulis form** of granular cell tumors occurs mainly in young adults, especially in blacks.

**K. Paragangliomas (chemodectomas)** can occur in the head or neck (see Chapter 25, section XII A).

**L. Nondental lesions of the jaw**

1. **Giant cell granuloma**
   a. This jaw lesion can occur in two forms:
      (1) **Central granulomas** occur within the jaw.
      (2) **Peripheral granulomas**, occurring on the gingival or alveolar mucosa, are four times more common.
   b. The mucosa is generally intact, but x-rays of the central lesions will show radiolucent areas.
   c. Excision or curettage is the treatment of choice.

2. **Fibrous dysplasia of the jaw** is noted early in life.
   a. It shows active growth in childhood and stabilization in adulthood.
      (1) Swelling of the bone is the most common sign, and may be either minor or significant enough to cause obvious facial asymmetry.

**(2)** The maxilla is more commonly involved than the mandible.
**b.** X-rays may reveal sclerosis, lytic lesions, or unilocular lesions.
**c.** Obvious deformity, pain, or interference with function suggests the need for surgery.
**d.** Malignant transformation is possible but uncommon, and conservative resection appears to be the best treatment.

**3. Torus** is a benign bony growth occurring at the midline of the palate (**maxillary torus**) or bilaterally lingual to the bicuspids (**mandibular torus**).
**a.** Tori are slow-growing and generally of no significance.
**b.** They may interfere with the fitting of dentures.

**4. Osteomas** are benign tumors with slow growth rates.
**a.** They can occur in the sinuses, the jaws, or the external ear canals.
**b.** Sinus osteomas may require excision if they produce headache or occlusion of drainage.

## M. Laryngeal lesions

**1. Laryngocele** is a dilatation of the laryngeal saccule, producing an air sac that communicates with the laryngeal ventricle.
**a.** Anything that increases intralaryngeal pressure will increase the size of a laryngocele (e.g., coughing, straining, and playing a wind instrument).
**b.** A **laryngopyocele** is an infected laryngocele. It can be fatal if it results in asphyxia or if the purulent contents drains into the tracheobronchial tree.
**c.** Laryngoceles may be unilateral or bilateral.
**d.** They may also be **internal** (within the larynx), **external** (presenting in the neck), or **both** (combined).
    **(1)** An internal laryngocele causes bulging of the false cord and aryepiglottic fold.
    **(2)** The external type appears as a neck swelling at about the level of the hyoid bone and anterior to the sternocleidomastoid.
**e. Symptoms**
    **(1)** Internal laryngoceles cause hoarseness, breathlessness, and stridor on enlargement.
    **(2)** External laryngoceles increase in size with coughing or the Valsalva maneuver.
        **(a)** They are tympanic to percussion.
        **(b)** A hissing may be heard as the laryngocele empties air into the larynx when the air pressure is reduced.
**f. Diagnostic studies**
    **(1)** Plain films may show cystic spaces that contain air.
    **(2)** Tomograms may help to demonstrate the continuity between the internal and external components.
    **(3)** CT and MRI scanning show these lesions well.
**g. Treatment**
    **(1)** Symptomatic laryngoceles are treated by surgical excision.
    **(2)** Laryngopyoceles should be treated by incision and drainage, with subsequent excision.

**2. Laryngeal webs** may be congenital or may follow bilateral vocal fold disruption.
**a.** When extensive, they present with stridor, weak phonation, and feeding problems.
**b.** Laser excision is now generally the preferred treatment.

**3. Vocal nodules** are bilateral benign masses that usually occur at the junction of the anterior and middle thirds of the true vocal cords.
**a.** They are associated with vocal abuse and are best treated by modifying the patient's speaking or singing technique.
**b.** Surgery is rarely necessary and may be contraindicated without a previous trial of speech therapy.

**4. Vocal polyps** are usually unilateral and often do not regress with speech therapy—two important points in distinguishing the polyps from vocal nodules.
**a.** The recommended therapy is careful excision with microscopic visualization and avoidance of injury to the underlying muscle.
**b.** In selected cases the laser may be helpful.

**5. Laryngeal granulomas** occur over the vocal processes of the arytenoid cartilages.
**a.** They are generally the result of trauma, usually from an endotracheal tube.
**b.** They are best treated by excision after a period of observation.

**6. Arytenoid dislocation** is also generally the result of endotracheal tube trauma.
**a.** A soft, breathy voice after extubation should arouse suspicion.

    **b.** Prompt reduction is essential; otherwise, the arytenoid will become fixed in the dislocated position.

    **7. Contact ulcers** are mucosal disruptions usually located posteriorly on the vocal cords.

        **a.** They sometimes result from trauma (e.g., from intubation), occasionally from vocal abuse, and often from gastric reflux esophagitis.

        **b.** Elevation of the head of the bed; avoidance of caffeine, chocolate, late-night snacks, and fried or fatty foods; and antacid therapy will usually result in prompt resolution of the ulcers.

**N. Common head and neck infections (otitis media, mastoiditis, and sinusitis)** are now controlled with antibiotics, which must be given at high enough doses and over long enough periods for these sequestered spaces.

**O. Tonsillar and adenoidal hypertrophy and infection.** Tonsillectomy with adenoidectomy—a "T and A"—once was the most common operation in the United States. It remains quite prevalent, but is now performed for specific **indications:**

    **1. Obstructive hypertrophy**

        **a.** Patients benefiting from T and A are those with airway obstruction, sleep apnea, cor pulmonale, dysphagia, or failure to thrive.

        **b.** Adenoidectomy is performed in children with chronic nasal obstruction, especially when they also demonstrate chronic serous otitis media or orthodontic problems.

    **2. Recurrent infection.** Patients with documented recurrent adenotonsillitis are improved after T and A. A history of 3 to 6 episodes yearly is a relative indication.

    **3.** Most authors suggest tonsillectomy after treatment for a **peritonsillar abscess** in patients with a history of previous tonsillitis.

# 25

# Malignant Lesions of the Head and Neck

Robert T. Sataloff
Joseph R. Spiegel
David A. Zwillenberg

## I. GENERAL PRINCIPLES

### A. Epidemiology

1. Primary malignant neoplasms of the head and neck account for 5% of new cancers per year in the United States, excluding skin cancer.

2. The male to female ratio is 3 to 1 to 4 to 1, and most lesions occur in patients over the age of 40 years.

3. Approximately 80% of primary head and neck malignancies are squamous cell carcinomas. The remainder are thyroid cancers, salivary neoplasms, and other, rarer, tumors.

4. The number of patients with a second primary at the time of initial presentation has been reported to be as high as 17%.

### B. Risk factors

1. Cigarette smoking, alcohol consumption, and exposure to radiation are etiologic factors in most squamous cell carcinomas of the head and neck.

2. Some 85% of patients with head or neck cancer presently smoke or formerly smoked cigarettes.

### C. Evaluation of the patient starts with a careful history and physical examination.

1. In the **history-taking**, the patient is particularly questioned about:
   a. Exposure to etiologic agents (tobacco, alcohol, irradiation)
   b. Associated symptoms (hoarseness or sore throat of more than 3 weeks' duration, dysphagia, dyspnea, nonhealing ulcers)
   c. Any history of prior head or neck malignancy

2. Information is also obtained about the patient's nutritional status, family history, and psychosocial status.

3. The **physical examination** must include inspection of all the skin and mucosal surfaces of the head and neck.
   a. An intranasal examination and indirect mirror examination of the nasopharynx and hypopharynx are included.
   b. A careful palpation of the oral cavity, base of the tongue, and oropharynx is mandatory.

4. Fiberoptic examination is performed whenever indirect mirror examination is inadequate.

### D. Therapeutic considerations

1. The patient's **nutritional status** is a prime concern in choosing therapy.
   a. Many patients are malnourished, either because of alcoholism or from an obstructive tumor.
   b. Treatment is sometimes delayed because of the need for hyperalimentation.
   c. In most patients this can be accomplished with tube feedings into the stomach, but parenteral nutrition is sometimes required.

2. Primarily, **treatment** is based on the site and pathology of the primary cancer and the extent of the local, regional, and distant disease.

3. **Surgery** is the indicated treatment for many patients with head and neck cancer.
   a. It permits a short treatment time, avoidance of radiation side effects, and the saving of

radiation for recurrent disease or other primaries, as well as allowing careful pathologic examination of the tissue removed.
   **b.** The choice of surgery can be influenced by many factors.
      **(1)** Malnourishment can increase the perioperative risk of morbidity and mortality.
      **(2)** The patient may have a coexistent systemic disease.
      **(3)** The necessary procedures can be disfiguring and can leave the patient with severe
         functional deficits.
         **(a)** Resection of the larynx, for example, alters communication; surgery on the tongue,
            oropharynx, hypopharynx, or mandible can alter or prevent swallowing.
         **(b)** Thus, the patient may refuse recommended surgery.
      **(4)** Surgery should be performed in institutions that have professionals trained to provide
         the intensive perioperative care and the rehabilitation that are needed.

**4. Radiation therapy**
   **a.** Given alone, radiation is adequate treatment for many early lesions.
      **(1)** It can provide cures without the functional or cosmetic deficits associated with surgery.
      **(2)** It can treat multiple primary lesions simultaneously, and can prophylactically treat
         regional nodes that are clinically negative.
   **b. Combined therapy** with radiation (usually postoperative) and surgery can significantly in-
      crease survival rates in advanced lesions.
   **c.** A careful dental examination is required prior to radiotherapy. Dental treatment during
      radiotherapy, or for up to 2 years afterwards, can be extremely hazardous due to de-
      creased vascularity and consequent delayed healing.
   **d. Complications of radiotherapy** include mucositis, xerostomia, loss of taste, dermal and
      soft tissue fibrosis, dental caries, and bone and soft tissue necrosis.

**5. Chemotherapy** is currently used palliatively for advanced, inoperable tumors. It is being
   tested in adjuvant therapy protocols.
   **a.** Methotrexate, bleomycin, and cisplatin are the most effective agents.
   **b.** Most palliative regimens utilize single agents or cisplatin-based multidrug combinations.
      Response rates range from 25% to 70%.
   **c.** In selected cases, chemotherapy can be delivered by intra-arterial infusion with an in-
      dwelling pump system via the external carotid.
   **d.** Trials are currently evaluating the role of chemotherapy as a pre- and postoperative adju-
      vant.
      **(1)** Initial studies are encouraging because tumor response rates have been high.
      **(2)** However, the studies have yet to show a significant impact on survival.

**6. Rehabilitation** should be planned at the same time as treatment.
   **a.** Cosmetic and functional defects are reconstructed at the time of the cancer resection
      whenever possible.
   **b.** The use of **surgical flaps** (see Chapter 30, section I E) has greatly facilitated reconstruction.
      The flaps may be:
      **(1)** Local flaps (nasolabial, forehead)
      **(2)** Distant pedicled skin flaps (deltopectoral, omocervical)
      **(3)** Myocutaneous flaps (pectoralis major, latissimus dorsi, trapezius)
      **(4)** Free flaps
   **c.** Prosthetic rehabilitation is necessary when portions of the maxilla, mandible, or palate are
      resected.
   **d.** When the larynx is removed, intensive rehabilitation is required to reestablish the voice.
      **(1)** Initially, patients are taught to speak with an electric larynx applied in the mouth or on
         the neck.
      **(2)** Later, they can learn to speak with regurgitated air (esophageal speech) or with a
         Blohm-Singer prosthesis (a one-way valve) placed in a surgically created tracheoesoph-
         ageal fistula.
   **e.** Many patients who undergo partial laryngectomy, pharyngectomy, or glossectomy require
      training to facilitate swallowing and to avoid aspiration.

## II. CANCER OF THE NECK

### A. Anatomy

**1.** The neck is divided into anterior and posterior triangles.
   **a.** The **anterior triangle** is bounded by the midline of the neck, the inferior border of the
      mandible, and the anterior border of the sternocleidomastoid muscle. It can be further
      subdivided into submandibular, submental, superior carotid, and inferior carotid triangles.
   **b.** The **posterior triangle** is bounded by the posterior border of the sternocleidomastoid mus-

cle, the anterior border of the trapezius, and the clavicle. It is further divided into supracla-vicular and occipital triangles.

**2. Lymphatic system**
  **a.** The lymphatic system is enclosed within the **fascial planes** of the neck.
   **(1)** The **superficial fascia** is subcutaneous and envelops the platysma.
   **(2)** The **deep fascia** has three parts:
      **(a)** A superficial layer which invests the sternocleidomastoid and trapezius muscles
      **(b)** The pretracheal fascia
      **(c)** The prevertebral fascia
  **b.** There are approximately 75 **lymph nodes** on each side of the neck.
   **(1)** Most lie within the deep jugular and spinal accessory chains.
   **(2)** The jugular chain is divided into superior, middle, and inferior groups.
   **(3)** Other nodal groups are the submental, submandibular, superficial cervical, retro-pharyngeal, paratracheal, anterior scalene, and supraclavicular.

**B. Evaluation of a neck mass.** A workup for malignancy should be undertaken in all adults with a persistent neck mass.

  **1.** A careful history is taken and the head and neck are examined for evidence of a possible pri-mary cancer (see section I C).

  **2.** If the "primary" is not identified on the initial examination, then **workup** includes:
   **a.** A chest x-ray, "barium swallow," and films of the sinuses
   **b.** A "GI series," intravenous pyelography, and other x-ray studies, if warranted by findings on the history and physical examination
   **c.** Panendoscopy (direct laryngoscopy, esophagoscopy, bronchoscopy, and nasopharyngos-copy)

  **3.** If the endoscopic survey is negative, random **biopsies** of the nasopharynx (right, middle, and left) are performed. A random biopsy of the tongue base or a tonsillectomy may also be worthwhile.

  **4.** If all biopsies are negative, the next step is to proceed with open neck biopsy and frozen sec-tion.

**C. Staging of metastatic neck disease**

  **1. Stage $N_0$:** No clinically positive node

  **2. Stage $N_1$:** A single clinically positive node homolateral to the primary tumor and 3 cm or less in its greatest diameter

  **3. Stage $N_{2a}$:** A single clinically positive homolateral node larger than 3 cm but less than 6 cm in its greatest diameter

  **4. Stage $N_{2b}$:** Multiple clinically positive homolateral nodes, with none larger than 6 cm in greatest diameter

  **5. Stage $N_{3a}$:** Multiple clinically positive homolateral nodes, with at least one larger than 6 cm in greatest diameter

  **6. Stage $N_{3b}$:** Bilateral clinically positive nodes

  **7. Stage $N_{3c}$:** Only contralateral clinically positive nodes

**D. Treatment**

  **1.** If a primary cancer is identified and confirmed with biopsy, the metastatic neck disease is treated in conjunction with the primary.

  **2. Types of neck dissection**
   **a. Radical neck dissection** is an en bloc dissection of the cervical lymphatics.
    **(1)** It includes the removal of the sternocleidomastoid muscle, internal jugular vein, and spinal accessory nerve.
    **(2)** Radical neck dissection is performed when squamous cell carcinoma is found in a neck mass with an unknown primary cancer.
   **b. Modified (functional, conservative) neck dissection** removes the cervical lymphatics within their fascial compartments.
    **(1)** It spares the sternocleidomastoid muscle, internal jugular vein, and spinal accessory nerve.

(2) Indications include:
    (a) Elective neck dissections
    (b) A single node less than 3 cm in diameter that is to be treated postoperatively with radiation
    (c) Differentiated thyroid cancers with neck metastases
    (d) Simultaneous bilateral neck dissections

3. **Elective neck dissection** refers to surgical treatment of $N_0$ disease.
    a. There is controversy about when and if to use elective neck dissections, since radiation therapy can provide prophylaxis for metastatic neck disease in many cases.
    b. The choice between surgery or radiation usually depends on the treatment of the primary tumor.
    c. In general, when elective neck dissection is performed, it is done for a primary cancer that has a 30% or greater rate of occult metastasis.

## III. CANCER OF THE NASAL CAVITY AND PARANASAL SINUSES

**A. Anatomy**

1. All sinuses come in pairs, and all are contiguous with the nasal cavity through their natural ostia.

2. The nose and sinuses are lined with a respiratory mucosa, which is pseudocolumnar, with goblet cells and cilia.

3. Primary lymphatic drainage is to the parapharyngeal or retropharyngeal nodes. Secondary lymphatics are the subdigastric nodes of the internal jugular chain.

**B. Classification of tumors**

1. Most tumors (59%) are in the maxillary sinus, 24% are in the nasal cavity, 16% in the ethmoid sinuses, and 1% in the frontal and sphenoid sinuses.

2. Some 80% of the malignancies are squamous cell carcinoma.
    a. Tumors that arise anteriorly tend to be well differentiated.
    b. Those arising from the posterior nasal cavity and ethmoids are generally poorly differentiated.
    c. Nasal and sinus cancers are locally invasive. Nodal metastases are unusual and tend to occur late, even with extensive local disease.

3. About 10% to 14% of the malignancies are adenocarcinomas, including adenoid cystic carcinoma.

4. Inverted papilloma (see Chapter 24, section IV D) has a 10% to 15% incidence of associated squamous cell carcinoma.

**C. Clinical evaluation**

1. **Presenting signs and symptoms** can include nasal obstruction; epistaxis; localized pain; tooth pain; cranial nerve deficits; a mass in the face, palate, or maxillary alveolus; proptosis; and trismus.

2. The **extent of the disease** is determined by physical examination and radiographic studies.
    a. Computed tomography (CT) is particularly useful for identifying bony erosions and orbital or intracranial extension.
    b. Arteriography is rarely needed.

3. Most biopsies can be performed under local anesthesia.

**D. Staging** is available for maxillary sinus cancer.

1. **Stage $T_x$**: Cannot be assessed

2. **Stage $T_0$**: No evidence of a primary cancer

3. **Stage $T_1$**: Tumor confined to the inferior antrum without bone erosion

4. **Stage $T_2$**: Tumor confined to the superior antrum without bone erosion of the inferior or medial walls

5. **Stage $T_3$**: Extensive tumor involving the skin of the cheek, the orbit, the anterior ethmoids, or the pterygoid muscles

6. **Stage $T_4$**: Massive tumor involving the cribriform plate, posterior ethmoids, sphenoid, nasopharynx, pterygoid plates, or base of the skull

### E. Treatment

1. For **maxillary sinus cancer**
   a. $T_1$ and $T_2$ tumors are treated with subtotal or radical maxillectomy. Radiation is used when cancer may have been left at the surgical margins and for recurrences.
   b. $T_3$ and $T_4$ tumors receive radiotherapy followed by reevaluation for surgical resection. Orbital exenteration and skin resection are performed when necessary.

2. Tumors restricted to the **ethmoid sinus** or **nasal cavity** are usually treated with radiation therapy followed by surgery for residual disease.

3. Combined craniofacial resection can be chosen for selected patients with **extensive cancers**.

4. **Inverted papillomas** are treated by en bloc resection that includes the lateral nasal wall and ethmoid sinus.

5. **Cervical lymph node metastases** are treated with radiotherapy followed by radical neck dissection for residual disease.

### F. Prognosis

1. There is an overall cure rate of approximately 30% to 35%.

2. The 5-year survival rate for patients with $T_1$ and $T_2$ lesions is 70%.

3. The 5-year survival rate for patients with $T_3$ and $T_4$ lesions is 15% to 20%.

## IV. CANCER OF THE NASOPHARYNX

### A. Anatomy

1. The nasopharynx is the most cephalad portion of the pharynx.
   a. Its roof is formed by the basioccipital and sphenoid bones, and its posterior wall is formed by the atlas.
      (1) These walls are covered by mucosa, and embedded within is the adenoid tissue.
      (2) The lateral wall contains the orifice of the eustachian tube, and, just posterior to that, the fossa of Rosenmuller.
   b. The choanae define the anterior limit, and the free edge of the soft palate provides the inferior limit.

2. Primary lymphatic drainage is to the lateral retropharyngeal, jugulodigastric (tonsillar), and high spinal accessory nodes.

### B. Epidemiology and etiology

1. There is a high incidence of nasopharyngeal cancer among persons from the Kwan Tung province of China.

2. There is a high incidence of elevated Epstein-Barr virus titers among persons with cancer of the nasopharynx.

3. Nasopharyngeal cancer occurs at younger ages than do most solid tumors.

### C. Classification

1. Some 85% of nasopharyngeal tumors are epithelial; 7.5% are lymphomas.

2. Epithelial tumors commonly arise in the fossa of Rosenmüller.

### D. Clinical evaluation

1. Common **presenting symptoms** are anterior or posterior epistaxis, cervical adenopathy, serous otitis media, and nasal obstruction. Headache, diplopia, facial numbness, trismus, ptosis, and hoarseness may also be present.

2. At presentation, 60% to 70% of patients will have nodal disease and 38% will have cranial nerve involvement.

3. Nasopharyngeal cancer can best be evaluated and monitored with CT and magnetic resonance imaging (MRI).

4. When a patient presents with an elevated Epstein-Barr virus titer, these titers can be monitored and can be expected to fall with successful treatment and to rise with recurrences.

### E. Staging

1. **Stage TIS**: Carcinoma in situ

    **2. Stage $T_1$:** Tumor is confined to one site, or no tumor is visible but random biopsy is positive

    **3. Stage $T_2$:** Tumor involves two sites (posterosuperior and lateral walls)

    **4. Stage $T_3$:** Tumor has extended to the oropharynx or nasal cavity

    **5. Stage $T_4$:** Tumor has invaded the skull or a cranial nerve

**F. Treatment**

    **1.** The primary treatment for all epithelial nasopharyngeal tumors is irradiation. The dose, usually 6500 to 7500 rads, is delivered to the nasopharynx and to both sides of the neck.

    **2.** Radical neck dissection is performed for residual nodes if the primary tumor is controlled.

**G. Prognosis.** The 5-year survival rate is 40% in patients without positive nodes; 20% in patients with positive nodes.

## V. CANCER OF THE ORAL CAVITY

**A. Anatomy**

    **1.** The oral cavity extends from the lip anteriorly to the faucial arches posteriorly. It includes the lips, the buccal mucosa, the gingivae, the retromolar trigones, the hard palate, the anterior two-thirds of the tongue (the oral tongue), and the floor of the mouth.

    **2.** Lymphatic drainage is to the submental, submandibular, and deep jugular nodes.

**B. Etiologic factors** include:

    **1.** Tobacco—90% of patients are heavy smokers or "snuff-dippers"

    **2.** Alcohol—80% of patients are heavy drinkers

    **3.** Syphilis

    **4.** Herpesvirus type 1—currently under investigation as a cause

**C. Clinical evaluation**

    **1.** The lip is the most common site of oral cavity carcinoma, followed by the oral tongue and the floor of the mouth.

    **2. Presenting symptoms** can include loose teeth, painful or nonhealing ulcers, odynophagia, otalgia (with posterior lesions), and cervical adenopathy.

    **3.** Mandibular x-rays should be taken, to assess bony involvement by adjacent tumors.

    **4.** Diagnosis is frequently delayed because pain is often a late symptom, occurring after ulceration develops.
        **a.** Nodal metastases (up to 30% of them occult, microscopic metastatic disease) are found in 50% of patients with squamous cell carcinoma of the anterior tongue, and in 58% of patients with cancer of the floor of the mouth (occult metastases in up to 12% of the cases).
        **b.** Metastases are uncommon and usually occur late in cancer of the lip or the buccal mucosa.

**D. Staging**

    **1. Stage $T_1$:** Tumor less than 2 cm in its greatest diameter

    **2. Stage $T_2$:** Tumor 2 to 4 cm in its greatest diameter

    **3. Stage $T_3$:** Tumor more than 4 cm in its greatest diameter

    **4. Stage $T_4$:** Massive tumor with involvement of the pterygoid muscles, antrum, root of the tongue, or skin

**E. Treatment**

    **1.** Stage $T_1$, $N_0$ tumors can be treated with either local excision or radiotherapy.

    **2.** Stage $T_2$ or larger lesions should be treated with combined surgery and radiation.
        **a. Surgery** involves an en bloc resection of the tumor and radical neck dissection.
        **b.** Either a partial mandibulectomy is included or else the tumor is "pulled through" medial

to the mandible, into the neck (i.e., the tumor is removed en bloc with the radical neck specimen, leaving the mandible intact).

3. Tumors attached to the mandible may be removed with a partial thickness of mandible (i.e., the lingual plate or alveolar process). The mandibular arch is kept intact when possible.

4. Tumors demonstrating bony erosion in the mandible are removed with a full-thickness portion of bone.

### F. Prognosis

1. The overall 5-year survival rate for cancer of all oral cavity sites is approximately 65%.

2. For lip cancer, 5-year survival rates as high as 90% have been reported.

3. The prognosis for tongue lesions is worse if the lesion is posterior. Posterior lesions involving the tongue base can invade the pre-epiglottic space, necessitating laryngectomy.

## VI. CANCER OF THE OROPHARYNX

### A. Anatomy

1. The oropharynx is bounded by the free edge of the soft palate superiorly, the tip of the epiglottis inferiorly, and the anterior tonsillar pillar anteriorly.

2. It contains the soft palate, the tonsillar fossae and faucial tonsils, the lateral and posterior pharyngeal walls, and the base of the tongue.

3. The parapharyngeal space lies directly lateral to the oropharynx.
   a. It contains the glossopharyngeal, lingual, and inferior alveolar nerves, the pterygoid muscles, and the internal maxillary artery.
   b. It is a site of early extension of an oropharyngeal tumor.
   c. It also provides a pathway for the tumor to spread to the base of the skull.

4. Lymphatic drainage is primarily to the jugulodigastric (tonsillar) nodes.
   a. Tumors of the soft palate, lateral wall, and tongue base also spread to the retropharyngeal and parapharyngeal nodes.
   b. Retromolar trigone lesions can drain to submaxillary nodes.

### B. Etiology

1. Alcohol and tobacco use are commonly found together in patients with oropharyngeal cancer. There appears to be a synergistic effect of the two substances, but it has not been defined.

2. Local mucosal irritation, malnutrition, and immune defects have also been implicated.

### C. Clinical evaluation

1. Diagnosis is often made late in the course.
   a. Many patients are asymptomatic until tumors are quite large and ulcerate.
   b. Others are treated conservatively for incorrectly diagnosed lesions.

2. The most common **symptom** is persistent sore throat.
   a. This is frequently accompanied by ipsilateral otalgia (referred pain via the tympanic branch of the glossopharyngeal nerve).
   b. A vague sensation of throat irritation, restriction of tongue motion ("hot potato voice"), odynophagia, and bleeding may also be noted.
   c. Most patients, especially those with large lesions, are significantly malnourished.

3. The **initial examination** must include careful palpation of the tonsils and base of the tongue. Many small tumors are difficult to see but may be easily palpated.

4. All lesions should be evaluated by endoscopy under general anesthesia before treatment is chosen.

5. Many patients present with cervical adenopathy.
   a. Nodal metastases are found in 76% of patients with cancer of the base of the tongue and in 60% of patients with tonsillar cancer.
   b. Most such nodes are palpable.

### D. Staging (Table 25-1)

1. **Stage TIS**: Carcinoma in situ

2. **Stage $T_1$**: Lesion of 2 cm or less in greatest diameter

3. **Stage $T_2$**: Lesion larger than 2 cm but less than 4 cm in greatest diameter

4. **Stage $T_3$**: Lesion larger than 4 cm in greatest diameter

5. **Stage $T_4$**: Lesion larger than 4 cm, with invasion of bone or of soft tissues of the neck or the root of the tongue

**Table 25-1.** International College of Surgeons Staging of Oropharyngeal Cancer

| Stage I | $T_1$ | $N_0$ | $M_0$ |
|---|---|---|---|
| Stage II | $T_2$ | $N_0$ | $M_0$ |
| Stage III | $T_3$ | $N_0$ | $M_0$ |
| | $T_4$ | $N_0$ | $M_0$ |
| | Any T | $N_1$ | $M_0$ |
| | Any T | $N_2$ | $M_0$ |
| Stage IV | Any T | $N_3$ | $M_0$ |
| | Any T | Any N | $M_1$ |

**E. Treatment**

1. $T_1$ and $T_2$ lesions are treated with radiotherapy.

2. Combined therapy offers improved survival rates for most large lesions.

3. Combined therapy is also indicated when nodal metastasis is present.

4. Composite resection (the "jaw-neck" or "commando" procedure) is the most common **surgical procedure**.
   a. It involves a radical neck dissection and partial mandibulectomy in continuity with excision of the tumor.
   b. A tracheotomy is routine.
   c. A laryngectomy is performed when either:
      (1) The tumor invades the pre-epiglottic space through the vallecula epiglottica
      (2) The entire tongue base and both hypoglossal nerves are removed
   d. Occasionally, the larynx is spared after total glossectomy in younger and otherwise healthy patients.

**F. Prognosis**

1. The generally poor prognosis of oropharyngeal cancers is directly related to their late diagnosis.

2. In tonsillar cancers, 5-year survival rates range from 63% for patients with $T_1$ tumors to 21% for those with stage IV disease.

3. Patients with tumors of the base of the tongue have 5-year survival rates of 40% to 60% for stage I disease, and 10% to 20% for stage IV disease. A high incidence of late presentation is reflected in the large number of stage IV patients.

4. For patients with tumors of the palatal arch, the 5-year survival rates range from 77% for stage I to 20% for stage IV.

5. The presence of nodal metastases reduces the 5-year survival rate significantly: for $N_0$ it is 75%; for $N_1$, 25%.

## VII. CANCER OF THE HYPOPHARYNX AND CERVICAL ESOPHAGUS

**A. Anatomy**

1. The hypopharynx extends from the pharyngoepiglottic fold to the inferior border of the cricoid, excluding the larynx.

2. It includes the pyriform sinuses, the postcricoid area, and the posterior pharyngeal wall.

3. There is a rich lymphatic network.
   a. The pyriform sinuses drain to jugulocarotid and midjugular nodes.
   b. The posterior pharyngeal wall drains primarily to retropharyngeal nodes.
   c. Lower hypopharyngeal areas drain to paratracheal and low jugular nodes.

**d.** The cervical esophagus additionally is drained by mediastinal nodes.

**B. Classification**

**1.** A good 95% of the tumors in this region are epithelial tumors.

**2.** About 60% to 75% arise in the pyriform sinuses and 20% to 25% on the posterior pharyngeal wall; rarely, tumors arise in the postcricoid area.

**C. Etiology.** As with other head and neck tumors, the tumors are related to heavy alcohol intake and tobacco use.

**D. Clinical evaluation**

**1.** The triad of throat pain, referred otalgia, and dysphagia is present in more than one-half of the patients.
  **a.** Hoarseness and airway obstruction signal laryngeal involvement.
  **b.** Small postcricoid tumors often present with mild symptoms of sore throat, a "lump in the throat," and throat clearing.

**2.** Cervical metastases (41% of them occult) are found in 75% of patients with pyriform sinus cancers and in 83% of pharyngeal wall tumors (66% occult).

**3.** A "barium swallow" and endoscopy with biopsy complete the workup.

**E. Staging**

**1. Stage TIS**: Carcinoma in situ

**2. Stage $T_1$**: Carcinoma confined to the site of origin

**3. Stage $T_2$**: Extension of the tumor to an adjacent site without fixation of the hemilarynx (vocal cord)

**4. Stage $T_3$**: Extension of the tumor to an adjacent site with fixation of the hemilarynx

**5. Stage $T_4$**: Massive tumor with invasion of bone, cartilage, or the soft tissues of the neck

**F. Treatment**

**1.** Most lesions are treated with laryngopharyngectomy and radical neck dissection, followed by radiotherapy.
  **a.** If the tumor is $T_1$ or $T_2$ and spares the apex of the pyriform sinus, a supraglottic laryngectomy can be considered.
  **b.** Some small $T_1$ tumors can be treated by radiation therapy alone or by surgical resection via a lateral pharyngotomy.
  **c.** Cancers of the cervical esophagus require removal of the pharynx, esophagus, and larynx.

**2. Reconstruction of circumferential defects** of the hypopharynx and cervical esophagus can be accomplished with:
  **a.** Regional skin flaps, such as deltopectoral or cervical (this requires multiple stages)
  **b.** Pedicled myocutaneous flaps
  **c.** Esophagectomy, followed by gastric "pull-up" (raising the stomach into the chest or neck to replace the esophagus)
  **d.** Colon interposition
  **e.** A free intestinal graft with microvascular anastomosis

**G. Prognosis** is poor because of extensive submucosal spread and the high incidence of cervical metastasis.

**1.** The overall 5-year survival rate is approximately 30% for patients with hypopharyngeal tumors.

**2.** It rises to 50% for those who qualify for supraglottic laryngectomy.

## VIII. CANCER OF THE LARYNX

**A. Anatomy**

**1.** The larynx is divided into three regions.
  **a.** The **supraglottis** extends from the tip of the epiglottis to include the false vocal cords and roof of the ventricle.

**b.** The **glottis** extends from the depth of the ventricle to 1 cm below the free edge of the true vocal cord.

**c.** The **subglottis** extends from 1 cm below the free edge of the true vocal cord to the inferior border of the cricoid cartilage.

**2. Lymphatic drainage**

**a.** The supraglottis has a rich network that crosses the midline and drains to the deep jugular nodes.

**b.** The glottis has poorly developed, sparse lymphatics.

**c.** The subglottis drains through the cricothyroid membrane to the prelaryngeal (delphian) and pretracheal nodes.

**B. Etiology**

**1.** Over 90% of patients have a significant smoking history.

**2.** Heavy alcohol consumption is common, but not a definite etiologic factor.

**C. Classification**

**1.** Some 95% to 98% of the tumors are squamous cell carcinomas.

**2.** Verrucous carcinoma is a variant of squamous cell carcinoma that is locally invasive but almost never metastasizes. It can undergo malignant degeneration.

**D. Clinical evaluation**

**1.** The most common symptom is hoarseness.
   **a.** Stridor, cough, hemoptysis, dysphagia, and aspiration also occur.
   **b.** Neck masses are uncommon at the time of presentation.

**2.** All patients require direct laryngoscopy and biopsy for **diagnosis**.

**3.** Laryngograms, a barium swallow, stroboscopic laryngoscopy, and CT may be helpful.

**E. Staging**

**1. Stage TIS**: Carcinoma in situ

**2. Stage $T_1$**: Tumor confined to the site of origin

**3. Stage $T_2$**: Tumor spread to an adjacent laryngeal site

**4. Stage $T_3$**: Tumor confined to the larynx with fixation of the hemilarynx

**5. Stage $T_4$**: Tumor with cartilage destruction or extension beyond the larynx

**F. Treatment**

**1.** Carcinoma in situ is treated by excision of the involved vocal çord mucosa, and is then closely monitored.

**2.** Radiation therapy is usually reserved for more extensive disease.

**3.** Most $T_1$ lesions are treated with radiation.
   **a.** Removal of the vocal cord by traditional techniques or by using a carbon dioxide laser is recommended by some authors, but cordectomy by laser is still controversial.
   **b.** Some glottic lesions that involve the anterior commissure may be treated by hemilaryngectomy (vertical laryngectomy).
   **c.** Some small lesions of the tip of the epiglottis can also be treated with limited surgical resection.

**4.** Supraglottic (horizontal) laryngectomy is the treatment for larger supraglottic tumors.
   **a.** This procedure removes the epiglottis, aryepiglottic folds, and false vocal cords, sparing the true vocal cords.
   **b.** For transglottic tumors (supraglottic tumors that spread to a true vocal cord), a supra-hemilaryngectomy may be considered.
   **c.** Radical neck dissection, radiation, or both, is often necessary, since nodal metastases (30% of which are occult) are found in 55% of supraglottic cancers.

**5.** All $T_3$ and $T_4$ lesions require total laryngectomy, often combined with radical neck dissection, radiation, or both.

**6.** Verrucous carcinoma is treated surgically, using a conservative laryngectomy when possible.

There is no need for elective radical neck dissection, and radiotherapy has been implicated in the causation of anaplastic transformation.

G. **Prognosis** is better in laryngeal cancer than with other head and neck sites. Five-year survival rates by stage are as follows:

1. $T_1$—85% to 90%, with surgery or radiation
2. $T_2$—80% to 85%
3. $T_3$—75%
4. $T_4$—30%

## IX. CANCER OF THE EAR

### A. Anatomy

1. The portions of the ear susceptible to tumors include the external ear (**pinna**), external auditory canal, and middle ear. The **tympanic membrane** separates the external canal from the middle ear.

2. Lymphatic drainage of the external ear and canal is anterior through the parotid, posterior to the mastoid nodes, and deep to the jugulodigastric nodes.

### B. Classification and etiology

1. Cancer of the ear is very rare.

2. The **etiology** has been related to thermal burns, chronic suppurative infection, and exposure to radium.

3. About 86% are epithelial cancers.
   a. Basal cell carcinomas comprise 8%, melanoma and adenocarcinoma comprise 2% each, and rhabdomyosarcoma and spindle cell sarcoma comprise 1% each.
   b. Other malignancies, such as osteogenic sarcoma, are extremely rare.

4. Approximately 80% of ear cancers arise on the auricle, 15% in the external canal, and 5% in the middle ear.

5. **Lytic lesions** deep in the temporal bone should be worked up as possible metastasis, and are usually from an adenocarcinoma or hypernephroma.

### C. Clinical evaluation

1. Most ear tumors present with a picture of an infected, painful, chronically draining ear.

2. If a mass is present in the external canal, it is usually friable.

3. When cancer is suspected, the mass is biopsied, under controlled conditions. Significant hemorrhage may occur.

4. Vertigo and facial paralysis are ominous signs.

5. CT is necessary in most cases to evaluate the extent of tumor invasion.

### D. Treatment

1. Cancers of the auricle can usually be treated with wedge excision.

2. In deeper, more advanced cancers, radical surgery provides the best chance for cure.
   a. Tumors of the canal that are at least 5 mm lateral to the eardrum can be treated by excision of the external canal.
   b. Cancers that impinge on the tympanic membrane without middle ear invasion are treated with partial (lateral) temporal bone resection. This removes the external canal, eardrum, incus, and malleus, while sparing the facial nerve.
   c. Cancers that involve the middle ear or pneumatized spaces are best treated by total en bloc temporal bone resection.

3. Radiation therapy is palliative and is utilized to treat recurrent or residual disease.

4. Combined therapy may be indicated in some cases.

**E. Prognosis.** Results are difficult to evaluate because of the small number of cases reported.

    **1.** For patients requiring temporal bone resection, 5-year survival rates have ranged from 25% to 35%.

        **a.** However, many of these operations transgressed the tumor, leaving gross tumor behind.

        **b.** Newly described en bloc procedures should improve these statistics.

    **2.** For lesions confined to the pinna, an 80% cure rate can be expected after treatment.

## X. CANCER OF THE SKIN (see also Chapter 30, section II C–F)

**A. Epidemiology.** Cancers of the skin account for 25% of all cancers, and fully 90% of skin cancers occur on the head and neck.

**B. Basal and squamous cell carcinomas**

    **1.** Basal cell carcinoma accounts for 60% of skin cancers, and squamous cell carcinoma for 30%.

    **2. Etiologic factors** include:

        **a.** Sunlight

        **b.** Radiation

        **c.** Arsenic

        **d.** Burns, scars

        **e.** Genetic disorders (xeroderma pigmentosa, basal-cell nevus syndrome, albinism)

    **3. Clinical evaluation**

        **a.** Skin cancers usually present as slowly enlarging cutaneous or subcutaneous lesions. Some form nonhealing ulcers.

        **b.** Nodal metastasis is uncommon.

    **4. Treatment.** The forms of therapy include electrodesiccation, curettage, cryosurgery, excision, Mohs' chemosurgery, radiation, and topical fluorouracil.

        **a.** Surgical excision is preferred for squamous cell carcinoma because it allows removal of a margin.

        **b.** Basal cell carcinomas of the nasolabial folds, medial and lateral canthi, or postauricular regions are especially aggressive. They can invade multiple tissue planes, and therefore require an extensive surgical resection.

        **c. Mohs' chemosurgery** involves the precise mapping and frozen-section control of the entire resection bed. It is especially useful for cancers in areas known for aggressive patterns of spread and recurrence.

        **d.** Radiation therapy is usually reserved for advanced lesions in areas where surgical excision leaves a cosmetically unacceptable defect (the nose, eyelid, lip).

            **(1)** Radiation probably should not be employed when tumors invade bone or cartilage.

            **(2)** These cases require radical excision.

        **e.** All positive nodes should be treated with radical neck dissection or radiotherapy.

**C. Malignant melanoma**

    **1. Epidemiology**

        **a.** Malignant melanoma accounts for 1% of all cancers.

        **b.** Some 20% to 30% of all melanomas arise in the head and neck.

        **c.** Melanoma occurs predominantly in whites. It commonly occurs in persons aged 30 to 60 and is rare in children.

    **2. Etiologic factors** include sunlight and heredity.

    **3.** Melanomas may arise from **junctional nevi** (see Chapter 30, section II D 2 a).

        **a.** These are usually present from birth.

        **b.** Nevi which undergo malignant transformation are usually in an irritated or exposed area.

    **4. Pathologic variants** include:

        **a.** Lentigo maligna melanoma

        **b.** Superficial spreading melanoma

        **c.** Nodular melanoma

    **5.** Melanomas can also arise on the mucosal surfaces of the head and neck.

    **6. Staging** is by depth of invasion:

        **a. Stage $T_1$:** Up to 0.75 mm deep

        **b. Stage $T_2$:** 0.76 to 1.5 mm

    **c. Stage $T_3$**: 1.51 to 3.0 mm
    **d. Stage $T_4$**: More than 3.0 mm

  **7. Treatment** is by wide excision of the melanoma.
    **a.** A radical neck dissection is performed for positive nodes.
      **(1)** A parotidectomy is added to the radical dissection for lesions of the anterior scalp, eyelids, auricle, and cheek because the first-level lymphatic drainage is to the periparotid nodes.
      **(2)** Elective radical neck dissection is usually performed on patients with $T_3$ and $T_4$ tumors.
    **b.** Radiation therapy is usually reserved for palliative treatment of recurrent disease.
    **c.** Chemotherapy, primarily with dacarbazine (DTIC), is used for disseminated melanoma.

  **8. Prognosis**
    **a.** This is related to the depth of invasion.
      **(1)** $T_1$ lesions have a 5-year survival rate of 90%; $T_4$ lesions, 10%.
      **(2)** $N_0$ lesions have a 90% 5-year survival rate; $N_1$ to $N_3$ lesions, 10%.
    **b.** The prognosis in mucosal melanoma is extremely poor.

## XI. LYMPHOMA OF THE HEAD AND NECK

### A. Epidemiology

  **1.** Some 80% of all malignant lymphomas arise from nodes, many in the head and neck.

  **2.** About 65% to 70% of patients with Hodgkin's lymphoma have cervical lymph node involvement.

  **3.** Extranodal presentation is rare in Hodgkin's disease but occurs in 20% of non-Hodgkin's lymphoma cases.

### B. Non-Hodgkin's lymphoma is really a group of diseases.

  **1.** They are classified into favorable and unfavorable types on the basis of therapeutic response.
    **a. Favorable types** include:
      **(1)** Nodular lymphomas
      **(2)** Well-differentiated lymphocytic lymphoma
    **b. Unfavorable types** include:
      **(1)** Diffuse poorly differentiated lymphocytic lymphoma
      **(2)** Diffuse histiocytic lymphoma
      **(3)** Diffuse undifferentiated lymphoma
      **(4)** Nodular histiocytic lymphoma

  **2.** The **histology** of a Hodgkin's lymphoma also influences prognosis:
    **a.** Lymphocyte-predominant—favorable
    **b.** Nodular sclerosing—favorable
    **c.** Mixed cellular—guarded
    **d.** Lymphocyte-depleting—unfavorable

### C. Clinical evaluation

  **1.** The usual presentation is of a single enlarged cervical node.
    **a.** Initial workup is aimed at discovery of an extranodal primary lesion.
    **b.** The enlarged node must be differentiated from squamous cell carcinoma.

  **2.** Most lymphomatous nodes are firm and rubbery.
    **a.** Non-Hodgkin's lymphoma typically presents in upper cervical nodes.
    **b.** Hodgkin's disease is discovered in nodes throughout the cervical chain.

  **3.** The most common **sites of extranodal involvement** in non-Hodgkin's lymphoma are in the head and neck.
    **a.** Most extranodal lesions arise in Waldeyer's ring.
    **b.** Other sites include the nasal cavity, paranasal sinuses, orbit, and salivary glands.

  **4.** About 40% of patients with Hodgkin's lymphoma have systemic symptoms of fever, sweats, weight loss, and malaise.

  **5.** Diagnosis is usually by excisional biopsy of a lymph node.
    **a.** If a possible extranodal source has been discovered, it should be biopsied first.
    **b.** Endoscopy should always precede lymph node biopsy to rule out a primary tumor.

**c.** For a node biopsy, one of the largest nodes should be removed in its entirety.

**d.** Frozen-section diagnosis is of little value, except to exclude squamous cell carcinoma.

**D. Staging** is aimed at determining the extent of spread of the lymphoma.

  **1.** After the diagnosis is made, all patients undergo chest x-ray, CT of the abdomen, and a bone marrow biopsy.

   **a.** CT of the chest, intravenous pyelography, and lymphangiography are sometimes added, depending on initial findings.

   **b.** All patients with non-Hodgkin's lymphoma should have a "GI series" because of the high incidence of gastrointestinal involvement.

  **2.** A **staging laparotomy** is often necessary for patients with an early stage of lymphoma when treatment with radiotherapy alone is contemplated. Laparoscopy can be substituted when patients will also receive chemotherapy.

  **3.** The **stages** are as follows:

   **a. Stage I**: Involvement of a single lymph node region or a single extralymphatic site

   **b. Stage II**: Either of the following:

     **(1)** Involvement of two or more lymph node regions on the same side of the diaphragm

     **(2)** Localized involvement of an extranodal site and of one or more lymph node regions on the same side of the diaphragm

   **c. Stage III**: Involvement of lymph node regions or extranodal sites on both sides of the diaphragm

   **d. Stage IV**: Diffuse or disseminated involvement of one or more distant extranodal organs

**E. Treatment**

  **1.** Patients with stage I or II Hodgkin's disease are treated with radiotherapy alone.

  **2.** Patients with more advanced stages are treated with **MOPP chemotherapy** [mechlorethamine, vincristine (Oncovin), procarbazine, and prednisone], usually combined with nodal irradiation.

  **3.** Treatment of non-Hodgkin's lymphoma is much less clear-cut.

   **a.** In general, early stages (I and II) are treated with radiotherapy, and later stages (III and IV) with chemotherapy.

   **b.** Combined radiation and chemotherapy are usually used for advanced unfavorable lesions.

**F. Prognosis**

  **1. Hodgkin's disease**

   **a. Favorable prognostic factors** include:

     **(1)** Localized disease

     **(2)** A limited number of anatomic sites

     **(3)** Absence of massive disease

     **(4)** A favorable histology (lymphocyte-predominant and nodular sclerosing)

   **b.** Stages I and II have 5-year relapse-free rates of 80% to 90%.

     **(1)** The rate falls to 60% to 80% in advanced disease treated with combined therapy.

     **(2)** Rates as low as 30% have been reported in stage IV lesions.

  **2. Non-Hodgkin's lymphoma**

   **a.** Radiation therapy for stages I and II patients yields 50% to 70% cure rates.

   **b.** In more advanced lesions, patients with favorable histology can have a 60% to 70% 5-year survival rate, and a 30% cure rate.

   **c.** Patients with an unfavorable histology face a 25% to 40% 5-year survival rate, with little chance for cure.

## XII. UNUSUAL TUMORS

**A. Chemodectomas (paragangliomas)** arise from chemoreceptor tissue.

  **1.** They are rarely malignant (2% to 6% are), but they have the propensity for extensive local invasion.

  **2.** Paragangliomas are often multicentric and associated with other malignancies.

  **3.** They are found in the carotid body, ganglion nodosum of the vagus nerve, aortic arch, jugular bulb, and within the middle ear, orbit, nose, nasopharynx, or larynx. Morbidity and mortality depend on the tumor type and extent.

a. **Carotid body tumors** usually present as a slowly growing, painless neck mass.
  (1) About 2.8% are bilateral. This increases to 26% in patients with a familial tendency for paragangliomas.
  (2) Large tumors can cause dysphagia, airway obstruction, and cranial nerve palsies.
  (3) The mass may be pulsatile and may have a bruit.
  (4) **Diagnosis** is by angiography, which shows a tumor blush at the carotid bifurcation that splays the internal and external carotids.
  (5) **Treatment** is by surgical excision. Large tumors may require carotid bypass.
b. **Glomus tumors**
  (1) **Glomus jugulare and glomus tympanicum tumors**
    (a) **Glomus jugulare tumors** arise in the jugular bulb.
      (i) They can invade the middle ear, the labyrinth, and the cranium.
      (ii) They commonly affect multiple cranial nerves, especially VII, IX, X, XI, and XII.
    (b) **Glomus tympanicum tumors** arise in the middle ear, along the tympanic nerve.
    (c) Most patients have pulsatile tinnitus and present with an aural "polyp" or a middle ear mass that can be seen with pneumatic pressure on the tympanic membrane. Hearing loss and vertigo are also common.
    (d) **Evaluation** includes angiography, retrograde jugular venography, and CT. Biopsy should be avoided.
    (e) The **treatment** of choice is surgical excision.
      (i) This is easily carried out for small tympanicum tumors, but can carry significant morbidity in patients with large jugulare tumors because of intracranial extension, hemorrhage, and recurrence.
      (ii) Glomus tumors are radiosensitive but not radiocurable.
      (iii) New skull-base surgical techniques have rendered essentially all lesions in this area resectable, and radiation should probably be reserved for recurrences, minimal residual disease, and patients physically unfit for surgery.
  (2) **Other rare sites of glomus tumor formation** are along the vagus nerve in the neck (**glomus vagale**), and in the larynx.
    (a) Up to 10% of patients with a glomus vagale will have associated bilateral glomus tumor, carotid body tumor, thyroid carcinoma, or other neural crest tumors.
    (b) The tumor is extremely rare in children.
    (c) Four-vessel carotid arteriography should be done.
    (d) Treatment is by surgical excision.

B. **Other rare malignant vascular lesions** are found in the head and neck.

1. **Angiosarcomas** arise from the vascular endothelial cells.
   a. They are rapidly growing, extend through the dermis, and frequently metastasize.
   b. The most common site on the head or neck is the scalp.
   c. The only chance for cure is complete excision.

2. **Hemangiopericytoma** arises from the pericytes of Zimmerman around capillaries.
   a. Approximately 25% are found in the head and neck.
   b. They are locally invasive and display an inconsistent malignant potential. Distant metastasis is not uncommon, but nodal spread is rare.
   c. Treatment is by surgical excision. Local recurrence is common.

3. **Kaposi's sarcoma** (see also Chapter 30, section II G 2 d) is a rare tumor that arises in the skin and presents as a bluish-red macule.
   a. It is receiving recent attention because a large percentage of patients with AIDS (acquired immune deficiency syndrome) present with Kaposi's sarcoma.
   b. Head and neck neoplasms in these patients tend to be multiple and have usually been treated with radiotherapy.

C. **Esthesioneuroblastoma (olfactory neuroblastoma)** is a rare neurogenic lesion that arises from the olfactory mucosa at the roof of the nose.

1. It presents as a nasal mass with the usual symptoms of epistaxis and obstruction.

2. Involvement of the cribriform plate is routine, and intracranial extension is common.

3. Pathologic diagnosis can be difficult.

4. Workup includes CT and occasionally angiography.

5. **Treatment** is with combined intracranial and intranasal resection, and radiotherapy in selected cases.
   a. Local recurrence rates are high (50%), but metastasis is uncommon (20%).

**b.** The 5-year survival rate is about 50%.

**c.** However, since most of the literature predates the current mode of therapy, recurrence and survival statistics should improve.

## D. Tumors of bone and soft tissue

1. **Osteogenic sarcoma**, the most common tumor of bone, occurs rarely in the head and neck.

   **a.** The most common site in the head and neck is the jaws. Only about a dozen cases have been reported that were primary to the temporal bone.

   **b. Etiologic factors** are unproven, although previous bone disease and prior irradiation have been implicated.

   **c. Treatment** is by radical excision.

      **(1)** The efficacy of adjuvant radiation therapy is controversial.

      **(2)** The most recent literature suggests that chemotherapy should be reserved for metastatic disease.

   **d.** The 5-year survival rate is extremely poor.

2. **Ewing's sarcoma**, in about 9% of the cases, occurs in the skull and facial bones.

   **a.** It is usually a painful, swollen lesion.

   **b.** Treatment is with radiation and adjuvant chemotherapy.

   **c.** The 5-year survival rate is about 50%.

3. **Ameloblastoma** is a locally invasive tumor arising from the odontogenic apparatus.

   **a.** It usually presents as a painless swelling and is much more common in the mandible than in the maxilla.

   **b.** Treatment is by conservative local excision. Radiation can be utilized for the rare malignant case.

4. **Rhabdomyosarcoma** (see also Chapter 30, section II G 2 c) is primarily a disease of children.

   **a.** It can occur in the orbit, oral cavity, pharynx, face, neck, ear, paranasal sinuses, or salivary glands.

   **b.** It is treated with radiation and chemotherapy.

   **c.** Except for tumors in the orbit, which have an 80% 2-year survival rate, the prognosis is poor.

5. **Soft tissue sarcomas [fibro-, lipo-, and chondrosarcomas** (see also Chapter 30, section II G)] are quite rare in the head and neck.

   **a.** They can be associated with prior irradiation.

   **b.** Treatment is with surgery and radiation. Local recurrence rates are high.

6. **Chordoma** is a rare tumor arising from the embryonic notochord.

   **a.** One-half of these tumors occur in the craniocervical region.

   **b.** They are slow-growing, locally invasive tumors that cause bone and soft tissue destruction.

   **c.** They can present as a nasopharyngeal mass.

   **d.** Treatment is with surgical excision, radiation therapy, or both. Local recurrence rates are high.

# 26

# The Parotid Gland

R. Anthony Carabasi, III

## I. ANATOMY

**A.** The parotid gland is the largest of the salivary glands.

**B.** It appears in the fourth week of gestation and originates from the epithelium of the oropharynx.

**C.** The gland covers the masseter muscle. It extends posteriorly beyond the vertical ramus of the mandible and abuts the external auditory meatus.

**D.** Enclosing the gland is a dense **fascial sheath**. The tightness of this fascia is responsible for the severe pain that accompanies acute swelling of the gland (acute parotitis).

**E.** **Drainage** is via Stensen's duct. This exits anteriorly, pierces the buccinator muscle, and enters the oral cavity opposite the second upper molar.

**F.** Classically, the parotid gland was thought to have two **lobes**, superficial and deep. Anatomically, this is probably not the case, but it is useful to think of the gland in this way when discussing the surgical treatment of parotid diseases.

**G.** The **facial nerve** enters the posterior part of the gland immediately after emerging from the stylomastoid foramen.

    **1.** It divides within the substance of the gland into two trunks. These eventually split into five major **branches**:
        **a.** Temporal
        **b.** Zygomatic
        **c.** Buccal
        **d.** Mandibular
        **e.** Cervical

    **2.** The nerve and branches separate the superficial and deep portions of the gland.

    **3.** The muscles of expression are supplied by the facial nerve on the ipsilateral side of the face.

## II. BENIGN NEOPLASMS

**A.** Approximately 80% of parotid tumors are benign. Although most are benign, these tumors require very careful identification and surgical treatment. Many are multicentric and have a high incidence of local recurrences.

**B.** **Types of benign neoplasms**

    **1. Mixed tumors** are so named because they contain both stromal and epithelial components.
        **a.** They are the most common benign salivary tumors, and account for 60% of all parotid tumors.
        **b.** Mixed tumors are slow-growing tumors, but may be quite large at the time of presentation.

    **2. Papillary adenocystoma (cystadenoma) lymphomatosum (Warthin's tumor)** occurs most often in men aged 40 to 60.
        **a.** These tumors are composed of both epithelial and lymphoid elements.
        **b.** They are soft (cystic) when palpated.

**c.** When cut, they are found to contain mucoid material which appears purulent. However, despite this appearance, the tumors are neoplastic and not inflammatory.

**3. Benign lymphoepithelial tumor (Godwin's tumor)**
   **a.** This uncommon tumor occurs most frequently in middle-aged or older women.
   **b.** It is characterized by slowly progressive lymphoid infiltration of the gland.
   **c.** Care must be taken not to confuse this lesion with a malignant lymphoma.
   **d.** Occasionally, Godwin's tumor is unencapsulated, and when this occurs it mimics an inflammatory process.

**4. Oxyphil adenomas** are made up of acidophilic cells called **oncocytes**.
   **a.** These tumors occur most frequently in elderly patients.
   **b.** They are slow-growing and do not usually become larger than 5 cm.

**5. Miscellaneous lesions** such as **hemangiomas** and **lymphangiomas** also occur.

**C. Surgical treatment of benign tumors**

   **1.** All of these tumors are treated by excision that includes a margin of normal gland.
      **a.** Tumors extending into the deep lobe of the gland will require total parotidectomy.
      **b.** At surgery, mixed tumors often seem to "shell out" easily; that is, they seem easy to remove from the surrounding normal tissue. However, this invariably leaves nests of residual tumor, resulting in recurrence that requires reexcision.
      **c.** Recurrences of Godwin's tumor may be treated with small doses of radiation.
      **d.** Hemangiomas that do not regress are treated by resection.

   **2.** During surgery, the facial nerve must be identified and preserved.

## III. MALIGNANT NEOPLASMS

**A.** Malignant tumors comprise 20% of all parotid neoplasms. They are often characterized by pain and facial nerve paralysis.

**B. Types of malignant neoplasms**

   **1. Mucoepidermoid carcinoma**
      **a.** This interesting tumor arises from the ducts of the gland.
      **b.** It is the most common parotid malignancy, and comprises 9% of all parotid tumors.
      **c.** It occurs in two forms:
         **(1) Low-grade tumors** are the more common form and are the tumors seen most frequently in childhood.
            **(a)** They are generally soft to palpation and appear encapsulated at surgery.
            **(b)** They are treated by excision of the tumor with preservation of those facial nerve branches that are not directly involved by the lesion.
            **(c)** When low-grade tumors are treated properly, the 5-year survival rate approaches 95%.
         **(2) High-grade tumors** are extremely aggressive, unencapsulated tumors which invade the gland widely.
            **(a)** Treatment must be radical and includes total parotidectomy, including the facial nerve, plus radical neck dissection (see Chapter 25, section II D 2). Neck dissection is done even without palpable nodes because there is a high incidence of microscopic nodal metastasis.
            **(b)** Surgery is usually supplemented by postoperative radiation.
            **(c)** The 5-year survival rate is 42% with optimal treatment.

   **2. Malignant mixed tumors**
      **a.** These comprise the second most common type of malignancy and are responsible for 8% of all parotid tumors.
      **b.** Treatment is total parotidectomy; a radical neck dissection is also done for either palpable adenopathy or a high-grade tumor.

   **3. Squamous cell carcinoma** is a rare tumor in the parotid gland.
      **a.** It is very hard on palpation and is usually accompanied by pain and nerve paralysis.
      **b.** It is important to differentiate this lesion from a metastasis arising from a primary tumor elsewhere in the head or neck.
      **c.** The 5-year survival rate is about 20%.

   **4. Other lesions** include **adenocystic carcinoma (cylindroma), acinic cell adenocarcinoma,** and **adenocarcinoma**.
      **a.** Treatment is total parotidectomy.

**b.** Neck dissection is added when obvious nodal disease is present and for high-grade lesions.

**c.** High-grade, recurrent, and inoperable tumors should be treated with postoperative radiation.

**5. Malignant lymphoma** may arise as a primary tumor in the gland. The treatment is the same as for other lymphomas (see Chapter 25, section XI).

## IV. PAROTID TRAUMA

**A. Lacerations** in the area of the parotid may damage the parenchyma of the gland, Stensen's duct, or the facial nerve.

**1. Parenchymal damage** without injury to Stensen's duct will usually heal spontaneously.

**2.** If **Stensen's duct** is lacerated or transected, it should be repaired over a small catheter. This is sutured to the oral mucosa and left in place for 10 days.

**3. Injuries to the facial nerve**
   **a.** These may recover spontaneously if only a distal branch is transected.
   **b.** If a main trunk is injured, it will require meticulous repair by primary anastomosis or nerve grafting.
   **c.** If the injured area is hard to expose, a superficial parotidectomy should be done to facilitate repair.

**B.** If a **foreign body** (e.g., a bullet) is present, it should be removed.

## V. INFLAMMATORY DISORDERS

**A. Acute suppurative parotitis** is usually found in patients who are debilitated and dehydrated and who have poor oral hygiene. Postoperative patients in this condition are particularly at risk.

**1.** *Staphylococcus aureus* is the usual **offending organism**.
   **a.** It most likely enters the gland from the mouth via Stensen's duct.
   **b.** The dehydrated patient whose salivary glands are not secreting actively is prone to rapid growth of the organism in this favorable environment.
   **c.** The bacterial proliferation leads to an intense inflammatory reaction in the gland, with edema and severe pain.

**2. Initial treatment** includes hydration, antibiotics, and measures to promote salivation, such as occasional sucking on a lemon.
   **a.** Cultures from Stensen's duct are taken.
   **b.** Antibiotics are initially directed against *S. aureus* and are later adjusted as indicated by the results of the cultures.

**3.** Small doses of radiation (e.g., 200 roentgens per day for 4 days) may be tried if these measures are not successful.

**4.** If the process is not arrested by the above measures, **surgical drainage** is required.
   **a.** An incision is made around the angle of the mandible, and multiple horizontal incisions are made in the parotid fascia.
   **b.** There are usually multiple abscesses, and each must be drained.
   **c.** The wound is left open to ensure adequate drainage.

**B. Sialadenitis** is a condition caused by stones in the salivary ducts.

**1.** Obstruction of the duct may occur, which causes inflammation and intermittent painful swelling of the gland.

**2.** Plain x-rays may show the stones. A **sialogram**, in which contrast is injected into the draining duct, will also show areas of obstruction and is useful in cases where the stone is not radiopaque.

**3. Surgery**
   **a.** When the stone is near the end of the duct it can be removed transorally.
   **b.** If it is deep in the gland, it can be removed by an external incision.
   **c.** If multiple stones are present and recurrent pain occurs, the entire gland should be removed.

**4.** A **variant of sialadenitis** can occur in which no stones are found.
   **a.** If there is a stricture of the duct on the sialogram, it should be dilated.
   **b.** If symptoms persist, surgery to remove the gland may be necessary.

## QUESTIONS

**Directions:** The question below contains five suggested answers. Choose the **one best** response.

1.  The most common benign tumor of the parotid gland is

(A) mixed tumor
(B) Warthin's tumor
(C) oxyphil adenoma
(D) hemangioma
(E) lymphangioma

**Directions:** Each question below contains four suggested answers of which **one or more** is correct. Choose the answer

    **A**  if **1, 2, and 3** are correct
    **B**  if **1 and 3** are correct
    **C**  if **2 and 4** are correct
    **D**  if **4** is correct
    **E**  if **1, 2, 3, and 4** are correct

2.  A knobby, bone-hard growth at the midline of the palate is discovered during a patient's physical examination. What can be stated about this finding?

(1) Biopsy is necessary
(2) Excision should be undertaken if the growth interferes with denture fitting
(3) Close follow-up is necessary
(4) This is not a malignant lesion

3.  A biopsy of a neck mass should be performed

(1) immediately upon discovery of the mass
(2) after local infectious causes have been ruled out
(3) whenever factors associated with malignancy are present
(4) after thorough endoscopic examination of the mouth, larynx, esophagus, and trachea

4.  True statements concerning treatment of traumatic injuries of the parotid gland include which of the following?

(1) Foreign bodies should be removed
(2) Lacerations of Stensen's duct usually heal spontaneously
(3) Transection of the main trunk of the facial nerve should be repaired by primary anastomosis or nerve grafting
(4) Minor damage to the superficial lobe should be treated by superficial parotid lobectomy

5.  Risk factors associated with the development of a head or neck malignancy include

(1) smoking
(2) radiation exposure
(3) alcohol ingestion
(4) drinking nonfluoridated water

6. Acute suppurative parotitis is an inflammatory disorder of the parotid gland that

(1) is usually found in debilitated, dehydrated patients with poor oral hygiene
(2) is usually caused by *Staphylococcus aureus*
(3) is usually treated by hydration, antibiotics, and measures to promote salivation
(4) may require surgical drainage if conservative measures fail

7. True statements concerning malignant tumors of the parotid gland include which of the following?

(1) Mucoepidermoid carcinoma occurring in childhood usually has a good prognosis
(2) Malignant mixed tumors are the most common malignant parotid tumors
(3) Malignant lymphoma of the parotid gland should be treated in the same way as lymphomas arising elsewhere
(4) Radical neck dissection is routinely performed for all malignant mixed tumors of the parotid gland

## ANSWERS AND EXPLANATIONS

**1. The answer is A.** (*Chapter 26 II A, B*) Mixed tumor accounts for 60% of all parotid tumors. It is so named because it contains both stromal and epithelial elements. Warthin's tumor contains both epithelial and lymphoid elements, and feels like a cyst when palpated. Oxyphil adenoma is composed of acidophilic cells and usually is small. Hemangioma and lymphangioma are uncommon benign parotid tumors.

**2. The answer is C (2, 4).** (*Chapter 24 IV L 3*) The patient has a maxillary torus, or torus palatinus. This benign, slow-growing bony mass is of little clinical significance and requires neither biopsy nor follow-up. Tori may interfere with dentures and in that case should be excised.

**3. The answer is C (2, 4).** (*Chapter 24 I C, D 4 c*) The workup for any head or neck lesion should follow a logical course beginning with a detailed history, a careful physical examination (including a search for signs of infection), appropriate laboratory tests, and relevant radiologic studies. Endoscopy and radiologic studies should precede any incision in the neck. A neck mass biopsy is the last step in a proper workup. The premature biopsy of a squamous cell carcinoma metastatic to the neck from a primary head or neck tumor worsens the overall prognosis by about 20%.

**4. The answer is B (1, 3).** (*Chapter 26 IV*) In the management of parotid gland injuries, bullets and other debris should be removed. Lacerations of Stensen's duct should be repaired over a small catheter, which is brought out into the mouth and returned to the oral mucosa. Minor damage to the parenchyma alone will usually heal spontaneously. Peripheral branches of the nerve may heal spontaneously but main trunk injuries must be repaired by primary anastomosis or nerve grafting.

**5. The answer is A (1, 2, 3).** (*Chapter 25 I B*) Smoking and drinking are significant risk factors in head and neck malignancies. Exposure to radiation is also an etiologic factor. In taking the patient's history, the patient should be questioned about exposure to any of these etiologic agents. As far as is known, the only disorder associated with a nonfluoridated water supply is dental caries.

**6. The answer is E (all).** (*Chapter 26 V A*) Acute suppurative parotitis is usually a staphylococcal infection that develops in debilitated patients who are dehydrated and who cannot maintain good oral hygiene. Elderly, debilitated postoperative patients are particularly at risk. If medical management with hydration, use of antibiotics, and measures to promote salivation are unsuccessful, irradiation is sometimes tried. When all of these conservative attempts have failed, multiple abscesses are commonly present, and each must be drained surgically.

**7. The answer is B (1, 3).** (*Chapter 26 III B*) Mucoepidermoid carcinoma of childhood is usually a favorable lesion, with a 5-year survival rate exceeding 90%. In adults the prognosis is much less favorable. Malignant lymphoma of the parotid is treated much the same as a lymphoma arising elsewhere. Mucoepidermoid carcinoma is the most common malignancy of the parotid; malignant mixed tumors are the second most common. Radical neck dissection is performed if a malignant mixed tumor is a high-grade tumor or if nodes are palpable.

# Part VIII
# Thoracic Disorders

# 27
# Pulmonary Disease
Scott M. Goldman
Bruce E. Jarrell

## I. GENERAL PRINCIPLES OF THORACIC SURGERY

**A. Anatomy of the thoracic cavity**

1. The **chest wall** (Fig. 27-1) is formed by ribs, intercostal muscles, vessels (which run on the undersurface of the ribs), and nerves, and is bordered inferiorly by the diaphragm. It is lined internally by the parietal pleura.

2. The **mediastinum** (Fig. 27-2) forms the compartment between the pleural cavities for the length of the thorax. **Superiorly**, its fascial planes communicate with the neck, thus allowing neck infection to extend into the mediastinum.
    a. The **anterior mediastinum** comprises the thymus gland, lymph nodes, ascending and transverse aorta, and great veins. It is bordered anteriorly by the sternum, posteriorly by the upper dorsal spine, and inferiorly by the anterior border of the heart.
    b. The **middle mediastinum** comprises the pericardium, heart, trachea, hilar structures of the lung, phrenic nerves, and lymph nodes. It is bordered superiorly by the anterior border of the heart, inferiorly by the diaphragmatic surface, and posteriorly by the anterior border of the dorsal spine.
    c. The **posterior mediastinum** comprises the sympathetic chains, vagus nerves, esophago-thoracic duct, descending aorta, and lymph nodes. It extends from the anterior border of the dorsal spine to the posterior rib cage.

3. The **lungs and tracheobronchial tree** (Fig. 27-3)
    a. The **right lung** has **three lobes**—the upper, middle, and lower—separated by two **fissures**. The **major (oblique) fissure** separates the lower lobe from the upper and middle lobes, and the **minor fissure** separates the upper lobe from the middle lobe.

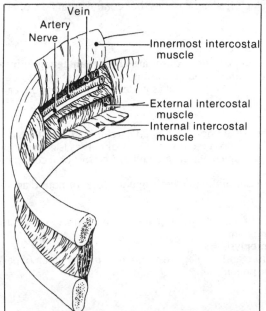

Vein
Artery
Nerve
Innermost intercostal muscle
External intercostal muscle
Internal intercostal muscle

**Figure 27-1.** The chest wall. (Adapted from Way L: Thoracic wall, pleura, lung, and mediastinum. In *Current Surgical Diagnosis and Treatment*, 6th ed. Los Altos, CA, Lange, 1983, p 268.)

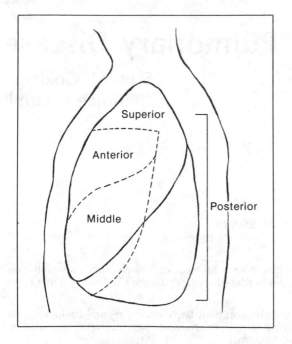

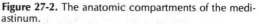

**Figure 27-2.** The anatomic compartments of the mediastinum.

**b.** The **left lung** has **two lobes**—the upper and the lower. The **lingula** is a portion of the upper lobe. The lobes are separated by a **single oblique fissure**.

**c.** **Bronchopulmonary segments** are intact sections of each lobe that have a separate blood supply, allowing segmental resection.

**d.** The **tracheobronchial tree** (see also section XII A) is formed of respiratory epithelium with reinforcing cartilaginous rings; the branching **bronchial tubes** are progressively smaller, down to a diameter of 1 to 2 mm.

**e.** The **blood supply** is dual.
  **(1) Pulmonary artery** blood is **unoxygenated**.
  **(2) Bronchial artery** blood is **oxygenated**.

**f. Lymphatic vessels** are present throughout the parenchyma and toward the hilar areas of the lungs.
  **(1)** Lymphatic drainage is cephalad, flowing toward the scalene nodal areas along the paratracheal areas.
  **(2)** Generally, lymphatic drainage affects ipsilateral nodes, but contralateral flow often occurs from the left lower lobe.

**B. General thoracic procedures**

  **1. Radiologic diagnostic procedures.** The standard procedures are **chest roentgenography** and **tomography** of a lesion. **Computed tomography (CT scanning)** has been shown to be extremely useful in localizing a process anatomically as well as in delineating cavitation, calcification, lymphadenopathy, or multiple lesions.

  **2. Endoscopy**
    **a. Laryngoscopy** is an important procedure to undertake when carcinoma of the lung is suspected. Tumor involvement of the left or both recurrent laryngeal nerves (signifying inoperability) can be diagnosed via laryngoscopy when suspicion is raised by vocal cord paralysis with resultant hoarseness.
    **b. Bronchoscopy** is useful in many diseases of the tracheobronchial tree for both diagnostic and therapeutic purposes.
      **(1) Diagnostic uses** include:
        **(a)** Confirming a lung or tracheobronchial tumor suggested by history, physical examination, or chest roentgenogram
        **(b)** Identifying the source of hemoptysis
        **(c)** Obtaining specimens for culture and cytologic examination from an area of persistent pulmonary atelectasis or pneumonitis
      **(2) Therapeutic uses** include:
        **(a)** Removal of a foreign body

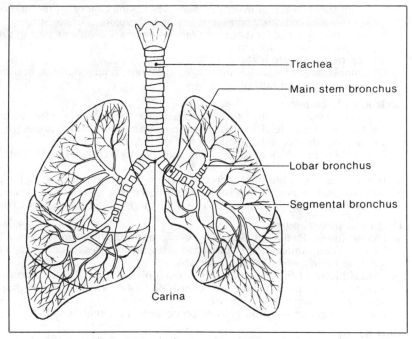

**Figure 27-3.** The lungs and tracheobronchial tree.

    **(b)** Removal of retained secretions (e.g., after administration of general anesthesia or from aspiration of gastric contents)

    **(c)** Drainage of lung infections such as abscesses

  **(3) Types**

    **(a) Rigid bronchoscopy** allows visualization of the trachea and main bronchi to the individual lobes.

      **(i)** It is excellent for biopsies of endobronchial lesions and for clearing of thick secretions postoperatively.

      **(ii)** The performance of rigid bronchoscopy under local anesthesia requires considerable skill.

    **(b) Flexible fiberoptic bronchoscopy** is used more frequently.

      **(i)** It is particularly helpful for visualizing lobar bronchi and the smaller bronchopulmonary segments and for the biopsy of lesions in that area.

      **(ii)** Although not as effective as rigid bronchoscopy, it may also be used for clearing secretions.

      **(iii)** It is especially useful when the patient is intubated, allowing the bronchoscope to be introduced through the endotracheal tube without removal of the airway.

  **(4) Specific advantages**

    **(a)** Bronchoscopically obtained specimens for cytology are positive for tumor in one-third to two-thirds of cases. However, cytologic findings are not adequate proof of a tumor; a tumor biopsy must still be obtained.

    **(b)** Biopsy for suspicion of endobronchial or parenchymal tumors may be performed successfully by bronchoscopy for about one-third to one-half of lung tumors.

      **(i)** As many as 10% of patients develop pneumothorax when biopsies are performed through the bronchus in an attempt to sample the pulmonary parenchyma; therefore, biopsy should not be performed as an outpatient procedure.

      **(ii)** Parenchymal biopsies are useful for suspicion of infection as well. Infections such as those due to *Pneumocystis carinii* can only be diagnosed with fixed-tissue specimens and so require biopsy.

    **(c)** Widening of the tracheal carina in patients with lung tumors can be seen on bronchoscopy. It suggests distortion of the tracheal anatomy by subcarinal nodes and is a poor prognostic sign.

**c. Mediastinoscopy** is a procedure in which a lighted hollow tube is inserted behind the sternum at the tracheal notch and directed along the anterior surface of the trachea.

  **(1) Indications**

    **(a)** It allows direct biopsy of paratracheal and carinal lymph nodes; the specimens are positive for tumor in 40% of cases where lung cancer is present. Positive nodes in this area indicate nonresectability and, therefore, obviate surgery.

**(b)** It is also useful for diagnosing other pulmonary problems such as sarcoidosis, lymphoma, and infections.

**(2)** The **mortality rate** is about 0.1%.

**(3) Complications** include hemorrhage, infections, pneumothorax, and injury to the recurrent laryngeal nerve.

**3. Scalene node biopsy**

**a.** The scalene node–bearing fat pad is located behind the clavicle in the region of the sternocleidomastoid muscle. This area should be palpated in patients suspected of having lung tumors, and should be biopsied if nodes are palpable.

**b.** Tumor is found in 85% of patients with palpable nodes but in only 15% with nonpalpable nodes.

**c.** The scalene nodes are surrounded by important structures, including the pleura, subclavian vessels, the thoracic and other large lymph ducts, and the phrenic and vagus nerves. The principal **complications** of scalene node biopsy result from injury to these structures.

**4. Diagnostic pleural procedures**

**a. Thoracentesis.** Pleural effusions are examined for organisms in suspected infections, and are examined cytologically in suspected malignancies. Positive cytologic findings prove a tumor to be inoperable and unresectable.

**b. Pleural biopsy.** Either percutaneous or open pleural biopsy yields a positive diagnosis in 60% to 80% of patients with tuberculosis or cancer when a pleural effusion or pleural-based mass is present.

**c.** The principal **complication** of these procedures is pneumothorax.

**5. Lung biopsy**

**a. Indications.** Percutaneous lung biopsy may be used for either a localized peripheral lesion or a diffuse parenchymal process.

**b. Types**

**(1) Needle biopsy** is an excellent means for obtaining tissue for tumor diagnosis. However, sampling errors do exist, and a biopsy negative for tumor does not necessarily rule out the existence of a tumor. Needle biopsy is also very useful for the diagnosis of infections and inflammatory processes.

**(a)** The needle can be guided by ultrasonography, fluoroscopy, or CT.

**(b)** The principal **complications** of needle biopsy are pneumothorax and hemorrhage.

**(2) Open lung biopsy** is necessary, with complete removal of the lesion, if needle biopsy fails to diagnose the problem. Open biopsies or resections are ultimately necessary for many lesions of the chest. Different **thoracic incisions** are necessary to expose different areas in the chest. These include:

**(a) Median sternotomy** (Fig. 27-4), for exposure of the heart, pericardium, and structures in the anterior mediastinum

**(b) Posterolateral thoracotomy** (Fig. 27-5), for exposure of the lung, esophagus, and posterior mediastinum

**(c) Axillary thoracotomy** (Fig. 27-6), for limited exposure of the upper thorax, for procedures such as upper lobe biopsy or sympathectomy

**(d) Anterolateral thoracotomy** (Fig. 27-7), for rapid exposure in patients with thoracic trauma or in patients with a very unstable cardiovascular status who cannot tolerate a lateral incision. This type of procedure also allows for excellent control of the airway during the incision.

**(e) Anterior parasternal mediastinotomy** (Chamberlain procedure), a 2- to 3-cm parasternal incision that allows insertion of a mediastinoscope into the mediastinum

## II. THORACIC TRAUMA

**A. Penetrating thoracic trauma**

**1. Pulmonary injury** due to penetrating trauma is usually via **gunshot wounds**; knife wounds are usually not as serious.

**a.** Civilian guns fire at low velocity, with resultant minimal injury to the tissue surrounding the missile tract. Intercostal drainage and thoracotomy, when indicated, are the treatment.

**b.** The military uses high-velocity weapons, which cause extensive damage to the surrounding lung tissue. Treatment is thoracic exploration with lung debridement.

**2. Injury to the upper thorax**

**a. Subcutaneous emphysema** may indicate tracheal injury.

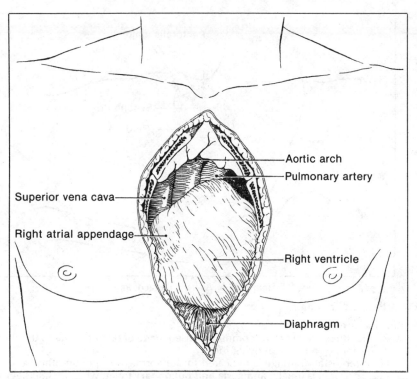

**Figure 27-4.** Median sternotomy. (Adapted from Bryant LR, Morgan CV, Jr: Chest wall, pleura, lung, and mediastinum. In *Principles of Surgery*, 4th ed. Edited by Schwartz SI, et al. New York, McGraw-Hill, 1984, p 612.)

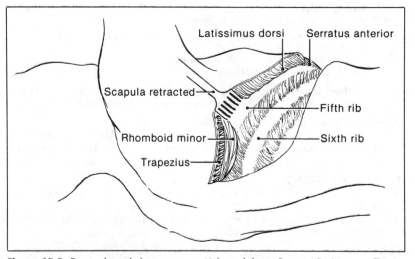

**Figure 27-5.** Posterolateral thoracotomy. (Adapted from Bryant LR, Morgan CV, Jr: Chest wall, pleura, lung, and mediastinum. In *Principles of Surgery*, 4th ed. Edited by Schwartz SI, et al. New York, McGraw-Hill, 1984, p 611.)

    **b.** A large **hemothorax** may indicate major vascular injury.
    **c. Esophageal injury** can often be ruled out by contrast esophagography.

**3. Treatment**
    **a. Intercostal drainage** is always necessary for penetrating thoracic injuries.
    **b. Indications for thoracotomy** include:
        **(1)** Continuing hemorrhage
        **(2)** Massive air leaks
        **(3)** Cardiac penetration
        **(4)** Esophageal injury

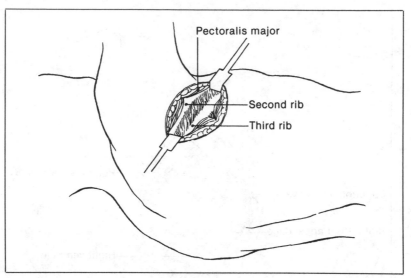

**Figure 27-6.** Axillary thoracotomy.

### B. Blunt thoracic trauma

1. **Rib fractures**
   a. Rib fractures are the most common consequence of blunt trauma to the thorax. They may cause injury to the underlying lung.
      (1) **Intercostal drainage** is indicated for hemorrhage or pneumothorax.
      (2) Treatment is usually **analgesia and pulmonary toilet**, which entails keeping the pulmonary tree free of secretions by suctioning.
   b. **Fractures of the first rib** result from great force, and **injury to the great vessels** may also be present.
      (1) **Angiography** is always indicated.
      (2) Signs of great vessel injury include:
         (a) Absent pulses
         (b) A large hemothorax
         (c) Evidence of brachial plexus injury
         (d) An expanding hematoma

2. In **sternal fractures**, an **underlying cardiac injury** must be suspected. Therapy is supportive, although it may require open reduction for painful nonunion.

3. **Pulmonary contusions**
   a. Contusions result from blunt trauma that causes capillary disruption of the lung, with consequent intra-alveolar hemorrhage, edema, and obstruction of the small airways.
   b. Therapy is supportive and may involve assisted ventilation, fluid restriction, and diuretics.

4. **Tracheobronchial injury**
   a. A tracheobronchial injury must be suspected if a collapsed lung fails to expand after insertion of an intercostal tube. The diagnosis is made by bronchoscopy.
   b. Esophagoscopy should be performed in order to rule out associated esophageal injury.
   c. Treatment is by primary repair.

5. **Flail chest**
   a. If blunt trauma causes extensive rib fractures **paradoxical chest wall movement** may occur.
   b. Paradoxical movement itself may cause **respiratory difficulty**, but the amount of respiratory difficulty is usually related to the underlying lung injury, which may be extensive.
   c. Therapy is supportive, and the patient may require assisted ventilation.

6. **Rupture of the diaphragm**
   a. Rupture is a result of blunt trauma. The **left diaphragm** is more frequently injured, and it tears from the esophageal hiatus radially. It is diagnosed by a chest roentgenogram showing evidence of the stomach above the left diaphragm.
   b. **Injuries of the spleen** are commonly associated with diaphragmatic rupture.
   c. **Treatment** is repair of the diaphragm through the abdomen and treatment of any associ-

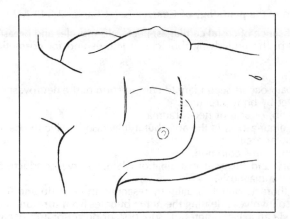

**Figure 27-7.** Anterolateral thoracotomy.

ated injuries. If the rupture is not diagnosed until very late after the injury, repair is under-taken via the chest, in order to free any adhesions from the lung.

**C. Traumatic pneumothorax**

1. **Open pneumothorax** indicates that an open wound in the chest wall has exposed the pleural space to the atmosphere. **Treatment** involves covering the wound and inserting an intercostal tube with underwater seal and suction. Later, debridement and closure of the wound may be necessary.

2. **Enclosed pneumothorax** indicates injury to the underlying lung. It is most often self-limited and is treated with intercostal drainage.

3. **Tension pneumothorax** implies that the pneumothorax has compressed the opposite lung, causing a mediastinal shift.
    a. It is caused by a check-valve type of mechanism in which air can escape from the lung into the pleural space but cannot be vented. It is **a cause of sudden death**.
    b. The collapsed lung results in chest pain, shortness of breath, and decreased or absent breath sounds on the affected side. Hypotension results from vena caval distortion.
    c. The thorax must be decompressed with a needle, which is replaced by an intercostal tube with underwater seal and suction.

**D. Traumatic hemothorax**

1. When blood collects in the pleural cavity due to trauma, the first step in treatment is inter-costal drainage.
    a. If the hemothorax is not drained adequately, the patient may develop an empyema or fi-brothorax and require thoracotomy and decortication.
    b. If the bleeding is from the lung parenchyma, the patient will rarely require thoracotomy.

2. **Continued hemorrhage** at a rate of 100 to 400 ml/hr may indicate intercostal arterial hemor-rhage and may require thoracotomy for repair.

## III. DISORDERS OF THE CHEST WALL

**A. Chest wall deformities**

1. **Pectus excavatum (funnel chest)**
    a. An exceedingly depressed sternum is the **most common chest wall deformity**. It is usually asymptomatic, but it may cause some functional impairment.
    b. **Surgery** is indicated for moderate to severe deformities and is performed at 4 to 5 years of age. The operation involves:
        (1) Excision of all involved costal cartilages
        (2) An osteotomy of the sternum
        (3) Overcorrection of the sternal defect with a bone wedge
        (4) The use of a supporting bar behind the sternum

2. **Pectus carinatum (pigeon breast)**
    a. An overly prominent sternum is less likely to cause functional impairment than a de-pressed sternum.
    b. The repair is similar to that for pectus excavatum.

3. A **distal sternal defect** occurs as part of the **pentalogy of Cantrell** (see Chapter 33, III A 2 d).

4. **Poland's syndrome** is a unilateral absence of costal cartilages, pectoralis muscle, and breast. **Surgery** is indicated for protection of the underlying thoracic structures and for cosmetic reasons.

5. **Thoracic outlet syndrome**
   a. In this condition, arm and neck pain occurs secondary to compression of the neurovascular structures at the thoracic outlet by bony structures.
      (1) The cause may be a cervical rib, or arm or neck trauma.
      (2) The pain usually involves the ulnar aspect of the arm, but it may also involve the back of the neck and the interscapular area.
      (3) Arterial or venous involvement is less common.
   b. **Diagnosis** is based on the history and physical examination. Ulnar nerve conduction studies are helpful in confirming the diagnosis.
   c. **Treatment** is to decompress the thoracic outlet, usually by resecting the first rib and the cervical rib, if present. Surgery also involves releasing the nerve bundles from surrounding scar tissue. It may be performed via an axillary, anterior, superior, or posterior approach.

B. **Chest wall tumors**

1. **Benign tumors**
   a. **Fibrous dysplasia of the rib** occurs posteriorly or on the lateral portion of the rib. It is not painful and is slow-growing. It may occur as part of Albright's syndrome.
   b. **Chondroma** is the most common benign tumor of the chest wall. It occurs at the costochondral junction.
   c. **Osteochondroma** occurs on any portion of the rib.

2. **Malignant tumors** include fibrosarcoma, chondrosarcoma, osteogenic sarcoma, myeloma, and Ewing's sarcoma.

3. **Treatment** of chest wall tumors involves wide excision and reconstruction, using autologous or prosthetic grafts, or both.

## IV. DISORDERS OF THE PLEURA

A. **Pleural effusions**

1. The most common **causes** of pleural effusions are congestive heart failure, infection, and neoplasm.

2. **Management** includes treatment of the underlying cause, thoracentesis (for either diagnostic or therapeutic purposes), and pleural drainage.

B. **Pleural empyema.** Pus in the pleural space usually accumulates secondary to pulmonary infection.

1. **Pathophysiology.** The infection leads to exudation of fluid, which gravitates to the dependent portion of the chest cavity. Fibrin and pleura fuse around the periphery of the fluid, and this becomes an **abscess**.

2. **Diagnosis** is made by thoracentesis in a patient with pleural effusion and fever.
   a. The aspirated fluid is sent for laboratory studies: If organisms are seen on Gram stain, if organisms are cultured out, or if the pH is below 7.4, the diagnosis is very probably an empyema.
   b. On gross examination, if the fluid is very cloudy or is foul-smelling, there is quite likely an empyema.

3. **Treatment**
   a. **Early empyemas** associated with pneumococcal pneumonia may be treated with repeated aspiration and antibiotics.
   b. An **established empyema**, which usually has thicker fluid, needs continuous closed drainage. If the empyema is not completely drained by the intercostal tube, then thoracotomy, debridement, and decortication are necessary.
   c. For **small dependent empyemas** that do not respond to tube drainage, open drainage may be preferred to thoracotomy, especially in poorer-risk patients.

C. **Pleural tumors. Mesothelioma** is related to asbestos exposure.

1. **Localized mesotheliomas** usually arise from the visceral pleura and are treated by local incision.

2. **Malignant mesothelioma** presents with a pleural effusion, and it is almost always a **fatal** disease. Patients may require palliative decortication.

## V. PULMONARY INFECTIONS

### A. Lung abscess

1. Abscess of the lung usually occurs secondary to aspiration. It occurs in the dependent or axillary segments of the lung (i.e., the posterior segment of the upper lobe or the superior segment of the lower lobe).

2. **Treatment**
   a. The usual treatment is **antibiotics**; over 90% of lung abscesses resolve with antibiotic therapy. The most effective antibiotic is **penicillin**.
   b. **Indications for surgery** include:
      (1) Failure of the abscess to resolve with adequate antibiotic therapy
      (2) Bleeding
      (3) Rupture with resulting empyema
   c. The surgery required is usually segmental resection or lobectomy.

### B. Bronchiectasis

1. Bronchiectasis is a complication of repeated pulmonary infections, which can cause bronchial dilatation. The disease usually affects the lower lobes. It occurs in adults and children, who present with a chronic illness with excessive sputum production.

2. **Bronchography** is the definitive diagnostic study.

3. **Treatment**
   a. Most cases respond to medical therapy.
   b. **Surgical therapy** involves segmental resection of the affected area, and best results are obtained in patients with localized disease.

### C. Tuberculosis

1. Approximately 25,000 new cases of tuberculosis are diagnosed each year in the United States.

2. **Treatment**
   a. The disease is now mostly treated with effective **chemotherapeutic agents**, and fewer than 5% of patients require pulmonary resection as part of their therapeutic regimen.
   b. Usually pulmonary resection is performed after a course of chemotherapy. Indications for surgery include:
      (1) Bronchopleural fistula with empyema
      (2) Persistent production of positive sputum
      (3) Persistent open cavities with positive sputum
      (4) Post-tubercular bronchial stenosis
      (5) Pulmonary hemorrhage
      (6) Suspected carcinoma
   c. A high percentage of patients with atypical mycobacteria are likely to have one or more indictions for pulmonary resection.

## VI. COIN LESIONS are solitary, well-circumscribed pulmonary nodules that are peripheral in the lung fields. They are manifestations of neoplastic disease (e.g., bronchogenic carcinoma) or of granulomatous or infectious processes (e.g., tuberculosis).

### A. General characteristics

1. Coin lesions are usually asymptomatic.

2. They occur more often in males than in females.

### B. Benign versus malignant etiology

1. When no other tumor is known to be present, the coin lesion is rarely a sign of metastatic disease.

2. If the patient is younger than 40 years old, there is a two-thirds chance that the lesion is benign.

3. The likelihood of cancer is higher in male than in female patients with coin lesions.

4. The **overall risk of carcinoma** in coin lesions is 5% to 10%.

5. In patients who are operated upon, the probability of cancer is about 33%, the probability of granuloma is about 33%, and the probability of tuberculous granuloma is about 20%. The lesions of the remaining surgical patients are due to other causes.

6. **Roentgenographic evidence** of a benign lesion includes the following.
   a. Calcification is present, particularly if the calcification is concentric, heavy, or has a popcorn-like appearance. If the calcification appears as small flecks, a malignant lesion should be suspected.
   b. Roentgenograms taken 1 year or more apart show no growth in the size of the lesion.
   c. The lesion size is less than 1 cm in diameter. The larger the lesion, the greater the chance of malignancy.
   d. CT scanning demonstrates a well-circumscribed lesion. Multiple lesions that are demonstrated on CT but are not seen on plain film suggest either metastatic disease or satellite lesions from carcinoma or granulomas.

C. Coin lesions should not be biopsied by the percutaneous needle technique because the procedure could result in chest wall seeding of an otherwise curable lesion.

D. The 5-year survival rate is between 70% and 90% with prompt surgical resection.

## VII. BRONCHOGENIC CARCINOMA

A. Incidence

1. Bronchogenic carcinoma is the **leading cause of cancer death in the United States**.

2. Approximately 130,000 new cases are diagnosed each year in this country.

3. About 95% of lung cancers occur in patients who are more than 40 years of age.

B. Etiology

1. **Seventy-five percent** of all lung carcinomas are **related to smoking**; affected individuals usually have a history of smoking 1 or more packs of cigarettes daily for 20 years.

2. There is no known environmental cause. However, chronic exposure to various substances may play a role; nickel, asbestos, arsenic, radioactive materials, and petroleum products have all been implicated.

C. Pathology

1. **Adenocarcinoma** is the **most common lung carcinoma**, representing 30% to 50% of all malignant lung cancers. It is less strongly associated with smoking and occurs more commonly in women.
   a. It arises from the subsegmental airways in the periphery of the lung.
   b. Growth is rapid, and the cancer metastasizes by a vascular route. It may spread diffusely throughout the lung via the tracheobronchial tree.
   c. The overall cure rates are somewhat better than those for squamous cell carcinoma. When the lesion is locally resectable, the cure rate is 50%.
   d. **Bronchioalveolar carcinoma** is a variant of adenocarcinoma.

2. **Squamous cell carcinoma** is the second most common carcinoma of the lung, representing 25% to 40% of all malignant lung tumors. It is associated with smoking.
   a. It is thought to arise from the squamous metaplasia of the tracheobronchial tree.
   b. The tumor is bulky and is associated with bronchial obstruction. It is characterized by slow growth and late metastasis.
   c. It undergoes central necrosis and cavitation.
   d. It may involve the chest wall or structures in the superior pulmonary sulcus (**Pancoast's tumor**).
   e. Approximately two-thirds of squamous cell carcinomas occur centrally in the lung hilus.

3. **Small cell anaplastic (oat cell) carcinoma**, which is highly malignant, represents approximately 15% to 25% of all malignant lung tumors.
   a. It is usually centrally located.
   b. It metastasizes early by lymphatic and vascular routes.
   c. It may be curable if it is resected in an early stage, and it does respond to combination chemotherapy.

**4. Large cell carcinoma** of the lung is highly malignant. It may be located either centrally or peripherally.

**5. Other tumors**, such as bronchial adenoma, papilloma, and sarcomas, are rare.

### D. Clinical manifestations

**1.** Patients may be **asymptomatic**, the only clue to the cancer being an abnormal chest x-ray.

**2. Pulmonary symptoms** include cough, dyspnea, chest pain, fever, sputum production, and wheezing.

**3. Extrapulmonary symptoms**
   **a.** These may be **related to metastasis**, such as weight loss, malaise, symptoms referable to the central nervous system, and bone pain.
   **b. Nonmetastatic extrapulmonary manifestations** are secondary to hormone-like substances that are elaborated by the tumor. These include Cushing's syndrome, hypercalcemia, myasthenic neuropathies, hypertrophic osteoarthropathies, and gynecomastia.

**4.** A **Pancoast tumor** involving the superior sulcus may produce symptoms related to brachial plexus involvement, sympathetic ganglia involvement, or vertebral collapse secondary to local invasion. This may result in pain or weakness of the arm, edema, or **Horner's syndrome** (i.e., ptosis, miosis, enophthalmos, and decreased sweating on the side of involvement).

### E. Diagnosis

**1.** The most common finding is an **abnormal chest x-ray**.
   **a.** The tumor may present as a nodule, as an infiltrate, or as atelectasis.
   **b.** An abnormal chest x-ray is more likely to represent carcinoma in patients over age 40.

**2. CT scanning** is performed in order to assess the extension of the tumor and to confirm the possibility of mediastinal metastasis.

**3. Bronchoscopy** is performed to assess the bronchial involvement and the resectability, and to obtain tissue for cytologic examination.

**4. Mediastinoscopy** is performed to obtain mediastinal lymph nodes for pathologic examination. Positive findings may or may not preclude a curative resection, depending on the pathologic cell type, the extent of nodal involvement, and the condition of the patient.

**5. Percutaneous needle biopsy** is used to obtain tissue for cytologic examination.

### F. Staging

**1.** Uniform staging of lung carcinoma is fundamental for the evaluation of treatment protocols.

**2.** Staging is based on information obtained during preoperative evaluation, findings at thoracotomy, and pathologic findings of the surgical specimens.

**3.** Definitions of tumor size (T), lymph node metastasis (N), and distant metastasis (M) comprise the **TNM classification** of carcinoma of the lung by the American Joint Committee of Cancer Staging.
   **a. T—primary tumors**
      **(1)** $T_0$: No evidence of primary tumor
      **(2)** $T_x$: Tumor proved by presence of malignant cells in bronchopulmonary secretions but not visualized radiographically or bronchoscopically; or any tumor that cannot be assessed
      **(3)** TIS: Carcinoma in situ
      **(4)** $T_1$: A tumor 3 cm or less in diameter, surrounded by lung or visceral pleura, and without invasion proximal to a lobar bronchus at bronchoscopy
      **(5)** $T_2$: A tumor more than 3 cm in diameter; or any size tumor with visceral pleural invasion, associated atelectasis, or obstructive pneumonitis extending to the hilar region but involving less than the entire lung. At bronchoscopy, the proximal extent of tumor must be within a lobar bronchus or at least 2 cm distal to the carina.
      **(6)** $T_3$: A tumor of any size with extension into an adjacent structure such as the parietal pleura, chest wall, diaphragm, or mediastinum and its contents; or a tumor demonstrated bronchoscopically to involve a main stem bronchus less than 2 cm distal to the carina; or any tumor associated with atelectasis or obstructive pneumonitis of an entire lung or with pleural effusion
   **b. N—regional lymph nodes**
      **(1)** $N_0$: No demonstrable metastasis to regional lymph nodes

      **(2)** $N_1$: Metastasis to lymph nodes in the peribronchial or ipsilateral hilar region, or both, including direct extension

      **(3)** $N_2$: Metastasis to mediastinal lymph nodes

    **c. M—distant metastasis**

      **(1)** $M_0$: No distant metastasis

      **(2)** $M_1$: Distant metastasis to regions such as the supraclavicular or contralateral hilar lymph nodes, liver, or brain

  **4. Stage grouping in cancer of the lung**

    **a. Occult carcinoma**—$T_x$, $N_0$, $M_0$: No evidence of the primary tumor, no evidence of metastasis to the regional lymph nodes, and no distant metastasis, but bronchopulmonary secretions contain malignant cells

    **b. Stage I**

      **(1)** TIS, $N_0$, $M_0$: Carcinoma in situ

      **(2)** $T_1$, $N_0$, $M_0$; $T_1$, $N_1$, $M_0$; or $T_2$, $N_0$, $M_0$: A tumor that can be classified $T_1$ without any metastasis or with metastasis to the lymph nodes in the ipsilateral hilar region only; or a tumor that can be classified $T_2$ without any metastasis to lymph nodes or distant metastasis

    **c. Stage II**—$T_2$, $N_1$, $M_0$: A tumor classified as $T_2$ with metastasis to the lymph nodes in the ipsilateral hilar region only

    **d. Stage III**—$T_3$ (any N or M); $N_2$ (any T or M); or $M_1$ (any T or N): Any tumor more extensive than $T_2$, any tumor with metastasis to the lymph nodes in the mediastinum, or any tumor with distant metastasis

**G. Treatment**

  **1. Surgical treatment**

    **a.** Bronchogenic carcinoma can only be cured by **pulmonary resection** (i.e., lobectomy, extended lobectomy, or pneumonectomy). The **surgical approach** is to resect the involved lung, regional lymph nodes, and involved contiguous structures, if necessary.

      **(1)** Lobectomy is used in disease localized to one lobe.

      **(2)** Extended resections and pneumonectomy are used when the tumor involves a fissure or is close to the pulmonary hilus.

      **(3)** Wedge resections or bronchial segmentectomy may be used in localized disease in high-risk patients.

    **b.** One-half of all patients with lung carcinomas are not candidates for thoracotomy at the time of diagnosis. **Contraindications for thoracotomy** include:

      **(1)** A malignant pleural effusion

      **(2)** Recurrent laryngeal nerve involvement

      **(3)** Contralateral mediastinal lymph node involvement

      **(4)** Poor pulmonary function (this is a relative contraindication)

      **(5)** Distant metastases

      **(6)** Phrenic nerve paralysis

      **(7)** Superior vena cava syndrome

      **(8)** Carinal or high paratracheal node involvement

  **2. Adjuvant therapy.** Further treatment using radiotherapy, chemotherapy, or both is indicated for some advanced-stage tumors.

    **a. Radiotherapy** is particularly helpful in patients with Pancoast's tumors. It has been helpful in the treatment of other tumors, but it is generally indicated in postoperative treatment of patients with positive mediastinal metastasis.

    **b. Chemotherapy**, in general, has not helped to prolong survival or to provide palliation in patients with lung carcinoma, whether combined with surgery or used alone. Chemotherapy with multiple agents has shown some success in controlling oat cell carcinoma, particularly when combined with radiation therapy.

**H. Prognosis**

  **1.** The prognosis is dependent on:

    **a.** The pathologic cell type

    **b.** The tumor size

    **c.** The extent of lymph node metastasis

    **d.** The extent of invasion of adjacent structures

    **e.** The presence or absence of distant metastasis

  **2.** The overall operative mortality rate is less than 5% when fair- to good-risk operative candidates are chosen.

    **a.** Fully 95% of patients with inoperable cancers will die within 2 years.

      **b.** About 25% to 35% of patients with resectable cancers will live 5 years if a lobectomy removes all visible disease. If pneumonectomy is required, the overall 5-year survival rate drops to 15% to 20%.

## VIII. CARCINOID TUMOR

### A. General considerations

1. The age of the average patient with carcinoid tumor is approximately 40 years.

2. There is no known environmental cause of this tumor.

### B. Pathophysiology

1. Bronchial carcinoid tumors **occur in the proximal bronchi**, arise from Kulchitsky-type cells, and histologically resemble carcinoid tumors of the small intestine.

2. The tumor is slow-growing and protrudes into the bronchial lumen to a degree, usually causing some **bronchial obstruction**.

3. It is a **vascular tumor**, and is red in color when visualized through a bronchoscope.

4. Regional lymph node metastases occur in 10% of the patients. Liver metastases are less common.

5. The tumor can excrete hormones, such as serotonin and adrenocorticotropic hormone (ACTH).

### C. Clinical manifestations

1. Patients may have symptoms of bronchial obstruction, with wheezing and atelectasis.

2. Chest roentgenography may reveal evidence of atelectasis or a pulmonary nodule.

3. Rarely, patients may present with carcinoid syndrome or Cushing's syndrome.

### D. Treatment. The only treatment for bronchial carcinoid tumor is **surgical resection**. The usual treatment is lobectomy with lymph node dissection. If the tumor is completely excised, the long-term survival rate is close to 90%.

## IX. BRONCHIAL GLAND TUMORS (BRONCHIAL ADENOMAS)

### A. Pathology

1. These tumors occur in the trachea and bronchi and arise from the bronchial glands.

2. There are two **histologic types**—adenoid cystic carcinoma (cylindroma) and mucoepidermoid tumors.

3. The neoplasms may show behavior that is benign, or they may be malignant, with both regional and distant metastases.

### B. Treatment. The only treatment is **surgical resection**, including lymph node resection. The tumors have a propensity for local recurrence.

## X. HAMARTOMAS

### A. Pathology. These are benign pulmonary tumors that histologically are adenochondromas. They occur within the substance of the lung and usually present as solitary pulmonary nodules.

### B. Treatment. They are usually removed during a diagnostic thoracotomy for evaluation of the solitary nodule.

## XI. METASTATIC TUMORS

### A. Metastatic tumors are common to the lung, which may be the only site of metastatic tumor from a nonpulmonary primary tumor.

### B. Treatment

1. Single or multiple metastatic tumors can be removed from the lung as part of the treatment protocol.

**2.** The best treatment results are obtained with tumors for which there is effective chemotherapy. This combination approach has been used frequently in patients with pulmonary metastases from osteogenic sarcoma and in some patients with metastases from colon carcinoma.

## XII. DISORDERS OF THE TRACHEA

### A. Anatomy

**1. Structure**

**a.** The trachea is 11 cm from the cricoid to the corona, with a range, in the adult, of about 10 cm to 13 cm in length and 2.3 cm to 1.8 cm in diameter.

**b.** The trachea is encircled by 18 to 22 cartilaginous rings. The **cricoid cartilage** is the only complete tracheal ring. The remaining rings are incomplete, with a membranous portion posteriorly.

**c.** The trachea is vertically mobile. When the neck is extended, one-half of the trachea is in the neck, and when the neck is flexed, all of the trachea is behind the sternum.

**2. Relationship to other organs**

**a.** The thyroid isthmus is at the second or third tracheal ring.

**b.** The innominate artery crosses the trachea in its midportion.

**c.** The aorta arches over the trachea in its distal portion.

**d.** The esophagus is posterior to the trachea throughout its course.

**3.** The **blood supply** is segmental and is shared with the esophagus. Blood is supplied by the inferior thyroid artery, the subclavian artery, the supreme intercostal artery, the internal mammary artery, the innominate artery, and the bronchial circulation.

### B. Congenital lesions

**1. Types**

**a. Stenosis.** There are three types of tracheal stenosis—generalized, funnel, and segmental. The bronchi may be small in congenital tracheal stenosis, and an associated pulmonary artery sling, in which the artery tethers the trachea, may be present. **Webs** may also be present.

**b. Congenital tracheomalacia**

**(1) Cartilaginous softening** is due to compression of the trachea by vascular rings, which are anomalies of the aortic arch. These anomalies include double aortic arch, right arch with left ligamentum arteriosum, aberrant subclavian artery, or aberrant innominate artery. The diameter of the trachea is normal, but the wall is collapsible.

**2. Diagnosis**

**a. Signs and symptoms** include:

**(1)** Inspiratory and expiratory wheezing, which may be paroxysmal

**(2)** Feeding problems

**(3)** Frequent infections

**b. Diagnostic studies** include:

**(1)** Air tracheography (tomography)

**(2)** Bronchoscopy

**(3)** Angiography, to assess vascular anomalies

**3. Treatment**

**a. Stenosis and webs** are usually **treated conservatively** because of the difficulty in performing tracheal reconstruction in infants.

**(1)** A web may be removed endoscopically.

**(2)** Tracheostomy may be helpful and should be performed in a narrow area to avoid injury to normal areas of the trachea.

**b. Chondromalacia** is treated by aortopexy, performed under bronchoscopic guidance to maximize the tracheal lumen. The patient may still have some airway problems for a period of time postoperatively.

### C. Neoplasms of the trachea

**1. Types**

**a. Primary neoplasms** are rare.

**(1) Squamous cell carcinomas** are the most common neoplasms of the trachea. They may be exophytic, and may cause superficial ulceration, or may be multiple lesions with interposed areas of normal trachea. The tumor spreads through the regional lymph nodes and by direct extension to mediastinal structures.

**(2) Adenocystic carcinoma** is slow-growing, with a prolonged course. It infiltrates airways beyond the gross tumor, and it spreads paratracheally.

**(3)** Other primary tracheal neoplasms include carcinosarcomas, pseudosarcomas, mucoepidermoid carcinomas, squamous papillomas, chondromas, and chondrosarcomas.

**b. Secondary tumors** to the trachea are usually from the lung, the esophagus, or the thyroid gland.

**2. Diagnosis**

**a. Radiographic studies** include chest roentgenography, air tracheography, and fluoroscopy for evaluation of the larynx. Instillation of contrast medium is not necessary for the evaluation of tracheal tumors.

**b. Bronchoscopy** is deferred until the final operation because the biopsy may be hazardous due to bleeding or obstruction of the airway. Frozen section examination is adequate for assessment of the tracheal tumor.

**c. Pulmonary function testing** is mandatory if carinal or pulmonary resection is contemplated.

**3. Treatment** is by tracheal resection.

**a. General considerations**

**(1) Preoperative antibiotics** are selected on the basis of preoperative tracheal cultures.

**(2)** When there is airway obstruction, **anesthesia** should be induced with halothane.

**(3)** High-frequency **ventilation** may be helpful, and it may be possible to pass a small tube beside the tumor.

**b. Incisions used**

**(1)** A neck incision is used for resection of the upper half of the trachea.

**(2)** A posterolateral thoracotomy is used for the lower portion of the trachea.

**(3)** To expose the entire trachea, it may be necessary to combine these incisions, along with an upper sternal split and a fourth interspace intercostal incision.

**c.** In the **resection procedure**, up to one-half of the trachea may be removed.

**(1)** Adequate mobilization can be obtained by flexing the patient's neck and releasing the larynx or the right lung.

**(2)** An end-to-end anastomosis is performed.

**d. Survival rates** are similar to those for resectable carcinoma of the lung (see section VII H 2 b).

# XIII. LESIONS OF THE MEDIASTINUM

**A. Anatomy** (see section I A 2)

**B. Lymphomas**

**1.** Fifty percent of patients with lymphomas (including those with Hodgkin's disease) have mediastinal lymph node involvement; however, only 5% of patients with lymphomas have *only* mediastinal disease.

**2. Symptoms** of mediastinal lymphoma include cough, chest pain, fever, and weight loss.

**3. Diagnosis** is by chest x-ray and lymph node biopsy, using either mediastinoscopy or anterior mediastinotomy.

**4. Treatment** is nonsurgical.

**C. Teratomas**

**1.** Teratomas occur most frequently in adolescents, and 80% of these tumors are benign.

**2.** They originate from the branchial cleft pouch, in association with the thymus gland. All tissue types are present in these tumors, including ectodermal, endodermal, and mesodermal elements.

**3.** Teratomas are **diagnosed** radiographically and may appear as smooth-walled cystic lesions or as lobulated solid lesions.

**4. Treatment** is total surgical excision.

**D. Germ cell tumors**

**1.** These are malignant tumors of **five distinct histologic types**:

**a.** Seminoma

**b.** Embryonal cell carcinoma

        **c.** Teratocarcinoma
        **d.** Choriocarcinoma
        **e.** Endodermal sinus tumor

    **2.** These tumors are very rare, occurring as less than 1% of all mediastinal tumors.

    **3.** They metastasize to pleural lymph nodes, the liver, bone, and retroperitoneum.

    **4.** They cause **symptoms** of chest pain, cough, and hoarseness due to invasion of the vagus nerves.

    **5.** They are **diagnosed** radiographically.

    **6. Treatment** is by as complete **surgical excision** as possible.

    **7. Adjuvant therapy.** Seminomas are very radiosensitive, and the other cell types may benefit from chemotherapeutic agents.

**E. Middle mediastinal lesions** are usually cystic in nature. The two most common are pericardial cysts and bronchogenic cysts.

    **1. Pericardial cysts** are usually asymptomatic and are found on chest roentgenography. They are smooth-walled and most commonly occur in the cardiodiaphragmatic angle. Surgery is usually performed as a diagnostic procedure, to identify the lesion.

    **2. Bronchogenic cysts** generally arise posterior to the carina. They may be asymptomatic, or they may cause pulmonary compression, which can be life-threatening, particularly in infancy. The usual **treatment** is excision.

**F. Posterior mediastinal lesions** are neurogenic tumors located in the paravertebral gutter. About 10% to 20% are malignant.

    **1.** Seventy-five percent of these neurogenic tumors occur in children under 4 years of age. Malignancy is most likely to occur if the tumor arises in childhood.

    **2.** There are five **histologic types:**
        **a.** Neurilemomas, which arise from the Schwann cells of the nerve sheath
        **b.** Neurofibromas, which can degenerate into neurosarcomas
        **c.** Neurosarcomas
        **d.** Ganglioneuromas, which originate from sympathetic ganglia
        **e.** Neuroblastomas, which also arise from the sympathetic chain

    **3. Pheochromocytomas** occur in the mediastinum, although rarely; they behave similarly to the usual intra-adrenal pheochromocytomas.

    **4. Symptoms**
        **a.** Symptoms include chest pain secondary to compression of an intercostal nerve. If the tumor grows intraspinally, it may cause symptoms of spinal cord compression. Rarely, these tumors have an endocrine function and can secrete catecholamines.
        **b.** The symptoms of neuroblastoma include fever, vomiting, diarrhea, and cough.

    **5. Diagnosis** is by chest roentgenography and CT scanning.

    **6.** Neuroblastomas may have **metastasized** to bone, liver, and regional lymph nodes by the time diagnosis is made. Also, direct extension to the spinal cord may occur.

    **7. Treatment** is by excision. Postoperative radiation is helpful in the treatment of the malignant tumors.

# 28
# Esophageal Disease

Scott M. Goldman
Bruce E. Jarrell

## I. GENERAL CONSIDERATIONS

### A. Anatomy

1. The esophagus is approximately 24 cm in length. It extends from the $C_6$ vertebral level to the $T_{11}$ level.

2. It starts at the **upper esophageal sphincter**, which is made up of the cricopharyngeal muscle, and then courses behind the arch of the aorta and descends into the thorax on the right.

3. It deviates anteriorly and enters the abdomen via the **esophageal hiatus**, which is formed by the right crus of the diaphragm.

4. The tubular esophagus meets the saccular stomach at the **gastroesophageal junction**, where the esophagus is anchored by the phrenoesophageal ligament.

### B. Blood supply

1. **Arterial supply** to the esophagus is from branches of the inferior thyroid artery, the bronchial arteries, and the intercostal arteries.

2. **Venous supply** is more complicated.
   a. An extensive subepithelial venous plexus empties superiorly to the hypopharyngeal veins and inferiorly to the gastric veins.
   b. This is an important portal-systemic connection, especially in patients with portal hypertension.

3. **Lymphatic drainage** is to the nearest lymph nodes, which are the cervical, mediastinal, and celiac nodes.

### C. Innervation. The esophagus is supplied by the sympathetic and parasympathetic system via the pharyngeal plexus and the vagus, upper and lower cervical sympathetic, and splanchnic nerves.

### D. Physiology

1. At the upper border of the esophagus, there is a high-pressure zone, approximately 3 cm to 5 cm in length, which makes up the **upper esophageal sphincter**, which functions in swallowing.

2. The central portion of the esophagus has active **peristalsis**. The waves pass down the body of the esophagus, becoming stronger toward the lower portion.

3. At the lower portion of the esophagus, there is another high-pressure zone, the **lower esophageal sphincter**. It is also 3 cm to 5 cm in length, and it functions to prevent esophageal reflux.

## II. DISORDERS OF ESOPHAGEAL MOTILITY

### A. Oropharyngeal dysphagia

1. **Pathophysiology**
   a. Oropharyngeal dysphagia is caused by **failure of the upper esophageal sphincter to relax** properly.
   b. The problem may be an incoordination between relaxation in the upper esophageal sphincter and simultaneous contraction of the pharynx. This is the cause of pharyngoesophageal

383

diverticulum, also known as **Zenker's diverticulum**, a false diverticulum composed of mucosa only, which pouches out between the fibers of the cricopharyngeal muscle.
c. Oropharyngeal dysphagia shows a frequent association with hiatal hernia and gastro-esophageal reflux.

**2. Symptoms** include dysphagia, reflux of undigested food, and a mass in the left side of the neck that occasionally causes tracheal compression.

**3. Diagnosis**
a. Oropharyngeal dysphagia is usually diagnosed by history and physical examination.
b. Roentgenographic studies are helpful to delineate the diverticulum.
c. Endoscopy is indicated to rule out other esophageal disorders, including significant gastro-esophageal reflux.

**4. Treatment**
a. Oropharyngeal dysphagia is treated by **cricoesophageal myotomy**.
b. Excision of the diverticulum is indicated when it is very long.

**B. Achalasia**

**1. Pathophysiology**
a. Achalasia is an esophageal disease of unknown etiology, although it may be secondary to ganglionic dysfunction. It consists of an absence of peristalsis in the body of the esophagus, a high resting lower esophageal sphincter pressure, and failure of the lower esophageal sphincter to relax during swallowing.
b. A similar symptom complex can be caused by **Chagas' disease**, which is due to the organism *Trypanosoma cruzi*.
c. Carcinoma of the esophagus is 10 times more common in patients with achalasia than in the general population.

**2. Symptoms** of achalasia include dysphagia followed later by regurgitation.

**3. Diagnosis**
a. Radiographic studies reveal a dilated esophagus with a beak-like extension into the lower narrowed segment.
b. Esophageal motility studies reveal the high resting lower esophageal sphincter pressure, failure of relaxation during swallowing, and lower than normal pressure in the body of the esophagus.

**4. Treatment**
a. The preferred method of treatment is **esophagomyotomy** by the **modified Heller procedure**.
 (1) Myotomy is confined to the narrowed lower portion of the esophagus, usually 5 cm to 7 cm in length.
 (2) It is carried out via a left thoracic approach, and care is taken not to disturb the phrenic attachments of the esophagus in order to prevent reflux.
b. Forceful pneumatic dilation may be helpful in patients in whom operation is contraindicated due to a concomitant medical disease.

**C. Diffuse esophageal spasm**

**1. Pathophysiology**
a. Diffuse esophageal spasm is a disorder of esophageal motility that consists of **strong nonperistaltic contractions**.
b. Unlike achalasia, this condition is associated with normal sphincteric relaxation. It may also be associated with gastroesophageal reflux.

**2.** The **symptoms** consist of pain in the chest, which can radiate to the back, neck, ears, jaw, or arms, and may be confused with typical angina pectoris. The pain usually occurs spontaneously, and many patients are considered to have a psychoneurosis.

**3. Diagnosis**
a. The diagnosis is made by manometry, which reveals high-amplitude repetitive contractions with a normal sphincteric response to swallowing.
b. Esophageal radiography is normal in one-half of the cases, but it may reveal esophageal diverticula, segmented esophageal spasms, and a corkscrew-appearing esophagus.

**4. Treatment**
a. **Surgical therapy** is moderately effective, with good results obtained in two-thirds to three-

fourths of the patients. The best results are obtained in emotionally stable patients with severe disease and without associated lower gastrointestinal problems.
  **b.** The surgery consists of a long **esophagomyotomy** that usually extends from the arch of the aorta to just above the lower esophageal sphincter.
  **c.** Care is taken to preserve lower esophageal sphincter function, because it is usually normal in these patients.
  **d.** If significant gastroesophageal reflux is present, an antireflux procedure is performed.

**D. Esophageal reflux**

1. **Etiology.** Esophageal reflux is secondary to **decreased function of the lower esophageal sphincter**, which results in recurrent reflux of the gastric contents into the lower esophagus.
   **a.** There is some evidence that decreased lower esophageal sphincter function may be related to **decreased endogenous gastrin production**.
      **(1)** Normal infants have decreased sphincter tone, which results in regurgitation; this condition usually corrects itself as the child grows.
      **(2)** Decreased function of the lower esophageal sphincter may occur after operations on or near the esophageal hiatus (e.g., vatogomy and gastrectomy).
   **b.** Many patients with esophageal reflux have sliding-type esophageal hiatal hernias. However, many patients with this type of hiatal hernia have no evidence of reflux, and many patients with normal lower esophageal anatomy suffer from esophageal reflux.
   **c. Scleroderma** is a systemic cause of lower esophageal sphincter dysfunction through weakening of the esophageal smooth muscle.
   **d. Exogenous causative agents** include tobacco and alcohol.

2. The **symptoms** of esophageal reflux are substernal pain, heartburn, and regurgitation. The symptoms worsen with bending and lying down.

3. **Diagnosis** is made by:
   **a.** Manometry, which reveals decreased lower esophageal sphincter pressure
   **b.** Esophagoscopy, which reveals varying degrees of esophagitis
   **c.** Placing a pH probe in the lower esophageal area, which demonstrates acid reflux
   **d.** Cineradiography, which reveals esophageal reflux via motion pictures of the lower esophagus.

4. **Treatment**
   **a. Medical therapy includes:**
      **(1)** Antacids
      **(2)** Metoclopramide, which increases both lower esophageal sphincter pressure and gastric motility, thus increasing the rate of gastric emptying
      **(3)** Histamine$_2$ (H$_2$)-receptor antagonists
      **(4)** Weight reduction
      **(5)** Abstinence from smoking and alcohol
      **(6)** Elevation of the head of the bed at night
   **b. Surgical therapy**
      **(1) Indications** for surgery include:
         **(a)** Symptoms that do not respond to medical treatment
         **(b)** Complications such as esophageal webs (see section VII B) or esophagitis with stricture formation or **Barrett's esophagus** (i.e., replacement of normal epithelium with columnar epithelium in the lower esophagus secondary to esophagitis)
      **(2) Antireflux operations** are designed to increase lower esophageal sphincter tone. All of the operations involve wrapping the lower esophagus with gastric fundus. The three most commonly used operations are:
         **(a)** The **Belsey Mark IV operation**, which is usually performed through a left thoracotomy
         **(b)** The **Nissen fundoplication**, which is performed through the abdomen
         **(c)** The **Hill repair**, also performed through the abdomen

## III. STRICTURES OF THE ESOPHAGUS

**A. Caustic stricture**

1. **Etiology.** Caustic stricture is caused by the ingestion of caustic agents such as lye, drain openers, and oven cleaners.

2. **Diagnosis** is made from a history of caustic ingestion and from the symptoms, which may be mild or may be very severe, including shock from severe burning of the esophagus. It is im-

portant to identify the etiologic agent. Endoscopy is indicated early on in order to determine the extent of damage.

3. **Treatment**
   a. A neutralizing agent (usually milk) is given as soon as possible to counteract the effects of the caustic agent.
   b. Corticosteroids and broad-spectrum antibiotics are administered for 3 to 6 weeks.
   c. Esophageal radiography is performed at 10 to 14 days to determine if **stricture formation** is occurring.
      (1) Strictures form in 5% to 10% of patients who have ingested lye.
      (2) If strictures have formed, a program of dilation, using esophageal dilators, is begun at 3 to 4 weeks after ingestion.
   d. In severe cases, it is not possible to maintain an adequate esophageal lumen, and the esophagus must be replaced with a segment of colon.

B. **Stricture secondary to esophagitis and reflux**

1. **Pathophysiology.** These strictures are caused by an alternating pattern of destruction and healing secondary to gastric acid reflux in the esophagus.
   a. The strictures may occur at the gastroesophageal junction, or they can occur in the middle or upper portion of the esophagus at the squamocolumnar junction in a patient with Barrett's esophagus.
   b. In severe cases a long stricture may result.

2. The **diagnosis** is suspected in a patient with reflux symptoms and dysphagia. It is confirmed by esophageal radiography, and esophagoscopy is performed to determine the extent of the disease and to rule out malignancy.

3. **Treatment**
   a. An attempt is made to dilate the esophagus and, if successful, an antireflux operation is performed.
   b. If dilation does not relieve the esophageal obstruction, a reconstructive procedure, using either stomach or colon for esophageal replacement, may be necessary to restore adequate swallowing function.

## IV. TUMORS OF THE ESOPHAGUS

A. **Benign tumors**

1. **Leiomyomas** account for two-thirds of all benign tumors of the esophagus.
   a. These tumors grow within the muscular wall, leaving the overlying mucosa intact. They only cause **symptoms** (chiefly dysphagia) when they exceed a diameter of 5 cm.
   b. **Diagnosis.** A history of dysphagia suggests leiomyoma. Esophageal radiography reveals a filling defect in the esophagus, and esophagoscopy is performed to confirm the diagnosis. The lesion should not be biopsied because this violates the mucosa, making subsequent surgical therapy much more difficult.
   c. **Treatment** of symptomatic patients involves surgically exposing the esophagus and enucleating the tumor from the esophageal wall without violating the mucosa. Occasionally, these tumors lie in the lower esophagus and cannot be enucleated. In this case, a limited esophageal resection is indicated.

2. **Intraluminal tumors** are usually **mucosal polyps**, **lipomas**, **fibrolipomas**, or **myxofibromas**.
   a. The usual **symptoms** are dysphagia, occasionally with regurgitation, and weight loss.
   b. The **diagnosis** is suggested by results on esophageal radiography, and esophagoscopy is performed to confirm the diagnosis and to rule out malignancy.
   c. **Treatment** is surgical and involves esophagotomy, removal of the tumor, and repair of the esophagotomy. These tumors should not be removed through an endoscope because of the possibility of esophageal perforation.

B. **Carcinoma**

1. **Incidence.** In the United States, the incidence of esophageal carcinoma ranges from 3.5 per 100,000 for whites to 13.5 per 100,000 for blacks. The highest incidence of esophageal carcinoma is noted in the Hunan Chinese population: As many as 130 per 100,000 are affected.

2. **Pathology**
   a. **Squamous cell carcinoma** is the most common form.
   b. **Adenocarcinoma**, the second most common, almost always occurs in patients with Bar-

rett's esophagus. Etiologic agents include tobacco, alcohol, and persistent esophageal reflux.
  c. **Rare tumors** of the esophagus include **mucoepidermoid carcinoma** and **adenocystic carcinoma**.
  d. **Tumor spread.** Esophageal malignancies metastasize through the lymph nodes as well as directly through the bloodstream, with liver, bone, and brain metastases occurring early.

3. **Diagnosis**
  a. There is almost always a history of dysphagia and weight loss.
  b. Esophageal radiography is performed to localize the tumor, and esophagoscopy is used to determine the resectability of the tumor and to obtain tissue for diagnosis. Bronchoscopy is also performed in order to assess the possibility of invasion of the tracheobronchial tree.
  c. A thorough search is made for distant metastasis.

4. **Treatment**
  a. **Surgical therapy** provides the only cure.
    (1) The operation involves a total thoracic esophagectomy and a gastroesophageal anastomosis. This is made possible by freeing the stomach and bringing it into the chest or neck while it is still vascularized by the gastroepiploic artery.
    (2) This operation is the best treatment for the patient and allows normal or near normal swallowing. For the patient whose stomach cannot be used to reconstruct the esophagus, an alternative procedure is to use a colon interposition to reconstruct the esophagus.
    (3) Overall, surgical therapy is associated with a 5% to 15% 5-year survival rate. As high as a 30% 5-year survival rate has been reported for patients who are in the early stages of disease with no demonstrable lymph node metastasis.
  b. **Radiotherapy** and **chemotherapy** are currently being investigated as adjuncts to surgery.
    (1) In some poor-risk patients, radiotherapy alone has been used for carcinoma of the esophagus with some palliative effects.
    (2) In patients who have advanced disease with either invasion of the tracheobronchial tree or advanced metastasis, some palliative effect may be obtained by placing a permanent, large-diameter tube through the area of esophageal obstruction, which allows swallowing of saliva and soft foods. However, patients usually survive less than 6 months following placement of such a tube.

## V. PERFORATION OF THE ESOPHAGUS

A. **Etiology**

  1. Perforations of the esophagus have two basic causes:
    a. **Instrumentation** (esophagoscopy or dilation)
    b. **Boerhaave's syndrome** (postemetic spontaneous rupture of the esophagus)

  2. Rupture of the esophagus results in **mediastinitis**, which, if not corrected, is almost always fatal.

B. **Diagnosis**

  1. **History.** The patient gives a recent history of severe vomiting or instrumentation of the esophagus. All patients complain of pain, which usually occurs in the area of the rupture.

  2. **Physical findings**
    a. Crepitations in the neck result from air escaping from the esophagus and dissecting into the tissue planes of the neck.
    b. Occasionally, a crunching sound can be heard over the heart (Hamman's sign), due to air in the mediastinum behind the heart.
    c. Shock also can occur.

  3. X-ray studies reveal air in the mediastinum and, possibly, a widened mediastinum. If the perforation is in the lower esophagus, air may be present under the diaphragm within the abdomen; if the pleura has been violated, a pneumothorax may occur.

C. **Treatment** includes adequate drainage of the mediastinum and prevention of further contamination.

  1. If diagnosed early, perforation can be treated with simple drainage and esophageal repair.

  2. However, if the diagnosis is delayed, it is impossible to repair the esophagus because of the massive infection in the area. In this case, drainage and esophageal diversion are performed first, and esophageal reconstruction is done later.

## VI. MALLORY-WEISS SYNDROME

  A. **Pathophysiology.** In this condition, bleeding from the lower esophagus occurs secondary to a partial-thickness tear of the lower esophagus which follows a prolonged period of severe vomiting and retching. The tear usually extends into the stomach and may involve the greater curvature of the cardia.

  B. **Diagnosis** is made by endoscopy in patients who present with upper gastrointestinal hemorrhage, usually after an episode of severe vomiting.

  C. **Treatment** is by supportive measures such as replacing blood volume, administering antacids, and evacuating clots from the stomach.

   1. In most cases, the bleeding subsides spontaneously.

   2. If bleeding persists, exploratory laparotomy is performed, and the tear of the esophagus is repaired from the stomach. The lacerations are closed using continuous nonabsorbable sutures, and recurrence is extremely rare.

## VII. ESOPHAGEAL WEBS

  A. **Upper esophageal webs** are part of the **Plummer-Vinson syndrome**, which presents in middle-aged, edentulous women with atrophic oral mucosa, anemia, and dysphagia. The web occurs just below the esophageal introitus. **Treatment** is usually by esophageal dilation.

  B. **Lower esophageal webs**, or **Schatzki's rings**, commonly occur in patients with reflux. Patients complain of dysphagia. **Treatment** consists of esophageal dilation and an antireflux procedure.

## QUESTIONS

**Directions:** Each question below contains five suggested answers. Choose the **one best** response to each question.

1. A 50-year-old man has a right upper lobe cavitary lesion that is 4 cm in diameter and of unknown age. Which one of the following tests is most likely to establish the diagnosis?

(A) Bronchography
(B) Computed tomography
(C) Bronchoscopy with biopsy brushings and washings
(D) Percutaneous needle aspiration of the cavity contents
(E) An immunologic skin test

2. Tension pneumothorax may cause all of the following problems EXCEPT

(A) hypoxia
(B) acidosis
(C) decreased venous return to the heart
(D) decreased cardiac output
(E) dullness to percussion on the side of the pneumothorax

3. All of the following symptoms and signs are indicative of a tension pneumothorax EXCEPT

(A) chest pain
(B) shortness of breath
(C) absent breath sounds unilaterally
(D) shifting of the trachea toward the pneumothorax
(E) hypotension

4. A patient undergoes a left scalene node biopsy to rule out carcinoma of the lung. One hour later the patient is cyanotic, dyspneic, and has a marked tachycardia with decreased breath sounds on the left. What is the maneuver that is most likely to improve the patient's condition?

(A) Blood transfusion
(B) Insertion of a right subclavian catheter and administration of intravenous fluids
(C) Endotracheal intubation
(D) Insertion of a left chest tube
(E) Reexploration of the wound

5. All of the following diagnoses in a 60-year-old man with a peripheral solitary pulmonary nodule (coin lesion) are likely EXCEPT

(A) bronchogenic carcinoma
(B) tuberculosis
(C) metastatic colon cancer
(D) hamartoma
(E) sarcoidosis

6. Which of the following findings indicates incurability of a lung cancer?

(A) Recurrent pneumonia
(B) Sputum cytology positive for cancer
(C) Shortness of breath
(D) Left vocal cord paralysis
(E) Clubbing of the digits

7.   Which of the following would be the most appropriate measure in the management of a patient with a spontaneous complete collapse of a lung for the first time?

(A) Observation with daily chest roentgenograms
(B) Aspiration of air with a needle, followed by observation
(C) Thoracotomy to biopsy the site of pneumothorax
(D) Chest tube drainage of the pleural space
(E) Thoracotomy and pleural abrasion to prevent recurrence

8.   The most acceptable measure in the management of a patient with a suspected carcinoma of the lung and with no evidence of spread is

(A) surgical resection of the lesion
(B) intense radiation therapy
(C) chemotherapy
(D) chemotherapy followed by resection
(E) reevaluation in 2 months to determine if the lesion is larger or has spread

9.   Hoarseness secondary to bronchogenic carcinoma is usually due to extension of the tumor into what structure?

(A) Vocal cord
(B) Superior laryngeal nerve
(C) Left recurrent laryngeal nerve
(D) Right vagus nerve
(E) Larynx

10. The lower esophagus of a patient is inadvertently perforated during esophagoscopy. A barium swallow done immediately after perforation demonstrates that a small amount of barium is leaking into the left pleural space. What is the most acceptable method of treatment?

(A) Observation alone
(B) Observation plus antibiotics
(C) Insertion of a left chest tube
(D) Prolonged esophageal intubation
(E) Drainage and surgical repair of the injury

**Directions:** The question below contains four suggested answers of which **one or more** is correct. Choose the answer

> **A**   if **1, 2, and 3** are correct
> **B**   if **1 and 3** are correct
> **C**   if **2 and 4** are correct
> **D**   if **4** is correct
> **E**   if **1, 2, 3, and 4** are correct

11. True statements regarding Barrett's esophagus include which of the following?

(1) It may reveal gastric columnar epithelium on biopsy
(2) It is almost always a malignant lesion
(3) It most commonly affects the distal esophagus
(4) It is treated by pneumatic dilation

## ANSWERS AND EXPLANATIONS

**1. The answer is C.** (*Chapter 27 I B 2 b*) Bronchoscopy is most likely to establish the diagnosis in a patient with a cavitary lung lesion. Aspiration of the cavity's contents usually yields necrotic debris and may not yield carcinoma.

**2. The answer is E.** (*Chapter 27 II C 3*) A tension pneumothorax results in collapse of the lung with decreased breath sounds and tympany on the ipsilateral side. This distorts the mediastinum, resulting in decreased venous return, and decreased cardiac output with resultant hypoxia and acidosis.

**3. The answer is D.** (*Chapter 27 II C 3*) Tension pneumothorax results from the trapping of air within the pleural space of the affected lung. The resultant total-volume (air and lung) increase on the affected side shifts the mediastinum away from that side. Hypotension results from impaired venous return, which is due to distortion of the vena cava by the mediastinal shift.

**4. The answer is D.** (*Chapter 27 I B 3*) The pleura of the lung lies immediately adjacent to the scalene fat pad. If the pleura is injured during scalene node biopsy, a pneumothorax can result, causing the symptoms that developed in the patient described in the question. Other nearby structures include the lymph duct structures, the brachial plexus, the vagus and phrenic nerves, and the subclavian vessels. Any of these structures can also be injured during scalene node biopsy, with corresponding symptoms.

**5. The answer is E.** (*Chapter 27 VI*) Sarcoidosis does not present as a solitary lung nodule. Bronchogenic carcinoma, tuberculosis, metastatic colon cancer, and hamartoma can all result in a coin lesion. The most likely diagnosis among those listed is bronchogenic carcinoma.

**6. The answer is D.** (*Chapter 27 I B 2 a*) Vocal cord paralysis is evidence of invasion of the recurrent laryngeal nerve by the cancer. Recurrent pneumonia, a positive sputum cytology, shortness of breath, and clubbing of the digits are general symptoms and signs that can be present in the absence of tumor extension or metastasis.

**7. The answer is D.** (*Chapter 27 II C*) Simple insertion of a chest tube will cure the majority of patients with a spontaneous pneumothorax. Observation or aspiration is usually not successful, and thoracotomy with pleural abrasion is reserved for recurrent cases.

**8. The answer is A.** (*Chapter 27 VII G*) The best chance for a cure in carcinoma of the lung is provided by expeditious thoracotomy with resection of the tumor. In a patient with no evidence of metastatic disease and with a less malignant histologic cell type, the likelihood of survival for 5 years postoperatively may be as high as 25% to 35%. Preoperative radiation therapy has only been useful for superior sulcus tumor.

**9. The answer is C.** (*Chapter 27 I B 2 a*) Bronchogenic carcinoma invades the left recurrent laryngeal nerve as it passes around the aortic notch; when this happens, hoarseness results. This finding indicates nonresectability of the tumor.

**10. The answer is E.** (*Chapter 28 V C*) Recognized perforation of the esophagus is most safely treated by thoracotomy and repair of the injury with wide drainage. Failure to carry out these measures may result in a life-threatening infection.

**11. The answer is B (1, 3).** (*Chapter 28 II D 4 b*) Barrett's esophagus involves replacement of the distal esophageal mucosa by columnar epithelium, of either the intestinal or gastric type. Gastric acid reflux is felt to be the usual etiology, and in many cases control of reflux, either by $H_2$-receptor blocking agents or by an antireflux procedure, will result in reversion back to normal mucosa. If the abnormal mucosa persists despite optimal therapy, adenocarcinoma develops in 10% of cases.

# Part IX
# Special Subjects

# 29
# Urologic Surgery
Demetrius H. Bagley

I. **INTRODUCTION.** Urology deals with disorders of the urinary tract in males and females as well as disorders of the male genital tract. In terms of the number of patient complaints and office visits, urology constitutes a major portion of any primary care practice, and urologic procedures constitute a major portion of most surgical schedules. Thus, all practitioners must be familiar with the major disease entities encountered in urologic care. Only certain aspects of major topics are considered in this chapter, and the reader is referred to general and specialized urologic texts for further information.

II. **URINARY TRACT INFECTIONS (UTIs)** are among the most common bacterial infections. In evaluating affected individuals, the physician must determine, in addition to the diagnosis and the treatment required for the acute episode, the value of follow-up studies and the need for referral for further evaluation.

A. **Diagnosis.** Urinary tract infection is usually considered on the basis of clinical findings. The diagnosis is further supported by the finding of **pyuria** and **bacteriuria** on urinalysis and is confirmed by **culture of the urine**.

1. **Clinical findings**
   a. The **major symptoms** of urinary tract infection are related to vesical irritation. These include:
      (1) **Urinary frequency**
      (2) **Urgency**
      (3) **Pain on voiding**
      (4) **Cloudy or foul-smelling urine**
   b. **Renal infection** may be indicated by the additional symptoms of:
      (1) **Fever**
      (2) **Chills**
      (3) **Flank pain**

2. **Urinalysis** is a valuable screening procedure that can be performed in the physician's office.
   a. Detecting bacteria on microscopic examination of the urine is strongly indicative of significant **bacteriuria**.
   b. **Pyuria**, the presence of white blood cells in the urine, indicates an inflammatory response within the urinary tract. The number of cells present can be affected by the technique of sample collection, by the handling of the specimen, and by the patient's state of hydration.

3. **Chemical studies.** Attempts have been made to use chemical studies to provide simple rapid screening for the presence of infection.
   a. **Nitrate reduction and urinary esterase detection**
      (1) Nitrate in the urine is reduced to nitrite in the presence of bacteria.
      (2) Leukocytes contain esterases, which can be detected in the urine.
      (3) Both nitrate reduction and urinary esterase can be indicated by a reagent, which changes color, and the two reactions have been combined on a dipstick as a nonspecific indicator of infection.
   b. **Other chemical tests** have included:
      (1) **Tetrazolium reduction**
      (2) **Urinary glucose reduction**
      (3) **Urinary catalase detection**

4. **Urine culture** can determine the presence of bacteria in the urine. Standard culture plates or slides coated with agar can be used, and selective media assist in identification of the bacteria present.

     5. **Antibiotic sensitivity testing.** Bacteria present in the urine at significant levels should be tested for their sensitivity to antibiotics.
       a. This is determined by culturing known quantities of bacteria on a plate containing disks impregnated with a known amount of antibiotic.
       b. The zone of inhibition around these disks is related to both the concentration of the antibiotic and the sensitivity of the organism.
       c. In most laboratories, the reported levels of sensitivity are related to serum antibiotic concentrations, which may be considerably less than the urinary concentrations.

**B. Treatment of bladder infection** consists of the administration of appropriate antibiotics. The duration of therapy has recently been of interest, and 1-day therapy appears to be as effective as therapy lasting 3, 7, or 10 days. In contrast, a longer course of therapy is necessary for **renal infections**.

## III. RENAL INFECTIONS

**A. Classification**

    1. Infections of the parenchyma include:
      a. Generalized **pyelonephritis**
      b. Localized forms called **lobar nephronia**, **renal carbuncle**, and **perirenal phlegmon**

    2. Abscesses include:
      a. **Intrarenal abscess**
      b. **Perinephric abscess**
      c. **Infected renal cysts**

**B. Pyelonephritis** usually has an acute onset and affects mainly young women.

    1. Patients may present with **high fever**, **chills**, and **flank or midback pain**, often with irritative lower tract symptoms.

    2. The most frequent **causative organism** is *Escherichia coli*.

    3. **Laboratory findings** include **pyuria** and **bacteriuria**. The urine culture should yield bacteria to substantiate a diagnosis of pyelonephritis, unless the patient has recently taken antibiotics.

    4. The patient usually responds to **antibiotic therapy** within 2 to 5 days.
      a. A patient needing a course longer than this should be evaluated further with radiologic studies.
      b. Any underlying complications such as calculus or obstruction can then be treated appropriately.

**C. Acute lobar nephronia** describes an acute focal infection with a renal or perirenal mass but without abscess formation.

    1. This illness is characterized by **fever**, **flank pain**, **and pyuria**, but there may be a more indolent course.

    2. **Therapy** consists of administration of appropriate **antibiotics**. Patients who do not respond to therapy or who deteriorate clinically should be evaluated further.

**D. Abscesses within the perinephric space** usually result from rupture of an intrarenal abscess.

    1. They are **associated with** other factors predisposing to the renal abscess, which include **calculi** and **diabetes mellitus**.

    2. *E. coli* and *Proteus mirabilis* are most frequently cultured from these abscesses.

    3. The **presentation** is usually less dramatic than that of pyelonephritis. The fever is usually lower and may persist for several days before diagnosis, and pain is milder and less frequent.

    4. **Radiologic studies** are often helpful in making the diagnosis.
      a. Chest x-ray reveals an effusion or elevation of the diaphragm.
      b. An abdominal mass may be detected on excretory urography, but ultrasonography and computed tomography (CT scanning) provide the most accurate localization of a perinephric abscess.

    5. **Therapy** consists of **drainage**, usually with **antibiotic administration**.

**E. Xanthogranulomatous pyelonephritis** is a chronic infection of the renal parenchyma and is a pathologic diagnosis.

1. *E. coli* and *P. mirabilis* are the organisms most frequently cultured from this infection.

2. Xanthogranulomatous pyelonephritis is usually **associated with obstruction**, and **calculi** are frequently present.

3. Women are affected more frequently than men, and the most common **symptoms** are **fever and flank or abdominal pain**.

4. **Excretory urography** may demonstrate a nonfunctioning kidney or the presence of renal calculi. A renal mass can be demonstrated in 60% of patients; it often cannot be distinguished from a renal tumor.

5. If xanthogranulomatous pyelonephritis can be diagnosed preoperatively, it can be **treated** by partial nephrectomy. Often, however, it is diagnosed as renal cancer and treated by nephrectomy.

## IV. PROSTATITIS

A. **General considerations.** Prostatitis, or inflammation of the prostate gland, is widely overdiagnosed.

1. Urinary frequency, urgency, dysuria, and perineal or suprapubic discomfort are symptoms of numerous other disorders, as well as prostatitis.

2. The various inflammatory and noninflammatory prostatic conditions should be distinguished in patients who have similar symptom complexes; treatment can then be based on an accurate diagnosis.

B. **Bacterial prostatitis** exists in both acute and chronic forms.

1. The **diagnosis** of bacterial prostatitis rests upon:
   a. Finding white blood cells within the prostatic fluid
   b. Detecting a significant number of bacteria in expressed prostatic fluid and distinguishing them from urethral organisms by differential cultures

2. Patients often respond to a course of **antimicrobial therapy** such as sulfamethoxazole-trimethoprim, tetracycline, or carbenicillin.

C. **Nonbacterial prostatitis** has also been called **prostatosis**, and the diagnosis depends upon finding prostatic fluid containing white blood cells but with cultures negative for bacteria. This diagnosis also includes patients with nonbacterial prostatic infections due to *Mycoplasma* and *Chlamydia* species.

D. **Prostatodynia** is a term describing symptoms similar to those of prostatitis but without inflammatory cells in the prostatic fluid and with cultures negative for microorganisms.

## V. URINARY CALCULI

A. **Phases.** The management of patients with urinary calculi within the kidney or ureter can be considered to have two phases.

1. In the **acute phase**, the patient has symptoms of obstruction or inflammation that result from the presence of the calculus.

2. In the **metabolic phase**, the metabolic basis for stone formation should be sought so that appropriate treatment will prevent the growth or formation of calculi.

B. **Diagnosis**

1. **Clinical findings**
   a. The most frequent **acute symptom** of upper urinary calculi is **pain**.
      (1) The site of the pain depends on the position of the calculus. The pain may be present in the upper back at the costovertebral angle, in the flank, or in the right lower quadrant. It may radiate into the testicle or vulva.
      (2) Pain results from dilation of the ureter or renal pelvis and can occur with a calculus of any size.
   b. Other symptoms include:
      (1) **Hematuria**
      (2) **Nausea and vomiting**
      (3) **Irritative bladder symptoms**
      (4) **General abdominal discomfort**, mimicking gastrointestinal disease

c. **Physical examination**

    (1) Most patients are clearly in severe distress, unable to find any position of comfort.

    (2) The abdomen should be examined closely. Bowel sounds may be decreased with a secondary ileus, and the costovertebral area is frequently tender.

2. **Urinalysis**

    a. **Hematuria** is usually present, although its absence does not rule out the presence of a calculus.

    b. Detection of **crystals** may give some indication of the presence and type of calculus.

3. **Radiologic findings**

    a. A **plain radiogram of the abdomen** can be very helpful in the evaluation of the patient suspected of having a calculus. Since most calculi are radiopaque, the presence of a calculus may be detected, although its exact identification as a urinary calculus cannot be made on a single plain x-ray.

    b. **Excretory urography** can usually locate a calculus accurately in the urinary tract. In the presence of obstruction, visualization of the kidney may be delayed, or dilation of the intrarenal collecting system may be apparent.

    c. **Other studies** are less frequently of value.

        (1) **Ultrasonography** may define hydronephrosis or demonstrate an acoustic shadow from a calculus.

        (2) **Retrograde urography** is occasionally valuable to provide contrast within the urinary tract, allowing opacification in the patient who is allergic to contrast medium.

        (3) **CT scanning** is not very helpful in the diagnosis of urinary calculi, but it has specific benefits in evaluating lucent intraluminal filling defects by differentiating soft tissue lesions from dense calculi.

## C. Surgical treatment

1. **Indications for intervention**

    a. Interventional procedures are not necessary in all patients with calculi or even in all patients with symptomatic calculi. The indications for the removal of calculi or for urinary drainage listed in Table 29-1 are not absolute.

    b. The patient must be actively involved in any decision for intervention:

        (1) Some patients tolerate pain much better than others and may prefer to wait for a ureteral calculus to pass by itself.

        (2) Others may find that any delay interferes with their life-style and may demand early intervention.

**Table 29-1.** Indications for Removal of Urinary Calculi

| |
| --- |
| Severe pain |
| Infection |
| Severe obstruction |
| Growth of calculus |
| Nonprogression |
| Interference with life-style |

2. **Open surgical procedures**

    a. Any renal or ureteral calculus can be removed by open surgical procedures. However, there has been a strong movement away from such procedures to endourologic and endoscopic techniques.

    b. Calculi throughout the kidney and in the ureter can be approached through a **percutaneous nephrostomy**.

        (1) Large calculi can be fragmented using ultrasonic or electrohydraulic lithotriptors, and smaller calculi can be withdrawn intact.

        (2) The percutaneous approach has been most effective for simple renal calculi, and less successful for branched renal calculi or for ureteral calculi.

3. **Transurethral procedures**

    a. Ureteral calculi that originated in the renal collecting system become symptomatic as they pass into the ureter and cause obstruction.

    b. Most ureteral calculi pass spontaneously.

        (1) Those measuring less than 4 mm in diameter and located in the distal ureter are the most likely (90%) to pass.

        (2) This probability declines to 50% as the calculus increases from 4 to 5.9 mm in diameter.

        (3) It drops to 20% for calculi greater than 6 mm.

**(4)** Proximal ureteral calculi are less likely to pass, but the frequency is also related to the size of the calculus.

**c.** **Surgical removal**

    **(1)** Calculi below the pelvic rim can be manipulated with a **"basket"** (a catheter with wires to trap the stone) from the level of the bladder.

    **(2)** Greater success has been achieved by visualizing the calculus with a **ureteroscope** passed directly into the ureter. Calculi can then be retrieved with various grasping instruments or fragmented for removal.

**4. Extracorporeal shock wave lithotripsy (ESWL).** Considerable success has been experienced with this treatment.

    **a.** The patient, under either epidural or general anesthesia, is placed in a tank of water, which serves as a conduction medium to carry shock waves from a generator.

    **b.** The generator has an ellipsoid reflector to focus the waves on a renal calculus in situ, thus fragmenting the calculus.

    **c.** The fragments must pass through the ureter. **Complications** requiring additional procedures such as percutaneous nephrostomy or ureteroscopy occur in 10% to 30% of cases.

    **d.** The appropriate role of ESWL in the United States remains to be clarified.

**D. Metabolic evaluation and prophylaxis.** It is of great importance to know the **composition** of any calculi removed from or passed by a patient, in order to direct appropriate metabolic study and eventual therapy. Table 29-2 lists the chemical types of calculi, in descending order of occurrence.

**Table 29-2.** Composition of Urinary Calculi

| Descending Frequency of Occurrence |
| --- |
| Calcium oxalate and calcium phosphate |
| Calcium oxalate |
| Struvite (magnesium ammonium phosphate) |
| Calcium phosphate |
| Uric acid |
| Cystine |

**1. Calcium-containing calculi.** The majority of calculi contain calcium in the form of **calcium oxalate, calcium phosphate, or both**. The frequency of calculi containing calcium is three times greater in men than in women.

    **a.** All patients who form a calcium calculus should be **screened** with a blood count, urinalysis, serum chemistry evaluation, excretory urography, and analysis of a 24-hour urine sample to check for calcium, phosphate, uric acid, and creatinine.

    **b.** Young women with a single calculus, men with a second calculus, and patients with calculi that are increasing in number or size should have **full metabolic evaluation**.

        **(1)** This can be performed as an outpatient procedure before and after calcium loading to distinguish patients with **renal hypercalciuria**, **absorptive hypercalciuria**, **hyperparathyroidism**, or **normocalciuric stone formation**.

        **(2)** **Treatment** can then be tailored to the patient and may include:

            **(a)** Thiazide diuretics

            **(b)** Orthophosphates

            **(c)** Dietary calcium restriction

            **(d)** Potassium citrate

            **(e)** Hydration to maintain a urine output of 3 to 4 L/day (in all patients)

    **c.** Conditions other than those listed above in section V D 1 b (1) resulting in calcium stone formation include:

        **(1)** Sarcoidosis

        **(2)** Renal tubular acidosis (type 1, distal renal tubular acidosis)

        **(3)** Hyperoxaluria

**2. Infection-related calculi**

    **a. Struvite (magnesium ammonium phosphate) stones** are associated with urinary tract infections and occur in women more often than in men.

        **(1)** Formation of struvite stones requires the presence of urea-splitting bacteria which maintain a low pH with increased concentrations of bicarbonate and ammonium ions.

        **(2)** *Proteus* species are the most common organisms causing stone formation.

    **b. Treatment** includes removal of the calculus and eradication of the urinary tract infection.

        **(1) Antibiotic therapy** pre- and postoperatively is essential.

        **(2) Urease inhibitors** have also been of value.

**3. Uric acid calculi** constitute only 5% to 10% of stones in the United States.
   **a.** Uric acid is insoluble in water, but the urate salt can be formed by alkalization of the urine.
      **(1)** The $pK_a$ of uric acid is 5.75, and therefore calculi can be dissolved and their formation prevented by maintaining the urinary pH at 6.5 to 7.0.
      **(2)** Allopurinol, which is a xanthine oxidase inhibitor, prevents the formation of uric acid and thus lowers the serum and urinary concentrations.
   **b.** Uric acid calculi are radiolucent and therefore must be demonstrated by x-ray studies using contrast medium or by other studies such as ultrasonography or CT.

**4. Cystine calculi**
   **a. Cystinuria** is an uncommon autosomal recessive disorder that results in decreased reabsorption of dibasic amino acids from the renal tubule. **Cystine calculi** form only because of the low solubility of cystine in urine with a pH of up to 7.0.
   **b.** Fluid diuresis and alkalization to a peak pH of 7.5 is the most important **therapeutic measure**. Cystine-binding drugs such as D-penicillamine or α-mercaptopropionylglycine have also been used in patients with recurrent calculi.

**VI. GENITOURINARY INJURIES** (see also Chapter 2, section I C 6 d). Injuries to the genitalia and urinary tract are often associated with other injuries, and a high index of suspicion for genitourinary injuries in the patient with multiple trauma should be maintained to avoid a potentially disastrous situation.

**A. Scrotal and testicular injury**

   **1.** Although the scrotum and its contents are mobile, they are subject to blunt and penetrating injuries.

   **2.** The patient's only complaint may be local pain, and physical examination may be difficult if a large hematoma is present.

   **3. Conservative treatment** is sufficient if the testicles are palpably normal or if there is a nonexpanding hematoma.

   **4. Surgical exploration**
      **a.** This should be undertaken in the following situations:
         **(1)** If a hematoma is enlarging
         **(2)** If the testicle has been fractured
         **(3)** If injury to the scrotum penetrates deeper than the dartos muscle
      **b.** Appropriate repair of the scrotal contents can be undertaken, and the wound can be closed with drainage.

**B. Urethral injury**

   **1.** The urethra is prone to damage when a "straddle" injury (e.g., from trauma while riding a bicycle) or pelvic fracture has occurred. The diagnosis rests upon proper evaluation in the patient in whom there is a suspicion of injury.

   **2.** The **classic signs of urethral damage** include:
      **a.** Blood at the urethral meatus
      **b.** Perineal ecchymosis or swelling
      **c.** Inability to void
      **d.** Palpable lower abdominal mass
      **e.** Associated pelvic fracture

   **3.** The most valuable technique for the **diagnosis** of urethral injury is **retrograde urethrography**. Contrast medium is injected into the urethra to fill the full length of the lumen.

   **4.** If a urethral injury is demonstrated, **cystotomy drainage** should be performed.

**C. Bladder injury**

   **1.** Injury to the bladder must be suspected in any patient with pelvic fracture or a history of lower abdominal trauma.

   **2.** Local or generalized abdominal pain and tenderness may be present on **physical examination**.

   **3. X-ray** may demonstrate an associated pelvic fracture, while **cystography** is the most definitive test for **bladder rupture**.
      **a.** The bladder should be filled to capacity with 300 ml of contrast medium.
      **b.** Films should be obtained with the bladder full and again after drainage.

**4.** A ruptured bladder is **treated** by **catheter drainage**. Surgical repair is necessary as well in the case of intraperitoneal rupture.

**D. Renal injury** should be suspected in patients with abdominal or lower thoracic trauma. Patients may have localized flank pain or may be free of symptoms. A **local flank contusion** should increase the suspicion of injury. **Hematuria** supports the diagnosis, but its absence does not rule out renal injury.

  **1. Classification.** Renal injuries can be grouped according to severity, and treatment can be tailored to the injury.
    **a. Minor injuries**
      **(1) Renal contusions** or **ecchymoses** constitute approximately 85% of renal trauma.
      **(2)** Minor injuries also include **subcapsular hematomas** and **superficial cortical lacerations**.
      **(3)** Surgical exploration is not necessary.
    **b. Major injuries**
      **(1)** Major renal trauma includes **deep lacerations of the kidney** extending into the collecting system. The value of immediate surgical exploration versus conservative **treatment is controversial**.
      **(2) Multiple lacerations** and **fragmentation of the kidney** are also considered major injuries and require early surgical intervention.
    **c. Vascular injuries** only constitute approximately 1% of blunt renal trauma.
      **(1)** The patient may **present** with massive bleeding or may be stable, with the kidney showing lack of perfusion upon excretory urography.
      **(2)** Prompt diagnosis and treatment are required in any attempt to save the kidney.

  **2. Diagnosis**
    **a.** Among the diagnostic modalities for renal injury, **excretory urography** has been used most frequently and should be performed very early in the patient with multiple trauma.
    **b. Arteriography** can accurately define the renal injury and has been essential for diagnosis of renal pedicle damage.
    **c. CT scanning** can accurately define parenchymal injuries.

# VII. UROLOGIC CANCER

**A.** The **diagnosis and treatment of neoplasms** constitute a large portion of urologic practice.

  **1.** In this field over the past 10 years, there have been dramatic advances in the treatment of certain neoplasms such as testicular tumors and superficial bladder tumors.

  **2.** Lesions such as renal carcinoma remain poorly responsive, amenable only to surgical extirpation.

  **3.** Knowledge of urologic cancer must include familiarity with the natural history and alternative forms of therapy of the major urologic neoplasms.

**B. Renal cell carcinoma**

  **1. Epidemiology**
    **a.** Renal cell carcinoma, also known as **renal adenocarcinoma** or **hypernephroma**, is the third most common urologic cancer and is by far the **most common malignant tumor of the kidney**.
    **b.** It occurs more frequently in men than women in a ratio of 3 to 1, and it achieves its **peak incidence in the fifth and sixth decades** of life.

  **2. Etiology.** Although the etiology of this lesion is not known, environmental chemicals, smoking, exogenous hormones, and viruses have been associated with occurrence of the tumor.

  **3. Diagnosis**
    **a. Clinical findings**
      **(1)** The classic triad consisting of **flank mass, gross hematuria**, and **flank or abdominal pain** is a late manifestation of renal tumors and occurs in only 5% of patients.
      **(2)** Hematuria is the most frequent finding, occurring in more than 38% of patients.
      **(3)** Fever, anemia, erythrocytosis, as well as evidence of metastases may be the presenting symptoms of this tumor.
    **b. Excretory urography with nephrotomography** is usually the first study obtained to indicate the presence of a renal tumor presenting as a renal mass. The pattern of the mass may be characteristic of a renal tumor, or the presence of calcification may suggest the diagnosis.

    **c.** Frequently, other studies are needed to differentiate among various renal masses.
        **(1) Ultrasonography** is extremely accurate in distinguishing classic renal cysts from solid mass lesions or complex cysts.
        **(2) Cystic puncture** is used in all cases but the classic cysts demonstrated by ultrasonography. The contents are examined, and the presence of blood, fat, or malignant cells is an indication for further evaluation and treatment.
        **(3) CT scanning** can help to differentiate cysts, including multilocular cysts, and angiomyolipomas from renal cell tumors.
    **d. Renal arteriography** has long been the standard for the diagnosis of renal cell carcinoma.
        **(1)** These tumors are usually quite vascular and have a distorted pattern, including pooling of contrast medium and a tumor "blush" characteristic of neoplasms.
        **(2)** Vascular encasement, arteriovenous fistulas, and parasitic vasculature from adjacent tissues may also be evident.

**4. Staging.** In order to determine the appropriate treatment of any neoplasm, the extent or stage of the disease must be determined.
    **a.** The most popular staging system remains that described by Robson. There is also a tumor, node, and metastasis (TNM) classification, which has been used more recently. Both are given in Table 29-3.

**Table 29-3.** Staging of Renal Cell Carcinoma

| | Staging System | |
|---|---|---|
| **Extent of Tumor** | **Robson** | **TNM** |
| Limited within the renal capsule | | |
|   Small tumor | A | $T_1$ |
|   Large tumor | A | $T_2$ |
| Perinephric fat | B | $T_{3a}$ |
| Renal vein | C | $T_{3b}$ |
| Renal vein and infradiaphragmatic | | |
|   vena cava | C | $T_{3c}$ |
| Adjacent organs | D | $T_{4a}$ |
| Renal vein and supradiaphragmatic | | |
|   vena cava | | $T_{4b}$ |
| Lymph nodes (regional) | C | $N_+$ |
| Distant metastases | D | $M_+$ |

    **b. Studies** to assist in the staging of renal tumors include serum liver function tests and chest x-rays and possibly tomography, bone scanning, and inferior venacavography. CT scanning and ultrasonography have both been valuable in the search for nodal and hepatic metastases and intravascular extension of the tumor.
    **c. Tumor markers** include renin and erythropoietin, although these have not been nearly as valuable nor as extensively studied as the markers for prostatic carcinoma and testicular tumors.

**5. Treatment**
    **a.** Treatment must be designed with consideration for the stage of the lesion.
        **(1) Stage I** tumors can be treated with surgical excision of the kidney and tumor by radical nephrectomy.
        **(2) Stage II** tumors can also be treated by radical nephrectomy alone.
        **(3) Stage III** tumors can be treated by radical nephrectomy with surgical excision of the intravascular extension of the tumor.
            **(a)** When nodal involvement is minimal, complete excision by radical nephrectomy with node dissection may be possible.
            **(b)** When nodal involvement is extensive, the prognosis is so poor that surgical removal may not be warranted unless the patient has a symptomatic primary tumor.
            **(c)** Invasion of the renal vein should be treated by excision since such extension does not adversely affect the prognosis.
        **(4) Stage IV** tumors are not excised except for palliative treatment of symptoms. Treatment with progestational agents has not shown a statistically significant benefit. Chemotherapeutic and immunologic agents have also been disappointing.
    **b. Results of treatment** of renal cell carcinoma show progressive deterioration with the increasing stage of the disease (Table 29-4).

**Table 29-4.** Survival of Patients with Renal Cell Carcinoma

| Stage | 5 Years (%) | 10 Years (%) |
|-------|-------------|--------------|
| I     | 67          | 49           |
| II    | 59          | 34           |
| III   | 30          | 19           |
| IV    | 7           | 2            |

**C. Transitional cell carcinoma of the renal pelvis and ureter**

1. **Epidemiology**
   a. Transitional cell carcinomas of the renal pelvis and ureter constitute fewer than 5% of urothelial neoplasms in the United States. The remainder are those of the bladder.
   b. The **frequency** of these lesions appears to be increasing, and in some countries the frequency of transitional cell carcinoma and renal cell carcinoma is nearly equal. Multiple tumors, including bilateral lesions, often occur.

2. **Etiology**
   a. **Environmental factors**, including cigarette smoking and occupational exposure to dyes and rubber products, are associated with an increased risk.
   b. **Analgesic nephropathy and Balkan nephropathy** (a familial disease prevalent in Yugoslavia) also result in an increased incidence.

3. **Pathology.** Transitional cell carcinomas, which represent 90% of renal pelvic tumors, may occur in situ or as papillary (85%) or planar lesions of the neoplastic type. Neoplastic lesions include squamous cell carcinomas (7%), adenocarcinomas, sarcomas, and metastatic lesions.

4. **Diagnosis**
   a. **Clinical findings**
      (1) **Gross hematuria** is seen in 70% to 95% of patients. **Microscopic hematuria** occurs in an additional 10%.
      (2) **Other symptoms** include flank pain or a palpable mass.
   b. **Urinalysis** can detect the presence of hematuria. It is necessary to note the urinary pH, since uric acid stones (which can also cause hematuria and appear radiologically as a filling defect) form only in the presence of an acidic urine.
   c. **Intravenous urography** is usually the initial study, and often shows a filling defect.
      (1) A filling defect must then be evaluated further.
         (a) The major distinction to be made is between a urothelial neoplasm and a radiolucent calculus.
         (b) Other diagnoses to be excluded are blood clot and a necrotic papilla.
      (2) In as many as 30% of patients the involved kidney does not visualize on the urogram, a finding often associated with a high-grade tumor.
   d. **Retrograde ureteropyelography** offers good radiologic definition of filling defects and is particularly useful in evaluating a nonfunctioning kidney.
   e. **Ultrasonography** may demonstrate a highly dense echo pattern, with an acoustic shadow behind a calculus; tumors show only a mass effect but no shadow.
   f. **CT scanning** can differentiate the very high density of uric acid calculi from tumors, which have essentially the same density as renal parenchyma. Tumors do not increase in density after intravenous administration of contrast medium.
   g. **Urine cytology** is particularly valuable in diagnosing transitional cell lesions of the ureter and renal pelvis. Voided urine, catheter-collected specimens, or brushed specimens can be used.
   h. **Ureteroscopy** is an endoscopic technique for the observation and direct biopsy of lesions that cause filling defects. Flexible ureteroscopy has been particularly valuable in the diagnosis of filling defects within the kidney.

5. **Treatment** of transitional cell carcinomas of the renal pelvis includes **nephroureterectomy** with a cuff of bladder included in the specimen.
   a. More conservative approaches such as local resection or partial nephrectomy can be undertaken in a patient with a solitary kidney.
   b. Conservative treatment should be considered for low-grade distal ureteral tumors.
   c. High-grade lesions and those located more proximally in the ureter necessitate nephroureterectomy.

### D. Carcinoma of the bladder

1. **Epidemiology.** Bladder cancer is of major importance throughout the world. The **incidence** in the United States is approximately 20,000 to 30,000 new cases, with 10,000 deaths per year.

2. **Etiology**
   a. Many **environmental and disease factors** have been associated with bladder cancer. These include cigarette smoking, exposure to aniline dyes, and ingestion of artificial sweeteners.
   b. Other risk-increasing agents include phenacetin and benzidine.
   c. Bilharziasis is associated predominantly with squamous cell carcinoma.

3. **Diagnosis**
   a. **Clinical findings**
      (1) Although presentation may vary widely, the majority of patients note hematuria among their symptoms. Others are found to have microscopic hematuria alone.
      (2) Irritative symptoms with disturbances of urination, pyuria, or a mass have also been presenting features.
      (3) The presence or absence of pain is not a distinguishing feature.
      (4) A new urinary tract infection with bleeding, particularly in an older patient with a history negative for infections, should be considered suspicious.
   b. **Excretory urography** is an essential study in any patient with gross hematuria. Although its sensitivity for vesical lesions is poor, filling defects in the bladder are often seen, and lesions of the upper urinary tract can be defined.
   c. **Endoscopy with cystoscopy** is absolutely essential to evaluate the urethra and bladder mucosa.
   d. **Urinary cytology** is valuable, with high sensitivity for high-grade neoplasms and carcinoma in situ.

4. **Staging.** The choice of the appropriate treatment for bladder carcinoma depends upon accurate staging of the disease (Table 29-5).

**Table 29-5.** Staging of Carcinoma of the Bladder

| Extent of Tumor | Staging System | |
| --- | --- | --- |
| | Jewett-Marshall | TNM |
| Carcinoma in situ | 0 | TIS |
| Lamina propria | A | $T_1$ |
| Superficial muscle | $B_1$ | $T_2$ |
| Deep muscle | $B_2$ | $T_3$ |
| Perivesical fat | C | $T_3$ |
| Adjacent organs | $D_1$ | $T_4$ |
| Lymph nodes (regional) | $D_2$ | $N_1$ |
| Lymph nodes (above aortic bifurcation) | $D_3$ | $N_2$ |
| Distant metastases | | M |

   a. **Endoscopic biopsy and resection of the bladder tumor** is the most important step in diagnosis and staging.
      (1) Histologic examination will reveal the **cell type** and the **grade** of the tumor as well as the **depth of invasion**. In general, the extent of infiltration of the primary tumor into the muscular wall of the bladder relates to the extent of regional and distant metastases.
      (2) The **gross appearance** of the mucosa is also important. In the presence of **carcinoma in situ** the bladder may appear entirely normal or diffusely erythematous and cobblestoned. Low-grade papillary tumors and high-grade solid-appearing tumors are also characteristic.
   b. **Bimanual examination** is essential to judge the extent of local disease. Papillary tumors may not be palpable, while a mass is suggestive of an invasive lesion. Any mass extending beyond the bladder must be evaluated further.
   c. **Ultrasonography** has been used to evaluate the extent of local disease. It has had some value in defining the depth of invasion of the primary tumor and in detecting nodal metastases.
   d. **CT scanning** has been most valuable in detecting nodal metastases. It has also been useful in examining the perirectal space for the extent of the primary tumor.

   e. **Lymphangiography** has not been found to be accurate enough to warrant routine use in bladder cancer patients.
   f. **Chest x-rays** must be obtained to screen for pulmonary metastases. Pulmonary tomography may increase the sensitivity in detecting pulmonary metastases; CT scanning is much less specific and may cause considerable confusion with benign pulmonary lesions when used on a routine basis.
   g. **Bone scans** are a satisfactory screening technique for bony metastases in patients being considered for major surgical procedures such as cystectomy. Although bony metastases are uncommon at tumor presentation, they do develop in high-grade invasive lesions and may be the first sign of metastases in these patients.
   h. **Cell surface antigens**
      **(1)** There are many antigens on the surface of urothelial cells just as there are on blood cells. These include the ABO (H) blood group antigens, T antigens, and tumor-associated antigens.
      **(2)** The loss or acquisition of these antigens by tumors has, in some cases, been shown to be related to the biologic behavior of the tumor.

5. **Treatment**
   a. **Carcinoma in situ** consists of mucosa with neoplastic degeneration of the cells but without invasion of the lamina propria.
      **(1)** Because of the frequent irritative symptoms, the diagnosis is often delayed. Urinary cytologic findings frequently indicate malignancy.
      **(2)** Because of the possible chronicity of carcinoma in situ and the unpredictability of invasion, **treatment has been controversial**.
         **(a)** **Topical chemotherapy** has been used as a primary treatment agent with encouraging results.
         **(b)** If the lesion is widespread and symptoms are prominent, or if the tumor extends into the urethra, the prostatic ducts, or the lower ureter, then early cystectomy and urinary diversion may be advisable.
   b. **Superficial bladder tumors** that have not invaded the muscle can be treated by local **transurethral resection**. Although these tumors seldom progress to invasive lesions, there is a high rate of recurrence or development of new tumors.
      **(1)** **Intravesical chemotherapy** has been effective in reducing the recurrence of superficial bladder tumors. Effective agents include thiotepa, ethoglucid (Epodyl), doxorubicin, and mitomycin C.
      **(2)** Local **immunotherapy** with bacille Calmette-Guérin (BCG) vaccine has also been effective in reducing recurrences, even in patients who have failed to respond to intravesical chemotherapy.
      **(3)** **Radiotherapy** by external beam has been shown to have poor long-term results (a 50% rate of recurrence within 5 years) and considerable complications, such as reduced bladder capacity. Interstitial radiotherapy in one series was more effective, but the true efficacy of this treatment awaits other studies.
      **(4)** **Cystectomy** remains a treatment possibility in patients with diffuse superficial lesions who have had a poor response to transurethral resection and intravesical chemotherapy.
   c. **Invasive bladder cancer** includes any lesion beyond the in situ or intraepithelial stage. Deeply invasive tumors extend more than halfway through the muscle layer or into perivesical fat.
      **(1)** The evaluation of affected patients is aimed at selecting those in whom **intensive local therapy** will eradicate an aggressive tumor, while withholding such treatment from those patients in whom the disease has already metastasized. It is in these patients that accurate staging is particularly valuable.
      **(2)** On occasion, an invasive tumor has infiltrated too deeply for local resection but is amenable to **partial cystectomy**.
         **(a)** There must be an adequate margin of normal bladder around the tumor, and selected-site biopsies from the remainder of the bladder should show no evidence of atypia or carcinoma in situ.
         **(b)** Preoperative radiotherapy and pelvic lymphadenectomy have often been employed as adjuvant therapy.
      **(3)** **Radiotherapy** has been an important factor in the treatment of invasive bladder cancer. Fractionated doses totaling 6000 to 7000 rads to the bladder have been effective in treating some tumors. There remains a significant failure rate; however, the possibility of successful preservation of bladder function without a major surgical procedure maintains radiotherapy as an option in treatment.
      **(4)** **Radical cystectomy** remains the primary choice of treatment for deeply infiltrating tumors.

    **(a)** Radical cystectomy includes removal of the bladder and prostate gland in men and the bladder, urethra, anterior vaginal wall, and usually the uterus in women.

    **(b)** Although the mortality rate due to this operation has been less than 5% in recent years, the morbidity rate remains at approximately 25%, and patients must endure urinary diversion.

    **(c)** The role of adjuvant radiotherapy has been controversial. Improved rates of survival have been seen only in patients who have exhibited downstaging of the primary tumor.

## E. Testicular tumors

### 1. Epidemiology

**a.** The major testicular tumors in terms of incidence are **seminomas** and **nonseminomatous germ cell tumors** (i.e., embryonal carcinoma with or without seminoma, teratoma, teratocarcinoma with embryonal carcinoma or choriocarcinoma, and pure choriocarcinoma).

**b.** Overall, testicular tumors are uncommon, constituting only 2% of all cancers.

**c.** Well over 50% of testicular tumors are found in men between 20 and 44 years of age.

**d.** The frequency of occurrence depends upon the population: The younger groups studied in reports from military institutions have a seminoma rate of 21% to 46%, while this rate may increase to 40% to 60% in older men.

**e.** Neoplasms of the testicle occur less frequently in blacks than in whites.

**f.** Cryptorchidism has been reported to increase the incidence of tumors.

### 2. Clinical findings.
Asymptomatic tumors occur frequently, which emphasizes the need for thorough physical examinations in men, including the genitalia, as well as the need for patient education and training in testicular self-examination.

**a.** The most common presenting complaint is **painless swelling** or enlargement of the testicle. This has been reported in 65% to 95% of patients, with an additional 10% to 15% noting a **painful swelling**, which is frequently confused with epididymitis.

**b.** A sense of **testicular heaviness** or dragging has also been reported.

**c.** Hydroceles have been associated with 2% to 8% of testicular tumors.

### 3. Diagnosis
of a scrotal mass is made by **physical examination**, possibly assisted by ultrasonography and surgical exploration via an inguinal approach.

### 4. Staging
is shown in Table 29-6.

**Table 29-6.** Staging of Testicular Cancer

| Extent of Tumor | Stage |
| --- | --- |
| Confined to the scrotum | I (or A) |
| Confined to the retroperitoneum | II (or B) |
| Beyond the retroperitoneum | III (or C) |

**a.** Procedures include chest tomography and CT scanning, inferior venacavography, lymphangiography, and abdominal CT.

**b.** The **major advance** in the staging of testicular tumors has been the use of **tumor markers**. Serum levels of human chorionic gonadotropin (HCG) and α-fetoprotein have been shown to be elevated in some patients with an existing tumor. The use of these markers has significantly decreased error in staging.

### 5. Treatment.
The treatment of testicular tumors varies with the cell type and with the disease stage.

**a. Seminoma** is generally sensitive to irradiation.

    **(1)** The treatment of **stage I seminoma** is fractionated doses totaling 2500 to 3000 rads to the periaortic and the ipsilateral pelvic and inguinal lymph nodes. Ipsilateral scrotal irradiation and contralateral inguinal nodal irradiation are considered in patients who have had previous scrotal surgery.

    **(2) Stage II seminoma** that has been detected radiographically or by elevation of β-HCG after orchiectomy is treated with 2500 to 3000 rads to the periaortic and the ipsilateral pelvic and inguinal lymph nodes.

        **(a)** Additional doses may be delivered to specific tumor masses.

        **(b)** Mediastinal irradiation has been routinely applied as well, although its use is being questioned due to the development of effective chemotherapy.

        **(c)** Retroperitoneal lymphadenectomy may be of value for histologic diagnosis in patients with bulky disease.

        **(d)** The survival rate for patients with stage I or II seminoma approaches 100%.

    **(3) Stage III seminoma** has not responded nearly as well to radiotherapy alone and should be treated with combination chemotherapy. A regimen of cisplatin, vinblastine, and bleomycin has been effective. Reduced dosage is necessary after previous radiotherapy.

**b. Nonseminomatous germ cell tumors**

    **(1) Stage I nonseminomatous testicular tumors** can be classified by finding no evidence of tumor spread upon retroperitoneal lymphadenectomy, in addition to a negative metastatic evaluation. Survival has been 100% in these patients.

    **(2) Stage II nonseminomatous testicular tumors**

      **(a)** Stage II tumors have been treated by lymphadenectomy.

      **(b)** Bulky disease benefits from preoperative combination chemotherapy. The role of adjuvant postoperative chemotherapy remains controversial.

      **(c) Retroperitoneal node dissection** for testicular tumor involves the surgical removal of tissue around the great vessels from the level of the diaphragm, including both renal hilar and ipsilateral perirenal tissue and extending to the common iliac artery contralaterally and to the inguinal ligament ipsilaterally.

    **(3) Stage III or disseminated testicular tumors**

      **(a)** The discovery of cisplatin and the development of combination chemotherapeutic regimens have markedly increased the response and survival rate of affected patients.

      **(b)** The response rate has been related to the extent of disease, with a 100% response seen among patients with elevated levels of tumor markers as their only indication of dissemination, and a 65% response in patients with advanced pulmonary or abdominal tumors.

**F. Prostatic tumors**

  **1. Epidemiology**

    **a.** Prostate cancer, over 95% of which is adenocarcinoma, is uncommon among men under the age of 50 years. The incidence increases rapidly with age, however, and the average patient age at diagnosis is 73 years.

    **b.** The rates of occurrence and mortality are higher among blacks than whites.

  **2. Etiology**

    **a.** Genetic and hormonal factors have been implicated.

    **b.** Exposure to cadmium is also a risk factor.

  **3. Diagnosis**

    **a.** Carcinoma of the prostate gland is frequently asymptomatic until it reaches an advanced stage.

    **b.** Low-stage tumors are most often found on routine rectal examination or on prostatectomy for benign indications. Induration or a firm nodule should be considered suspicious for cancer.

    **c.** The diagnosis of carcinoma can be confirmed by needle biopsy of the suspicious area.

  **4. Tumor grading.** Various grading systems for prostatic tumors have considered the histologic appearance—both cytologic characteristics and glandular morphology. Survival has been shown to be affected adversely by loss of differentiation.

  **5. Staging** is shown in Table 29-7.

**Table 29-7.** Staging of Prostatic Cancer

| Extent of Tumor | Stage |
|---|---|
| Incidental, focal | $A_1$ |
| Incidental, diffuse | $A_2$ |
| Prostatic nodule | $B_1$ |
| Large or multiple nodules, within prostate | $B_2$ |
| Localized to periprostatic area | C |
| Distant metastases | D |

    **a. Local tumor extension** is staged by **physical examination.** The extent of the tumor mass within the prostatic capsule or its extension beyond the capsule can be determined by **digital rectal examination.**

    **b.** Although ultrasonography and CT scanning may assist in determining local tumor extension, any superiority of these techniques over physical examination remains in question.

    **c.** The search for metastatic disease should be conducted by **chest x-ray**, **excretory urography**, **bone scanning**, and **CT scanning.**

    **d. Acid phosphatase** produced by the prostate gland is an extremely valuable **tumor marker.**

It is elevated in the serum in 70% to 85% of patients with metastatic disease but in fewer than 10% to 30% of patients with local disease alone.

6. **Treatment**
   a. Therapy for prostatic carcinoma is related both to the extent of disease and the status of the patient.
      (1) In approximately 40% of patients, metastases are present at the time of diagnosis.
      (2) In another 40%, the tumor extends beyond the prostatic capsule; in turn, nearly 50% of these patients have clinically undetectable metastases.
      (3) Only in the remaining 20% can cure be obtained by local treatment of the disease.
   b. **Stage A**
      (1) If adenocarcinoma of the prostate gland is localized to a focus involving only a few prostatic chips on transurethral resection of the prostate (stage $A_1$), survival without recurrence can be expected in over 90% of patients.
      (2) However, if the tumor is diffuse (stage $A_2$) or of a high grade early on, undetected metastases are likely in approximately 30% of patients.
      (3) Because of this important differentiation between stages $A_1$ and $A_2$, some authors have recommended a repeat of transurethral resection in a search for residual tumor.
   c. **Stage B** tumors are the most controversial in terms of treatment. These lesions respond to local ablative therapy, and it has been difficult to determine the most successful treatment. Radical prostatectomy, interstitial radiation with lymph node dissection, and external beam radiation all have their advocates and supporting data.
      (1) The selection of patients for **radical prostatectomy** depends on the patient's status as well as on the tumor. Candidates should be in good medical condition and should have an expected survival of 10 to 15 years.
         (a) The procedure includes removal of the prostate gland, seminal vesicles, and usually the pelvic lymph nodes.
            (i) Although the operative mortality rate is less than 1%, **morbidity** occurs, with impotence in up to 90% of patients. However, a new modification appears to have lessened this rate by avoiding section of the periprostatic autonomic nerves.
            (ii) Early urinary incontinence occurs in some patients but clears within 6 months in approximately 90% of those affected.
         (b) The survival rate in patients with $B_1$ lesions has been excellent. When the tumor has increased from stage $B_1$ to $B_2$, the 15-year survival has dropped from 27% to 18%.
      (2) **Interstitial radiation**
         (a) Interstitial radiation by implantation of iodine 125 ($^{125}$I) seeds has recently been popular for the control of prostatic carcinoma. Lymph node dissection is usually performed as well.
         (b) Long-term survival studies are not yet available, although at 5 years, persistent tumor has been noted in nearly two-thirds of patients initially staged with B or C disease.
      (3) **External beam radiation**
         (a) Tumoricidal doses of 6500 or 7000 rads can be delivered in fractionated doses to a locally confined prostatic tumor.
         (b) The 5-year survival rates have been shown to be 75% for stage B and 52% for stage C tumor. Ten-year survival rates decreased to 47% and 28%, respectively.
         (c) Local control, again, is related to the size and grade of the tumor. Histologic evidence of persistent tumor has been seen in significant numbers of patients after any form of radiotherapy, but the biologic significance of these findings remains unclear.
   d. **Treatment of metastatic carcinoma of the prostate gland** cannot rely on local ablative therapy alone. Symptomatic urinary obstruction may be treated by resection, but metastases must be treated systemically.
      (1) **Castration** and **estrogen administration** have long been established as effective therapeutic regimens.
         (a) Orchiectomy rapidly reduces the serum testosterone concentration from normal levels of 500 to 700 ng/dl to less than 50 ng/dl.
         (b) Estrogen administered in the form of **diethylstilbestrol** suppresses the release of pituitary gonadotropins in a dose-dependent fashion. Doses of 3 mg are necessary. Additionally, the diethylstilbestrol may have a direct effect on the prostate gland.
      (2) **Antiandrogen therapy** has proved to be useful.
         (a) Androgen synthesis can be obstructed by inhibitors such as aminoglutethimide, cyproterone, medrogestone, or spironolactone.
         (b) Gonadotropin release can be inhibited by luteinizing hormone-releasing hormone (LH-RH) analogs such as leuprolide.

(3) Chemotherapy for the treatment of metastatic carcinoma of the prostate gland has generated considerable interest recently. Some improvement has been demonstrated with single agents, and combination regimens have also been studied.

## VIII. BENIGN PROSTATIC HYPERTROPHY AND URINARY OBSTRUCTION. Enlargement of the prostate, resulting in urinary obstruction, has long been recognized as a process affecting the aging male. The central glandular portion of the prostate undergoes stromal and epithelial hyperplasia with well-defined nodular growth. The etiology of this hyperplasia remains unknown.

A. **Diagnosis** relies on the patient's symptoms, the finding of an enlarged prostate gland, and histologic confirmation.

1. The major symptoms result from bladder outlet obstruction and, as a group, constitute **prostatism**. The patient may notice a **decrease in the force** of the urinary stream, **hesitancy** in initiating the stream, an **intermittent stream**, or **dribbling** after voiding. **Hematuria** and **calculus formation** can occur. The patient may progress to total **urinary retention**.

2. On physical examination, differentiation from carcinoma of the prostate rests to a large extent on the presence or absence of nodules or firm areas within the gland.

B. **Treatment** may be indicated in patients with severe symptoms, obstruction, or damage extending to the upper urinary tract, and is certainly indicated in those with acute retention.

1. Agents producing α-adrenergic blockade have had some effect in decreasing outlet obstruction and increasing urinary flow rates in patients with benign prostatic hypertrophy.

2. Although hormonal therapy has aroused considerable interest, no regimen has been uniformly beneficial or outweighs the potential side effects.

3. **Treatment remains surgical** by transurethral resection or open prostatectomy to remove the obstructing intraurethral prostatic tissue.

## IX. NEUROGENIC BLADDER. Damage to the bladder's nerve supply, either motor or sensory, can hinder normal bladder function. Damage may occur from spinal cord trauma, congenital anomalies, or disease states such as diabetes mellitus or multiple sclerosis.

A. **Diagnosis by urodynamic studies**

1. **Urinary flow rate.** The normal urinary flow rate is approximately 20 to 25 ml/sec in men and 25 to 30 ml/sec in women. Many factors can operate together or independently to alter the flow rate, but obstruction should be considered when a flow rate of less than 15 ml/sec is seen in a patient with a full bladder.

2. **Bladder function** can be evaluated by **cystometry**. The bladder is filled at a known rate with water or carbon dioxide, and the intravesical pressure is recorded and plotted against the volume of fluid introduced. Thus, the contractility of the detrusor muscle and the patient's ability to inhibit this contraction can be monitored.

3. Responses of the **urinary sphincter** can be studied by measuring the intraluminal pressure of the sphincter and the electrical activity of the muscle via electromyography.

B. **Patterns of neurogenic bladder dysfunction**

1. A **spastic neurogenic bladder** can be the outcome of either partial or complete injury of the spinal cord above the sacral level.
   a. There may be spasms with resultant obstruction of the external urinary sphincter, and frequent involuntary contraction of the bladder can be observed.
   b. In affected patients, functional changes result in diminished bladder capacity, with urinary incontinence and with increased intravesical pressure that can be transmitted to the kidneys as well.

2. **Uninhibited neurogenic bladder** can result from incomplete lesions of the cortex or the pyramidal tracts. Patients experience urinary frequency, urgency, and nocturia. Uninhibited contractions can be noted on the cystometrogram. The patient empties the bladder completely, and there is a sensation of both fullness and emptying of the bladder.

3. A **flaccid or atonic bladder** can be caused by injury to the sacral portion of the spinal cord or to the nerves within the cauda equina, with resultant loss in the reflex arc to the bladder. Trauma, tumors, and congenital anomalies are the most frequent causes. The patient exhibits a large bladder capacity with low pressures and has no spontaneous detrusor contractions. The most frequent urinary symptom is overflow incontinence.

## C. Treatment

1. **Pharmacologic manipulation** can be used to affect the bladder directly and reverse the neurologic effect.
   a. Bethanechol has been used for the atonic bladder, often with an $\alpha$-adrenergic blocking agent, to decrease bladder neck and posterior urethral tone.
   b. Propantheline or oxybutynin have been used for the spastic or uninhibited bladder.

2. **Intermittent catheterization** has become the preferred method for mechanical emptying of the bladder. It has major advantages in decreasing the infection and long-term complications that are seen with chronic catheterization.

3. **Bladder stimulators** have been used experimentally, with encouraging results.

## X. MALE SEXUAL DYSFUNCTION

### A. General considerations

1. Male impotence can be defined as the inability to obtain or maintain an erection that is satisfactory for sexual intercourse.

2. With an increase in public awareness of the options for evaluation and treatment, impotence is no longer accepted as a part of growing old and has been recognized increasingly as a medical problem.

3. As with many disorders that are manifested by a loss of functional capability, there may be a wide spectrum of sexual disability. Although some patients may have a total loss of erectile ability, others may have intermittent difficulty or problems with maintaining an erection.

### B. Diagnosis

1. Since the therapy for male sexual dysfunction is rather sharply divided between organic and psychological approaches, a search for the major cause of the dysfunction is extremely important.

2. The diagnosis of sexual dysfunction necessarily relies almost entirely on the **history** given by the patient. Tact and completeness in taking a sexual history are of major importance.
   a. Affected patients are embarrassed by their problem, are often desperate, and are almost apologetic in seeking medical attention.
   b. The history must include the nature of the present problem, its onset and development, contributing psychological and medical factors, the effects of any prior treatment, and the patient's expectations.

3. Thorough consideration of **psychological factors** is of paramount importance.

4. The patient should have a thorough **physical examination**, with particular emphasis on the genitalia and the vascular and neurologic systems.

5. **Laboratory studies**
   a. **Blood studies** should include screening tests for the patient's general health, including a complete blood count and evaluation of the renal, hepatic, and metabolic status.
   b. **Hormonal studies** should include serum levels of testosterone (total and free), luteinizing hormone (LH), follicle-stimulating hormone (FSH), and prolactin.
   c. In addition, specific studies should be undertaken as indicated.
      (1) Blood flow can be studied by Doppler determinations of the penile blood pressure, ultrasonic evaluation of the vessels, or blood flow scans.
      (2) Perineal electromyography will indicate the status of the pudendal nerves.

6. **Monitoring of nocturnal penile tumescence (NPT)**
   a. Men normally have erections during periods of rapid-eye-movement (REM) sleep, which has been recognized as a major distinguishing factor between psychogenic and organic erectile failure.
   b. Many techniques have been developed for evaluating these erections, and there is a major advantage of in-hospital evaluation where a laboratory technician can observe and evaluate the quality of each erection.
      (1) NPT can be monitored with **gauges** evaluating the extent and firmness of an erection.
      (2) **Stamps or plastic bands** graded to break at specific forces also have proven useful.

### C. Treatment.
A major division in treatment exists between patients with predominantly psychological dysfunction and those with organically based dysfunction. There are, in addition, many patients with both factors who require combination therapy.

1. **Psychological treatment** may include sex therapy, individual psychotherapy, marital therapy, and pharmacologic treatment. In a few patients relatively uncommon techniques such as hypnosis may be helpful.

2. **Treatment of organic impotence** is often directed toward the specific etiology.
   a. **Hormonal abnormalities** can be corrected in some patients by the replacement of testosterone.
   b. Impotence related to **diabetes** can occasionally be improved by better control of the diabetes.
   c. **Vascular insufficiency** usually results from diffuse involvement of the small arteries to the penis. Success with revascularization has been limited mainly to those patients with a single, usually traumatic, lesion. Obstruction of the larger pelvic vessels such as the iliac arteries can often be treated surgically.
   d. **Neurologic disorders** have generally not responded to direct treatment.

3. **Penile prostheses**
   a. Implantation of a penile prosthesis to provide sufficient rigidity for intercourse has become an increasingly prevalent treatment.
   b. Three general **types** of prostheses are available: a semirigid type, an inflatable type contained within the corpora, and a fully inflatable type, which continues to have the largest number of mechanical failures but provides the most normal-appearing and normal-functioning erection.

4. **Other treatment techniques**
   a. Recently there has been considerable interest in the injection of vasodilators directly into the penis. This technique has provided satisfactory rigidity for many patients. Short- and long-term complications are not known, and the eventual role of this treatment remains to be determined.
   b. **Transrectal stimulation** of the nerves to the corpora cavernosa has produced erections in nonhuman primates and has been demonstrated with varying success in human volunteers.
   c. A **suction device** has recently been introduced, which can be placed over the penis, causing penile engorgement with blood that can be contained by means of a rubber band at the base of the penis. Although this technique has been effective in many patients, fear of complications such as ischemia from prolonged compression at the base of the penis has limited its widespread recommendation.

# 30
# Plastic Surgery and Skin and Soft Tissue Surgery

R. Anthony Carabasi, III
John H. Moore, Jr.

## I. PLASTIC SURGERY

A. **Introduction.** As an art and science, plastic surgery deals with the reconstruction of body parts altered by trauma, birth defects, or advanced age. It is one of the oldest fields of surgery, having first been described in 700 BC, in India. In 1818, von Graefe used the term "plastic" in his monograph on nasal reconstruction, and throughout the years since, this term has been associated with surgery that is concerned with form and function.

B. **The skin.** The skin, or **integumentary system**, is the largest organ in the body.

1. The skin has three **properties** that are essential for understanding reconstruction—elasticity, extensibility, and resilience.
   a. **Elasticity** keeps skin in constant tension, owing to underlying collagen fibers. The function of elasticity becomes apparent by its absence in "wrinkle lines" on the face.
   b. **Extensibility** refers to the skin's ability to stretch, which can be seen on abdominal skin during pregnancy.
   c. **Resilience** is noted by the skin's resistance to infection and puncture.

2. **Anatomically**, the skin has two principal **layers**, each with a specialized **function**.
   a. The **epidermis** is composed of stratified squamous epithelium, which covers the entire body and provides **protection**. Living cells migrate from the innermost level of the epidermis to the surface, to form a dead desquamating layer. The migration takes approximately 19 days.
   b. The **dermis**, which serves in a nutritive capacity to the epidermis, is itself composed of two layers.
      (1) The **papillary layer** is composed of fine collagen fibers, ground substance, and capillaries.
      (2) The **reticular layer** is composed of dense collagen, hair follicles, sebaceous glands, sweat glands, and the subdermal plexus.
   c. Beneath the dermis lies the **hypodermis, or subcutaneous tissue**, which may contain hair follicles, sweat glands, and nutrient vessels.

C. Various **suture materials and wound closure techniques** are available to the surgeon, and proper closure requires knowledge of them.

1. **Suture material** can be **classified** according to the body's ability to absorb it.
   a. **Absorbable sutures**
      (1) **Catgut** is made from the small intestine of sheep or cows. It is absorbed by phagocytosis in 2 weeks to 6 months. If it is treated with chromium salts, the rate of resorption is slower.
      (2) **Polyglycolic acid** is a braided polymer of glycolic acid and is stronger than comparably sized catgut. It is absorbed by enzymatic degradation, generally in 2 weeks to 2 months.
      (3) **Polydioxanone** is a monofilament which is useful for extended wound support. Absorption is by enzymatic degradation and is usually complete by 6 months.
   b. **Nonabsorbable sutures**
      (1) **Organic sutures** include **silk** and **cotton**, which are both braided. They are the most reactive of the nonabsorbable sutures.
      (2) **Synthetic sutures** include **nylon, polypropylene,** and **Dacron**. They evoke minimal tissue reaction.
      (3) **Stainless steel wire and clips** are the most inert of the nonabsorbable sutures.

**2. Suture marks** are imprints of the sutures themselves. They result from pressure on the skin during the time that the suture is left in place. They are exacerbated by tension on the wound, large bites of tissue, and infection.

**3.** A **cosmetically acceptable appearance** is a major goal of all closures.
   **a. Atraumatic handling of tissue** minimizes necrosis and decreases scarring.
   **b. Buried sutures** reduce dead space and decrease tension along skin edges.
   **c. Eversion of the wound edges** results in a level scar with time, while inversion of the edges may result in a concave scar.

**4. Techniques of wound closure** (Fig. 30-1)
   **a.** A **simple interrupted suture** results in equal full–thickness bites of skin and subcutaneous tissue. As the knot is secured, the underlying subcutaneous tissue helps to draw the skin edges into opposition.
   **b.** A **vertical mattress suture** is similar to a simple suture, but an additional bite through the wound edge is used to ensure edge eversion.
   **c.** A **horizontal mattress suture** is similar to a simple suture, but an additional bite is taken laterally on the opposite side so that eversion takes place in wounds under tension.
   **d.** A **subcuticular suture** is an intradermal closure that can be continuous or interrupted; suture material can be absorbable or nonabsorbable. The main advantage is the avoidance of suture marks on the skin.
   **e. Continuous over-and-over sutures** result in a secure closure. They are most commonly used on the scalp, where suture-line marks will be hidden by hair.
   **f. Skin tape** is useful for areas such as the face where suture-line scars must be minimized. In addition, it is a useful adjunct for subcuticular closure and for bolstering a wound following early suture removal.

**D. Skin grafts** are segments of epidermis and dermis that have been detached from their native blood supply in order to be transplanted to another area of the body. A skin graft may be an **autograft** (from the same person), an **allograft** (from a genetically dissimilar individual of the same species), or a **xenograft** (from a different species) [see also Chapter 16, section I B].

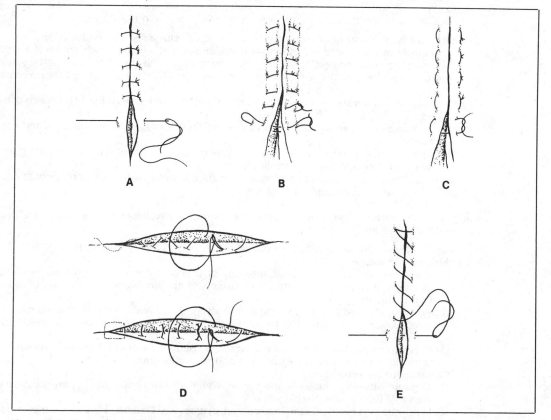

**Figure 30-1.** Types of wound closures: (*A*) simple interrupted suture, (*B*) vertical mattress suture, (*C*) horizontal mattress suture, (*D*) subcuticular suture, and (*E*) continuous over-and-over suture.

**1. Types of skin grafts.** Skin grafts are classified according to thickness.

    **a. Split-thickness skin grafts** contain the epidermis and a portion of the dermis. They are further subdivided into thin, medium, and thick, based upon the amount of dermis included in the graft (0.010 inch to 0.025 inch).

        **(1)** The abdomen, buttocks, and thighs are common donor sites.

        **(2) Advantages** of split-thickness skin grafts include:

            **(a)** A large supply of donor areas

            **(b)** Ease of harvesting

            **(c)** Availability of donor site for reuse in 10 to 14 days

            **(d)** Decreased primary contracture

            **(e)** Coverage of large surface areas

            **(f)** Ability to be stored for later use

        **(3) Disadvantages** of split-thickness skin grafts include:

            **(a)** Cosmetic inferiority to full-thickness skin grafts

            **(b)** Decreased durability

            **(c)** Hyperpigmentation

            **(d)** Increased secondary contracture

    **b. Full-thickness skin grafts** contain the epidermis and the full thickness of dermis without subcutaneous fat.

        **(1)** Full-thickness skin grafts are most useful for covering defects on the face or hand that are not amenable to coverage with a skin flap (see section I E).

        **(2)** A good match of skin color can be obtained from donor sites in the postauricular or supraclavicular areas. The forearm and groin can also serve as donor sites.

        **(3) Advantages** of full-thickness skin grafts include:

            **(a)** Cosmetic superiority to split-thickness skin grafts

            **(b)** Decreased secondary contractures (grafts may be cut as required to fill the defect)

            **(c)** Increased durability

        **(4) Disadvantages** of full-thickness skin grafts include:

            **(a)** Limited donor sites

            **(b)** Increased primary contracture

    **c.** A **composite graft** is one that is formed of multiple tissues (e.g., a fingertip containing skin, subcutaneous fat, and bone or a segment of ear containing skin and cartilage). These grafts may be effective in younger patients or where the distal portion of the graft is less than 1 cm from the blood supply.

**2. Grafting procedures**

    **a. Split-thickness skin grafts**

        **(1)** Split-thickness grafts are best obtained with specifically designed instruments rather than being taken freehand. **Methods of obtaining the graft** include the following.

            **(a) Knives**, such as the Humby or Weck, are fitted with an adjustable roller or gauge to determine thickness. The knife is slowly advanced as cutting proceeds in a back-and-forth direction.

            **(b)** The **drum** (Reese) **dermatome** fixes the epidermis to the drum with glue, which allows the graft to be cut as the drum is rolled back. Grafts cut are of uniform thickness.

            **(c)** The **electrical dermatome**, such as the Brown or Padgett, has a rapidly oscillating knife and a gauge to adjust depth. Long strips of skin can be removed with this instrument.

        **(2)** Proper **care of the donor site** following the cessation of capillary oozing will aid in re-epithelialization.

            **(a) Meshed, nonadherent gauze** allows the scab to be incorporated into the dressing. In 2 days the dressing is dry, and the covering, with the incorporated scab, falls from the wound by 2 weeks.

            **(b) Semipermeable membranes** trap leukocyte-rich fluid to form an artificial blister, which hastens epithelialization. Patients note diminished pain at the donor site.

        **(3) Care of the recipient (grafted) site** (see also section I D 3)

            **(a)** Hemostasis is necessary to ensure adequate tissue contact.

            **(b)** When excessive wound drainage or potential infection may be a problem, the graft can be cut and a meshing device can be used in order to ensure adequate drainage. This technique is also useful for expanding the surface area of a graft. Epithelialization quickly occurs in the meshed interstices following graft ''take.''

            **(c)** The graft may be fixed to the recipient site by sutures or tapes. External fixation with a ''tie-over bolus'' dressing (i.e., a large dressing made of gauze or cotton) may be required in areas where immobilization is difficult or where shear forces are expected. The open method, in which the graft is left exposed, may be useful for large surface areas in burn patients, where daily inspection for infection is important.

**b. Full-thickness skin grafts**
  **(1) Method of obtaining the graft.** The grafts are "harvested" with a freehand technique using a #10 or #15 knife blade. A portion of subcutaneous fat is also harvested, which needs to be excised carefully prior to grafting.
  **(2) Care of the donor site** involves primary skin closure in most instances. Split-thickness skin grafts may be necessary in some cases.
  **(3) Care of the recipient site** is similar to that in split-thickness skin grafts. Tie-over bolus dressings are frequently used.

**3. Survival of skin grafts**
  **a.** A **vascular recipient bed** is necessary to provide nourishment for the transplant tissue.
    **(1) Imbibition of plasma** supports survival during the first 48 hours. In addition, **fibrin** is laid down, which helps to hold the graft in place.
    **(2) Inosculation** (vascular budding) occurs, and the graft is usually supported by a true circulation by the fourth to seventh day. Generally, a graft begins to turn pink at this time. Lymphatic connections are formed by the fifth day.
  **b. Contact of the skin graft is essential** for inosculation to take place. Factors that can lead to **loss of contact** include:
    **(1) Tension** on the graft
    **(2) Fluid** (blood, serum, or pus) underneath the graft
    **(3) Movement** between the graft and its bed
  **c.** The **wound to be grafted** must be properly **prepared**.
    **(1)** Bone denuded of periosteum, cartilage denuded of perichondrium, and exposed tendon do not support skin grafts; these require a flap procedure.
    **(2) Infected wounds** do not support skin grafts. The critical bacterial concentration appears to be $10^5$ organisms per g of tissue, and bacterial counts are useful in determining a wound's suitability for grafting. Mechanical debridement and use of a biologic dressing (i.e., an allograft or a xenograft) help to reduce the bacterial count.

**E. Flaps**

  **1.** A **flap** is a segment of skin and subcutaneous tissue that is moved from one part of the body to another, either retaining or transplanting its vascular supply.
    **a.** The vascular supply is via a segmental artery through a perforating artery to a cutaneous artery supplying the dermal-subdermal plexus.
    **b.** Because of its intrinsic blood supply, a flap is useful for healing and for covering defects that require padding.

  **2. Types of flaps**
    **a. Skin flaps**
      **(1)** A **random flap** receives its blood supply from the dermal-subdermal plexus. This flap lacks an anatomically recognized arterial and venous system. Examples include:
        **(a)** Z-plasty
        **(b)** V-Y advancement flap
        **(c)** Rotation flap
        **(d)** Transposition flap
      **(2)** An **axial flap** has a direct cutaneous artery and vein supplying its subdermal plexus. Thus, the blood supply is more reliable than with a random flap, and a flap of greater length may be obtained. An axial flap may be detached as a free flap and transplanted to other areas of the body, provided that the vessels are large enough. Examples of axial flaps include:
        **(a)** Forehead flap
        **(b)** Groin flap
        **(c)** Deltopectoral flap
    **b. Myocutaneous flaps** involve the transfer of skin, subcutaneous tissue, and the underlying muscle.
      **(1)** The blood supply is predictable, and the flaps can be anatomically outlined. The flaps contain muscle with a named artery which must be identified and preserved.
      **(2)** Myocutaneous flaps have been most useful in reconstruction of the lower extremity and in areas of poor vascularity.
    **c. Free flaps** are those in which the native blood supply is completely severed, with transplantation of the flap to a separate body area. Revascularization is accomplished by microvascular anastomosis. Axial flaps and myocutaneous flaps may be transferred in this manner.

  **3. Uses of flaps** include:
    **a.** Wound closure in areas of poor vascularity (e.g., wounds overlying bare bone, cartilage, nerves, or tendons)

   **b.** Facial reconstruction (e.g., the nose or lips)
   **c.** Areas over bone where padding is needed (e.g., the ischial tuberosity in a patient with pressure sores)

   **4. Vascular patency** may be assessed by color, temperature, Doppler flowmetry, and fluoroscanning.
   **a.** In fluoroscanning, a fluorescent dye is injected so that the blood flow in the flap can be assessed (e.g., under a Wood's light).
   **b.** Fluoroscanning is the most useful technique in determining the adequacy of both the arterial and venous circulation.

**F. Reconstructive breast surgery.** Techniques are available for treating micromastia (small breasts), macromastia (oversized breasts), and gynecomastia and for reconstruction following mastectomy. Because the breast is frequently viewed as a symbol of femininity, there is much emotional overlay in this type of surgery. Careful planning and realistic goals are necessary for patient satisfaction.

   **1. Micromastia** is present when a patient feels she lacks development of one or both breasts.
   **a. Treatment** is by augmentation with a **silicone implant**. Usually this is placed under the pectoralis major muscle with either local or general anesthesia.
   **b. Complications** include infections and hematoma formation. A capsule may form around the prosthesis. Subsequent contracture of the capsule around the implant may occur, but this is a more common situation when the implant is in the submammary position.

   **2. Macromastia** is present when the patient feels she has abnormally large breasts, and it is usually associated with obesity or an endocrine imbalance. Frequently, macromastia can be debilitating because of neck and back pain. **Ptosis** is present when the nipple has extended below the inframammary fold.
   **a. Treatment.** A variety of techniques have been described. All involve resecting breast tissue and the inferior breast skin, transposition of the nipple-areolar complex superiorly, and closure of the resultant flap defects. All resected specimens should be examined histologically because occult carcinoma may be present, although rarely.
   **b. Complications** include hematoma formation, infection, and necrosis. Frequently, decreased sensation in the nipple-areolar complex is noted postoperatively.

   **3. Gynecomastia** is enlargement of the male breast. In adolescents, the problem is often transient and regresses spontaneously. It can also occur with various endocrine abnormalities and in association with hepatic disease. Treatment by excision is aimed at restoring normal contour to the breast.

   **4. Reconstruction of the breast following mastectomy** is an alternative to the use of external prosthetic devices. Reconstruction may be performed at the time of mastectomy or delayed for several months; however, the percentage of women who request reconstruction diminishes with increasing time following mastectomy.
   **a.** If there is **adequate soft tissue coverage** and if muscle has been preserved, Silastic implants may be placed subpectorally to increase fullness. The nipple-areolar complex may be resonstructed with tissue taken from the opposite breast or from the labia. Reduction mammoplasty may be necessary for the opposite breast to achieve symmetry.
   **b.** If there is **inadequate soft tissue coverage**, a latissimus dorsi or rectus abdominis myocutaneous flap may be necessary. A silicone implant is rarely required. Reconstruction of the nipple-areolar complex and procedures for the opposite breast are the some as described above.

**G. Reconstruction of congenital anomalies** (see also Chapter 33)

   **1.** Congenital anomalies may result from genetic or environmental factors. In most instances, an initiating environmental factor acts on a genetically predisposed individual. The inheritance risk for most anomalies remains low.

   **2.** The repair and reconstruction of many congenital anomalies do not fall within the scope of plastic surgery; examples include the gastrointestinal anomalies discussed in Chapter 33.

   **3. Maxillofacial deformities** can be reconstructed by craniofacial surgery.
   **a.** Both soft tissue and bony abnormalities can be reconstructed by a specialized team approach. Examples include:
      **(1)** Hypertelorism
      **(2)** Orbital dystopia
      **(3)** Treacher Collins syndrome
      **(4)** Facial clefts

      **(5)** Crouzon's disease

      **(6)** Apert's syndrome

   **b. Cleft lip** may be unilateral, bilateral, or incomplete. It is seen in 1 in 1000 births and is more common in Orientals and males.

      **(1)** Reconstruction is generally performed at about 3 months of age; the age for surgery is determined by the **"rule of tens"**: 10 lb, 10 weeks of age, and 10 g of hemoglobin.

      **(2)** The goal is to approximate normal anatomy, and this is accomplished best by means of local flap reconstruction.

   **c. Cleft palate** may occur as defects in the primary or secondary palate or both. It occurs in 4 in 10,000 births.

      **(1)** Reconstruction is performed before 2 years of age to aid in normal speech development and commonly involves local flap advancement.

      **(2)** Early attention to nutrition is important, as sucking is impaired.

**H. Facial trauma** frequently accompanies other major trauma. After ensuring adequate ventilation and circulation, attention should be directed initially to areas where trauma is more life-threatening (i.e., the chest and abdomen) [see Chapter 2, section I]. Once the patient is stabilized, the facial structures can be systematically examined.

   **1. Soft tissue**

     **a. Lacerations of the face** bleed readily because of its rich blood supply. Bleeding is controlled by direct pressure and never by "blind" clamping. Control in the operating room may be necessary.

     **b.** Lacerations may involve deeper structures such as the facial nerve and parotid duct.

     **c.** Most lacerations can be repaired by primary closure, following thorough debridement of all devitalized tissue.

   **2. Blunt trauma** may result in **contusions or associated fractures.**

     **a.** Many injuries of this type can be initially diagnosed by inspection, noting facial asymmetry, if present.

      **(1)** Dental malocclusion may signify a mandibular or maxillary fracture.

      **(2)** Instability of the upper jaw may signify a maxillary or midface fracture.

      **(3)** Pain on palpation at the nose, depression, or asymmetry may signify a nasal fracture.

      **(4)** Diplopia, malar deformity, enophthalmos, or hypoesthesia of the cheek may signify an orbital blow-out fracture.

     **b.** Complete radiologic examination is essential. Operative stabilization is usually required.

**I. Genitourinary anomalies** may interfere with normal urinary function and result in severe psychological problems if not corrected. These congenital anomalies are apparent at birth, and treatment should be initiated at an early age.

   **1. Hypospadias** is a condition in which the urethral meatus opens on the ventral surface of the penis, scrotum, or perineum.

     **a.** It occurs in 1 in 300 live male births and is usually associated with downward curvature of the penis caused by fibrous tissue, a condition called **chordee.**

     **b.** Evaluation of the upper urinary tract is essential, as 10% of patients have associated abnormalities.

     **c.** If present, the chordee is resected, and reconstruction is completed by local skin flap advancement, full-thickness skin grafts to create a urethra, or both.

   **2. Epispadias** is failure of closure of the dorsal surface of the penis. **Exstrophy of the bladder** occurs when the anterior bladder wall opens on the abdomen. Both represent degrees of the same abnormality.

     **a.** These are unusual disorders, occurring in 1 in 40,000 births.

     **b.** Associated upper urinary tract abnormalities are rare.

     **c.** Treatment is aimed at preserving renal function, which may be accomplished by closure of the bladder defect or excision of the bladder and urinary diversion.

   **3.** Vaginal reconstruction in patients with **vaginal agenesis** may be performed with split-thickness skin grafts. Myocutaneous flaps are used for reconstruction following ablative surgery.

   **4. Gender dysphoria** is treated surgically by altering sexual appearance to coincide with personality. After careful preoperative evaluation, ablative surgery is performed followed by reconstruction with flaps and skin grafts.

**J. Aesthetic surgery** is an attempt to improve on nature or to control the body's aging process by surgical means. Changes that occur secondary to aging are the result of decreased elasticity of the skin and loss of subcutaneous fat. Most commonly, procedures are performed on the more noticeable areas of the body (face, neck, abdomen, extremities, and breast). The expectations of the patient must be realistic; he or she must understand that surgery will alter appearance but not the person.

1. **Rhytidectomy** ("**facelifting**") involves plication of the underlying facial superficial musculoaponeurotic system and removal of excess facial skin. Dermabrasion and chemical face peeling are useful for diminishing fine facial wrinkles.

2. A **blepharoplasty** is used to treat **baggy eyelids**. This is accomplished by excision of varying amounts of skin and fat.

3. A **rhinoplasty** is performed to correct congenital or acquired **nasal defects**. The procedure involves a controlled nasal fracture with excision of varying amounts of bone and cartilage.

4. **Abdominoplasty** is the excision of excess abdominal fat and skin. It is frequently performed following weight loss or pregnancy.

5. Excessive amounts of skin and fat in the **extremities** usually are associated with weight loss and may be excised to improve appearance.

6. Reconstructive **breast surgery** is discussed in section I F, above.

## II. SKIN LESIONS

### A. General considerations

1. Many skin tumors can be **diagnosed at an early stage** because of their obvious difference from adjacent skin. They frequently have a **characteristic appearance**, which can aid in planning appropriate therapy.

2. **Examination should be systematic** and based on the gross appearance of the lesion. Inspection can reveal color changes and ulceration. Palpation can reveal fixation to underlying tissues or the involvement of adjacent lymph nodes.

3. **Biopsy** is usually required for accurate diagnosis and can either be **excisional** for smaller lesions or **incisional** for larger ones. In all instances, the biopsy should be carefully planned, as a more radical resection may be necessary. Additionally, cosmetic considerations must be kept in mind.

### B. Benign conditions are common, and frequently the patient seeks medical attention for cosmetic reasons or from fear of cancer. Only the more common lesions are discussed in this chapter.

1. **Common warts** (verrucae vulgaris) occur most frequently in the second decade of life and may be transmitted by direct or indirect contact.
   a. **Etiology.** They are caused by a member of the papovavirus family, which invades the stratum spinosum epidermidis, causing papillomatosis.
   b. **Clinical findings.** The fingers are the most common location. The lesions have a characteristic rough and elevated surface and can become tender.
   c. **Treatment** involves minimal destruction of normal tissue. In many cases, the warts will resolve spontaneously. Problematic lesions can be treated by:
      **(1)** Curettage and electrodesiccation
      **(2)** Freezing with liquid nitrogen
      **(3)** Chemotherapy with caustic agents

2. **Cysts** are fluid-filled cavities in the subcutaneous tissues; they may resemble solid tumors.
   a. **Epidermal inclusion cysts** develop when epidermal cells are trapped in the subcutaneous tissue. Desquamation leads to the creation of a cavity. Excision is curative.
   b. **Sebaceous cysts** result from blockage of a sweat gland, which causes the accumulation of sebum and the creation of a cyst. Excision is curative and prevents recurrence. If infection is present, the cyst should be incised and drained prior to excision.
   c. **Dermoid cysts** are congenital lesions that manifest themselves later in life. They commonly occur on the head and body. Treatment is by excision.
   d. **Ganglia** can occur in areas of weakened retinaculum with outpouching of underlying synovial structures. They occur most commonly on the hands and feet in areas subjected to trauma or inflammation. Excision is curative, but there can be recurrences which are most probably due to inadequate resection of the ganglion's stalk and base.

3. **Vascular tumors** (see also Chapter 24, section III E) are frequently disturbing to the patient and family because they are cosmetically deforming. Hemangiomas and pyogenic granulomas are more commonly seen during childhood.

    **a. Capillary hemangiomas (port-wine stains)** are found on the face, chest, and extremities and may be associated with Sturge-Weber and Klippel-Trenaunay-Weber syndromes. There is dilatation of capillaries in the subpapillary, dermal, or subdermal layer. If the tumor is small, excision is curative. Treatment of larger lesions requires careful planning for optimal results. The laser has recently proved to be helpful in treatment.

    **b. Immature hemangiomas (strawberry marks)** are found on the head, neck, chest, and extremities of infants. They are elevated, red, soft, and compressible tumors, which frequently enlarge during the first year of life. Almost all lesions undergo spontaneous regression during the next 2 to 7 years. Hemorrhage is not common, and usually there is minimal residual scarring.

    **c. Cavernous hemangiomas** involve a matrix of mature vessels in the subcutaneous tissues; frequently they involve deeper tissues, including muscle or central nervous system tissue. These congenital lesions may sequester platelets. After careful preoperative planning, treatment involves wide excision with attention to the involved structures. High doses of prednisone have been helpful in some cases.

    **d. Pyogenic granulomas** are papular lesions, commonly located on the face, chest, and fingers, which develop rapidly and then stop growing after variable periods of growth. The lesions tend to bleed freely. After curettage and electrodesiccation, satellite lesions or a recurrence may be seen.

    **e. Spider nevi (telangiectasias)** occur in all age-groups and are commonly located on the face, chest, and extremities. They may arise during pregnancy and in cirrhosis. The lesion consists of a central arteriole with vessels resembling venules radiating from the center. They rarely bleed, and treatment (electrodesiccation or cryotherapy) is undertaken primarily for cosmetic reasons.

    **f. Glomus tumors** (see Chapter 25, section XII A 3 b), which are extremely painful, are located most frequently in the nail beds. Treatment is by excision.

**4. Lipomas (fat tumors)** can be found in any area of the body where fat is normally found, but are most common on the neck, shoulders, back, and thighs. Malignant transformation is uncommon, and excision is curative.

**5. Nerve tumors** (see also Chapter 24, section IV I) are of two varieties.

    **a. Neurilemomas** arise from the Schwann cell sheath, do not cause much pain, and are treated by excision.

    **b. Neurofibromas** involve masses of nerve and fibrous tissue and are related to **von Recklinghausen's disease**. They may undergo malignant degeneration.

**6. Seborrheic keratosis** is a light- to dark-brown raised papular lesion which must be differentiated from malignant skin lesions. Treatment is by biopsy followed by curettage and electrodesiccation.

**7. Keloids** are abnormal accumulations of fibrous tissue which extend above and beyond an area that was initially traumatized. They occur more commonly in black persons. Treatment is by excision and closure, occasionally with adjuvant corticosteroid therapy.

**8. Hidradenitis suppurativa** may be confused with a tumor, but it is an **infection** of the apocrine sweat glands and subcutaneous tissue most frequently occurring in the axilla or groin. Treatment involves controlling the infection with antibiotics and (if indicated) incision and drainage, followed by excision with either primary closure or a split-thickness skin graft.

**C. Premalignant skin lesions** are benign lesions with a high likelihood of progressing to invasive squamous cell carcinoma.

**1. Actinic keratosis** is a rough, scaly epidermal lesion that occurs in areas of the body subjected to chronic sun exposure.

    **a.** It may appear in the third or fourth decade of life, and approximately 10% to 20% of the lesions will undergo malignant transformation.

    **b.** If biopsy proves the lesion to be benign, it is treated by excision or cryotherapy. Topical chemotherapy with 5-fluorouracil has been useful in patients with many keratoses.

**2. Bowen's disease** is intraepidermal squamous cell carcinoma or carcinoma in situ of the skin. It appears as a well-defined, erythematous plaque covered by an adherent scaly yellow crust.

    **a.** There are no lymphatics in the layer affected, and there is no potential for metastasis.

    **b.** Bowen's disease occurs mainly in the fourth to sixth decade of life, and arsenical ingestion and viruses have been implicated as etiologic agents. Treatment is similar to that for actinic keratosis.

**3. Keratoacanthoma** is a locally destructive skin lesion most commonly found in the head, neck, and upper extremities.

   **a.** Rapid progression of the tumor occurs within a 2- to 8-week period, followed by spontaneous resolution.
   **b.** Treatment is excision and biopsy of the lesion; squamous cell carcinoma is found in approximately 1/4 of the lesions biopsied.

**D. Nevi (moles)**

**1. General considerations**
   **a.** Nevi are pigmented lesions of the skin that frequently concern the patient because of the fear of malignancy.
   **b.** Because the average white male has 15 to 20 nevi, total excision is unreasonable.
   **c.** Clinical diagnosis is of prime importance because **malignant transformation** can occur. In general, however, malignant transformation is rare in children. Also well-circumscribed lesions and lesions with a uniform color rarely progress to malignancy.
   **d.** Suspicious looking lesions should be biopsied by excision with a margin of normal skin.

**2. Benign pigmented lesions**
   **a. Junctional nevi** are dark, flat, smooth lesions, which range generally from 1 mm to 2 cm in diameter. They are occasionally hairy and develop from the basal layer of epidermis. Nevi that are located on the palms and soles are usually junctional. They can develop into malignant melanoma, but this rarely occurs before puberty.
   **b. Compound nevi** are brown-to-black, well-circumscribed lesions, usually less than 1 cm in diameter. They may be elevated and are frequently hairy, arising from the epidermal–dermal interface and within the dermis. Malignant transformation is rare.
   **c. Intradermal nevi** are light-colored, well-circumscribed lesions less than 1 cm in diameter. Hairs are usually present, and the cell distribution is in the dermis. Malignant transformation is rare.
   **d. Giant pigmented nevi**
      **(1)** These are brown-to-black, hairy lesions with an irregular nodular surface. They frequently involve more than 1 square foot of body surface and arise from the dermis and junctional areas. The lesions are frequently described, in terms of distribution, as ''bathing trunk,'' ''vest,'' ''sleeve,'' or ''stocking.''
      **(2)** Malignant degeneration has been estimated at approximately 10%.
      **(3)** Excision with a margin of normal tissue is indicated, either in stages or with flap reconstruction.
   **e. Blue nevi** are smooth, hairless lesions measuring less than 1 cm in diameter. They arise in the dermis, and malignant degeneration is rare.
   **f. Spitz nevi (benign juvenile melanomas)** are smooth, round, pink-to-black lesions measuring 1 cm to 2 cm in diameter. They have increased cellularity and occur in nests within the upper dermis. Malignant degeneration is rare.

**3.** Nevi must be distinguished from **freckles (ephelides)**. These pigmented lesions occur in the basal and upper dermis and have no malignant potential.

**4. Treatment of nevi**
   **a.** Treatment is indicated for **junctional and giant pigmented nevi** because of their malignant potential.
   **b. Indications for excision** of any pigmented lesion include:
      **(1)** Changes in color, size, shape, or consistency
      **(2)** Pain
      **(3)** Satellite nodules
      **(4)** Regional adenopathy
   **c.** Except for large lesions, **excisional biopsy**, with a margin of normal skin, should be performed. Further therapy may be indicated, depending upon the histologic diagnosis and location of the lesion.
   **d.** For large lesions, a full-thickness wedge biopsy, including a small area of normal skin, should be taken.

**E. Malignant melanoma** (see also Chapter 25, section X C) is a melanoblastic tumor which may develop in the skin or eye.

**1. Epidemiology.** The incidence is approximately 13 new cases per 100,000 population per year, representing an increase of 50% in the past decade. The tumor occurs most commonly in the fifth decade of life, and the incidence is approximately equal in males and females.

**2. Etiology. Exposure to sunlight** appears to be an initiating event in the development of melanoma, and fair-skinned whites with frequent direct (overhead) exposure to the sun are most often affected.

3. Men are most frequently affected on the back, chest, and upper extremities, while women are most frequently affected on the back, lower extremities, and upper extremities.

4. The **detection** of melanoma is determined by changes in the color, size, or shape of a nevus.

5. **Classification** of melanomas is based on their gross and histologic appearance.
   a. **Superficial spreading melanoma** accounts for 70% of all melanomas. It can be present on any area of the body but is most frequently found on the back and legs. The median age at diagnosis is the fifth decade. The tumor has irregular borders with a varied color pattern. Cell distribution is in the upper dermis with lateral junctional spread. Generally, the prognosis is good.
   b. **Nodular melanoma** accounts for 15% of melanomas and occurs most commonly in the sixth decade of life. The tumor is blue-black and may be found on any area of the body. Spread is primarily vertical, with rapid dermal invasion, and the prognosis is poor.
   c. **Acrolentiginous and mucosal melanomas** comprise 10% of all melanomas. They most commonly occur in the fifth decade of life and are distributed on the mucous membranes, palms, and soles. Irregular borders are common, and lesions generally are black but may be amelanotic. Growth occurs slowly in a radial direction; cells are mainly in the upper dermis with occasional deep invasion. The prognosis depends on the depth of invasion and is between that of superficial spreading and nodular melanomas.
   d. **Lentigo maligna** (melanotic freckle of Hutchinson) is the least common of the melanomas, and it appears most frequently in the seventh decade of life. The lesions are brown-black and contain elevated nodules within a smooth freckle. They occur most frequently on the head, neck, and hand. Growth is slow and in a radial direction, with cells in the upper dermis; vertical extension is infrequent. The prognosis is excellent.

6. **Staging.** Classification of the lesion is imperative for optimal treatment. Histologic evaluation with regard to the depth of invasion as well as the type of tumor is important for determining prognosis.
   a. **Clark's classification** assesses the **level of invasion** and has been adopted by the American Joint Committee for Cancer Staging and End Results.
      (1) **Level I:** The tumor is confined to the epidermis.
      (2) **Level II:** The tumor invades the papillary dermis.
      (3) **Level III:** The tumor fills the papillary dermis but does not invade the reticular dermis.
      (4) **Level IV:** The tumor invades the reticular dermis.
      (5) **Level V:** The tumor invades the subcutaneous fat.
   b. The **Breslow method** is an additional method that is sometimes used. It involves measuring the depth of invasion precisely in millimeters. However, erroneous estimates of the depth of invasion can occur if ulceration is present.
      (1) Patients with Clark's level I, II, or III lesions and with a depth of invasion that is less than 0.76 mm are at low risk for metastasis.
      (2) Patients with lesions at level IV or V and with a depth of invasion greater than 1.5 mm are at high risk for distant spread.
   c. In order to complete the staging, a thorough history and physical examination are necessary, including a complete blood count, 12-test sequential multiple analysis (SMA-12), urinalysis, and chest x-ray.

7. **Treatment** depends upon the depth of invasion and the tumor level.
   a. **Excision**
      (1) For Clark's level I lesions, excision along with a cuff of normal tissue is all that is required.
      (2) When the tumor is level II, III, IV, or V, excision with a 5-cm margin, and possibly the underlying fascia, is required. The only exception would be for lesions of the face, for which at least a 2.5-cm margin is necessary.
   b. **Resection**
      (1) Clinically involved regional lymph nodes with level II, III, IV, or V disease should be resected.
      (2) Prophylactic resection of clinically benign nodes is controversial.
         (a) Some authors recommend prophylactic resection only for patients who are expected to be problems in follow-up, for patients whose tumor overlies a lymph node basin, or for level V disease.
         (b) Other authors have advocated prophylactic resection with invasion greater than 0.75 mm or with Clark's level III, IV, or V disease, feeling that this aids in staging and may enhance survival.
      (3) Postoperative morbidity from lymph node resection needs to be considered when lesions involve the face or lower extremities.
   c. **Adjuvant therapy** is recommended by some authors in order to prolong the disease-free interval.

        **(1) Regional hyperthermic perfusion** involves isolating the blood supply of a limb with a pump-oxygenator, enabling high doses of chemotherapy at elevated temperatures (40° C) to be delivered to the limb without the side effects of systemic toxicity. The role of this treatment has yet to be clarified.

        **(2) Chemotherapy** with dacarbazine (DTIC), carmustine (BCNU), and lomustine (CCNU) has not significantly altered the course of disease.

        **(3) Immunotherapy** is useful for the control of cutaneous metastases, but visceral metastases have not responded to any significant degree.

        **(4) Radiotherapy** is strictly palliative and has been used for brain and bone metastases.

    **8. Prognosis** is related to the status of the regional lymph nodes. When disease is confined at the primary site, the 5-year survival rate approaches 80% to 90%. If regional lymph nodes are involved, this figure drops to 30% to 50%. Patients with distant or visceral metastases are usually dead within 12 months.

**F. Other malignant tumors of the skin** commonly occur in exposed areas. Generally, they are low-grade and metastasize late. For this reason, they are highly curable.

    **1. Basal cell carcinoma** (see also Chapter 25, section X B) is the most common skin tumor seen. It is localized and slow-growing, and it generally occurs in the head and neck. It is found most commonly in individuals of northern European descent.

      **a. Etiology. Exposure to sunlight** is the principal etiologic factor. Basal cell carcinoma has also been associated with xeroderma pigmentosum, basal cell nevus syndrome, nevus sebaceous, and unstable burn scars. With the advent of radiation therapy, basal cell carcinomas are being seen with increasing frequency in areas of dermatitis.

      **b. Clinical findings.** The lesion has pearly translucent edges, which may become erythematous or pigmented. Frequently, a visible telangiectasia is present. As the lesion grows, it may ulcerate and eventually invade underlying structures.

      **c. Treatment** involves complete removal of the tumor to achieve cure. **Biopsy is mandatory** to establish a pathologic diagnosis.

        **(1) Curettage and electrodesiccation** results in a 95% cure rate, and the technique is acceptable for lesions less than 2 cm in diameter. The disadvantage is the lack of a specimen for determining the adequacy of resection.

        **(2) Radiation therapy** can be used in areas where tissue preservation is important (e.g., the eyelids). The cure rate is approximately 90%. The disadvantages are that depigmentation and skin atrophy can occur with time.

        **(3) Excision with primary closure** results in a cure rate approaching 95% and allows inspection of the specimen for adequate margins. Lymph nodes should be excised in continuity if they are clinically positive. If necessary, reconstruction can be performed at the same sitting.

        **(4) Other methods** that have been successful include **Mohs' chemosurgery** and **cryotherapy.** 5-Fluorouracil cream has an unacceptably high recurrence rate.

      **d. Recurrent disease** requires wide reexcision.

    **2. Squamous cell carcinoma** (see also Chapter 25, section X B) is second to basal cell carcinoma in occurrence. It may grow rapidly and has the capacity to metastasize via the blood and lymphatic system.

      **a. Etiology. Exposure to sunlight** appears to be a causative factor in that the tumor is more common on the head and hands. Squamous cell carcinoma may develop from the premalignant lesions already mentioned (see section II C) or from old burn scars; it may also occur in people exposed to arsenicals, nitrates, or hydrocarbons.

      **b. Clinical findings.** The lesion may have satellite nodules or a central area of ulceration that may become encrusted, obscuring deeper invasion. The tumor is common on the lips, in the paranasal folds, and on the axilla. It can be classified as well-differentiated or poorly differentiated squamous cell carcinoma, based upon the histologic examination.

      **c. Treatment**

        **(1)** Treatment is based upon examination of the biopsy specimen.

          **(a) Excisional biopsy** with a cuff of normal tissue is preferred for lesions less than 1 cm in diameter.

          **(b) Incisional biopsy** can be performed for larger lesions or those on the face.

        **(2) Treatment methods**

          **(a) Electrodesiccation** can be used to treat lesions less than 1 cm in diameter. It can also be used in older individuals and in patients with a history of repeated tumors.

          **(b) Excision with primary closure** offers the advantage of histologic examination of the specimen. Reconstruction following the excision of larger lesions may be required.

            **(i)** Regional lymph node dissection should be performed only if there is clinical evidence of nodal disease.

(ii) Frequently, regional adenopathy may accompany ulcerated lesions. In this case the lymph nodes should not be excised at the same sitting as the primary tumor, because the nodes will resolve with time if the adenopathy is inflammatory in nature.

(c) **Radiation therapy** can result in cure with improved cosmetic results in certain instances.

(d) **Mohs' chemosurgery** (see Chapter 25, section X B 4 c) has also been successful in treatment.

3. **Sweat gland tumors** are rare lesions arising from the eccrine or apocrine glands. They occur in later life and present as a soft tissue mass that has been present for years. Metastases to regional lymph nodes are common, and consideration should be given to regional node dissection at the time of initial excision. The overall 5-year survival rate approaches 40%.

### G. Sarcomas of the soft tissue

1. **General considerations.** Sarcomas of the soft tissue constitute only 1% of malignant tumors, and they may occur at any location in the body. Roughly 20 different types have been described, each with a slightly different tendency to metastasize or to invade locally.

   a. These tumors usually **present** as an enlarging mass which is frequently painless. If they occur in deeper locations, such as the retroperitoneum, they are often quite large at the time of diagnosis.

   b. The **diagnosis** is made on permanent sections of a representative **biopsy**. If the lesion is smaller than 3 cm, the biopsy is excisional. A wedge (incisional) biopsy is used for a larger lesion.

   c. These tumors are frequently **treated** inadequately because they have a pseudocapsule, which may lead the surgeon to assume falsely that all of the tumor has been removed. In reality, these tumors extend along tissue planes well beyond their apparent margins.

   (1) **Wide excision** is the most important aspect of treatment. In an extremity, this may require removal of muscle groups from origin to insertion. More proximal lesions of the extremities may require amputation.

   (2) The combination of a more **limited type of surgery** with **high-dose radiotherapy** is also an acceptable form of treatment. The local recurrence rate for combination therapy appears to be similar to that for radical surgery (i.e., 20% to 25%).

   d. The **route of metastasis** is usually **hematogenous**, and the lungs are the most frequent site of involvement. Lymphatic spread occurs less often and usually later in the course of the disease. Metastatic lesions in the lungs should be resected if the primary tumor is under good control and there is no evidence of other sites of involvement.

2. **The major soft tissue sarcomas**

   a. **Liposarcoma** is the most common of the soft tissue sarcomas.

   (1) Only 1% arise from preexisting benign lipomas.

   (2) Liposarcomas can occur in any area, including the retroperitoneum.

   (3) They are **treated** by wide excision. The tumors are radiosensitive, and radiotherapy may be helpful in locations where wide excision is not possible.

   (4) Well-differentiated lesions have a 70% 5-year survival rate, while poorly differentiated lesions have only a 20% survival rate at 5 years.

   b. **Fibrosarcoma** is the second most common soft tissue sarcoma.

   (1) These lesions are usually found in an extremity, where they present as a hard, round mass. They are more common in men than in women and are the most common sarcoma found in black persons.

   (2) They are radioresistant, and the **treatment** is wide excision. Fibrosarcomas are very prone to local recurrence and must be treated aggressively at the time of presentation.

   (3) Adequately treated fibrosarcomas have a 5-year survival rate of 77%.

   c. **Rhabdomyosarcoma** arises from skeletal muscle and occurs in both a juvenile and an adult form.

   (1) **Embryonal rhabdomyosarcoma** usually occurs in children under 15 years of age.

   (a) The head, neck, and genitourinary system are most frequently involved.

   (b) This tumor has recently enjoyed a spectacular increase in the 5-year survival rate. The combination of surgery, radiotherapy, and multidrug chemotherapy now achieves a 70% 5-year survival rate for patients with isolated lesions. If metastases are present, the survival rate is lower but still approaches 40%.

   (2) **Pleomorphic rhabdomyosarcoma** is the histologic type usually found in adults.

   (a) **Wide excision** (including amputation, if necessary) is the **treatment** of choice. Chemotherapy is much less effective in this form of the tumor.

   (b) Although lymph node dissections are not done in most cases of sarcoma, they should be done for pleomorphic rhabdomyosarcoma because 25% of patients have regional nodal metastasis.

    **(c)** The 5-year survival rate is 30%.

**d. Kaposi's sarcoma**, which has attracted attention recently in connection with acquired immune deficiency syndrome (AIDS), is a malignant lesion of vascular origin.

    **(1)** Until recently it was usually seen in the lower extremities of older men. Now it is often seen in the perianal area in connection with AIDS.

    **(2)** It usually begins as a single bluish-red macule, and gradually multiple nodules appear and may ulcerate.

    **(3)** A solitary nodule should be excised, and widespread disease should be treated with radiotherapy. Although there is no cure for systemic Kaposi's sarcoma, patients may live many years.

**e. Lymphangiosarcoma** is a peculiar tumor that develops in areas of chronic lymphedema (e.g., in the arm of women with postmastectomy edema, particularly if radiotherapy has also been used). The prognosis is dismal, and there is no effective treatment.

# 31
# Neurosurgery
## Bikash Bose

**I. INTRODUCTION.** Neurosurgery involves the surgical management of diseases of the nervous system. In the past two decades, rapid strides have been made in the field with the development of computed axial tomography (CAT or CT scanning) for detecting lesions of the brain and spinal cord, and with the introduction of operative tools like the operating microscope, the laser, and the ultrasonic aspirator. The **goal of neurosurgical intervention** is to prevent and, if possible, to reverse the loss of neurologic function.

**II. EMBRYOLOGY.** The entire nervous system is ectodermal in origin.

- **A.** First, there is formation of the **neural folds**, which are thickened ridges on either side of the midline in front of the primitive streak in the embryonic disk.

- **B.** The area between the neural folds is called the **neural groove**.

- **C.** With the descent of the primitive streak, there is elongation of both the neural folds and the neural groove. The neural folds rise into ridges and finally close around the neural groove, forming the **neural tube**.

    - **1.** The neural tube closes first in the region of the future hindbrain and then progresses both cranially and caudally.

    - **2.** With the closure of the neural folds, a narrow angular interval is left along the neural tube between it and the primitive body of the ectoderm. Cells at the top of the neural tube at this junction push out into the groove, forming the **neural crest**.
        - **a.** The **cranial end** of the neural tube forms the future **forebrain (prosencephalon), midbrain (mesencephalon),** and **hindbrain (rhombencephalon)**.
        - **b.** The **walls** develop into the **neuronal tissue** and **neuroglia** of the **brain**, and the **cavity** gives rise to the **ventricular system**.
        - **c.** The **caudal end** of the neural tube is modified by the formation of a longitudinal groove called the **sulcus limitans** along the middle portion of each side. This marks the subdivision of the tube into:
            - **(1)** An **alar** (dorsal) **lamina**, which gives rise to the **sensory elements** of the **spinal cord**
            - **(2)** A **basal** (ventral) **lamina**, which gives rise to the **motor elements**

**III. ANATOMY.** The brain constitutes only 2% of the body weight but requires 18% of the **cardiac output** and 20% of the **oxygen** utilized by the body. The normal **cerebral blood flow** is about 50 ml per 100 g of brain tissue per minute.

- **A.** The **arterial supply to the brain** (see Chapter 13, Fig. 13-3) can be divided into an anterior and a posterior circulation.

    - **1.** The **anterior circulation** is derived from the two **internal carotid arteries**, each with its terminal branches, the larger **middle cerebral** and the smaller **anterior cerebral** arteries. These vessels supply mainly the **frontal, temporal,** and **parietal lobes** as well as the **deep gray matter**.

    - **2.** The two **vertebral arteries** give rise to the **posterior circulation**.
        - **a.** At the caudal margin of the pons the vertebral arteries unite to form the **basilar artery**.
        - **b.** The basilar artery gives off branches supplying the **pons, cerebellum, thalamus,** and (via the **posterior cerebral arteries**) the **occipital lobes**.

**3.** An arterial circle, the **circle of Willis**, is formed at the base of the brain between branches of the internal carotid and basilar arteries.
  **a.** This arterial circle is fully developed in only about 55% of the population and is of great clinical significance.
  **b.** In the event of occlusion of a cerebral vessel (see section XII), the blood supply to its territory may be taken over by another vessel via the circle of Willis.

**B. Venous drainage of the brain** can be divided into two parts.

  **1. Superficial cerebral veins** drain the cortex and subcortical white matter and finally end in the superior sagittal sinus or other basal sinuses (i.e., the transverse, petrosal, or cavernous sinuses).

  **2. Deep cerebral veins** drain the deeper structures (nuclei). The deep veins consist of the paired **internal cerebral** and **basal (Rosenthal) veins**, which finally form the **great vein of Galen** before emptying into the straight sinus.
  **a.** All venous blood from the brain returns to the heart via the internal jugular vein.
  **b.** Thus, sampling of the jugular bulb blood provides an estimate of cerebral metabolism.

**C. Arterial supply to the spinal cord.** The spinal cord is supplied by the **anterior spinal artery** and the paired **posterior spinal arteries**, reinforced by the **segmental radicular arteries**.

  **1.** The **anterior spinal artery** gives off the **anterior sulcal artery**, in the anterior sulcus, which supplies the anteromedial gray matter.

  **2.** The **segmental radicular arteries** follow the anterior and posterior roots and join the spinal arteries, forming an arterial circle or **arteria coronae**.
  **a.** A large segmental artery at the $C_5$–$C_6$ vertebral level, called the **artery of Lazorthes**, has been described, and a similar artery exists at the thoracolumbar area, termed the **artery of the lumbar enlargement** or the **artery of Adamkiewicz**.
  **b.** These segmental arteries are important because their interruption by trauma or surgery can lead to vascular infarction of the spinal cord.

**D.** The **venous drainage of the spinal cord** is similar to the arterial supply.

  **1. Anterior longitudinal venous trunks**, consisting of anteromedian and anterolateral veins, drain corresponding areas of the cord. These in turn are drained by 6 to 11 radicular veins draining into the epidural venous plexus.

  **2. Posterior longitudinal venous trunks**, consisting of one posteromedian and paired posterolateral veins, drain the posterior funiculus, the posterior horns, and the white matter in the lateral funiculi. These in turn are drained by 5 to 10 radicular veins into the epidural venous plexus.

  **3.** The **epidural venous plexus** is located between the vertebral periosteum and the dura mater.
  **a.** The plexus consists of two or more anterior and posterior longitudinal veins interconnected at various levels.
  **b.** At each intervertebral space there is an extensive anastomosis with intercostal, thoracic, and abdominal veins.
  **c.** None of these venous channels have valves, and thus blood from these plexuses may directly enter the systemic circulation and vice versa.

**E. Cerebrospinal fluid (CSF)**

  **1.** The CSF is the third major component within the intracranial compartment, the others being brain tissue and blood.

  **2.** Normally the total volume of the CSF is about 150 ml, with 25 ml located in the ventricles. The CSF is formed at the rate of 0.35 ml/min. About 80% of the CSF is produced by the choroid plexus, with another 10% to 20% formed in the interstitial spaces of the brain.

  **3.** The **CSF flows** through the **ventricles** from the lateral to the third and then to the fourth, and **exits** by the **foramina of Magendie** (midline) **and Luschka** (lateral).
  **a.** The fluid may then circulate around the spinal cord or pass via the arachnoid villi into the posterior part of the superior sagittal sinus.
  **b.** The **arachnoid villi** act as one-way valves, allowing only CSF to drain into the venous sinus, and they open at a pressure of 5 mm Hg.
  **c.** Some of the CSF is absorbed around the spinal nerve roots.

**F. Functional anatomy of the nervous system.** The following **principles** form the basis for evaluating and treating neurologic disease.

1. Three aspects of the nervous system contribute to pathophysiologic processes unique to diseases of the nervous system. These include:
   a. The **complexity of the functional anatomy** of the nervous system
   b. The **rigidity of the bony enclosures** of the brain and spinal cord
   c. The **responses of the nervous system** to injury

2. In general, **focal lesions** affect local neurologic function by:
   a. **Local destruction** of brain tissue
   b. **Tissue distortion**, with functional loss attributable to axonal stretching and consequent damage
   c. Changes in **local blood flow**, causing ischemia or venous congestion
   d. Alterations in the **electrical or metabolic activity** of a local area, producing an epileptic focus

3. The **location of the lesion** is also important.
   a. A small focal lesion in the **brain stem** can produce devastating effects.
   b. A similar lesion in the **frontal (silent) area** may produce no significant neurologic deficit.

## IV. PATHOPHYSIOLOGY

A. **Cerebral edema.** The brain reacts to different insults by developing edema.

1. Three **types of cerebral edema** have been described:
   a. **Cytotoxic edema**
      (1) Cytotoxic edema is usually seen in the gray matter as a result of a metabolic derangement within the astroglia, leading to an intracellular accumulation of water.
      (2) The blood-brain barrier is preserved.
      (3) This type of edema is common following anoxia and ischemia, and in association with Reye's syndrome.
   b. **Vasogenic edema**
      (1) Also called extracellular white matter edema, vasogenic edema results from a breakdown of the blood-brain barrier and the leakage of plasma into the extracellular spaces.
      (2) This is the **most common type of edema seen clinically**, and it occurs around tumors, abscesses, surgical sites, and areas of ischemia or trauma.
   c. **Interstitial edema.** The protein content is low in situations of interstitial edema, which is usually seen in the periventricular region in patients with acute hydrocephalus.

2. Edema causes alterations in neuronal and axonal function by various mechanisms. Those proposed include:
   a. Ischemia as a result of increased intracranial pressure and decreased cerebral perfusion pressure (CPP)
   b. Decreased oxygen diffusion
   c. Lipid peroxidation in membranes

3. Investigators have reported that **acute edema** causes more deterioration in neurologic function than does **chronic edema**. That is, the **rate of formation** of edema is directly proportional to the neurologic deficits.

B. **Intracranial pressure (ICP)**

1. The **skull** is a rigid box with a volume of approximately 1900 ml and containing three **types of tissue**.
   a. About 85% is **brain** (5% is extracellular fluid, 45% is glial tissue, and 35% is neuronal tissue)
   b. About 7% is **blood**
   c. About 7% is **CSF**

2. According to the **Monro-Kellie hypothesis**, under normal conditions these three components are in equilibrium, and the ICP is the sum of the pressure exerted by each one of them.
   a. Hence, in order to maintain a normal ICP, a change in one compartment must be followed by **compensatory changes** in the other compartments.
   b. Moreover, the **rate of the added volume** is important.
      (1) Thus, a slow-growing tumor (e.g., a meningioma) can become quite large before there is any evidence of a change in the ICP or in neurologic function.
      (2) In contrast, a smaller but acute mass lesion (e.g., an acute epidural or subdural hematoma) can cause a tremendous increase in the ICP and severe neurologic deficits.

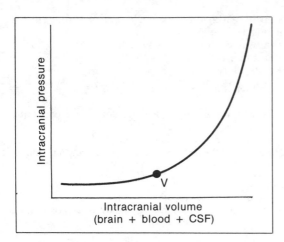

**Figure 31-1.** The pressure–volume relationship within the intracranial space can be represented by a pressure–volume curve. The intracranial pressure stays within normal limits until a critical volume (V) is reached, above which the pressure rises steeply.

**3.** The relationship between ICP and intracranial volume is described by an exponential curve (Fig. 31-1) with an initial flat portion and a later steep portion.
  **a.** As the volume of one compartment increases, the volumes of the other compartments must decrease in order to maintain normal ICP.
  **b.** Beyond a certain point (i.e., beyond the end of the flat portion of the curve), a slight increase in intracranial volume produces a very large increase in ICP (as evidenced by the steep portion of the curve).
  **c.** Equilibrium is maintained mainly by CSF buffering. With continued volume changes, CSF buffering becomes exhausted and the elastic properties of the brain substance and the blood vessels play the major buffering role (represented by the steep portion of the pressure–volume curve).

**4.** The upper limit of normal ICP is considered to be 15 mm Hg.

**5. Symptoms and signs of increased ICP (intracranial hypertension)** include:
  **a.** Headache
  **b.** Nausea
  **c.** Vomiting
  **d.** Clouding of mentation
  **e.** Papilledema
  **f.** Paralysis of upward gaze (**Parinaud's syndrome**)
  **g.** Sixth nerve palsy
  **h.** Bulging fontanelles and splitting of sutures (in infants)

**C. Herniation.** When all compensatory mechanisms have been exhausted and the ICP continues to rise, the brain "herniates" or shifts towards the lower-pressure compartment (the falx and the tentorium divide the interior of the skull into compartments). Various **herniation syndromes** are recognized.

**1. Subfalcial herniation** is a displacement from one supratentorial compartment to another underneath the falx. It may lead to loss of function in the opposite leg, loss of bladder control, or both.

**2. Transtentorial (uncal) herniation**
  **a.** This is the **most common type of brain herniation seen clinically** and occurs when the parahippocampal gyrus and uncus of one or both hemispheres is forced down the tentorial notch.
  **b.** Uncal herniation may occur as a result of diffuse brain swelling or a supratentorial mass lesion.
  **c.** The **neurologic signs** are:
    **(1)** Progressive deterioration of consciousness
    **(2)** Ipsilateral pupillary dilatation as a result of third nerve compression
    **(3)** Contralateral hemiparesis as a result of compression of the cerebral peduncles
  **d.** Hemiparesis is ipsilateral in 50% of the cases, while pupillary dilatation is ipsilateral in 80%. Thus, pupillary dilatation is much more reliable in localizing the lesion. In 20% of the cases, the pupillary dilatation occurs on the side opposite to the lesion—a false localizing sign known as the **Kernohan-Woltman notch phenomenon**.

### 3. Trans–foramen magnum herniation
   a. The cerebellar tonsils may herniate through the foramen magnum.
   b. The resultant medullary compression may elicit a Cushing response (i.e., hypertension, bradycardia, and apnea) and ultimately lead to death.

## D. Cerebral blood flow, autoregulation, and cerebral perfusion pressure

### 1. General considerations
   a. Normally the **average cerebral blood flow** is about **50 ml per 100 g of brain tissue per minute**, with the gray matter having a higher flow (i.e., 75 ml/100 g/min) than the white matter (25 ml/100 g/min).
   b. The blood flow is coupled to the local metabolic demands and is highest where the density of synapses is greatest (this is termed **metabolic autoregulation**).
   c. The flow is directly proportional to the **mean arterial pressure (MAP)** and the radius of the vessel raised to the fourth power (**Poiseuille's law**), and it is inversely proportional to the blood viscosity and the length of the blood vessels. Thus, increasing the caliber of the vessels or decreasing the blood viscosity can increase the flow markedly, and these factors are manipulated in clinical situations to improve cerebral blood flow.

### 2. Pressure autoregulation describes the observation that normally over a wide range of MAP (50 mm Hg to 150 mm Hg) the cerebral blood flow remains unchanged at 50 ml per 100 g of brain tissue per minute.
   a. This may change focally or globally as a result of head injury, subarachnoid hemorrhage, stroke, or a brain tumor.
   b. If the patient has an ICP monitor and an arterial line, autoregulation can be tested simply by elevating the systolic blood pressure by 10 mm Hg to 15 mm Hg and observing the changes in ICP.
      (1) If autoregulation is intact, the ICP should remain unchanged.
      (2) However, if the ICP passively follows the arterial pressure it is indicative of impaired autoregulation (vasoparalysis) and is usually a terminal event.
   c. The **cerebral perfusion pressure (CPP)** is equal to the MAP minus the ICP; that is, **CPP = MAP − ICP**. A CPP as low as 50 mm Hg can maintain an adequate cerebral blood flow; below 50 mm Hg the cerebral blood flow decreases steeply. Hence, it is the goal of neurosurgical intervention to **maintain the CPP above 50 mm Hg**.

# V. EVALUATING THE NEUROSURGICAL PATIENT

## A. Personal and family history

### 1. The **patient's history** is an important part of the diagnostic armamentarium.
   a. A good history may be the only clue to the diagnosis of either a transient ischemic attack (TIA), which causes no neurologic signs, or a subarachnoid hemorrhage.
   b. It may also help to ascertain the severity of a head injury by identifying periods of anterograde and retrograde amnesia.

### 2. However, it may be necessary to delay taking the history in the event of a life-threatening emergency that requires the physician's immediate attention.

### 3. The **family history** helps to rule out congenital lesions, metabolic disorders, neurofibromatosis, Huntington's chorea, and various degenerative central nervous system (CNS) disorders.

## B. General physical examination

### 1. Vital signs. Simple observations of blood pressure, pulse rate, and respiration can be helpful in localizing a lesion because the vital signs are controlled by CNS mechanisms.

### 2. Hypertension (the Cushing response)
   a. Cushing first pointed out that compression of the medullary centers by increased intracranial pressure results in hypertension, bradycardia, and short, shallow respirations.
   b. The **Cushing response** is, however, generally considered to be a **terminal response**; when it is noted, irreversible neurologic changes have already taken place.

### 3. Hypotension
   a. Hypotension in the neurosurgical patient may be produced by interruption of the sympathetic innervation of peripheral vessels, leading to venous pooling.
   b. This may be secondary to a hypothalamic, medullary, or spinal cord injury.

### 4. Respiration patterns
   a. **Lesions in the forebrain** can lead to **posthyperventilation apnea (PHVA)**.

(1) In normal individuals, following a period of hyperventilation, there is a resumption of regular breathing without a delay, although there is a reduction of the tidal volume until normal carbon dioxide partial pressure ($PCO_2$) is restored.

(2) Patients with **structural or metabolic forebrain damage** do not resume their regular breathing rhythm following hyperventilation and undergo a period of apnea. Regular respirations are resumed after the $PCO_2$ returns to the normal level.

b. **Lesions deep in the cerebral hemispheres** and involving the **basal ganglia** are associated with **Cheyne-Stokes respiration.**

(1) This pattern of breathing is characterized by regular periods of hyperpnea alternating with apnea.

(2) The breathing gradually rises in a smooth crescendo and then wanes in a smooth decrescendo.

c. **Lesions in the midbrain** can cause **central neurogenic hyperventilation (CNH)**—deep breathing at a very fast rate, which may lead to severe **alkalosis.**

d. **Lesions in the lower pons** can cause **apneustic breathing**—complete cessation of involuntary breathing, leading to respiratory arrest during sleep (**Ondine's curse**).

e. **Medullary lesions** can lead to various types of abnormal breathing patterns, which include:

(1) **Cluster breathing** (a disorderly sequence of clusters of breaths with irregular pauses in between)

(2) **Ataxic breathing** (**Biot's breathing**—periodic breathing in which apneic periods are punctuated by a few irregular deep breaths, lacking the waxing and waning pattern of Cheyne-Stokes respiration)

(3) **Cheyne-Stokes respiration**

(4) **Gasping** (breathing in which both deep and shallow breaths occur randomly, with haphazard intervening pauses and a slow respiratory rate, and which may finally lead to apnea)

f. **Kussmaul's respiration**, deep rapid breathing similar to CNH, usually occurs as a result of diabetic or uremic acidosis.

5. **Hyperthermia**

a. Neurologic disorders can cause severe hyperthermia, with body temperatures exceeding 105° F.

b. The most common **causes** are:

(1) Hyperthyroidism

(2) Heat stroke

(3) Lesions involving the posterior hypothalamus

(4) Status epilepticus

(5) Drug intoxication [e.g., due to isoniazid, amitriptyline, phenothiazines, or carbidopa-levodopa (Sinemet)]

(6) Malignant hyperthermia [idiopathic or as a result of a hereditary (autosomal dominant) muscle disease]

(7) Intraventricular hemorrhage

6. **Hypothermia.** Cold coma may be a result of:

a. Lesions involving the anterior hypothalamus

b. Myxedema

c. Alcohol intoxication

d. Severe hypoglycemia

e. Hepatic and renal failure

C. **Neurologic evaluation.** A detailed neurologic evaluation may not be possible in some emergency situations, such as trauma, in which case it may be necessary to do a **brief examination** to assess the neurologic damage.

1. The level of consciousness is determined initially. The different **levels of consciousness** are:

a. Alert, awake, and oriented

b. Lethargic (i.e., sleepy but easily arousable)

c. Stuporous (i.e., responsive only to noxious stimuli)

d. Comatose (i.e., not responsive to noxious stimuli)

2. The **pupils** are examined for their size and reaction to light, and the **position and movement of the eyes** are noted. A few general **rules** may be of help **in localizing a lesion:**

a. When a **cortical** lesion is present, the size of the pupil may be 6 mm or larger, and there may be wandering or roving eye movements.

b. With a lesion in the **basal ganglia**, the pupils may range from 2 mm to 3 mm in size and the eyes are deviated downward and inward.

**c.** A lesion in the midbrain may be associated with pupils that are 4 mm to 5 mm in size (midrange), and convergent nystagmus or nystagmus retractorius may be present.

**d.** A lesion in the **pons** may be associated with pinpoint pupils (1 mm) and with ocular bobbing.

**e.** When a **medullary** lesion is present, the pupils may be slightly small (2 mm), and there is downbeat nystagmus.

**3.** Other **brain stem reflexes**, such as the oculocephalic (doll's eye) reflex, and the caloric (oculovestibular) responses are checked to rule out irreversible brain stem damage.

**4.** A **motor examination** is then performed. In a comatose patient, it may only be possible to assess the response to painful stimuli.

**5. Sensory level determination** is important in patients with spinal cord lesions (see section VII C).

**6.** Finally, checking the deep tendon reflexes and plantar responses helps in distinguishing a lower motor neuron lesion from an upper motor neuron lesion.

**D. Special diagnostic tests**

**1. Selective angiography (arteriography)** [See Fig. 31-7 (section XII C 3) for an example of an angiogram.]

**a.** This study involves the introduction of a catheter via the transfemoral route (currently the most common route) into one of the major cerebral vessels (carotids or vertebrals) and the injection of a contrast agent while rapid-sequence x-rays are taken. A definitive picture of the cerebral circulation is obtained.

**b.** In most major neurosurgical centers this is a relatively safe procedure with a morbidity rate that is less than 1%.

**2. Myelography**

**a.** A contrast agent (usually the water-soluble metrizamide) is instilled in the thecal space through a $C_1$–$C_2$ tap or a lumbar puncture.

**b.** By the movement of this dye column or its appearance on the x-ray, the nature of the intraspinal lesion can be determined.

**3. CT scanning** has been a major breakthrough in the past decade. The new scanners provide anatomically precise images of the brain and the spinal cord. [See Figures 31-2 to 31-5 (section VI C 5) for examples of CT scans.]

**4. Magnetic resonance imaging (MRI)**

**a.** Because it enables one to look through bone, this new technique is very helpful in the diagnosis of intraspinal lesions. However, its role is not fully established.

**b.** MRI is based on the **principle** that the nuclei of certain elements [e.g., $^1$H (proton), $^2$H, $^{13}$C, $^{19}$F, $^{31}$P, and $^{127}$I] respond to the application of electromagnetic pulses by absorbing energy and reemitting it as detectable radio waves.

**(1)** These waves can be analyzed by computer and used to obtain morphologic or chemical information about body constituents, or to generate detailed anatomic images.

**(2)** Several studies have proved the sensitivity of MRI to pathologic changes seen in a broad spectrum of neurologic diseases, especially CNS tumors and ischemic lesions.

**c.** MRI has rapidly emerged as an **imaging technique** with the potential for providing more diagnostic information in certain situations than any other imaging modality, including CT. The main **advantages of MRI over CT** include:

**(1)** Superior contrast between gray and white matter

**(2)** Multiplanar or three-dimensional imaging

**(3)** Absence of bone artifacts

**(4)** High sensitivity to pathologic change

**(5)** Absence of any known risks

**5. Electromyography**

**a.** Electromyography involves the recording and study of neuromuscular transmission such as nerve conduction velocities and the response of muscle to stimulation.

**b.** It can help in the evaluation of patients recovering from peripheral nerve injuries and in the diagnosis of entrapment neuropathies.

**6. Ultrasonography**

**a.** This is a very helpful tool in infants, as the fontanelle affords easy access to ultrasound imaging.

**b.** Currently, ultrasonography is used frequently in the intraoperative diagnosis of lesions located deep within the spinal cord or brain.

## VI. HEAD INJURIES

**A. Incidence.** There were 7,560,000 head injuries in the United States in 1976. Of these, 1,255,000 were classified as major head injuries, which included concussion, intracranial hemorrhage, cerebral laceration, cerebral contusion, and crushing of the head.

**B. Classification**

1. Brain injuries following trauma can be classified as:
   a. **Primary**, occurring instantaneously at the time of impact
   b. **Secondary**, resulting from a chain of events triggered by the initial injury. If not controlled, secondary injuries lead to further damage as a result of ischemia, hypoxia, or both.

2. Primary and secondary injuries can be either:
   a. Nonhemorrhagic focal or diffuse **edema**
   b. **Hemorrhages**
      (1) Intra-axial (i.e., intracerebral—within the brain substance)
      (2) Extra-axial [i.e., extracerebral—outside the brain parenchyma (e.g., epidural and subdural hematomas)]

**C. Initial management and assessment**

1. The **immediate care** of a head trauma victim is no different from that of any other injured patient (see Chapter 2, section I C 5).
   a. Priority is given to the following:
      (1) **Establishment of adequate ventilation**
      (2) **Control of hemorrhage**
      (3) **Maintenance of peripheral vascular circulation**
   b. When **volume replacement** with intravenous fluid is necessary, colloid or blood products are used if at all possible, in order to reduce the risk that cerebral edema will develop or worsen.
   c. The patient's **neck is stabilized** with a hard cervical collar (Philadelphia collar) or by sandbags placed on either side of the head.
      (1) Fully 10% of patients with severe head injuries have **associated spinal cord injuries**, and consequently all patients with head injuries should be transported as if they had a spinal cord injury.
      (2) Precautions include immobilization of the spine on a hard board and use of a cervical collar until further investigation for spinal cord injury is carried out.
   d. **Blood is drawn** for typing and crossmatching, and for other laboratory studies.

2. **Initial examination** of the patient can provide information regarding the **type and magnitude of the injuries**.
   a. Examples include:
      (1) A closed head injury—injury inflicted to the brain without any evidence of scalp laceration
      (2) An injury resulting from a high-speed, nonimpact acceleration-deceleration
      (3) Blunt trauma with or without a scalp laceration or contusion (all scalp lacerations should be checked manually for an underlying skull fracture)
      (4) A penetrating wound from a knife or a bullet (entrance and exit wounds must be sought)
   b. Specific signs can point to the location of a fracture. For example:
      (1) Fractures traversing the base of the skull (**basilar fractures**) often cause ecchymosis behind the ear (**Battle's sign**).
      (2) Anterior basilar fractures often result in periorbital ecchymosis (raccoon's eyes) and subconjunctival hemorrhage.
      (3) Hematotympanum is associated with fractures of the middle fossa.

3. **History.** After the initial management, and if the patient is awake, a quick history should be obtained. The severity of a head injury and the final outcome are directly related to the duration of the unconsciousness, which the history may reveal.

4. **Neurologic evaluation**
   a. A rapid assessment of the patient is performed (see section V C).
   b. The **Glasgow coma scale (GCS)** is now used almost universally in the assessment of the head injury victim. This scale measures three responses:
      (1) **Eye opening:**
         (a) Spontaneous = 4
         (b) In response to command = 3

(c) In response to pain = 2
(d) None = 1
**(2) Motor response:**
(a) Obeys commands = 6
(b) Localizes pain = 5
(c) Withdraws from pain = 4
(d) Shows flexion (decorticate) response to pain = 3
(e) Shows extension (decerebrate) response to pain = 2
(f) None = 1
**(3) Vocal response:**
(a) Oriented to person, place, and time = 5
(b) Confused = 4
(c) Shows inappropriate speech = 3
(d) Makes incomprehensible sounds = 2
(e) None = 1
**c.** The GCS score ranges from 3 to 15.
(1) The GCS score at 6 hours after trauma is a good predictor of the long-term outcome in head injury (i.e., recovery, disability, vegetative state, or death).
(2) Adult patients with a 6-hour GCS score below 7 are likely to have a poor outcome; the prognosis is much better in the pediatric population.
**d.** Neurologic examinations are repeated periodically; a change of 2 or more in the GCS score is considered to be significant.

**5. Radiologic studies**
**a. CT scans** are preferable to skull x-rays in severely injured patients.
**(1) Diagnostic findings**
(a) A **hematoma** (Figs. 31-2 and 31-3) can be easily diagnosed because fresh blood appears hyperdense on a CT scan.
(i) **Epidural hematomas** appear as semilunar dense collections with a convexity towards the brain (see Fig. 31-2).
(ii) **Acute subdural hematomas** have a concavity towards the brain.
(b) The subarachnoid spaces appear denser if there is any **subarachnoid hemorrhage**.
(c) **Hemorrhages in the white matter**, such as the corpus callosum, internal capsule, and midbrain, suggest a diffuse axonal type of injury (Fig. 31-4).
(d) **Cerebral edema** (Fig. 31-5) can be indicated by the size of the ventricles and basal subarachnoid cisterns.
**(2)** If the CT scan is positive, the patient is taken immediately to the operating room for evacuation of hematomas or to the intensive care unit for ICP monitoring and management of brain swelling.
**b. X-rays**
**(1) X-rays of the cervical spine** are taken to rule out associated spinal injuries.
**(2) Skull x-rays** are used instead of CT scans **to screen for skull fractures** in patients with less severe injuries.
(a) Intracranial air or clouding of the sinuses suggests a CSF leak.

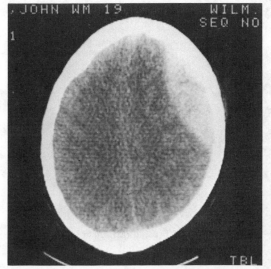

**Figure 31-2.** CT scan of the head showing a large right frontotemporal epidural hematoma. Acute epidural hematomas have a convexity towards the brain in contradistinction to acute subdural hematomas, which have a concavity towards the brain. Chronic subdural hematomas may resemble acute epidural hematomas but are much less dense.

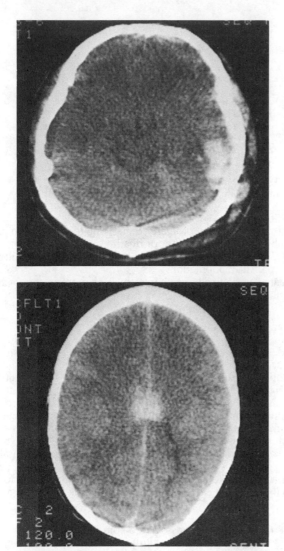

**Figure 31-3.** CT scan showing a right temporal intracerebral hematoma following a head injury.

**Figure 31-4.** CT scan showing evidence of a "bleed" in the corpus callosum. This type of hemorrhage deep in the white matter is seen in diffuse axonal (closed-head) injuries.

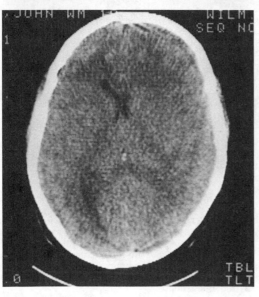

**Figure 31-5.** CT scan showing diffuse swelling of the right cerebral hemisphere with effacement of the right lateral ventricle and a midline shift.

**(b)** If a fracture line crosses the groove of the middle meningeal vessels, an epidural hematoma should be suspected.

**(c)** Basilar skull fractures are very poorly visualized on x-ray, and even a CT scan can miss them unless they are searched for carefully. However, clouding of the mastoid air cells or the sphenoid sinus is suggestive of a basilar skull fracture.

### D. Management of increased ICP

1. The **main goal** in the treatment of increased ICP is to **maintain an adequate perfusion pressure** (see section IV D 2 c), in order to **prevent irreversible ischemic injury** to the brain (which is a secondary type of post-traumatic brain injury). The patient's CPP is maintained above 50 mm Hg by manipulation of the ICP and the mean arterial pressure.

2. Aggressive control of ICP requires the placement of an ICP monitor.
   a. **Criteria for placement of an ICP monitor** include one or both of the following:
      **(1)** A score of 5 or less on the GCS
      **(2)** Associated systemic complications such as severe hypotension or hypoxia
   b. **ICP measuring devices** (monitors) are of two types:
      **(1) Intraventricular catheter**
         **(a)** This gives the most accurate measurement and provides the option of removing CSF to lower the ICP in an emergency.
         **(b)** However, the placement of an intraventricular catheter can be difficult in the presence of diffuse brain swelling with slit-like ventricles.
      **(2) Subarachnoid bolt** (Richmond screw or Philly bolt)
         **(a)** The subarachnoid bolt is easy to place, gives accurate readings, and is associated with a low infection rate.
         **(b)** Most head trauma centers use this type of ICP monitoring device.

3. **Intracranial hypertension** can be managed by a variety of methods. The following therapies can be used in sequence.
   a. **Elevation of the patient's head.** This promotes venous drainage and thereby decreases ICP.
   b. **Hyperventilation.** The cerebral vessels respond quickly to a change in the arterial $P_{CO_2}$. A low $P_{CO_2}$ causes vasoconstriction, while an elevated $P_{CO_2}$ causes vasodilatation.
      **(1)** The $P_{CO_2}$ is not lowered below 25 mm Hg because the consequent decrease in cerebral blood flow could be counterproductive and also because a problematic respiratory alkalosis develops.
      **(2)** Thus, if the ICP is not sufficiently lowered by hyperventilation other therapies have to be used.
   c. **Increasing the serum osmolality** (to around 300 mOsm)
      **(1) Fluid restriction**
         **(a)** The patient is given only two-thirds of the calculated volume of maintenance fluid (5% dextrose in one-half normal saline solution), in order to increase the serum osmolality and reduce the transcapillary fluid movement.
         **(b)** This helps in reducing the cerebral edema and thus in lowering ICP.
      **(2) Hyperosmolar agents**
         **(a)** The diuretic most commonly used is mannitol, which is administered intravenously in a bolus of 1 to 1.5 g/kg or by continuous infusion of 0.05 to 0.15 g/kg per hour. Its effect can be seen in 5 to 20 minutes. Bolus doses are usually given every 6 hours or if there is a dangerous rise in ICP.
            **(i)** Mannitol is an osmotic diuretic and acts by withdrawing water from the cerebral interstitial spaces if the blood-brain barrier is intact.
            **(ii)** Repeated use can lead to severe dehydration, hypernatremia, and hyperosmolality. In a patient with hypovolemia, mannitol can cause renal tubular damage.
         **(b) Glycerol** can be administered, either as an intravenous bolus or by continuous infusion, if the patient is refractory to mannitol.
      **(3)** Serum osmolality and electrolytes have to be measured every 6 to 8 hours.
   d. **Loop diuretics. Furosemide** is the drug most commonly used and is administered intravenously. The effect of the drug is rapid.
   e. **Corticosteroids**
      **(1)** Steroids have not been shown to lower the ICP, but they improve the compliance of the brain (i.e., they shift the pressure–volume curve to the right) and prevent a steep increase in pressure (Fig. 31-6).
      **(2)** Some head injury centers use megadose steroid therapy (i.e., 1 mg/kg of dexamethasone administered intravenously followed by 0.5 mg/kg per day in four divided doses).
   f. **Barbiturates** can be used if all of the previously mentioned efforts fail to lower the ICP.

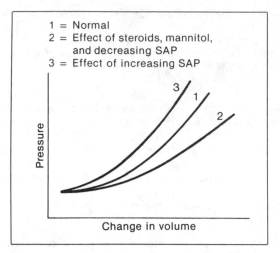

1 = Normal
2 = Effect of steroids, mannitol, and decreasing SAP
3 = Effect of increasing SAP

Pressure

Change in volume

**Figure 31-6.** Changes in pressure–volume curves. *Curve 1* represents a baseline. It has an initial flat portion, which becomes very steep. Steroids, mannitol, and decreasing systemic arterial pressure (SAP) improve the cerebral compliance, and the curve moves to the right (*curve 2*). An increase in SAP, on the other hand, causes a stiffening of the brain—that is, a decrease in cerebral compliance (*curve 3*).

    **(1)** An initial dose of 3 mg/kg of sodium pentobarbital is given intravenously, followed by a maintenance dose of 0.5 to 3 mg/kg per hour. The effect of the drug occurs within minutes, and an adequate serum level (25 to 40 mg/L) is maintained. A burst suppression pattern on the electroencephalogram suggests that a therapeutic serum level has been reached.

    **(2)** Barbiturates cause myocardial depression leading to hypotension, and vasopressor agents may be necessary to elevate the MAP in order to maintain an adequate CPP.

    **(3)** Although the exact mechanism of action is not known, it is suggested that barbiturates may act by:

        **(a)** Decreasing cerebral blood flow

        **(b)** Reducing the metabolic activity of the brain

        **(c)** Reducing synaptic transmission

  **g. Hypothermia** may be used as an adjunct to other therapies. The core temperature of the body is lowered from normal to a temperature that ranges from 89.6° to 93.2° F (32° to 34° C), which probably decreases the ICP by reducing cerebral metabolism.

**E. Management of intracranial hemorrhages**

  **1. Subarachnoid hemorrhage**, the most common type of post-traumatic intracranial hemorrhage, usually requires no immediate surgical intervention. However, there is a risk of developing hydrocephalus, and thus follow-up CT scans are necessary.

  **2. Epidural hematomas**

    **a.** Epidural hemorrhages (those between the skull and dura mater) arise from tears in the middle meningeal artery or vein or in a dural sinus.

    **b.** The initial impact may result in a temporary loss of consciousness, which is followed by a lucid interval in which the patient is fully awake.

    **c.** As bleeding continues, a stage is reached when the ICP rises steeply and there is uncal herniation, causing loss of consciousness, an ipsilateral dilated pupil, and contralateral hemiplegia.

    **d.** Prompt surgical evacuation makes the difference between a good prognosis and death.

  **3. Subdural hematomas**

    **a.** Subdural hematomas are **classified** according to the **interval of time** between the trauma and the onset of symptoms:

        **(1) Acute** (up to 48 hours)

        **(2) Subacute** (48 hours to 12 days)

        **(3) Chronic** (more than 12 days)

    **b.** Subdural hematomas arise from tears in the dural sinuses or bridging veins, and they are bilateral in 15% of the cases.

    **c.** Acute subdural hematomas with a rapid progression of symptoms have a poor prognosis unless they are surgically evacuated.

**F. Management of intracerebral hematomas and cerebral contusions**

  **1. Intracerebral hematomas** result from the tearing of small vessels in the white matter and are due to penetrating trauma or acceleration-deceleration injuries.

**2. Cerebral contusions.** Superficial hemorrhages most commonly occur when the anterior temporal and frontal lobes strike the rough edges of the tentorium (**contrecoup contusion**).
   **a.** A **coup injury** occurs where the skull strikes the brain underlying the site of impact.
   **b.** A **contrecoup injury** occurs directly opposite to the impact site.
   **c.** Thus, if a person is struck on the back of the head, the coup injury would be to the occipital lobe while the frontotemporal tips would sustain the contrecoup injury.

**3. Surgical decompression** of intracerebral hematomas and cerebral contusions may be necessary when increased ICP (caused by a mass effect from the accumulated blood and the secondary edema) becomes refractory to medical management.

**G. Management of scalp injuries**

   **1. The scalp** is made up of **five layers**:
      **S** —skin
      **C** —dense subcutaneous tissue
      **A** —aponeurosis
      **L** —loose areolar tissue
      **P** —pericranium

   **2.** The scalp is a **highly vascular** structure, and much blood can be lost from scalp lacerations before they are sutured.
      **a.** The scalp wound is thoroughly cleansed, debrided, and sutured as soon as possible.
      **b.** In general, any laceration greater than 6 to 8 inches should be closed in the operating room.

**H. Management of skull fractures**

   **1. Classification**
      **a. Skull fractures are described as linear, stellate, or comminuted**, depending upon the complexity of the fracture line.
      **b.** If a portion of the vault is displaced inward, the fracture is termed **depressed**.
      **c.** A **compound** fracture is present if the overlying scalp is lacerated.
      **d.** Fractures traversing the base of the skull are called **basilar**.

   **2. Operative intervention** is necessary to deal mainly with a depressed skull fracture and a compound comminuted skull fracture with underlying cerebral damage.
      **a. Depressed skull fractures** are usually associated with dural tears and may or may not be accompanied by underlying brain damage. If they are left untreated, scarring may lead to an epileptogenic focus, and hence it is necessary to elevate these fractures.
      **b. Compound comminuted fractures** with damage to the underlying brain are handled by removal of all bony fragments (including those embedded in the brain), thorough debridement, and closure. Failure to remove all bony fragments may lead to the later development of a brain abscess.

**I. Management of CSF leaks**

   **1.** Leaks of the CSF, if mixed with blood, can be **diagnosed** by the **ring (halo) sign**: If drops of CSF mixed with blood are placed on gauze, a lighter halo forms around a central bloodier area.

   **2.** Most **post-traumatic CSF fistulas** close spontaneously with **conservative management**, which includes elevating the head to reduce both the ICP and the CSF leakage.
      **a.** In some cases, a drain may have to be placed in the lumbar theca to drain CSF preferentially through it and allow the fistula to heal.
      **b.** In extreme cases, operative closure of the leak may be necessary.
      **c.** The administration of antibiotics in cases of CSF leaks is controversial, but most surgeons who do use them choose a narrow-spectrum drug such as nafcillin.

**VII. SPINAL CORD INJURIES** (see also Chapter 32, section III B 3 a)

**A. General considerations**

   **1.** Most spinal cord injuries are **caused** by automobile accidents, sports injuries, and falls.

   **2.** The common **sites of injury** to the vertebral column are the junctions between relatively fixed and mobile segments. These are:
      **a.** The lumbosacral junction

      **b.** The thoracolumbar junction

      **c.** The cervicothoracic junction

  **3.** The **aims of neurosurgical intervention** are:

      **a.** Preservation of neuronal function

      **b.** Restoration of bony alignment

      **c.** Rehabilitation

  **4.** The presence of **associated injuries** must be sought. These include:

      **a.** Hemo- or pneumothorax

      **b.** Damage to the thoracic aorta

      **c.** Intra-abdominal or head injuries

**B. Initial management**

  **1.** Great care must be taken to **immobilize the spine** during transfer of the patient to the hospital from the trauma site.

      **a.** This can be done by transferring the patient on a firm surface, by use of a hard cervical collar (Philadelphia collar), or both.

      **b.** It cannot be overemphasized that the **paramedic plays a critical role** in the initial evacuation of patients with spinal cord injuries. Spinal cord injuries can be worsened if proper precautions are not taken during transfer.

  **2. Stabilization**

      **a.** The stabilization procedures that are essential for trauma management (see Chapter 2, section I C) should be carried out. These are:

         **(1)** Airway assessment and control

         **(2)** Establishment of ventilation

         **(3)** Circulatory support

      **b.** Patients with **cervical cord injury** may lose their vascular sympathetic tone as a result of the injury and develop **hypotension**. Fluid replacement restores normal blood pressure.

      **c.** Mannitol, sodium bicarbonate, and dexamethasone are given intravenously to reduce cord edema and lactic acidosis.

**C. Neurologic evaluation**

  **1.** A **motor and sensory examination** is performed rapidly to determine:

      **a.** The **level of the injury**. Sensory level determination can be done easily by running a sharp pin lightly across the body to elicit the **triple response of Lewis (reflex erythema**—a red line, then a flush, then a wheal), which is diminished or absent below the level of the lesion.

      **b.** The **type of injury** (i.e., **complete**, with no function below the level of the injury, or **incomplete**). Important **examples of incomplete injuries** include:

         **(1) Central cord injury**, which involves the central portion of the cord (the upper extremities are affected more often than the lower extremities)

         **(2) Anterior cord injury**, which involves the anterior segment of the cord, resulting in muscular weakness, hypoesthesia, and hypalgesia below the level of the lesion

         **(3) Brown-Sequard syndrome** (hemisection of the cord), which causes contralateral sensory loss and homolateral paralysis

  **2.** An examination of the sacral segment of the cord (i.e., the bulbocavernosus reflex, the anal twitch, and sacral sensations) must be carried out, because the prognosis is better in patients with preserved sacral reflexes.

**D. Radiologic studies**

  **1.** It must be emphasized that in a case of suspected spinal cord injury, the **entire spine must be visualized** with films of good quality before a diagnosis is made.

  **2. X-ray studies and CT scans** are done to determine the site and extent of bony injury.

  **3. Myelography** is performed if the bony lesion and the neurologically determined level do not match or if there is a deterioration in the patient's neurologic status.

**E. Treatment**

  **1. Skeletal traction.** In cases of cervical injuries with fracture dislocations of the spine, skull tongs (such as Gardner-Wells, the most commonly employed) are attached and weights are used to apply traction to the spine. These procedures restore the normal alignment of the vertebral column and relieve the compression of the neural structures.

    **2. Surgical intervention**
      **a.** Previously, patients with spinal cord injuries were managed by immobilization and postural reduction, but there has been a change towards more aggressive surgical management.
      **b.** The **aim** of surgical management is to stabilize the spine and allow early rehabilitation.
      **c.** The **indications** for surgery may be acute or subacute.
        **(1)** Immediate surgical intervention is needed in cases of marked neurologic deterioration with myelographic evidence of block.
        **(2)** Surgery is needed subacutely in patients with incomplete injuries when there is evidence of continued neural compression and the patient, having reached a plateau, fails to show any further neurologic recovery.

  **F.** The **long-term complications** of spinal cord injuries include:

    **1. Pressure sores**, the incidence of which is reduced by the use of a Stryker frame or a rotokinetic (e.g., Rotorest) bed

    **2. Flexor spasms**, which can be managed medically with muscle relaxants (e.g., diazepam or baclofen) or in extreme cases by rhizotomy (sectioning the nerve root)

    **3.** Renal stones, pyelonephritis, and renal failure:

    **4.** Deep vein thrombosis, which is the most deadly complication and is diagnosed by:
      **a.** Maintaining a high index of suspicion
      **b.** Performing routine impedance plethysmography, iodine 125 ($^{125}$I)-labeled fibrinogen scanning, and venography, if necessary (see Chapter 14, section I C 3 c)

# VIII. PERIPHERAL NERVE INJURIES (see also Chapter 32, section III B 3 b)

  **A. Classification**

    **1. Neurapraxia** is focal contusion of a nerve, resulting in loss of function. There is continuity of the axons, and the myelin sheaths remain intact.
      **a.** This type of injury may be due to:
        **(1)** A direct blow
        **(2)** Prolonged compression
        **(3)** Stretching
        **(4)** A gunshot wound
        **(5)** A blast injury
      **b.** Function returns spontaneously in about 6 weeks.

    **2. Axonotmesis** is disruption of axons with intact myelin sheaths. The distal axon degenerates. Since the myelin sheaths are in continuity, return of function can be anticipated, because the axon grows back at the rate of 1 mm per day or 1 inch per month.

    **3. Neurotmesis** is complete disruption of both the axons and the myelin sheaths. The divided nerves must be approximated for optimal recovery, and there are residual neurologic deficits.

  **B. Treatment**

    **1.** The only **indications for immediate surgical repair** are:
      **a.** Digital nerve injuries
      **b.** Clean and sharp lacerations

    **2.** In **open injuries of peripheral nerves**, the final extent of the injury is not known for a few weeks.
      **a.** Nerve repair is therefore delayed for 3 to 4 weeks.
      **b.** At the time of primary wound repair, the divided ends of the nerves are identified and a suture is tied around the stumps to make identification easier in subsequent repair.

    **3.** In cases of **deep wounds** (e.g., gunshot wounds or deep lacerations), recovery of function is monitored by serial neurologic examinations and electromyography. Surgical intervention is necessary only when there is lack of optimal recovery.

# IX. TUMORS OF THE CNS

  **A. Incidence**

    **1.** Three percent of all cancer deaths are due to brain tumors, which have an incidence of 5 per 100,000 of the population. The frequency peaks in the sixth decade of life.

    **2.** About 85% of CNS tumors are intracranial, while 15% are intraspinal.

**3.** Fully 25% of CNS tumors are metastatic, and 30% of all metastasizing tumors (i.e., lung, breast, skin, gastrointestinal, and urinary tract) have multiple brain metastases.

**4.** Fifteen percent of all brain tumors occur in children. Among the malignancies of children, CNS tumors are second only to leukemia in prevalence.

**5.** Sixty-five percent of brain tumors in children are infratentorial, and thirty-five percent are supratentorial. This ratio is reversed in adults.

### B. Brain tumors

**1. Classification.** Brain tumors can be broadly classified as glial and nonglial, depending upon the cell of origin.
  **a. Glial tumors (gliomas)** constitute 40% to 50% of brain tumors.
    **(1)** They include astrocytomas (grades I through IV, depending upon their malignancy), oligodendrogliomas, and ependymomas.
    **(2)** Grade IV **astrocytomas (glioblastomas)** that arise in the hemispheres are **the most common brain tumors** in adults. Low-grade (i.e., grades I and II) midline astrocytomas are the most common brain tumors in children.
  **b. Nonglial cell tumors**
    **(1)** This classification is made up of meningiomas (arising from arachnoidal cells), neurilemomas (arising from nerve sheaths), medulloblastomas (of neuroectodermal origin), pituitary tumors, pineal tumors, tumors arising from blood vessels (e.g., hemangioblastomas and endotheliomas), congenital tumors (e.g., dermoid tumors and teratomas), and metastatic tumors.
    **(2)** Meningiomas account for 15% to 20% of brain tumors; neurilemomas account for 10% to 15%; and metastatic tumors account for 5% to 10%.

**2. Clinical findings**
  **a. Focal neurologic deficits** result from destruction or compression of neuronal tissue either directly by the tumor or indirectly by a decrease in the blood supply.
  **b. Seizures** may occur due to the alteration of neuronal function.
  **c.** Signs and symptoms of **raised ICP** may occur, including headache, nausea, vomiting, loss of consciousness, papilledema, and sixth nerve palsy.
  **d.** A tumor may cause a **mass effect** by one or all of the following mechanisms:
    **(1)** Growth of the neoplasm
    **(2)** Edema formation
    **(3)** Obstruction of CSF pathways, leading to enlargement of the ventricles and hydrocephalus
  **e. Abnormal endocrine function** may result from a pituitary tumor.

**3. Neurologic evaluation**
  **a.** A history of progressive neurologic deficits and the neurologic examination give a clue to the diagnosis of brain tumors.
  **b.** Additional studies may be necessary to pinpoint the lesion. These include:
    **(1)** Skull x-rays
    **(2)** CT scans
    **(3)** Angiography
    **(4)** MRI

**4. Treatment**
  **a. Medical management** consists of dehydration and administration of large doses of dexamethasone to reduce cerebral edema.
  **b.** The aim of **surgical therapy** is cure. However, this is not always possible, and the **main objectives** are:
    **(1)** To obtain tissue for diagnosis
    **(2)** To debulk the tumor in order to reduce its mass effect and make it curable by radiotherapy, chemotherapy, or both
    **(3)** To prolong survival
  **c. Radiation therapy and chemotherapy** (intravenous, intra-arterial, or intrathecal) are useful adjuncts in tumor management.

### C. Spinal cord tumors

**1. Classification**
  **a. Extradural tumors**
    **(1)** Extradural tumors are mostly malignant. These grow rapidly and destroy the spinal column.

(2) Rarely, benign extradural tumors occur, such as meningiomas, neurofibromas, and osteomas.

**b. Intradural-extramedullary tumors.** Neurofibromas and meningiomas constitute 90% of these tumors.

**c. Intramedullary tumors** are mainly (95%) gliomas. Histologically, they are benign.
   (1) The majority of these tumors are ependymomas (50%) and astrocytomas (45%).
   (2) Ependymomas have a predilection for the conus medullaris and filum terminale.

**d. Metastatic tumors** constitute 50% of intraspinal tumors and are commonly from the lungs, breast, lymphoid tissue, prostate gland, kidneys, and thyroid gland.

**2. Clinical findings**
   **a. Pain** is commonly associated with spinal tumors. **Nocturnal pain** that awakens the patient from sleep, along with a history of progressive weakness, is highly suggestive of an intraspinal neoplasm.
   **b.** The **presenting signs** are usually those of **cord compression**:
      (1) Sensory changes below the level of involvement
      (2) Motor weakness
      (3) Bowel and bladder incontinence

**3. Radiologic studies** include spinal x-rays, myelography, CT scans, and MRI.

**4. Treatment**
   **a. Primary tumors**
      (1) Medical management includes:
         (a) Intravenous administration of furosemide or mannitol to promote diuresis and reduce cord edema
         (b) Dexamethasone, which also helps in decreasing edema
      (2) **Surgical intervention** is aimed at:
         (a) Obtaining tissue for diagnosis
         (b) Tumor removal
         (c) Decompression
      (3) The availability of laser surgery and ultrasonic aspirators has made the radical removal of many tumors feasible and safe.
   **b. Metastatic lesions**
      (1) If they are radiosensitive, metastatic tumors are initially managed with diuretics, dexamethasone, and radiation therapy.
      (2) **Surgery** is indicated if:
         (a) The tumor is radioresistant
         (b) Radiation therapy fails
         (c) The patient who previously had received a full dose of spinal radiation develops another lesion
      (3) Radiation therapy and chemotherapy are helpful in palliation and in tumor control.

## X. CONGENITAL LESIONS OF THE NERVOUS SYSTEM

**A. Dysraphism.** Usually, defective fusion of a raphe is associated with some findings on general physical examination. For example, examination of the back may reveal a tuft of hair, a nevus, a lipoma, abnormal blood vessels, a dimple, or a sinus tract. All of these are highly suggestive of an underlying dysraphic state.

**1. Spina bifida**
   **a.** This lesion results from failure of fusion of the vertebral arches.
   **b.** It may be totally asymptomatic and be found incidentally on spinal x-ray (spina bifida occulta), or it may be symptomatic.
   **c.** Spina bifida can be associated with other congenital anomalies such as a dermal sinus, diastematomyelia (splitting of the cord into halves), or neurenteric cysts.

**2. Meningocele**
   **a.** This rare lesion is a saclike posterior midline herniation of the dura mater and is usually not associated with any neurologic deficits.
   **b.** Repair is indicated primarily for cosmetic reasons.

**3. Myelomeningocele**
   **a.** Myelomeningocele is herniation of the dura mater and neural elements posteriorly as a result of incomplete closure of the spine.
   **b.** Neurologic defects are common, and their severity is related to the location of the lesion. Patients with high lesions have a worse prognosis.

      **c.** Surgical treatment is aimed at closure of the defect.

      **d.** This lesion may be associated with hydrocephalus secondary to an Arnold-Chiari malformation (i.e., an abnormally low position of the cerebellar tonsils).

  **B. Hydrocephalus** literally means "water head," and the abnormality may be congenital or acquired. It is usually caused by an obstruction of the flow of CSF.

    **1. Etiology.** The most common causes are:

      **a.** Sequelae of intraventricular hemorrhage in the premature baby

      **b.** Aqueductal stenosis

      **c. Arnold-Chiari malformation**

        **(1)** In **type I** the fourth ventricle is above the foramen magnum but the upper part of the cervical cord is displaced caudally.

        **(2)** In **type II** (most commonly seen), there is a downward herniation of the fourth ventricle and the cerebellar tonsils.

        **(3)** In **types III and IV** there is progressive caudal displacement of the cerebellar vermis, pons, and medulla below the foramen magnum.

      **d.** Dandy-Walker syndrome, in which there is agenesis of the foramina of Luschka and Magendie, resulting in the filling of the posterior fossa with a large cyst and enlargement of the lateral and third ventricles

    **2. Clinical findings.** Patients may present with bulging fontanelles, scalp vein dilatation, a rapidly increasing head circumference, decreased upward gaze (Parinaud's syndrome), papilledema, lethargy, irritability, nausea, and vomiting.

    **3. Treatment.** A CT scan is done first to confirm the diagnosis, and then a shunt is placed to divert the ventricular fluid.

      **a.** A **ventriculoperitoneal shunt** is most commonly used.

      **b.** However, **in very small infants**, the absorptive surface of the peritoneum may be inadequate, and this situation may warrant the placement of a **ventriculoatrial shunt**.

      **c.** In some special situations, the CSF may need to be shunted to the pleural space.

## XI. LESIONS OF THE INTERVERTEBRAL DISKS

  **A. Etiology.** The intervertebral disks are subjected to everyday wear and tear.

    **1.** In **young adults**, tears in the posterolateral portion of the anulus fibrosus lead to extrusions of the nucleus pulposus, which may result in **nerve root compression**.

    **2.** In the **elderly**, desiccation of the disk material results in osteophyte formation, and this leads to **nerve root or spinal cord compression**.

  **B.** Disk herniations produce **signs and symptoms** by causing either root compression or cord compression.

    **1.** In the lumbar area, compression may lead to shooting pains along the distribution of the sciatic nerve. Stretching the nerve root, as is done by straight-leg raising, exacerbates the symptoms.

    **2.** Careful neurologic examination helps in localizing the level of the lesion.

    **3.** Diagnostic tests include:

      **a.** Plain spinal x-rays

      **b.** Myelography

      **c.** Electromyography

      **d.** CT scan

  **C. Treatment**

    **1.** Management is **initially conservative** and consists of **bed rest**, **traction**, and **analgesics** in the acute phase. Once the patient is relieved of the acute pain, **exercise** may help to strengthen the muscles.

    **2. Indications for surgical therapy** include:

      **a.** Significant motor involvement

      **b.** Bowel or bladder incontinence

      **c.** Poor response to conservative therapy

      **d.** Relapse upon resumption of routine activities following initial pain relief by conservative treatment

## XII. CEREBROVASCULAR DISEASE

### A. General considerations

1. **"Stroke"** is a term broadly used to describe a category of disorders characterized by a relatively acute onset and an etiology referable to the cerebrovascular system (see also Chapter 13, section VIII).

2. The main part of a stroke (paralysis or other deficit) is preceded by **warning ischemic attacks** in approximately 80% of cases. Such episodes rarely precede a cerebral embolism or intracerebral hemorrhage but very frequently precede the development of a thrombotic stroke.

### B. The various **subgroups** are:

1. **Thrombotic stroke**
   a. **General considerations**
      (1) Atheromatous narrowing, thrombotic occlusion, or medial hypertrophy of the arteries supplying the brain results in a cessation of blood flow, or a decrease of blood flow below a critical threshold, leading to infarction. It is characterized clinically by a fluctuating course over minutes to days.
      (2) A patient may or may not have warning episodes, that is, **transient ischemic attacks (TIAs)**, prior to a full-blown stroke. An individual suffering from TIAs develops one or more neurologic deficits which may range from blindness (amaurosis fugax) to hemiplegia and which are sudden in onset and brief in duration, lasting minutes to hours (see also Chapter 13, section VIII C 1).
   b. **Lacunar infarction**
      (1) The small deep penetrating vessels are occluded as a result of degenerative changes.
      (2) The **sites** that are affected most often are the internal capsule, the thalamus, the pons, and the cerebral white matter.
      (3) Clinically, lacunar infarction can be manifested as pure motor stroke, pure sensory stroke, dysarthria (slurred speech), "clumsy hand" syndrome, crural paresis and ataxia, ataxia with hemiparesis, or extrapyramidal syndrome.
   c. **Carotid circulation thrombosis**
      (1) Thrombosis at the **internal carotid artery bifurcation in the neck** commonly results from atherosclerotic degenerative changes, trauma, or fibromuscular dysplasia. Clinical symptoms include amaurosis fugax, headache, and hemispheric dysfunction.
      (2) **Internal carotid artery siphon occlusion** differs from bifurcation occlusion by the absence of ophthalmic signs and symptoms.
      (3) **Anterior cerebral artery occlusion** leads to paresis and cortical sensory loss in the contralateral inferior extremity.
      (4) **Middle cerebral artery occlusion**
         (a) The middle cerebral artery is occluded more frequently by emboli than by an in situ stenosis or occlusion.
         (b) **Occlusion of the superior trunk of the artery** leads to hemiparesis and hemisensory loss which affect the face and hands more than the legs. Motor aphasia (Broca's aphasia) results if the left hemisphere is involved.
         (c) **Occlusion of the inferior trunk of the artery**
            (i) **Left-sided** occlusion leads to Wernicke's aphasia (receptive aphasia) and to right homonymous hemianopia or right superior quadrantanopia.
            (ii) **Right-sided** occlusion results in constructional dyspraxia, spatial disorientation, and left homonymous hemianopia or left superior quadrantanopia.
   d. **Vertebrobasilar circulation occlusion** (see also Chapter 13, section VIII C 3)
      (1) **Vertebral artery occlusion** leads to lateral medullary infarction, with ataxia, decreased pain and temperature sensations, contralateral Horner's syndrome, and hoarseness. It also causes cerebellar infarction, with hemiplegia and dizziness.
      (2) **Basilar occlusion** results in pontine infarction and is incompatible with life.
      (3) **Basilar tip occlusion** causes:
         (a) **Midbrain and thalamic infarction**, leading to pupillary, oculomotor, and motor abnormalities
         (b) **Posterior cerebral artery occlusion**, resulting in hemianopia, alexia without agraphia (i.e., inability to read without loss of the ability to write), and, occasionally, hemisensory loss and ataxia

2. **Embolic stroke**
   a. Embolic occlusion of an artery results in infarction.
   b. **Etiology**
      (1) Eighty percent of the causative emboli are **cardiac in origin**. The cardiac disorders that

give rise to emboli are atrial fibrillation, rheumatic heart disease, myocardial infarction, mitral valve prolapse (Barlow's syndrome), and subacute bacterial endocarditis.
   **(2)** Emboli may also arise from an **atherosclerotic plaque** in the proximal portion of the vessel (these are called artery-to-artery emboli).
   **c.** Symptoms and signs depend on the vessel occluded.

**3. Intracerebral hemorrhage**
   **a.** The **etiology** of intracerebral hemorrhage (bleeding into the brain parenchyma) may be hypertension, arteriovenous malformations, a bleeding diathesis, drug use (anticoagulants, platelet inhibitors), or trauma.
   **b.** The **hemorrhages are located**, in order of frequency, in the putamen (50%), thalamus (20%), pons (10%), cerebellum (10%), and hemispheres (10%).
   **c.** The **onset is usually gradual**.
   **d.** The **signs and symptoms result from**:
      **(1)** Focal destruction, leading to neurologic deficits
      **(2)** Increased ICP (see section IV B)
      **(3)** Herniation (see section IV C)

**4. Subarachnoid hemorrhage**
   **a.** Bleeding in the subarachnoid space is usually **secondary to a congenital lesion**, such as a berry aneurysm or an arteriovenous malformation.
   **b.** The **onset is sudden**, with evidence of meningeal irritation (e.g., nuchal rigidity, headache, vomiting, and clouding of consciousness).
   **c.** Neurologic deficits are related to the location of the aneurysm or arteriovenous malformation.
   **d.** Vasospasm may develop later on, leading to ischemia and increasing the neurologic deficits.

**5. Severe systemic hypotension** causes decreased cerebral blood flow, leading to ischemia and infarction in the watershed areas (i.e., the arterial border zones—the area supplied by the distal ends of two or more arteries).

**C. Management of stroke**

**1.** The initial management of stroke involves the taking of an adequate **history** and a **neurologic evaluation**.

**2.** A **CT scan** is then done.
   **a.** The CT scan can rule out or suggest:
      **(1)** Hemispheric infarction
      **(2)** Intraparenchymal hemorrhage
      **(3)** Subarachnoid hemorrhage
      **(4)** Any mass effects
   **b.** The **blood-brain barrier** can be checked by doing a CT scan following a double-dose injection of contrast medium.
   **c.** If the **CT scan is negative in the face of frequent TIAs**, the patient is given anticoagulant therapy.
      **(1)** This may be with heparin, dextran, or even, in some centers, simply aspirin and dipyridamole orally.
      **(2)** Frequent TIAs (**crescendo TIAs**) are managed more aggressively with heparin (anticoagulant) and dextran (to decrease blood viscosity) in order to increase the cerebral blood flow.
   **d.** If there is evidence of **intraparenchymal hemorrhage**, the patient is treated for increased ICP and cerebral edema (see section VI D) to reduce the mass effect. **Surgical evacuation** of the hematoma may be necessary if conservative therapy fails.
   **e.** The patient is treated with an **antifibrinolytic agent** such as aminocaproic acid if there is any evidence of **subarachnoid hemorrhage** on the CT scan.

**3.** An **angiogram** is obtained as soon as possible to identify the pathology.
   **a.** According to some investigators, the risks of angiography preclude its use in cases of advanced stroke. However, in most major centers, the risks of angiography have been decreased considerably, so that the benefits far outweigh the risks.
   **b.** If angiography reveals carotid stenosis or occlusion, middle cerebral artery occlusion, or decreased blood flow in the vertebrobasilar distribution, **surgical therapy** may be necessary to augment the blood supply.
      **(1)** This may be either a **carotid endarterectomy** (see Chapter 13, sections VIII E 2 and 3) or an extracranial artery to intracranial artery (EC–IC) bypass (Fig. 31-7).
      **(2)** A recent international study concluded that EC–IC bypass has no significant benefit

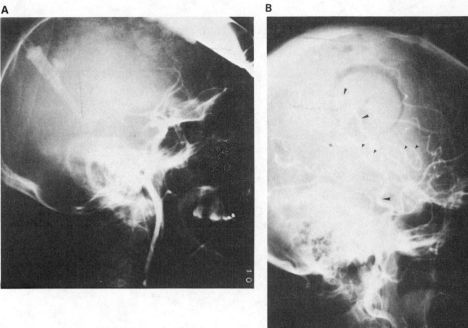

**Figure 31-7.** (A) Cerebral arteriogram showing poor arterial circulation in the territory of the right middle cerebral artery. (B) Following a superficial temporal artery to middle cerebral artery (EC–IC) bypass, there is a markedly improved blood supply in the right middle cerebral artery distribution.

over aspirin plus dipyridamole in reducing the risk of stroke. Thus, this procedure is now indicated only when a major cerebral vessel has to be occluded for trapping an aneurysm.

   **c.** Aneurysms and arteriovenous malformations require surgical correction.

## XIII. CNS INFECTIONS

**A. General considerations.** Infections of the CNS and its coverings are surgically important only if they produce a mass effect, hydrocephalus, or osteomyelitis.

   **1. Brain abscesses** and **subdural empyemas** can cause a mass effect.

   **2. Osteomyelitis** of the skull and spine can lead to chronic inflammation, abscess, and continued infection of adjacent structures.

**B. Management of CNS infections** involves:

   **1.** Identification of the organism

   **2.** Appropriate antibiotic therapy

   **3.** Evacuation of pus

   **4.** Treatment of the source of infection

   **5.** Treatment of the complications of infection, such as mycotic aneurysms, subdural effusions, and hydrocephalus

# 32

# Orthopedic Surgery

Eric L. Hume

## I. GENERAL PRINCIPLES

**A.** Orthopedics encompasses the care of the musculoskeletal system. Disease processes that the orthopedic surgeon must deal with include degeneration, tumor, trauma, metabolic disorders, and infections.

**B. Bone healing**

  **1. Endochondral ossification.** By recapitulation of embryologic bone formation, primitive cells of hematogenous origin undergo the following **stages**:
  **a. Metaplasia** from an initial primitive inflammation
  **b. Maturation of cartilage**
  **c. Necrosis of cartilage** with **calcification**
  **d. Replacement** by primitive woven bone
  **e. Remodeling** of the woven bone into mature organized trabecular and cortical bone

  **2. Primary bone healing** occurs when rigid fixation of a fracture allows cell-to-cell cortical contact.
  **a.** A cutting cone composed of an advancing front of osteoclasts, followed by a vascular bud, and osteoblastic proliferation behind that, can directly remodel a fracture gap without the progression of endochondral ossification.
  **b.** This process proceeds much more slowly than does endochondral ossification.

  **3. Failure of bone healing**
  **a.** A **nonunion** is the result of inadequate primary bone healing or endochondral ossification at a fracture site.
  **b. Etiologies** include:
    **(1)** Excessive motion at the fracture site
    **(2)** Infection
    **(3)** Severe soft tissue damage with loss of local vascularity
    **(4)** Soft tissue interposition within the fracture gap
  **c.** Autogenous bone transplantation (bone grafting) or electrical stimulation of the fracture site are the main **management** options.

## II. INFECTIONS

**A. Acute infections**

  **1. Osteomyelitis**
  **a. Hematogenous osteomyelitis** is not uncommon in childhood.
    **(1)** In the metaphysis of children's bones, there is a unique capillary venous sinusoid underneath the growth plate. This sinusoid is predisposed by minor trauma to allow organisms from minor bacteremia to initiate an infection.
    **(2)** The inflammation evoked about this focus devascularizes the surrounding bone and allows the infection to progress.
    **(3)** The infection can then track to the periosteum and cause a periosteal elevation or, if the metaphysis is intra-articular, as in the hip or shoulder, it can cause a septic arthritis.
  **b. Causative organisms**
    **(1)** *Staphylococcus aureus* and gram-negative rods predominate as the causative organisms in neonates.

**(2)** Osteomyelitis in young children is most commonly caused by *Hemophilus* species from ear infections.

**(3)** *S. aureus* resumes the role of most likely cause in older children and adolescents.

**(4)** Adults whose immune system is suppressed, drug addicts, and patients with sickle cell anemia are predisposed to osteomyelitis from the hematogenous spread of unusual organisms.

**(a)** Those with immune suppression and drug addicts are prone to gram-negative infections.

**(b)** In sickle cell anemia, the osteomyelitis is most commonly due to *S. aureus*; however, a particularly high incidence of *Salmonella* osteomyelitis is noted.

**c.** A child with a history of minor trauma who does not get better rapidly must be suspected of having osteomyelitis.

**d.** A careful physical examination, needle aspiration, a complete blood count, the sedimentation rate, and a bone scan confirm the **diagnosis**.

**e. Treatment** includes appropriate antibiotics and sometimes surgical drainage. Antibiotics for initial treatment are selected to cover the most likely causative organisms.

**2. Septic arthritis**

**a.** Spontaneous joint infections can occur in children or adults, again by the hematogenous spread of the same organisms that cause osteomyelitis in the different age groups.

**b.** Joint disease, as well as immune suppression such as occurs in rheumatoid arthritis, can predispose the patient to these joint infections.

**c. Physical examination** shows exquisite tenderness, effusion, and pain with minimal motion of the joint.

**d.** The **diagnosis** is confirmed by needle aspiration of the synovial fluid and by finding that the white cell count and sedimentation rate are elevated.

**e. Treatment** includes decompression of the joint and appropriate intravenous antibiotic therapy.

**(1)** Most of the joints of the body except the hip, shoulder, and spine can be decompressed satisfactorily by means of needle aspiration.

**(2)** The excepted joints, and any joint that does not respond promptly to needle aspiration, should be surgically incised, debrided, and drained.

**3. Penetrating wounds** that reach a bone or joint can lead to infection. The magnitude of the wound is the main factor related to the severity of the infection.

**B. Chronic osteomyelitis**

**1.** In today's antibiotic era, chronic osteomyelitis is a different problem from that seen in the past.

**a.** Most cases are due to postoperative infection following a surgical procedure involving a bone.

**b.** The cases that are seen in children may result in limb deformity and growth arrest.

**2.** Osteomyelitis involving the **bony cortex** is a particularly frustrating problem.

**a.** Cortical bone, which has minimal vascularity at best, is even more poorly vascularized as a result of the osteomyelitis.

**b.** Therefore, white cells, as well as antibiotics, have only limited access to the site of the infection.

**3. Treatment.** Attempts to cure chronic osteomyelitis involve removal of foreign material, a thorough debridement of infected bone, good local wound care, and prolonged use of intravenous antibiotics.

**a. Tetracycline bone labeling** with a Wood's lamp illumination in the operating room may aid in the debridement of devascularized bone, since well-vascularized bone incorporates the tetracycline, which fluoresces under the Wood's lamp.

**b. Bone defects** can be managed with either an open Papineau type of bone graft, in which morselized cancellous bone is packed into an open wound without any soft tissue coverage, or a vascularized bone graft.

**c.** The use of muscle flaps and split-thickness skin grafts, employed after the control of infection, completes the treatment.

## III. TRAUMA

**A. General principles**

**1.** The extent of an injury to the musculoskeletal system varies according to the age of the patient, the direction of the causative violence, and the magnitude of the violence.

      **a.** The **age of the patient** suggests the weak link in the musculoskeletal system.
- **(1)** The weak link in the **skeletally immature patient** is the growth plate in the ends of the long bones.
- **(2)** **Young but skeletally mature patients**, in the age range of 16 to 50 years, are more likely to sustain ligamentous injuries because the strength of the mature bone exceeds the strength of the soft tissue supporting the joints.
- **(3)** This situation reverses in **late middle age**, so that **elderly patients** with significant osteoporosis rarely injure the ligaments, but instead sustain fractures of the metaphyseal portion of the bone. The metaphysis is usually injured because, as osteoporosis occurs, much of the bone loss is from this metabolically active area.

      **b.** The **direction of violence** determines which structures are injured.
- **(1)** An example is the typical "clipping" injury of the knee, with the violence applied to the lateral aspect of the knee.
- **(2)** This stretches the soft tissue in the medial side of the knee, causing a medial collateral tear.

      **c.** The **magnitude of the violence** is related to its velocity.
- **(1)** **High-velocity injuries**, as in motor vehicle accidents, tend to cause comminuted complex skeletal injuries.
- **(2)** **Lower-velocity injuries**, as occur in sports, are more likely to cause simple, isolated injuries of ligaments, muscles, or bones.

**2. Evaluation of the patient**
      **a.** The **history** must take into account the above factors.
- **(1)** A **fall from a height** can frequently lead to calcaneus fracture, hip dislocation, and fracture of the thoracolumbar spine.
- **(2)** A **motor vehicle accident** in which the patient is thrown forward, with knees striking the dashboard, frequently causes patellar fracture, femur fracture, and hip fracture or dislocation.
- **(3)** A **fall on the outstretched upper extremity** will frequently cause fracture of the distal radius, the radial head, or the metaphysis of the humerus at the shoulder.

      **b. Physical examination**
- **(1)** Musculoskeletal injuries make their presence known by the findings of bony crepitus at the fracture site, gross limb deformity, or dislocations and local swelling and tenderness at the specific point of injury.
- **(2)** The integrity of the skin, neural function, and circulatory status must be carefully evaluated when the patient is initially seen and also during the course of treatment. (Specifics are addressed in section III B.)

**3. Principles of management**
      **a. Indications for open reduction and fixation**
- **(1) Intra-articular fractures.** The smooth painless function of a joint demands an absolutely smooth contour on the articular surfaces. This is best obtained with direct surgical visualization.
- **(2) Extremity function requiring perfect reduction.** A typical example is a fracture of both bones of the forearm.
  - **(a)** The shape of the radius and ulna must be anatomic to allow smooth supination and pronation.
  - **(b)** To achieve this requires open reduction and surgical fixation.
- **(3) Unsatisfactory results after closed reduction.** If closed care does not give adequate results, open techniques are required.
- **(4) Metastatic tumors** (see section IV B)
- **(5) Multiple trauma**
  - **(a)** Patients with multiple-system injuries have a better prognosis if the extremity injuries can be internally fixed or splinted so that the patient can be mobilized at an early date.
  - **(b)** Early mobilization improves pulmonary function and facilitates nursing care and further diagnostic evaluation of the patient.
- **(6) Injuries in elderly patients**
  - **(a)** The elderly patient is poorly able to withstand the complications of prolonged bed rest and does not have the cardiovascular reserves or muscular stamina to allow ambulation after a prolonged period of bed rest.
  - **(b)** Fractures of the weight-bearing bones in the elderly should be surgically fixed, if necessary, to allow early mobilization and ambulation.

      **b. Indications for external fixation**
- **(1)** External fixation of fractures is carried out when the soft tissue injuries about the fracture prevent casting or when there is a risk of infection with internal fixation.

    **(2)** External fixators maintain bone alignment and permit access to the skin for wound care and dressing changes, but at the expense of potential infection from the percutaneous pins held with external clamps.

   **c. Cast immobilization** is the most widely applied and most varied method of fracture care.

    **(1)** With the increasing awareness of the problems associated with immobilization of the joints, casting techniques have come to include hinges and designs that allow early weight bearing and joint motion.

    **(2)** These techniques should not be used at the expense of adequate fracture immobilization.

## B. Orthopedic emergencies

**1. Open fractures**

   **a.** An open fracture is a surgical emergency for several reasons:

    **(1)** In part, because of the relative susceptibility of bone to infection

    **(2)** Even more, because of the associated devitalized soft tissue wounds, which may be extensive and which carry a high risk of life-threatening anaerobic infection

   **b. Surgical management includes:**

    **(1)** Prophylactic antibiotics, including those effective against gram-positive and anaerobic organisms

    **(2)** Thorough surgical debridement, ideally within 8 hours after injury

    **(3)** Inoculation against tetanus, unless this is known to be unnecessary

**2. Vascular injuries.** Arterial and venous compromise must be given careful consideration in association with orthopedic trauma. The patient is also at risk for developing **compartment syndromes** especially in the lower extremities. The circulation to the muscles and nerves is compromised by increased tissue pressure (e.g., due to a cast).

**3. Neural compromise**

   **a. Spinal cord injuries** (see also Chapter 31, section VII). Injuries to the spinal column take a very high priority in the initial management of the injured patient.

    **(1)** Any patient with significant head or face injuries and any patient who is comatose after trauma must be assumed to have a cervical spine fracture.

    **(2)** Appropriate cross-table lateral x-rays must be obtained. These include x-rays of the cervical spine from the occiput down to and including the first thoracic vertebral body.

    **(3)** Reduction of any deformity is a surgical priority of the highest order.

   **b. Peripheral nerve injuries** (see also Chapter 31, section VIII)

    **(1)** Peripheral nerves are frequently injured in association with trauma to the extremities.

    **(2)** Any such injury must be carefully noted before treatment, both for medicolegal reasons and to restore the anatomic alignment of the extremity in order to relieve pressure on the peripheral nerve.

    **(3)** Most peripheral nerve injuries associated with closed injuries to the extremities will recover without nerve exploration. While the nerve is recovering, careful attention must be directed to the muscles and joints in order to prevent contraction or stretching of the muscles.

    **(4)** Penetrating wounds have a high incidence of nerve transection and therefore should be surgically explored when the patient is stable and an appropriate surgical environment (i.e., a rested staff, magnification, and appropriate instruments) can be obtained.

## C. Fractures in children

**1. General principles**

   **a.** The **growth plate** is weaker than the rest of the long bone in the child.

    **(1)** Therefore, a relatively large number of fractures in children disrupt the growth plate with the associated risk of growth problems.

    **(2)** The patient should be treated with careful, accurate closed reduction of the growth plate, and both patient and parents should be warned about the potential problems.

   **b. Buckle fractures**

    **(1)** Because children's bones are relatively flexible in comparison with those of the adult, buckle fractures occur. These fractures are incomplete, with more plastic deformation than in adults.

    **(2)** Buckle fractures can be treated with simple cast protection to prevent further displacement.

   **c. Greenstick fractures**

    **(1)** Again because of the flexibility and plasticity of children's bones, some shaft fractures extend through only one portion or one aspect of the cortex.

    **(2)** Because of the potential for recurrent angulation despite an initial excellent closed reduction, the remaining cortex of the fractured bone should be disrupted so that the alignment of the bone can be easily obtained.

   **d. Child abuse** is appropriately suspected If the child has unusual oblique fractures or spiral fractures of long bones; fractures of various ages in different extremities; skin bruises, burns, or scrapes of various ages; or a history that is suspicious.

**2. Supracondylar fracture of the humerus.** This is associated with a high incidence of injury to the brachial artery and compartment syndromes.
   **a.** In **treatment**, traction for several weeks may be indicated. However, these fractures may be amenable to closed reduction and casting.
   **b.** The **neurovascular status** of the extremities should be carefully examined both before and after closed reduction of these injuries. The patient should be admitted to the hospital for these evaluations.

**3. Fractures of both forearm bones**
   **a.** In children, these are usually managed with closed reduction and plaster immobilization.
   **b.** The cast must be carefully molded and the patient observed to ensure that the interosseous space is preserved in order to maintain forearm supination and pronation after healing.

**4. Distal radius fractures**
   **a.** The distal radial metaphysis is a frequent site for buckle fractures.
   **b.** The distal radial epiphyseal plate is a frequent site for growth plate fractures. The growth plate fracture, if displaced, should have a closed reduction, usually under general anesthesia, with cast immobilization.

**5. Femur fractures**
   **a.** In young children aged about 2 to 10 years, these can most often be managed with closed reduction and plaster spica immobilization.
   **b.** Usually a small amount of femoral overlap is acceptable.
      **(1)** The increased vascularity that occurs in response to the injury usually causes overgrowth of the epiphysis on the involved side.
      **(2)** Without the overlap, the limb is likely to end up longer than the opposite, uninjured extremity.

**6. Supracondylar fractures of the femur and fractures of the proximal tibia**
   **a.** Both of these injuries, on physical examination, can be easily confused with a ligamentous knee injury.
   **b.** It is important to remember that skeletally immature individuals almost never have injuries to the ligaments, but instead fracture through the growth plates.
   **c.** Therefore, when a child's knee is unstable on physical examination, a stress x-ray of the knee should be taken to verify the exact cause and location of the false motion.

**7. Tibia fractures**
   **a.** These are frequently open because of the subcutaneous position of the bone. They are also associated with a relatively high incidence of compartment syndromes.
   **b.** Therefore, all patients with tibial fractures should be examined for any skin disruption, and the neurovascular status of the leg should be evaluated.
   **c.** These fractures are well managed in children with plaster immobilization.

**D. Fractures in adults**

**1.** In **elderly persons with osteoporosis**, fractures of the hip, the proximal humerus, and the distal radius at the wrist are all quite common.
   **a.** In general, the upper extremity fractures can be managed with cast immobilization, with an attempt to prevent stiffness, especially at the shoulder.
   **b.** Because of the weight-bearing function of the hip, open reduction and internal fixation of the fracture or hemiarthroplasty is actually the conservative management, associated with better long-term function and survival of the patient.

**2. Humeral shaft fractures** are associated with a relatively high incidence of radial nerve palsies.
   **a.** In general, the palsy will recover with immobilization. However, careful attention must be paid to the hand, to prevent stiffness and contractures until the radial nerve recovers.
   **b.** The fracture may be treated with a sling and humeral cuff, with early range-of-motion exercises of the shoulder and elbow, and with isometric exercises of the biceps and triceps.

**3. Fractures of both forearm bones**
   **a.** Because of the precise functional requirements of the forearm, these fractures require open reduction and internal fixation for maximal functional results.

**b.** Especially in crushing injuries, the consideration of a compartment syndrome is important.

**4. Finger fractures**
   **a.** Because of the precise, fine function of the fingers and the problem of stiffness in adults, early range-of-motion exercise of the fingers has a high priority.
   **b.** Percutaneous pin or plate fixation or early splinting with "buddy" taping are all acceptable methods, assuming that the goal of early motion can be obtained to avoid finger contracture and dysfunction.

**5. Spinal fractures** are associated with high-velocity, high-energy mechanisms of injury. Automobile accidents, motorcycle accidents, and falls from heights are the frequent mechanisms in spinal (and pelvic) fractures.
   **a. Management** of the spinal fracture includes:
      **(1)** Decompression of the central nervous system as well as peripheral nerves
      **(2)** Spinal stability for early rehabilitation
   **b.** Early mobilization is especially important in paraplegics and quadriplegics so that the overwhelming task of rehabilitation can begin promptly.

**6. Femur fractures**
   **a.** Treatment traditionally has been via traction for 4 to 6 weeks, until enough healing allows cast immobilization for the duration of the patient's care.
   **b.** However, improved intramedullary rodding techniques may allow better quadriceps, hip, and knee function, with shorter hospital stays.
   **c.** The decision must be individualized, and the pros and cons of the two options must be carefully explained to the patient.

**7. Tibia fractures** are frequently open and frequently associated with compartment syndromes.
   **a.** These two associated problems must be anticipated and managed appropriately.
   **b.** Fractures of the tibia are generally best managed with plaster immobilization and early weight bearing.
   **c.** The incidence of delayed union or nonunion of tibial fractures is high. In selected instances, plate fixation or intramedullary nail fixation has an important role.

**8. Ankle fractures** are classified according to the degree of instability of the ankle. If ankle fractures are treated successfully, post-traumatic osteoarthritis and delayed ankle instability can be avoided.

**E. Dislocations**

**1. Shoulder**
   **a.** Dislocations of the glenohumeral joint are especially common in young adults.
   **b.** Glenohumeral dislocations frequently recur, especially when management does not include careful immobilization.
   **c.** These injuries are also associated with axillary nerve palsy.

**2. Hip**
   **a.** Dislocations of the hip occur in high-velocity injuries, especially automobile accidents.
   **b.** They are associated with fractures of the ipsilateral femur and patella, and with contralateral hip fractures or dislocations.

**3. Knee**
   **a.** Dislocations of the knee are extreme cases of ligamentous injuries about the knee.
      **(1)** Ligamentous knee injuries occur more commonly in sports-related activities.
      **(2)** Total ligamentous disruption and dislocation are associated with violent injuries.
   **b.** The most important consideration is the common occurrence of injuries to the popliteal artery and vein, and to the peroneal nerve.
   **c.** Therefore, with dislocations of the knee the first step in management is to evaluate the neurovascular status of the lower leg, followed by evaluation of the ligaments and capsule about the knee.

**F. Musculotendinous injuries**

**1.** Disruptions of the musculotendinous unit are most commonly associated with overuse.
   **a. Tear of the rotator cuff**
      **(1)** Middle-aged and older patients with intermittent shoulder pain may have an episode of acute pain when the weakened tendon tears.
      **(2)** Most tears are small and may be treated symptomatically initially.
      **(3)** However, after resolution of the acute symptoms, if the shoulder demonstrates poor muscular function, repair must be undertaken.

    **b. Quadriceps disruptions**
- **(1)** Middle-aged and older patients, especially those with diabetes mellitus, may acutely disrupt the quadriceps mechanism at a level just superior to the patella.
- **(2)** Physical examination shows minimal swelling and tenderness.
- **(3)** The patient will complain only of weakness in the leg after hearing a "pop," and may be able to raise the leg if the knee is straight. However, the patient will be unable to initiate extension against gravity with the knee at 90° of flexion.
- **(4)** Surgical repair is necessary.

    **c. Achilles tendon disruptions**
- **(1)** The usual patient is middle-aged or older and may have had heel pain. Typically, the patient was trying to bend or to push a heavy object forward, when an audible "pop" was heard.
- **(2)** The patient is usually able to walk, and the symptoms are minimal. Physical examination reveals a palpable defect in the Achilles tendon.
- **(3)** The **Thompson test** may aid in diagnosis. This is performed by squeezing the calf and looking for plantar flexion of the foot. This response is absent with Achilles tendon ruptures.
- **(4)** The treatment is surgical repair or cast immobilization.

  **2. Acute muscle ruptures**
- **a.** Any musculotendinous unit may be disrupted by a forced lengthening of the muscle.
- **b.** The disruption usually occurs at the musculotendinous junction but may be within the muscle belly.
- **c.** These injuries may be very difficult to repair, and the results are variable.

## IV. TUMORS

  **A. Primary bone tumors**

    **1. General considerations**
- **a. Clinical presentation.** The patient with a neoplastic bone lesion presents with pain, swelling, or, occasionally, a pathologic fracture induced by minimal trauma. This is true for bony metastases as well as for benign and malignant tumors of bone.
- **b. Diagnosis**
  - **(1)** In addition to differentiating a primary from a metastatic tumor of bone, some metabolic processes such as hyperparathyroidism and infection must be carefully considered.
  - **(2)** **Physical examination** demonstrates the tumor mass, allowing the selection of appropriate x-rays.
  - **(3)** **Plain x-rays** alone will often suggest whether a tumor of bone is benign or malignant.
    - **(a)** A **malignancy** can be expected if the films show:
      - **(i)** A tumor of large size
      - **(ii)** Aggressive destruction of bone
      - **(iii)** Ineffective reaction of the bone to the tumor
      - **(iv)** Extension of the tumor into soft tissue
    - **(b)** At the opposite extreme, the lesion is almost surely **benign** if the films show:
      - **(i)** A small, well-circumscribed lytic lesion
      - **(ii)** A thick, sclerotic rim
      - **(iii)** No extension into soft tissue
  - **(4)** If there is any question whatsoever that the tumor is malignant, a careful **workup** must be performed.
    - **(a)** An incomplete workup or a poorly thought out biopsy is likely to be fatal for the patient or may cost the patient a deforming radical amputation.
    - **(b)** An **appropriate workup** includes **computed tomography** (CT scanning) and **technetium-99m ($^{99m}$Tc) scanning** of the involved bone to stage the tumor and delineate its extent and anatomic relationships.
    - **(c)** If **malignancy** is suspected, then **CT scanning of the chest** is important to rule out pulmonary metastases. No other metastatic workup is required, since sarcomas metastasize to the lung first.
  - **(5)** Only after staging has been completed should a **biopsy** be performed.
    - **(a)** All biopsy incisions should be:
      - **(i)** Longitudinal
      - **(ii)** Made through a muscle belly to avoid contaminating intermuscular planes
      - **(iii)** Directed away from neurovascular structures
      - **(iv)** Directed through structures that can be safely and successfully resected to leave a functional limb if radical excision will be carried out

**(b)** The biopsy should be carefully planned so that the biopsy material can be removed with a definitive surgical resection. The biopsy is best planned and performed by the surgeon who will ultimately carry out the definitive surgical procedure.

**c. Treatment**

**(1) Surgical therapy**

**(a)** Surgery continues to be the mainstay of management for both benign and malignant tumors.

**(b)** The **surgical margin**, obviously, varies significantly.

**(i) Benign tumors** can be adequately treated by intralesional or intracapsular excision of the tumor with or without chemical cautery or electrocautery, and with or without bone grafting of the defect.

**(ii) Malignant tumors** require at least a 2-cm margin.

**(c)** One or two isolated pulmonary metastases of sarcoma, especially osteosarcoma or chondrosarcoma, should be considered for surgical resection, since the literature shows that this will result in an occasional cure, and certainly a prolonged life span, in these patients.

**(2) Adjuvant therapy for malignant tumors**

**(a) Radiation therapy**

**(i)** Some tumors, such as Ewing's tumors, are very sensitive to radiotherapy.

**(ii)** Some protocols include radiation therapy initially, but in general radiation therapy is not an important part of the protocol.

**(b) Chemotherapy**, like radiation therapy, has limited use.

**(i)** Ewing's tumors are well known to be very sensitive to various chemotherapeutic regimens.

**(ii)** Osteosarcoma appears to be sensitive to some chemotherapeutic agents, and work is under way to delineate the benefits.

**2. Types of primary bone tumors**

**a. Tumors of bone cell origin**

**(1) Benign osteoid osteoma** is a painful lesion commonly affecting the femur or the tibia.

**(a)** It occurs in adolescents, with more than 50% of the tumors presenting in patients aged 10 to 20 years.

**(b)** The lesions are benign and are not prone to malignant degeneration. Pathologic examination demonstrates a nidus of disorganized, dense, calcified osteoid tissue which histologically is benign.

**(c)** Typically, aspirin offers excellent relief.

**(d)** Surgical management is indicated for lesions that are painful. A bone graft may be necessary.

**(2) Osteoblastoma** is a benign, rare, painful lesion that histologically appears very similar to osteoid osteoma. One distinguishing feature is its size: An osteoblastoma is defined as a benign bone-forming lesion greater than 2 cm.

**(a)** It occurs most often in the second decade of life.

**(b)** Osteoblastomas are cured by surgical excision if symptoms warrant. Bone grafting may be necessary.

**(3) Osteosarcoma** is a malignant tumor of adolescence.

**(a)** Over 60% of patients with these tumors are aged 10 to 20 years.

**(b)** At least 60% of osteosarcomas occur about the knee at either the distal femur or proximal tibia.

**(c)** Typically, the patient **presents** with pain and tumefaction.

**(d) Radiographically**, the lesion is typically lytic, but it may be a blastic lesion of the bone. CT shows that the lesion is ill-defined, with soft tissue extension.

**(e) Histologically**, the tumor may be predominantly fibrogenic, chondrogenic, or osteogenic; each of the three types predominates in approximately equal numbers of patients.

**(f)** The **sine qua non** of osteosarcomas is that somewhere within the tumor the tumor stroma is forming bone.

**(i)** Although the tumor may look predominantly like a chondrosarcoma or a fibrosarcoma, if bone is being formed by even one small part of the tumor, then by definition the tumor is an osteosarcoma.

**(ii)** The distinction is important because the **prognosis** differs significantly for chondrosarcoma and for osteosarcoma: The 5-year survival rate for an osteosarcoma is around 10% to 20%. Early pulmonary metastases occur.

**(g)** The principal treatment is surgical resection; amputation or limb salvage surgery may be required.

**(h)** Adjuvant chemotherapy does seem to have a potentially beneficial effect and its use is being actively investigated.

**b. Tumors originating in cartilage**
  **(1) Enchondromas** frequently are asymptomatic findings on x-rays, although some present as pathologic fractures.
   **(a)** The tumor occurs in patients aged 10 to 50, and is commonly found in the hand.
   **(b)** It is typically an intraosseous lytic lesion marked by characteristic "popcorn" calcifications and surrounded by reactive sclerosis.
   **(c)** A tumor that appears radiographically to be an enchondroma must be suspected of being a sarcoma if it presents with pain but no pathologic fracture.
   **(d)** When an enchondroma causes a pathologic fracture, curettage and bone grafting are required.
  **(2) Osteochondromas** are benign, easily palpable tumors of bone. They are quite common.
   **(a)** They grow during adolescence, as does any cartilage portion of bone. If pain or growth occurs after skeletal maturity, malignant degeneration must be suspected and excisional biopsy is warranted.
   **(b)** Osteochondromas may be symptomatic because of their prominence, or because of a resultant fracture or neurovascular compression.
   **(c)** If symptoms warrant it, osteochondromas can be excised, including the soft tissue covering and cartilage. Bone grafting is generally not necessary.
  **(3) Chondroblastomas** are less common cartilage tumors that almost always occur within the epiphysis of long bones.
   **(a)** Over 70% of these tumors occur during the second decade of life. They are very rare if the growth plates have closed.
   **(b)** They are benign lesions, but a very small percentage undergo malignant degeneration.
   **(c)** They frequently require excision and bone grafting.
  **(4) Chondromyxoid fibromas** are relatively rare tumors that usually occur in the first and second decades of life.
   **(a)** The tumor is a relatively large, well-defined lytic lesion with a sclerotic rim, found in the metaphysis juxtaposed to the growth plate. It may present with pathologic fracture.
   **(b)** Curettage and bone grafting may be required for treatment.
  **(5) Chondrosarcoma** is a primary malignant tumor of adulthood that sometimes develops in preexisting benign cartilage lesions.
   **(a)** It occurs with an essentially constant incidence in patients of all ages from 10 to approximately 70 years.
   **(b)** Typically, the tumor presents with pain and tumefaction.
   **(c)** X-rays may show a lytic lesion with or without stippled calcification.
   **(d)** The tumor is locally recurrent, rather than showing early pulmonary metastases as does osteosarcoma.
   **(e)** Treatment is surgical, with the goal of obtaining a 2-cm margin of tumor-free tissue.

**c. Other primary tumors**
  **(1) Giant-cell tumors** occur in the epiphyseal–metaphyseal region of long bones, especially about the knee in the femur and tibia. The lesions are benign, but are problematic because of their propensity to recur locally.
   **(a)** Giant-cell tumors occur in young adults, with the peak occurrence in patients between the ages of 20 and 30. The patient almost always is skeletally mature.
   **(b)** The lesion usually extends to the subchondral plate of the joint. It is a lytic lesion, fairly well circumscribed, with some ballooning of the cortex.
   **(c)** The lesion is characterized **histologically** by the giant cells found in a benign stroma. The giant cell nuclei and the stroma nuclei are identical in appearance.
   **(d)** In **treatment**, curettage is often accompanied by cryotherapy, phenol chemocautery, or electrocautery. The lesion may be packed with polymethylmethacrylate bone cement, or bone grafting may be done. Recurrence usually requires wide resection of the involved bone.
  **(2) Unicameral bone cysts** are lytic lesions of bone that occur in older children in the metaphyseal region that extends to the growth plate. The proximal end of the humerus is the most common site.
   **(a)** Typically, the patient presents with a pathologic fracture, and ultimately the cyst may resolve in response to this trauma.
   **(b)** Unicameral bone cysts may be managed with intralesional steroid injections administered under radiographic control. Multiple injections may be required, which presents a problem in growing children.
  **(3) Ewing's sarcoma** is a disease of childhood and adolescence. It occurs evenly among individuals under the age of 20 years.

       (a) Typically, the patient presents with significant tumefaction and pain in the involved area.

       (b) The history, physical examination, and x-ray findings mimic those of osteomyelitis.

       (c) **Radiologically**, the lesion is seen to be a lytic bone lesion with some periosteal reaction around it.

       (d) **Histologically**, this is a tumor of small round cells, which may form pseudorosettes reminiscent of neuroblastoma.

       (e) In **treatment**, the relative roles of chemotherapy, radiation therapy, and surgical therapy are being evaluated.

          (i) These tumors are sensitive to both chemotherapy and radiotherapy, and together these modalities have a significant cure rate.

          (ii) However, new information suggests that patients are at risk of forming osteosarcoma in the radiated bone during early adulthood.

    (4) **Fibrosarcoma** is a tumor that occurs in adulthood, between the ages of 20 and 70.

       (a) It is predominantly a lytic lesion occurring in the femur and tibia about the knee.

       (b) It presents with pain and an x-ray appearance of a purely lytic lesion of bone.

       (c) **Histologic examination** shows sheets of spindle cells in a herringbone pattern and with various amounts of atypism.

       (d) **Treatment** is wide surgical excision.

    (5) **Multiple myeloma**

       (a) Whether this lesion is a primary tumor of bone or of bone marrow is argued. Whatever its classification, it is a common tumor that occurs in patients aged 30 years and older, with a peak in incidence at 50 to 60 years.

       (b) Multiple myeloma is characterized by overproduction of monoclonal immunoglobulins or immunoglobulin subchains (Bence Jones protein).

       (c) The initial presentation is often a pathologic fracture, frequently of the spine or long bones.

       (d) The diagnosis should be suspected when lytic lesions are found in a patient with anemia, an elevated sedimentation rate, and elevated serum calcium levels.

       (e) The diagnosis can be made by serum or urine electrophoresis or immunophoresis in 95% of cases, but 5% of myeloma patients are nonsecretors of M protein (immunoglobulins or Bence Jones protein).

       (f) Biopsy of the bone marrow to identify secreting and nonsecreting tumors shows plasma cells replacing the marrow. The percentage of bone marrow replacement offers some prognostic information.

       (g) Treatment is by a combination of chemotherapy and radiation therapy, with surgical fixation of pathologic fractures, to improve the quality of life.

## B. Metastatic disease

  **1.** Tumors metastatic to the skeletal system are far more common than primary musculoskeletal tumors. Primary tumors that metastasize to bone include carcinomas of the breast, lung, prostate, thyroid, and kidney, or, indeed, almost any type of tumor.

  **2. Diagnosis**

    **a.** Most bony metastatic disease presents with pain in the involved bone. Metastatic bone disease may be the initial presentation of a malignancy.

    **b. Radiographs** show most bone lesions to be lytic. With some breast tumors and most prostatic tumors, the bone has a blastic appearance.

    **c.** A **bone scan** is helpful when a single symptomatic lytic lesion is found on initial x-rays.

      **(1)** If the bone scan shows multiple lesions, the likelihood of metastatic disease is high.

      **(2)** Bone scanning may also demonstrate a lesion that is more surgically accessible for biopsy.

  **3. Treatment**

    **a.** The likelihood of pathologic fracture is relatively high, and **prophylactic fixation** of long bones with metastatic lesions should be considered in the following situations:

      **(1)** If the lesion involves more than half of the circumference of the long bone

      **(2)** If the length of the lesion in the long bone is greater than the diameter of the bone

    **b.** The **treatment** of most metastatic lesions in bones is radiation therapy.

    **c.** If the pain does not respond to irradiation, a pathologic fracture has probably occurred, and it should then be fixed.

    **d.** Pathologic fractures in general should be fixed internally, using a combination of metal implants plus methylmethacrylate bone cement to manage bone loss.

## V. ARTHRITIS

### A. Classification

1. **Degenerative disease** includes:
   a. **Osteoarthritis** with Heberden's nodes and symmetric hip, knee, and spine involvement
   b. **Post-traumatic arthritis** of the isolated joint

2. **Rheumatoid arthritis and its variants** include the autoimmune group of inflammatory diseases in which the hyaline articular cartilage is attacked by a local invasive pannus.

3. **Crystal deposition diseases** include **gout** and **calcium pyrophosphate deposition disease**. These usually present as an isolated hot, inflamed joint.

4. **Infectious arthritis** (see also section II A 2) also presents as an isolated hot, inflamed joint.
   a. This is the one form of arthritis that requires immediate emergency care.
   b. Diagnosis can be made by aspirating the joint fluid and examining it microscopically and by cell count, sugar determinations, and culture.

### B. Nonoperative management

1. **Nonsteroidal anti-inflammatory drugs (NSAIDs)**
   a. These are especially important in rheumatoid arthritis, which requires a long-term maintenance regimen.
   b. The crystalline and degenerative joint diseases require NSAIDs during acute flare-ups, but do not respond to long-term management with these drugs.

2. **Gold** and **antimalarial agents** have an important place in the rheumatoid arthritis armamentarium.
   a. In general, these drugs provide the "second level" of management.
   b. They are indicated when the rheumatologist caring for the patient has not been successful with the NSAIDs.

3. **Corticosteroids**
   a. These provide the "third level" of care for rheumatoid arthritis when NSAIDs have failed to quiet the inflammation. They can be used:
      (1) Systemically if multiple joint involvement or generalized disease is the problem
      (2) Locally by instillation into a single joint that has been identified as the most bothersome one
   b. Degenerative joint disease occasionally benefits from local instillation of corticosteroid into the joint.

4. **Immunosuppressants** are a last level of drugs for uncontrolled rheumatoid arthritis.

5. **Exercise** has an important place in all forms of arthritis after the acute joint inflammation has been controlled. The exercise is designed to maintain a full range of joint motion as well as to maintain muscle strength by exercising the joint through a painless arc of motion.

### C. Operative management

1. **Types of surgical procedures**
   a. **Arthroplasty**, or **total joint replacement**, is the newest addition to the surgical management of joint disease.
      (1) It can be used for joints destroyed by any of the arthritides.
      (2) However, postinfectious arthritis is a relative contraindication to arthroplasty because of the increased risk of infection around the implant.
      (3) Arthroplasty is indicated for the relief of pain predominantly in patients over age 65.
      (4) At the present state of the art, the "life expectancy" for an arthroplasty implant is about 10 to 12 years, depending on the joint and the functional requirements of the patient.
   b. **Arthrodesis**
      (1) In this procedure, the joint surfaces are excised and the extremity is immobilized so that the joint heals in a fixed position.
      (2) Arthrodesis is indicated for the relief of pain, especially in the younger individual.
         (a) The results of arthrodesis are very durable and long-lasting.
         (b) Therefore, any patient who is young or has a high functional demand should be considered for arthrodesis rather than arthroplasty.
   c. **Osteotomy**
      (1) Cutting a bone and realigning a joint may alter the mechanics enough to give significant, although incomplete, relief of pain.

**(2)** To be successful, the procedure must not completely destroy a joint, but must leave some remaining articular surface.

**(3)** Osteotomy is designed to transfer weight-bearing onto this relatively normal articular surface.

**2. Specific examples**

**a. Hip**

**(1) Total hip arthroplasty** was the first successful replacement and is by far the most common hip procedure done today.

**(2)** However, for the young individual, **hip arthrodesis** is a very successful means of providing a functional joint.

**(3) Osteotomies about the hip** are becoming more popular again and have a place, albeit limited, in the surgical management of the hip.

**b. Knee**

**(1) Arthroplasties** have become more durable and more widely accepted.

**(2)** The standard of care for early degenerative disease is still the **Coventry type of osteotomy**, in which the weight-bearing axis of the body is transferred to the usually more normal lateral condyle of the knee.

**(3) Arthrodesis** is a reliable procedure for the unstable, painful knee in the younger individual.

**c. Foot and ankle.** In general, **arthrodesis** of the midfoot joints is indicated for painful involvement of the subtalar or midfoot joints. Ankle arthrodesis is also the standard of care, although ankle **arthroplasty** has a place for certain conditions in patients with extremely limited functional requirements.

**d. Shoulder.** The shoulder is not a weight-bearing joint, and degenerative disease of this joint is less common. However, total shoulder **arthroplasties** are beginning to show promise in the treatment of degenerative disease and rheumatoid arthritis.

**e. Elbow. Arthroplasty** with prosthetic components is still a procedure with limited indications. Elbow **arthrodesis** affords good pain relief, as does excisional arthroplasty without the addition of prosthetic components.

**f. Wrist and hand. Arthroplasty** with Silastic implants often allows functional, painless motion of wrist and hand joints, especially in patients with rheumatoid arthritis. Patients with severe wrist involvement, especially from post-traumatic degenerative disease, are well managed by **arthrodesis** of the involved joint.

# VI. PEDIATRIC ORTHOPEDICS

**A. Congenital dislocation of the hip** is most common in female neonates, especially if the child is the firstborn and was in the breech presentation. The condition is bilateral in 10% of the patients.

**1.** The **diagnosis** can be made within the first 2 weeks after birth, once relaxin is gone from the child's circulation.

**a. Physical examination**

**(1)** The examiner can feel a click on reduction of the dislocated hip **(Ortolani's sign)**.

**(2)** The examiner is able to dislocate the hip with the hip flexed to 90° **(Barlow's test)**.

**(3)** Other physical findings, especially if the dislocation is unilateral, include asymmetry of the gluteal fold and asymmetric leg lengths, demonstrated by the height of the knee when the hips are flexed to 90°.

**b.** X-rays confirm the diagnosis.

**2.** A hip that is still dislocatable after 2 weeks should be treated.

**a.** Initial **management** is with a Pavlik harness.

**b.** Double and triple diapering probably has no significant effect on the dislocation.

**B. Scoliosis**

**1. Etiology**

**a.** The most common form of scoliosis in the United States is the **idiopathic scoliosis** that occurs in adolescent females, beginning at the age of about 11 or 12 and progressing until growth is completed.

**b.** Scoliosis can also be the result of neuromuscular paralysis, painful lesions, radiation, thoracic surgery, and congenital anomalies.

**2. Clinical presentation**

**a.** Scoliosis most commonly occurs as a right thoracic curve, but thoracolumbar, lumbar, and double curves can occur.

**b.** Thoracic curves are most noticeable because of the associated chest rotation and deformity, creating a rib hump.

**c.** If the scoliosis is severe, exceeding about 60°, significant cardiopulmonary complications can occur.

**3. Treatment**

**a. Braces.** The **Milwaukee** and **Boston braces** are relatively recent additions to the management of scoliosis. They may eliminate the need for surgery in many patients.

(1) The brace is not expected to correct a curve that is already established when the diagnosis is made, but is meant to prevent the scoliosis from advancing into a cardiopulmonary or serious cosmetic problem.

(2) Typically, patients are placed into braces:

(a) If the curve measures about 20° in a patient with significant growth still remaining

(b) If the scoliosis, even with a smaller angle, is clearly progressing during a period of observation

**b. Surgery**

(1) A variety of surgical techniques are available, but the one most commonly performed is **Harrington rod fixation** with bone graft fusion of the spine over the area of the curve.

(2) Significant, although never complete, correction is obtained, and the long-term results are maintained by the bone graft's healing and fusing the spine in the corrected position.

**c. Electrical stimulation**

(1) Recent work suggests that using electrodes to stimulate the muscles on the convex side of the curve can prevent the progression of scoliosis, much as a brace would.

(2) Clinical trials are under way to allow further assessment of the initial encouraging results of this technique.

**C. Foot deformities** constitute a large part of pediatric orthopedic practice.

**1. Etiology**

**a.** Idiopathic foot deformities are quite common and include **metatarsus adductus, talipes equinovalgus (clubfoot)**, and **planovalgus**.

**b.** However, a careful neurologic evaluation must be done to make sure that the foot deformity is not due to a **neuromuscular disorder**. Poliomyelitis, cerebral palsy, myelomeningocele, diastematomyelia, and Charcot-Marie-Tooth muscular atrophy can all present with foot deformities.

**c.** In addition, **congenital dislocated hips** must be ruled out whenever a child presents with a foot deformity.

**2. Flatfoot** seldom represents a significant problem, and does not need treatment unless it causes symptoms or unless the neurologic examination is abnormal.

**3. Clubfoot** requires early treatment.

**a.** Repeated manipulation and casting will correct the deformity in some cases.

**b.** However, if the foot is relatively resistant to manipulation and casting, surgery is needed.

(1) In recent years, surgical soft tissue releases before age 1 year have shown a better prognosis than manipulation and casting.

(2) Recurrence of the clubfoot despite correction remains a problem until the cartilaginous anlage of the child's foot has become the fixed osseous bone of the adolescent.

**4. Neuromuscular foot disorders**

**a.** Treatment of the "neuromuscular foot" includes initial correction to a plantigrade neutral foot, either by manipulation of the very immature foot or by osteotomy and fusion of the more mature adolescent foot.

**b.** Once the foot alignment is corrected, then muscle transfers are carried out to prevent deformity. Tendons are transferred to replace the function of a paralyzed foot or to weaken the function of a spastic foot.

# 33
# Pediatric Surgery

Bruce E. Jarrell
Charles W. Wagner

## I. INTRODUCTION

**A.** Pediatric surgery has evolved as a subspecialty for several reasons.

1. Infants and children differ from adults physiologically as well as anatomically.
   **a.** For example, their nutritional needs and fluid and electrolyte management are not the same as for adults.
   **b.** Thus, specialized knowledge is required for the care of pediatric surgical patients.

2. Infants and children also differ to some extent in the types of disorders that require surgical management. For example, in infants, many such disorders are congenital malformations requiring prompt correction, and again specialized knowledge is needed.

**B.** The full discussion of specialized pediatric considerations is far too extensive to be covered in this book. Therefore, only certain topics have been touched on. For more complete information, the reader is referred to standard textbooks on pediatric surgery.

## II. CONGENITAL HERNIAS (see also Chapter 1, section X)

### A. Inguinal hernia

1. Repair of an inguinal hernia remains the most common general surgical procedure in the child. The defect is due to nonfusion of the processus vaginalis, not to a breakdown of the floor of the inguinal canal.

2. **Incidence**
   **a.** Inguinal hernia occurs in 1% to 3% of all children.
      **(1)** The hernia is on the right about 60% of the time, on the left about 30% of the time, and bilateral between 10% and 15% of the time.
      **(2)** The male to female ratio is 6 to 1.
   **b.** In premature infants the incidence is one and one-half to two times greater.
   **c.** There is also an increased incidence of hernias in patients with hydrocephalus who are treated by ventriculoperitoneal shunts.

3. **Clinical presentation**
   **a.** The age at diagnosis is in infancy, with about 35% of patients presenting before the age of 6 months.
   **b.** The classic history and clinical presentation is that of a mass or bulge in the groin, scrotum, or labia, usually occurring at times of abdominal pain. The mass usually disappears after the straining or crying has been resolved.

4. **Physical examination** may reveal the mass in the groin or scrotum. It is for the most part easily reducible.
   **a.** If no mass is present, one may feel the thickened spermatic cord, which represents the nondistended hernia sac. This has been described as the "silk glove" sign.
   **b.** If no hernia is identified but the patient's history is both classic and reliable, then most surgeons feel that surgery is indicated.

5. **Incarceration**
   **a.** In the male, the risk associated with a hernia is the chance of incarceration of the intestine.
      **(1)** Intestinal ischemia and obstruction can occur.
      **(2)** Also, with time, the entrapped bowel becomes edematous enough to compress the spermatic vessels and cause testicular ischemia with resultant necrosis.

   **b.** In females, the intestine does not usually incarcerate into the hernia, but the ovary may. While ischemia of the ovary may result, this is not usually the case.

   **c. Treatment** includes reduction of the incarcerated hernia, hydration of the patient, and herniorrhaphy.

    **(1)** These steps should all be done within 48 to 72 hours.

    **(2)** Reduction is performed, with or without sedation, by gentle, continuous pressure on the incarcerated intestine.

    **(3)** Almost all hernias in children will reduce. However, the chance of reducing necrotic intestine is very low.

  **6. Herniorrhaphy**

   **a.** A hernia should be repaired soon after it is diagnosed unless there is a major medical reason not to use general anesthesia.

   **b.** In most children, the repair can be done as daytime surgery without hospitalization.

   **c.** Herniorrhaphy in the child consists of identifying the sac, dissecting the spermatic structures free, and ligating the sac high at the internal ring of the inguinal canal. Very rarely is there a need for a floor repair.

   **d. Complications** of the procedure include damage to the vas deferens, vascular injury to the testes, recurrence of the hernia, and iatrogenic cryptorchidism.

    **(1) Recurrence** can be associated with both Hunter's syndrome and Elhers-Danlos syndrome.

    **(2) Iatrogenic cryptorchidism** occurs when the testicle has been mobilized from the scrotum but not properly replaced. The point to remember is that unlike regular cryptorchidism, in which the testes may later descend, the testes will remain in the abnormally high position with iatrogenic cryptorchidism.

**B. Diaphragmatic hernias** are communications through the diaphragm that allow abdominal contents to migrate into the thoracic cavity. The incidence of this defect is 1 in 4000 births.

  **1. Etiology.** Two underlying anatomic defects are common; both result from the failure of the surrounding tissues to fuse in utero.

   **a. Foramen of Bochdalek** is a posterolateral diaphragmatic defect.

    **(1)** This hernia (Fig. 33-1) is the most common congenital hernia.

    **(2)** It occurs most often in the left hemidiaphragm. It is bilateral in fewer than 10% of infants.

   **b. Foramen of Morgagni** is an anterior diaphragmatic defect. It is much less common and generally results in less severe problems.

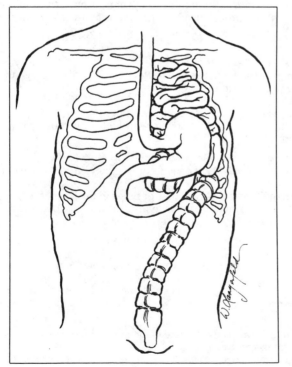

**Figure 33-1.** Bochdalek hernia.

    **2.** The **diagnosis** of herniation of abdominal contents into the thorax is based primarily on impaired ventilatory capacity.

        **a.** The earlier that respiratory distress is noted in the infant, especially if it occurs during the first 24 hours, the more severe the impairment and the worse the prognosis.

        **b. Physical examination** reveals the following:

            **(1)** Tachypnea, dyspnea, use of accessory muscles for ventilation, cyanosis, and nasal flaring

            **(2)** Decreased or absent breath sounds on the affected side

            **(3)** Heart sounds that are shifted away from the affected side

            **(4)** Bowel sounds in the affected hemithorax

            **(5)** Scaphoid abdomen, due to the migration of abdominal contents into the chest

        **c.** The **chest roentgenogram** has signs typical of herniation:

            **(1)** A loculated gas pattern in the affected hemithorax

            **(2)** A mediastinal shift away from the hernia

            **(3)** Atelectasis of the unaffected lung

            **(4)** The presence of the nasogastric tube in the affected hemithorax after passage of the tube through the nose or mouth

    **3. Preoperative management**

        **a.** Gastrointestinal decompression should be performed via nasogastric or orogastric tube.

        **b.** A pneumothorax in the unaffected hemithorax should be sought and, if present, treated with a chest tube.

        **c.** Attempts to correct the respiratory insufficiency preoperatively will be futile until the herniated contents are returned to the abdomen.

    **4. Operative management** is based on the following principles:

        **a.** Surgical reduction of the herniated contents back into the abdomen (through an abdominal incision); this can immediately relieve the distress

        **b.** Repair of the hernia defect

        **c.** Exploratory laparotomy to diagnose associated congenital anomalies; intestinal malrotation is often associated with this hernia

        **d.** Insertion of a chest tube into the affected hemithorax

        **e.** Careful monitoring of the infant's acid-base balance and respiratory function

        **f.** Creation of a gastrostomy for decompression of the gastrointestinal tract

    **5. Postoperative management** is aimed primarily at maintaining adequate ventilation and perfusion, and includes the following:

        **a.** Respiratory support on a ventilator as needed, with monitoring of arterial blood gases

        **b.** Treatment of atelectasis of either lung and the prevention of retained secretions

        **c.** Use of chest tube suction on the affected side to stabilize the mediastinum in the midline

        **d.** Observation for contralateral pneumothorax and rapid treatment if it occurs

        **e.** Adequate gastrointestinal compression

            **(1)** The abdomen is small and may not be able to hold all of the contents after reduction.

            **(2)** The loss of the "right of domain" of the abdominal contents will greatly distend the abdomen and raise intra-abdominal pressures.

            **(3)** Abdominal distention will significantly impair both thoracic excursion and venous return from the lower body.

    **6.** The **prognosis** for the infant with a diaphragmatic hernia remains a function of the hernia's preoperative severity and the time of its presentation.

        **a.** The immediate mortality rate is 50% or more.

        **b.** The resolution of respiratory insufficiency in the postoperative period depends on the maturity of the contralateral lung.

            **(1)** The ipsilateral lung is almost always hypoplastic when a diaphragmatic hernia is present, and therefore does not aid in respiratory function during the immediate postoperative period.

            **(2)** If the infant survives, the lung will eventually develop.

        **c.** No permanent respiratory difficulties have been noted in later life once the acute pulmonary insufficiency has resolved.

## III. ABDOMINAL WALL DEFECTS

    **A.** These can be divided into two categories, gastroschisis and omphalocele. Although the abdominal contents are located outside of the peritoneal cavity in each type, the similarities, both developmental and therapeutic, end at that point.

    **1. Gastroschisis** is an opening in the abdominal wall, usually immediately adjacent to the umbilicus, which is located in the normal position.

    **a.** During fetal development, the abdominal wall is completely formed, but the peritoneal cavity does not enlarge enough to hold the abdominal contents.

    **b.** The protruding viscera, which consists of the midportion of the small intestine, the spleen, stomach, colon, and occasionally the liver, has no protective covering.

    **c.** The intestine is edematous, semirigid, leathery, and matted together as a result of chemical peritonitis.

    **d.** Associated anomalies and syndromes are rare.

  **2. Omphalocele** is an opening in the abdominal wall at the umbilicus.

    **a.** It is due to incomplete closure of the somatic folds of the anterior abdominal wall in the fetus.

    **b.** Unless ruptured, a sac covers the extruded visceral contents, and there are no signs of chemical peritonitis.

    **c.** The liver and small bowel are the most common organs to protrude through the defect.

    **d.** The omphalocele may be a part of the **pentalogy of Cantrell**, which consists of:

      **(1)** Omphalocele

      **(2)** Diaphragmatic hernia

      **(3)** Cleft sternum

      **(4)** Absent pericardium

      **(5)** Intracardiac defects

    **e.** If the caudal folds are involved, there will be exstrophy of the bladder or exstrophy of a cloaca.

    **f.** Approximately 50% of these infants will have one or more **associated anomalies**, including trisomies 13 and 18, Beckwith's syndrome, and cardiac, neurologic, and genitourinary malformations.

**B. Diagnosis** of either gastroschisis or omphalocele is obvious.

  **1.** Further studies may be required on an infant with omphalocele to define any associated problems.

  **2.** The associated anomalies may dictate the approach in management of these patients.

**C. Preoperative management** is similar in both disorders.

  **1.** Gastrointestinal decompression is instituted, as well as intravenous fluids and antibiotics.

  **2.** Both disorders are associated with hypoproteinemia, and the infant should be given albumin.

  **3. Protection of the abdominal contents** is imperative, especially because the escape of moisture and heat is considerable in these patients.

    **a.** In the unruptured omphalocele this is done by wrapping antibiotic-soaked gauze around the sac to prevent it from drying out.

    **b.** A gastroschisis or a ruptured omphalocele is protected with moist antibiotic-soaked gauze under a plastic covering (Saran wrap, an intestinal bag, or a plastic tracheostomy bag).

  **4.** When the patient with gastroschisis has a small defect and a swollen intestine, kinking of the vascular supply may occur at the edge of the defect. This vascular compromise may be prevented by placing the infant on its side.

**D. Surgical management** differs somewhat for the two disorders. However, the goal in both conditions is to cover the abdominal viscera, either with prosthetic material or with the abdominal wall itself.

  **1.** For a **gastroschisis**, primary closure involves decompressing the gastrointestinal tract and stretching the abdominal wall over the defect.

    **a.** If the closure is excessively tight, the blood supply to the intestine, abdominal wall, or lower extremities will be compromised.

    **b.** To avoid this complication, it is better to cover the exposed organs temporarily with prosthetic materials.

      **(1)** Currently, Silastic sheeting is used because it is nonreactive and allows the gradual reduction of the viscera into the abdominal cavity.

      **(2)** This **staged repair** requires daily reduction under sterile conditions. Reduction should be completed within 10 days to minimize the risk of infection.

    **c.** A gastrostomy is placed for decompression in either method of treatment.

  **2.** For an **omphalocele**, the choice of procedures includes primary closure, staged repair, or, for an unruptured omphalocele, nonoperative management. The important factor is the size of the defect.

        **a.** The greater the size of the defect, the less the peritoneal cavity has enlarged, and with a large defect, primary closure may involve too much tension

            **(1)** An alternative method of treatment is to cover the defect with skin flaps, leaving the resultant ventral hernia to be repaired at a later date.

            **(2)** A Silastic-sheet covering can be used to stage the repair; by keeping tension on the prosthetic sac, the Silastic will stretch the abdominal wall enough to accommodate the herniated viscera.

            **(3)** As with a staged repair of a gastroschisis, closure must be accomplished within 10 days.

        **b. Nonoperative management** offers an alternative in those patients with complex associated anomalies.

            **(1)** The sac is coated with tincture of merbromin (Mercurochrome).

            **(2)** An eschar will form, with subsequent coverage by granulation tissue.

            **(3)** Repair of the resultant ventral hernia can be done at a later date.

            **(4)** The risks associated with this method are rupture of the sac, requiring subsequent repair in an infected area; sepsis; undiagnosed intestinal atresia; mercury poisoning; and a prolonged hospitalization.

        **c.** As with gastroschisis, a gastrostomy is placed for decompression.

### E. Postoperative management

    **1.** With primary closure, respiration may be inhibited if the reduced abdominal contents compress the diaphragm. Patients may require muscular paralysis and mechanical ventilation until the abdomen stretches enough to accommodate the viscera.

    **2.** Venous return may be compromised due to compression of the inferior vena cava.

        **a.** For vascular access, upper extremity veins should be used.

        **b.** The legs may show signs of venous obstruction and resultant edema.

    **3.** With staged repair, the patient needs to be observed after each daily reduction, for both respiratory compromise and decreased venous return due to increased abdominal pressure.

    **4.** With both primary and staged repairs, patients will require hyperalimentation because intestinal motility and absorption are slow to return.

    **5.** After repair of an unruptured omphalocele, intestinal function is not as delayed as in gastroschisis; however, hyperalimentation may still be needed.

### F. Results

    **1. Gastroschisis**, while more difficult to manage initially, has very few long-term problems.

        **a.** Intestinal strictures may occur at the site of evisceration and will require resection at a later date.

        **b.** The mortality rate, formerly around 30%, has improved greatly with the use of hyperalimentation and is now around 10%. Mortality is related to sepsis and the viability of the gastrointestinal tract at the time of surgery.

        **c.** With resection for intestinal gangrene, short-bowel syndrome may develop.

    **2.** The outcome for **omphalocele** is related to the size and location of the defect and to the presence of associated anomalies. The overall mortality rate ranges from 20% to 60%.

## IV. ESOPHAGEAL ATRESIA AND TRACHEOESOPHAGEAL MALFORMATIONS

  **A.** These anomalies occur once in every 3000 live births.

    **1.** They encompass a spectrum of lesions that can vary greatly in their time of presentation and in their treatment.

    **2.** There is a high incidence of associated maldevelopments in other organ systems that may complicate the treatment of these patients.

  **B.** There are **four types of lesions** (Fig. 33-2)

    **1.** The most common type is an **esophageal atresia** (proximal pouch) **with a distal tracheoesophageal fistula**; it occurs in 86% of the cases.

    **2.** The next two occur almost equally (in 6% of cases); they are:

        **a. Pure esophageal atresia** (proximal and distal blind pouches) **without fistula**

        **b. Tracheoesophageal fistula without atresia** (H fistula)

    **3.** The most uncommon type (in 2% of cases) combines **both a proximal and a distal tracheoesophageal fistula with a proximal atresia**.

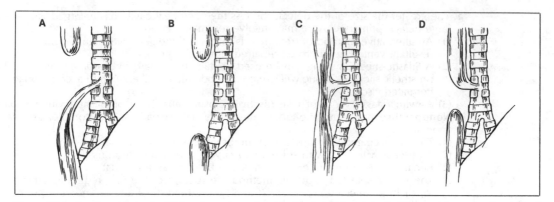

**Figure 33-2.** Esophageal atresia. (*A*) Esophageal atresia with distal tracheoesophageal fistula, (*B*) proximal and distal blind pouches without fistula, (*C*) H fistula, and (*D*) esophageal atresia with proximal tracheoesophageal fistula. (Adapted from Altman RP, et al: Pediatric surgery. In *Principles of Surgery*, 4th ed. Edited by Schwartz SI, et al. New York, McGraw-Hill, 1984, p 1644.)

 **C. Associated anomalies.** In approximately 40% of these patients other malformations are present in one or more organ systems.

  **1.** The **heart** is the most common single involved organ, usually by an endocardial cushion defect.

  **2.** A well-recognized anomaly complex is called the **VATER complex**. This involves **v**ertebral and **a**nal defects, **t**racheoesophageal fistula, and **r**adial limb dysplasia or **r**enal abnormalities.

   **a.** The complex may be fully or partially demonstrated; that is, one or any combination of lesions may occur.

   **b.** If it seems to be partial, the complete complex must be ruled out.

 **D.** The **diagnosis** of esophageal atresia and tracheoesophageal fistula is usually made soon after birth, when the affected infant exhibits some form of respiratory distress.

  **1.** Some symptoms are caused by **aspiration of material from the upper pouch**.

   **a.** The infant may appear to be salivating excessively, and may show continuous drooling.

   **b.** The aspiration may also cause coughing spasms or intermittent choking, or cyanosis that develops when the infant is feeding.

  **2.** If a fistula is present, the patient also suffers from continuous **aspiration of gastric secretions**. This aspiration is more severe and more harmful than that from the upper pouch.

  **3.** Tachypnea and signs of pneumonia may develop.

  **4.** With a pure atresia, the abdomen will be scaphoid due to the unused gastrointestinal tract.

  **5.** Attempts to pass a tube through the nose into the stomach will fail, since the tube will stop in the blind pouch of the esophagus, confirming the suspicion of esophageal atresia.

 **E. Roentgenograms** of both the chest and the abdomen are important, both in diagnosis and in preparation for treatment.

  **1.** The chest film will show the blind upper pouch with the failure of passage by the gastric tube.

  **2.** A gas-free abdomen speaks for a pure atresia.

  **3.** Hyperventilation, atelectasis, or pneumonia must be evaluated so that the proper surgical approach (i.e., immediate versus delayed repair) can be chosen.

  **4.** Identification of the aortic arch is also necessary for proper surgical management.

  **5.** The length of the esophageal defect can be measured on a lateral film.

 **F.** In the **choice of operative management**, surgical judgment is based on the various factors mentioned above.

  **1. Primary repair** at the time of presentation can be done if the defect is less than 2 cm and there are no signs of pneumonitis.

  **2.** If the defect is greater than 2 cm, or extends the length of 2½ vertebral bodies, **delayed repair** may be needed.

**G. Preoperative management**

1. **With any surgical approach**, several steps are taken once the diagnosis is made.
   a. The patient requires constant **decompression** of the proximal pouch. This is done by means of a sump tube with constant suction (Replogle tube).
   b. The infant is also kept in an **upright position**. A "chalasia chair" is convenient for this.

2. If a **delayed repair** is decided upon, a **gastrostomy** is performed.
   a. This prevents further gastric aspiration.
   b. It also provides a route for preoperative feedings in cases where surgery is delayed for an extended period.

3. If a **pure atresia** is present, daily **stretching** of the proximal pouch will shorten the defect in preparation for eventual repair.

**H. Surgical approach.** At the time of surgery, the approach is the same for either immediate or delayed repair.

1. Broad-spectrum antibiotic therapy is begun.

2. If not previously done, a gastrostomy may be performed, although this measure is controversial.

3. An extrapleural dissection is currently favored.
   a. The purpose is to prevent the complication of an empyema from occurring as the result of an anastomotic leak.
   b. The repair is done through the hemithorax opposite the aortic arch.

4. The tracheoesophageal fistula is repaired.

5. A primary esophagostomy is performed.
   a. Care is taken during dissection of the distal esophagus, as the blood supply here is tenuous.
   b. An adequate length of esophagus is necessary to create a tension-free anastomosis, and is obtained by dissecting the proximal pouch.

6. A drain is placed in the extrapleural space.

**I. Postoperative care** is directed at potential pulmonary and esophageal problems.

1. The infant is extubated as soon as possible to protect the tracheal repair.

2. Vigorous pulmonary toilet is necessary in order to clear up any previous pneumonia and to prevent the need for reintubation.
   a. Reintubation may disrupt either the esophageal repair or the tracheal repair, or both.
   b. There is also a degree of tracheal malacia which compromises pulmonary function.

3. The infant is kept in a chalasia chair because esophageal functions at first will not be adequate to control secretions.

4. Esophagotracheal suction is done carefully and with a specifically defined length of tubing. Disruptions of the esophagus can occur during placement of a suction catheter through the anastomotic line.

5. The esophagus is evaluated in 7 to 10 days by means of a "barium swallow."
   a. If no leak is present, oral feedings are started and, if tolerated, the extrapleural drain is removed.
   b. Prior to this, the gastrostomy, if present, may be used for feedings.

**J. Surgical follow-up** is critically important. There are well-recognized **problems that can develop** which can have a drastic effect on the outcome in these patients.

1. The major concern is **esophageal dysmotility** and its concomitant problems.
   a. The patient may develop a **dilated proximal pouch**, with resultant aspiration or tracheal compression.
   b. The patient may also have severe **gastroesophageal reflux** and aspiration.
      (1) **Anastomotic stricture**, once thought to be solely related to ischemia at the suture line, is now considered to be a consequence of esophagitis from gastroesophageal reflux.
      (2) Currently, if gastroesophageal reflux can be implicated in postoperative problems, an **"antireflux" procedure**, usually a Nissen fundoplication, is recommended.

2. **Recurrent fistulas** were formerly considered to be a relatively common potential problem, but in recent studies they have been rare.

K. The **prognosis** is related to the size of the patient, the condition of the lungs, and the presence or absence of associated anomalies. Patients have been grouped into three **categories**:

1. **Group A**—100% survival: Patients weigh over 2500 g, have no associated anomalies, and no signs of pneumonitis.

2. **Group B**—80% survival: Patients either:
   a. Weigh 1800 to 2500 g
   b. Weigh over 2500 g but have mild pneumonitis
   c. Have one or more associated anomalies that are not life-threatening

3. **Group C**—43% survival: Patients either:
   a. Weigh less than 1800 g
   b. Have severe pneumonitis
   c. Have a life-threatening anomaly

## V. DISORDERS OF INTESTINAL ROTATION

A. **Malrotation** is the abnormal placement and fixation of the midgut into the peritoneal cavity (Fig. 33-3).

1. The **involved portion of the gut** includes all of the small intestine from the ampulla of Vater to the proximal two-thirds of the transverse colon.

2. There are two **potential problems** with this lesion.
   a. **Intestinal obstruction** can result from adhesive bands across the second portion of the duodenum fixing to the right upper quadrant.
   b. More serious, a **midgut volvulus** can occur.
      (1) This develops when the intestine twists on its vascular pedicle (the superior mesenteric artery) and causes ischemia as well as obstruction of the entire midgut.
      (2) The result can be catastrophic, with gangrene of the entire small bowel.

3. Because of the seriousness of the potential problem, the lesion must be handled expeditiously.

B. **Embryonic development**

1. During **normal in utero development**, the midgut develops extra-abdominally. It then migrates intraperitoneally, where it undergoes a 270° rotation. The results are as follows.
   a. The cecum ends up in the right lower quadrant.
   b. The right colon becomes fixed in the right paracolic gutter.
   c. The duodenum becomes fixed in the retroperitoneal location, with the superior mesenteric artery passing over the duodenum.

2. **Malrotation** causes several **displacements.**
   a. The cecum is not in the right lower quadrant, and the duodenum does not pass posterior to the superior mesenteric artery.
   b. Instead of the base of the small bowel being fixed from the ligament of Treitz to the cecum

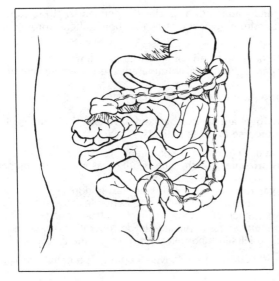

**Figure 33-3.** Malrotation and volvulus of the midgut.

in the right lower quadrant, the whole midgut is anchored on the superior mesenteric artery.
   c. Various stages of fixation of the cecum can be seen, but it usually is fixed to the right upper quadrant with fibrinous bands (Ladd's bands) that extend across the second portion of the duodenum.

   3. Malrotation can occur independently or can be associated with **other malformations** such as a diaphragmatic hernia and omphalocele or gastroschisis.

C. **Early diagnosis** of malrotation is crucial to prevent the development of a volvulus with resulting intestinal gangrene. Therefore, when malrotation in an infant is suspected, all efforts are made to confirm the diagnosis rapidly.

   1. Bilious vomiting is the usual presenting symptom.

   2. Passage of a bloody stool is a late occurrence and implies ischemia with necrosis of the bowel mucosa, bowel wall, or both.

   3. The infant may appear normal, with hemodynamic stability, or may be dehydrated and in shock.

   4. **Roentgenograms** are very useful in diagnosis.
      a. The plain film may demonstrate the **"double-bubble"** sign, produced by intestinal gas confined to the stomach and duodenum with no gas in the residual, unused gastrointestinal tract.
      b. The "upper GI series" may demonstrate an abnormally located ligament of Treitz, the presence of the duodenum to the left of midline, duodenal obstruction, or a "beaked" end in the barium column at the point of the intestinal twist.

   5. If the diagnosis of malrotation is made, or, more importantly, if the diagnosis is entertained but cannot be ruled out, prompt **surgical exploration** is imperative, because approximately 50% of infants with obstructive malrotation will have a volvulus.

D. The **surgical procedure** for malrotation will vary with the presence or absence of volvulus and the status of the intestine.

   1. **Simple malrotation** is treated by the **Ladd procedure**.
      a. This consists of releasing the adhesive bands and mobilizing the duodenum.
      b. The cecum is placed in the left lower quadrant and the duodenum in the right lateral abdomen so that both organs will be in positions that should prevent intestinal obstruction or ischemia.
      c. An appendectomy is performed and the remaining abdominal contents are examined for other anomalies, such as a duodenal web.

   2. The presence of a **volvulus** requires several **preliminary steps**.
      a. The first step is counterclockwise detorsion of the midgut volvulus.
      b. The bowel is then examined for viability and for areas of necrosis.
         (1) If small areas of gangrene are present, resection is performed, followed by the Ladd procedure.
         (2) If large amounts of the midgut appear necrotic, long lengths of bowel are not resected.
            (a) Instead, the bowel is untwisted and the abdomen is closed and then reexplored 24 hours later.
            (b) This second look allows marginally viable tissue to recover, hopefully minimizing the amount of bowel to be resected.

E. **Prognosis**

   1. The recurrence of a **midgut volvulus** following surgical exploration and a Ladd procedure occurs in as many as 10% of cases, usually in the immediate postoperative period.

   2. The long-term sequelae are minimal after repair of **simple malrotation**.

   3. When **extensive intestinal resection** is required, the result depends strongly on the amount of intestine remaining. Extreme resections result in severe malabsorption and even in death.

## VI. INTESTINAL ATRESIA

A. **Duodenal atresia and stenosis** occur because the second portion of the duodenum fails to recanalize in the early embryonic stages.

**1.** The lesion may be complex, partial, or in the form of a web.

**2.** Because the lesion develops early in gestation, there is a high rate of **associated anomalies**.
   **a. Trisomy 21** occurs in 30% of infants with duodenal malformations.
   **b.** Many infants have **cardiac lesions** and various elements of the **VATER complex**.
   **c.** An **annular pancreas** may be present, with the pancreas forming a ring around the duo-denum. This anomaly is now thought to result from the malformation, rather than being a cause of duodenal stenosis.

**3. Diagnosis**
   **a.** This is usually made from two simple findings.
       **(1)** The first is bilious vomiting that occurs soon after birth in a nondistended infant. This speaks for a high obstruction.
       **(2)** The second, confirmed with abdominal roentgenography, is the classic **double-bubble sign** (air in the stomach and proximal dilated duodenum).
           **(a)** This speaks for duodenal obstruction, but can also be seen with malrotation.
           **(b)** While duodenal atresia or stenosis in itself is not life-threatening, malrotation is (see section IV).
               **(i)** Therefore, if delay in treatment is being considered in the patient with a double-bubble x-ray, a barium contrast study to rule out malrotation is necessary.
               **(ii)** This may be a barium enema to localize the cecum or an upper gastrointestinal study to see the duodenal sweep.
   **b.** With an upper gastrointestinal study, a duodenal web may be identified.

**4.** Once the diagnosis is made, the patient is **prepared for surgery**.
   **a.** Gastric decompression and fluid resuscitation are performed as needed.
   **b.** Broad-spectrum antibiotic therapy is begun.
   **c.** Since these lesions have a high association with other more critical anomalies, stabilization and evaluation of these lesions may be done prior to surgery.
   **d.** However, this can only be done if malrotation is ruled out as the cause of duodenal obstruction.

**5. Operative management** has as its goal the reestablishment of a patent gastrointestinal tract.
   **a.** The site of obstruction is identified.
   **b.** Usually a duodenoduodenostomy can be performed. If not, a duodenojejunostomy is a good alternative. Gastrojejunostomy is contraindicated.
   **c.** If a **web** is present, the duodenum is opened at the site of obstruction, the web is excised, and the duodenum is closed. Care must be taken to identify the ampulla of Vater, for it is also located on the mesenteric side of the web.
   **d.** If an **annular pancreas** is present, care is taken not to damage this structure.
       **(1)** In no circumstance is the pancreas divided.
       **(2)** The annular pancreas is not the obstructing lesion (the duodenal stenosis is), and the mortality rate is extremely high among patients in whom division of the annular pancreas is performed.
       **(3)** The annular pancreas can usually be bypassed by a duodenoduodenostomy.
   **e.** Because 15% of the patients have other gastrointestinal atresias, a thorough search is undertaken to ensure the patency of the entire gastrointestinal tract.
   **f.** A gastrostomy is performed for gastrointestinal decompression.

**6. Postoperative care** is simple but requires patience.
   **a.** Gastrointestinal decompression is important, to protect the suture line and prevent possible aspiration.
   **b.** The return of gastrointestinal function is slow because of duodenal dysfunction and because the distal intestine is small due to disuse.
   **c.** Nutritional support by hyperalimentation may be needed.

**7. Long-term results** of surgery are good. Mortality in these patients is related to prematurity of the infant and to associated anomalies.

**B. Jejunal, ileal, and colonic atresias** are caused by in utero vascular accidents that result in ischemia of a segment of bowel, with consequent stenosis or atresia.

**1.** The **ileum** is most commonly affected; the **jejunum** and **colon** less often.
   **a.** The severity of the lesion is related to the size of the vascular arcade that was affected in utero.
   **b.** Since these are not embryonic maldevelopments, **associated anomalies** are much less common than with duodenal atresia. However, approximately 10% of patients will be found to have **cystic fibrosis**.

**2.** The **diagnosis** is suspected when an infant develops bilious vomiting after 24 hours of life.
   **a.** The degree of abdominal distention will vary with the level of the obstruction.
   **b.** The passage of meconium does not rule out an atresia, since the gastrointestinal tract was intact before the vascular accident.
   **c.** Abdominal **roentgenograms** will show various degrees of obstruction, depending on the level of the atresia or stenosis.
      **(1)** The picture can be confused with meconium ileus.
      **(2)** However, in atresia, air–fluid levels are present, whereas with a meconium ileus there is only distended bowel, without fluid levels, and a soap-bubble appearance.
   **d. Contrast studies** are helpful in both diagnosis and management.
      **(1)** A barium enema will reveal colonic lesions and perhaps low ileal lesions.
      **(2)** Hirschsprung's disease, meconium ileus, and other congenital disorders may also be ruled out, making diagnosis of the atresia more certain.
   **e.** All patients with small bowel or colonic atresia should have an early evaluation for cystic fibrosis.

**3. Preoperative treatment** includes gastrointestinal decompression and fluid replacement. Broad-spectrum antibiotics are begun.

**4. Surgery** is performed to reestablish intestinal continuity.
   **a.** The current **procedure of choice** is an end-to-end intestinal anastomosis.
      **(1)** This may be difficult because of the marked size disparity of the bowel, with the proximal bowel dilated and the distal, unused bowel small in size.
      **(2)** Because of this, tapering of the proximal bowel may aid in the repair.
   **b.** The distended bowel has been found to have varying degrees of impaired motility. Thus, gastrointestinal function may be extremely slow to return.
   **c.** A gastrostomy is placed to allow decompression, prevent aspiration, and protect the suture line.
   **d.** A thorough abdominal examination for **multiple atresias** is performed. Their overall occurrence rate is 6%, but the frequency is higher with ileal atresia, and very low with colonic atresia.
   **e.** In a patient with **both an atresia and meconium ileus**, the distal intestine may contain inspissated small bowel secretions. In this case, the site of inspissation should be irrigated with a 4% Mucomyst (acetylcysteine) solution to relieve any potential obstruction before the atresia is repaired.

**5. Postoperative management** involves decompression and patience.
   **a.** Hyperalimentation may be needed until the gastrointestinal tract begins to function.
   **b.** Malabsorption, if present, may prolong recovery time.

**6. Prognosis.** Since associated anomalies are few, survival is a function of the prematurity of the infant. Current results show a survival rate of nearly 100%.

**C.** A severe form of small bowel atresia is known as **"apple-peel" atresia** because of its appearance.

   **1.** This occurs when there is a large vascular accident to one or more of the mesenteric arcades in utero.

   **2.** There is loss of intestinal length and atresia of the remaining distal intestine.

   **3.** In these patients, return of gastrointestinal function is very prolonged and malabsorption is common.

## VII. IMPERFORATE ANUS (Fig. 33-4)

**A.** Abnormal termination of the anorectum has a clinical spectrum that ranges from a fistulous opening in the perineal area or a colourethral fistula to a completely blind ending of the rectum.

   **1.** The incidence of these malformations ranges from 1 in 1500 live births to 1 in 5000.

   **2.** The male to female ratio is 2 to 1.

**B.** While there are many proposed **classifications** for imperforate anus, the simplest is to divide them on the basis of sex and the relationship to the levator ani.

   **1.** With the **infralevator (low) type**, the rectum passes through the puborectalis sling.

   **2.** With the **supralevator (high) type**, the rectum does not pass through the puborectalis sling.

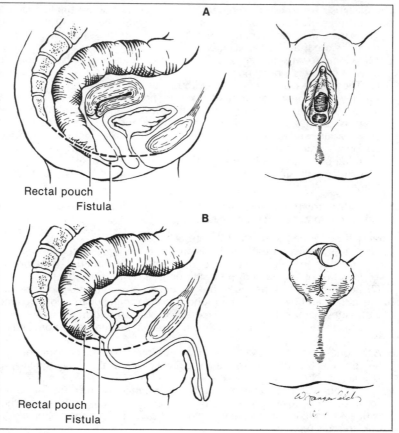

**Figure 33-4.** Imperforate anus. (*A*) In the female, (*B*) in the male.

3. The infralevator type is more common in females, while the supralevator type is more common in males.

C. **Associated anomalies** are common in patients with imperforate anus.

1. The **genitourinary tract** is the most commonly involved organ system.
   a. Malformations include renal agenesis, renal dysplasia, hypospadias, epispadias, and bladder exstrophy.
   b. These findings have been reported in up to 40% of patients with imperforate anus.

2. **Other organ systems** involved are:
   a. The **gastrointestinal tract** (in 15%), most often as a tracheoesophageal fistula
   b. The **heart** (in 7%)
   c. The **skeletal system** (in 6%)
      (1) Defects include hemivertebrae, sacral agenesis, and spina bifida.
      (2) While sacral agenesis may not physically affect the patient, it may have some implications for the successful function of the surgically created anus.

D. While the **diagnosis** of imperforate anus would appear to be easy, determining the **level of the lesion** is critical for appropriate management.

1. The first step is a thorough examination of the perineum and, in females, the vaginal vault.
   a. A fistula in the perineal area may be found.
   b. The patient may have a fistulous tract which opens:
      (1) In the case of the female, to the apex of the vagina
      (2) In the case of the male, to the posterior urethra

2. If no external fistula is identified, one must attempt to determine if the rectum has traversed the puborectalis sling.
   a. Using a cross-table lateral x-ray of the pelvis, one may identify the extent of the rectum by visualizing the end of the infracolonic air.

(1) A line drawn from the posterior portion of the symphysis pubis to the tip of the coccyx (the **pubococcygeal line**) aids in differentiating the infralevator from the supralevator type.

(2) Air visible in the bladder suggests a posterior urethral fistula, which implies a supralevator type.

(3) If the distance from the tip of the colonic air column to the anal dimple is greater than 2 cm, the lesion is supralevator in type.

b. In the male, meconium in the urine should be sought. This occurs only if there is a fistula between the rectal pouch and the urinary tract.

**E. Surgical management**

1. If an **external fistula** is identified, there are several alternatives in the initial management.
   a. If the fistula can be dilated, it may function satisfactorily until the patient is older, at which time the opening can be relocated to the correct site (**Pott's anal transfer**).
   b. If the mucosa is close to the opening, the fistula may be enlarged by a procedure known as a **Denis Brown cutback**.
   c. These procedures are more common in females because the **infralevator type** of imperforate anus occurs more often in females.

2. The treatment for the **supralevator type** of imperforate anus is initially the formation of a colostomy, followed by formation of a neorectum and anus at about 1 year of age.

**F. Postoperative care**

1. In part, this will depend on the type of imperforate anus.
   a. **Infralevator types** will require constant dilations until the stool obtains bulk.
   b. **Supralevator types** will require colostomy care until the definitive procedure can be performed. With the formation of the new anus, the patient may require dilations to prevent strictures.

2. The **goal of treatment** in these patients is to have a socially accepted, continent child. These children require patience during toilet training; they usually are trained between 3 and 5 years of age.

**G.** Two **problems** may develop in patients with a **fistula**.

1. They may develop symptomatic **urinary tract infections**.

2. They may also develop a **hyperchloremic acidosis** due to reabsorption of chloride by the colonic mucosa.
   a. This is characterized by lethargy, tachypnea, and elevation of the serum chloride and the blood urea nitrogen.
   b. While the condition may resolve with time, treatment with bicarbonate may be required and, if the condition is severe or not correctable, division of the rectal pouch–urinary tract fistula may be necessary before the time of the definitive procedure.

**H. Prognosis**

1. The mortality rate among patients with imperforate anus is directly related to the associated anomalies.

2. Functional morbidity is directly related to:
   a. Inappropriate management
   b. Associated neurologic dysfunction due either to spina bifida or to sacral agenesis

## VIII. HIRSCHSPRUNG'S DISEASE

**A. General information**

1. Hirschsprung's disease is caused by the congenital absence of parasympathetic ganglia cells in the wall of the gastrointestinal tract.
   a. As a result, the affected portions of the bowel are unable to relax and allow effective peristalsis to occur.
   b. Hirschsprung's disease always involves the rectum and extends proximally with no skip areas. Any other part of the gastrointestinal tract, or even the entire tract, may also be involved.

2. There is a male predominance of 4 to 1, except when the entire colon is involved. In that situation, the frequency ratio is reversed, with females predominating.

**3.** Some 30% of patients with Hirschsprung's disease have a relative afflicted with the disease.

**B. Clinical presentation**

**1.** The **newborn** with Hirschsprung's disease presents with a history of nonpassage of meconium.
   **a. Meconium** is usually passed within 24 hours after birth in term infants and within 48 hours in premature infants.
   **b.** Distention and bilious vomiting are common.

**2. Infants and older children** have a history of obstipation and constipation as well as a failure to thrive.
   **a.** Bouts of diarrhea, vomiting, and abdominal distention may herald the development of enterocolitis.
   **b. Enterocolitis** is sometimes associated with Hirschsprung's disease. If untreated, it has a high mortality rate.

**3.** Hirschsprung's disease may go **undiagnosed** for years following birth. It should be **suspected** in any patient with a chronic unexplained illness who has an abnormal bowel pattern dating back to early infancy.

**C. Physical examination** in the newborn reveals a distended abdomen.

**1.** Occasionally, loops of stool-filled bowel may be palpated.

**2.** Rectal examination shows the ampulla or rectal vault to be empty and the sphincter tone to be increased. Classically, on removal of the examining finger there is an explosion of watery stool.

**D. Diagnosis** is confirmed by roentgenography and tissue studies.

**1. Abdominal roentgenograms** reveal air–fluid levels and a distended bowel. Often no air is seen in the rectum.

**2.** A **barium enema** shows spasm and a narrowed lumen in the affected bowel.
   **a.** A **transition zone** is present, showing a dilated proximal gut and a narrowed distal gut.
      **(1)** This represents the most distal area in which ganglia cells are present.
      **(2)** In the majority of patients, this zone will be in the rectosigmoid segment of the colon.
   **b.** In total colonic Hirschsprung's disease or with a longer segment involving the small bowel, the findings may not be as clear and the transition zone may not be identified.

**3.** When the barium enema is inconclusive in a newborn with suspected Hirschsprung's disease, a 24-hour follow-up roentgenogram is obtained. The appearance of residual barium in the bowel is very suggestive of Hirschsprung's disease.

**4. Tissue confirmation**
   **a.** Usually, a **biopsy specimen** is examined for the presence of Auerbach's plexus in the muscular layer.
      **(1)** The specimen can be obtained by either of two procedures:
         **(a)** Seromuscular biopsy of the bowel wall at laparotomy
         **(b)** Full-thickness transrectal biopsy
      **(2)** Both of these require bowel preparation and general anesthesia.
   **b.** More recently, a **suction biopsy technique** has been developed.
      **(1)** With this procedure, the biopsy specimen is examined for Meissner's plexus in the submucosal layer.
      **(2)** The procedure can be performed at the bedside with little risk to the patient.
      **(3)** While the procedure is simple, it produces small specimens and requires an experienced pathologist for a correct interpretation.

**E.** Once the diagnosis is made, the patient is prepared for **surgery**.

**1. Preoperatively**, if enterocolitis is present, the patient will require parenteral antibiotics and gastric decompression. In addition, rectal decompression and irrigations with saline or an antibiotic solution are performed.

**2.** The usual **surgical approach** is to perform a colostomy in an area of intestine that has ganglia cells. Failure to perform this will result in a patient who will be functionally obstructed.

**3.** Once the gastrointestinal tract is patent, the child can be fed orally.

**F. Definitive corrective surgery** is usually done at the age of at least 1 year or at a weight of 20 lb or more.

1. While there are different operative procedures for the definitive repair, all have two goals in common:
   a. Removal of most or all of the involved intestine
   b. Reestablishment of a functional, continent anus

2. The three operations most commonly performed are the Swensen, Duhamel, and Soave procedures.
   a. The **Swensen procedure**
      (1) This is the standard operation, but it is difficult to perform and today is not done by the majority of pediatric surgeons.
      (2) The involved colon is excised to within 1 cm of the anal mucocutaneous margin.
      (3) The bowel is then sutured to the cuff of distal anorectal segment, thus establishing gastrointestinal continuity.
   b. The **Duhamel procedure**
      (1) The involved colon is excised to the level of the peritoneal reflection within the abdomen.
      (2) The proximal normal bowel is tunneled between the sacrum and rectum, and is then anastomosed end-to-side to the low anorectum.
   c. The **Soave procedure**
      (1) In this operation the involved colon is also excised to the level of the peritoneal reflection.
      (2) The mucosa is removed in the remaining rectum.
      (3) The proximal normal bowel is pulled through the stripped anorectal segment and sutured to the anorectal junction.

3. **Enterocolitis** may occur following these operations.
   a. Although it occurs rarely, the mortality rate is as high as 60%.
   b. Therefore, early diagnosis and treatment are critical.

**G.** The **prognosis** for infants properly treated for Hirschsprung's disease is excellent.

1. Anal dilation may be intermittently necessary if constipation occurs secondary to the retained aganglionic internal anal sphincter.

2. Problems of incontinence and fecal soiling occasionally occur.

## IX. AGNOGENIC DISORDERS OF INFANCY

**A. Pyloric stenosis**

1. In this condition, there is hypertrophy of the muscular layer of the pylorus, which causes gastric outlet obstruction.

2. The hallmark symptom is nonbilious projectile vomiting.

3. The etiology of the condition is unknown. However, there are consistent elements that imply a hereditary, genetic basis.
   a. It is a male-predominant disease; the male to female ratio is 4 to 1.
   b. However, the offspring of a female with pyloric stenosis stand a 10-fold greater than normal chance of developing pyloric stenosis.
   c. The condition is more common in whites than in blacks.

4. **Clinical presentation.** Pyloric stenosis occurs early in life, usually between the ages of 2 weeks and 2 months.
   a. The history is one of nonvomiting at birth, a gradual onset of vomiting, and final progression to nonbilious projectile vomiting.
   b. The vomiting may lead to dehydration.
   c. A hypochloremic, hypokalemic metabolic alkalosis may be present; this varies with the degree of dehydration.
   d. Jaundice is present in 10% of the infants. It is felt to be due to a deficiency of glucuronyl transferase, and resolves after surgical treatment of the pyloric stenosis.

5. **Diagnosis**
   a. **Physical examination** can often provide the diagnosis.
      (1) Palpation of a midepigastric mass in the right upper quadrant of an infant with projectile vomiting is the sine qua non of pyloric stenosis.

**(2)** However, finding the mass may require experience, persistence, and patience.
**(3)** Complete evacuation of the stomach by nasogastric tube may aid in finding the mass.
   **b.** An **upper GI series** may be helpful in diagnosis.
   **(1)** The findings include:
      **(a)** Gastric retention of 3 to 4 hours
      **(b)** Elongation and narrowing of the antrum
      **(c)** A "string" sign or "railroad track" sign (one or two thin barium tracts, respectively, through the pylorus)
   **(2)** A mass effect on the antrum must also be sought.
   **(3)** On fluoroscopy, the most important sign is the nonprogression of a peristaltic wave through the pylorus to the duodenum.
   **c.** The diagnostic value of ultrasonography is being investigated.

**6. Preoperative preparation**
   **a.** Correction of the alkalosis and volume deficits is necessary.
      **(1)** This is done by fluid replacement and potassium supplementation.
      **(2)** Adequate hydration is determined by voiding patterns (the normal infant voids four to five times per day).
      **(3)** Alkalosis correction is measured by the serum bicarbonate, which should be less than 28 mEq/dl before surgery is considered.
   **b.** Gastric decompression may also be instituted to protect against aspiration.

**7.** The **surgical procedure** is pyloromyotomy. This involves incision of the serosa over the pylorus and division of the hypertrophic muscle of the antrum but not the duodenum. The stomach is not entered.

**8. Postoperative care**
   **a.** The patient may be started on feedings of glucose and water or an electrolyte infant formula (e.g., Pedialyte) 4 to 6 hours after surgery.
   **b.** Vomiting will occur in 50% to 80% of the patients due to gastric atony or acute gastritis.
      **(1)** This is usually self-limited.
      **(2)** Occasionally the patient will benefit from gastric lavage with half-strength bicarbonate solution.
   **c.** Feedings are advanced on a prescribed schedule, with full feedings usually being reached by 24 hours after surgery. The patient may be discharged at this point.

**9. Complications**
   **a.** The major complication is duodenal perforation.
      **(1)** Its danger is not so much its occurrence as overlooking the problem at the time of surgery.
      **(2)** The perforation is handled by simple repair, nasogastric decompression for 48 hours, and antibiotics.
      **(3)** If it is recognized and handled appropriately, the major difficulty is an extended hospital stay.
      **(4)** If it is missed, the morbidity is severe and the incidence of mortality is significant.
   **b.** **Apnea** may also occur in the early postoperative period.
      **(1)** The patient should therefore have an apnea monitor in place for the first 24 hours postoperatively.
      **(2)** Postoperative apnea is associated with a serum carbon dioxide level greater than 28 ml/dl.

**10. Prognosis.** Once treated, pyloric stenosis does not recur, and long-term studies indicate no sequelae such as ulcer disease, food intolerance, or hiatal hernia. There are also no problems with growth and development.

**B. Biliary atresia** is a disease that affects the development of the biliary duct system both intra- and extrahepatically. It occurs once in every 25,000 births.

**1.** The **etiology** of the disease is unknown. Many possible causes have been implicated but not confirmed, including viral infections, hereditary factors, neonatal hepatitis, and malformation of the extrahepatic ductal system.

**2.** Biliary atresia appears to develop after birth. While isolated fetal cases have been described in Japan, none has been reported in the United States.

**3. Classification**
   **a.** Classically, biliary atresia is divided into correctable and noncorrectable types.
      **(1) Correctable biliary atresia** occurs in 20% of the cases.
         **(a)** There is a **normal common bile duct** that becomes atretic at some distal point.

**(b)** It is called "correctable" because the duct can be anastomosed to a jejunal conduit.

**(2)** In noncorrectable biliary atresia there is no macroscopic biliary system in the portal triad. Until the Kasai operation, there was no successful procedure to establish bile drainage of the liver.

**b.** The current feeling is that biliary atresia represents a progressive spectrum of disease and that the above divisions have little bearing on the eventual outcome.

4. **Clinically**, the child presents from 4 weeks to 4 months of age as a healthy but jaundiced infant with few other complaints. Some patients have associated light stools.
   **a.** Laboratory studies will show a conjugated hyperbilirubinemia.
   **b.** Liver function studies may or may not be abnormal, depending on the degree of liver damage from the cholestasis.

5. In **diagnosis**, the most important rule of thumb is that **persistent jaundice** beyond the first month of life must be evaluated.
   **a.** This may not affect the outcome in patients with medical causes of conjugated hyperbilirubinemia (for whom no effective therapy may exist). However, the prognosis of surgery for biliary atresia is related to the age at diagnosis.
   **b.** The workup is designed to differentiate true anatomic obstruction of the biliary tree from other causes of hyperbilirubinemia.
      **(1)** **TORCH** (**t**oxoplasmosis, **o**thers, **r**ubella, **c**ytomegalovirus, and **h**erpes simplex virus) titers are checked for possible infection.
      **(2)** Serum electrophoretic patterns are examined for $\alpha_1$-antitrypsin deficiency.
      **(3)** However, the results of these tests should not delay the consideration of more aggressive diagnostic procedures.
         **(a)** **Ultrasonography** is performed to examine for dilation of the biliary ducts and for the presence or absence of a gallbladder.
         **(b)** Also available are the newer **nuclear scans** employing technetium-99m ($^{99m}$Tc)-labeled iminodiacetic acid derivatives (PIPIDA, HIDA, DECIDA) to look for biliary excretion into the gastrointestinal tract.
         **(c)** **Percutaneous liver biopsy** is very helpful in experienced hands. If it shows bile duct proliferation in the face of hepatocellular necrosis, one should suspect biliary atresia.
   **c.** If biliary atresia cannot be ruled out by these methods, the child should undergo **diagnostic laparotomy**.
      **(1)** If **intraoperative cholangiography** demonstrates a normal patent biliary system, a **wedge biopsy** of the liver is taken and the surgical procedure is ended.
      **(2)** If patency cannot be demonstrated, the porta hepatis is explored in an effort to find the atretic duct.
      **(3)** If an extrahepatic duct can be found, a Roux-en-Y loop of jejunum is anastomosed to it. This is the so-called **correctable biliary atresia**.
      **(4)** If the common duct cannot be found, the dissection is then carried to the hilus of the porta hepatis and a **Kasai procedure** (hepatoportal enterostomy) is performed. This involves anastomosing a loop of jejunum to the liver hilus, incorporating the area where the common bile duct should be.

6. **Prognosis**
   **a.** Two factors influence the outcome of the Kasai operation:
      **(1)** The **age** of the patient at surgery
         **(a)** The best results are obtained in patients 8 to 12 weeks old.
         **(b)** To date there have been no long-term survivors among patients who were repaired when more than 20 weeks old. This is due to the irreversible liver damage that results from the cholestasis.
      **(2)** The **microscopic stage** of the biliary tree examined from the hilar dissection specimen
         **(a)** Patients with ductules greater than 120 $\mu$ in diameter have a good prognosis.
         **(b)** Patients with ductules smaller than 70 $\mu$ have a very poor prognosis.
         **(c)** A "gray zone" occurs when the ductules are between 70 and 120 $\mu$. While bile drainage may occur, resolution of the jaundice and reversibility of the liver disease may or may not occur.
   **b.** Currently, about 60% of the patients with biliary atresia undergo a **surgical repair**.
      **(1)** However, only a little more than one-half of these patients will have a resolution of jaundice and a return to normal liver function.
      **(2)** Therefore, one-third of all patients with biliary atresia who undergo surgery will be successfully treated by current surgical techniques. (These are United States results.)
   **c.** Until recently, if initial surgery failed to reverse the liver changes, no alternative was available.

**(1)** However, now **liver transplantation** allows one-half of the patients with failed hepatoportal enterostomies to be treated more successfully.

**(2)** More recently, the question of liver transplantation as primary therapy for biliary atresia has been raised for debate. The answer is still to be arrived at.

**C. Necrotizing enterocolitis** is an ischemic disorder of the intestine in the newborn.

**1.** While the etiology and underlying mechanism of the disease are unknown, many **causes** have been implicated, including bacterial infection, hypoxia, umbilical artery catheterization, aortic thrombosis, and hyperosmolar feedings.

**2.** The **basic defect** is an ischemic or hypoxic insult which causes intestinal mucosal sloughing. This may lead to bacterial invasion with subsequent intestinal gangrene and perforation.

**3.** Although the disease is primarily a medical disorder, approximately 25% of all infants who develop necrotizing enterocolitis will require surgery for its complications (perforation, gangrene, or intestinal stricture).

**4.** The **diagnosis** is made from both clinical and laboratory findings.
   **a.** The patients are usually born prematurely or have a low birth weight (75% weigh less than 2000 g at birth).
   **b. Associated perinatal problems** include premature rupture of the membranes, prolonged labor, amnionitis, umbilical artery catheterization, respiratory distress, apneic episodes, cyanosis, or delivery-room resuscitation.
   **c.** The disease usually occurs within the first 2 weeks of life.
   **d.** The first signs are usually formula intolerance and abdominal distention. These may be associated with the passage of either heme-positive or grossly bloody stools.
   **e.** Laboratory findings include leukopenia, thrombocytopenia, a low hematocrit, low serum sodium levels, metabolic acidosis, and coagulation defects.

**5. Abdominal roentgenograms** are used to aid in diagnosis and to follow the patient's clinical course. Initial findings include distended, edematous intestines, intramural air (pneumatosis), portal vein gas, an isolated persistent distended loop of bowel, or free intraperitoneal air.

**6.** The **primary management** remains medical. This includes gastrointestinal decompression with a large oral or nasal tube, parenteral antibiotics, fluids, and nutritional support.

**7. Surgical therapy** is instituted in the following situations.
   **a.** The only **absolute indication** for surgery in the **acute stage** is **intestinal perforation**.
      **(1)** This can usually be documented by the abdominal roentgenogram.
         **(a)** A cross-table lateral or left lateral decubitus position is used.
         **(b)** Films are obtained every 4 to 6 hours or as clinically indicated.
      **(2)** If perforation occurs, it is **treated** by resection of the involved intestine.
         **(a)** The gastrointestinal tract is diverted with either a jejunostomy or an ileostomy and colostomy.
         **(b)** A gastrostomy is performed to allow gastric decompression and nutritional support.
      **(3)** Primary reanastomosis of the normal bowel is done only in patients with limited disease or an isolated perforation.
      **(4)** In the severely ill patient with perforation, a major resective procedure may not be tolerated. In this situation, placement of peritoneal drains (using local anesthesia) may be acceptable treatment.
   **b. Relative indications** for surgery include:
      **(1)** Increasing signs of peritonitis (erythema or edema of the abdominal wall)
      **(2)** Failure of the patient to stabilize after 12 hours of optimal medical treatment (the patient shows persistent acidosis, apnea, or hypothermia)
      **(3)** A persistent distended loop of bowel seen on serial roentgenograms
      **(4)** Palpation of an abdominal mass
   **c.** The development of a **stricture** with subsequent intestinal obstruction requires surgical intervention.
      **(1)** This problem usually occurs 3 to 6 weeks after the acute episode.
      **(2)** Strictures are treated by resection and primary anastomosis once the patient is nutritionally prepared for surgery.

**8. Postoperative care** includes continued medical management of the primary disease as well as routine postsurgical care.
   **a.** The infant is treated with antibiotics, gastrointestinal decompression, and hyperalimentation.
   **b.** Progression of the disease may occur, requiring further surgery for additional perforations.
   **c.** Oral feedings are not started until 10 to 14 days after resolution of the acute disease.

Dietary adjustments may be necessary until the mucosa has regenerated and undergone functional maturation.
  **d.** The enterostomy can be closed during the initial hospitalization or at a later date.
  **e. Management of the stoma** can be difficult.
    **(1)** Local problems include prolapse, degeneration of the surrounding skin, or mucosal irritation.
    **(2)** Physiologic problems include fluid losses, electrolyte abnormalities, and intolerance of the diet.
    **(3)** Early recognition and treatment of these difficulties are necessary in order to prevent further complications.

**9. Prognosis**
  **a.** The mortality rate is 20% among patients who require only medical management for necrotizing enterocolitis.
  **b.** The mortality rate among patients requiring surgery is 50%, reflecting the greater severity of the disease in this group.
  **c.** The **long-term morbidity** is relatively low after recovery from necrotizing enterocolitis.
    **(1)** It is principally related to concomitant problems such as intraventricular cerebral hemorrhage, chronic pulmonary insufficiency, or associated cardiac problems.
    **(2)** A patient who has had an extensive bowel resection may develop a short bowel syndrome (see Chapter 6, section VII) requiring a change of diet or nutritional support.

## X. SOLID TUMORS

**A.** The two most common solid tumors of childhood are Wilms' tumor and neuroblastoma.

  **1.** While **other tumors** occur (rhabdomyosarcoma, Ewing's tumor, osteogenic sarcoma, and various brain tumors), neuroblastoma and Wilms' tumor illustrate the multidisciplinary approach that is currently used in the management of childhood tumors.

  **2.** They also illustrate an outstanding example of successful management (Wilms' tumor) and the need for continued research to improve current poor results (neuroblastoma).

**B. Wilms' tumor**

  **1.** Wilms' tumor can involve either the entire kidney or a part of it.
    **a.** Bilateral involvement occurs in 3% to 10% of the cases.
    **b.** Mesodermal, mesonephric, and metanephric origins have been proposed for this tumor.

  **2.** It has been estimated that there are 500 new cases of Wilms' tumor per year in the United States.

  **3.** The most common **presentation** is an asymptomatic flank mass that is usually discovered by the parents or on routine physical examination.
    **a.** Other complaints or findings include abdominal pain, hematuria, and anorexia.
    **b.** Hypertension occurs in about 10% of the patients.
    **c.** The age at presentation is between 1 and 4 years; most patients are between 1 and 3 years old.

  **4.** Wilms' tumor has been **associated** with congenital **anomalies** such as aniridia, hemihypertrophy, Beckwith's syndrome, sexual ambiguity, cryptorchidism, urinary tract anomalies, and abnormal karyotypes.

  **5. Physical examination** reveals a flank mass that is smooth, lobulated, and commonly mobile. The tumor rarely crosses the midline but may appear to do so because of its size.

  **6. Diagnostic studies**
    **a.** Findings on **intravenous pyelography** may range from compression of the collecting system to complete nonfunction of the kidney. Calcifications are seen in 10% of the patients.
    **b.** The most common **site of metastasis** is the lung, and a **chest x-ray** will reveal metastasis.
    **c.** A **venogram** may be indicated, to identify tumor extension into the vena cava.
    **d. Ultrasonography** and **computed tomography (CT)** may both identify the tumor and define the vena cava, but greater refinement of these structures is needed for accuracy.

  **7.** The **staging** of Wilms' tumor is as follows.
    **a. Stage I:** The tumor is limited to the kidney, and can be resected with the capsule intact.
    **b. Stage II:** The tumor extends beyond the kidney; when resected the capsule is found to be involved.

    **c. Stage III:** There is residual nonhematogenous tumor in the abdomen; the capsule is ruptured; implants are not completely resected.

    **d. Stage IV:** There is hematogenous metastasis to the liver, lungs, bone, or brain.

    **e. Stage V:** Bilateral involvement is present.

**8. Treatment** of Wilms' tumor involves a **multidisciplinary approach**.

    **a.** The mainstay of treatment is **surgery**.

        **(1)** The timing of surgery depends on the stage of the tumor (i.e., stage IV or V)

        **(2)** The operation includes:

            **(a)** An exploratory laparotomy

            **(b)** Examination of the opposite kidney

            **(c)** Resection of the tumor

            **(d)** Periaortic node dissection or sampling

        **(3)** Because of the relatively good prognosis, even with extensive disease, resection of other organs in an effort to remove the tumor is acceptable.

    **b. Chemotherapy** currently involves the use of dactinomycin (actinomycin D) and vincristine.

        **(1)** These are given after surgery in patients with stage II or III Wilms' tumor, and in some patients with stage I tumor.

        **(2)** They are given preoperatively in stage IV and V disease.

        **(3)** Adriamycin is added to the chemotherapy regimen for patients with advanced disease.

    **c. Radiotherapy** is used to treat extensive disease.

        **(1)** Currently, studies are under way to evaluate the need for radiation in stages I and II.

        **(2)** There are many **complications** after high-dose radiotherapy, including secondary cancers; interference with growth and development of bones, joints, and muscles; radiation pneumonitis; and cardiotoxicity.

**9.** Current 2-year **survival statistics** are as follows:

    **a. Stage I:** 90%

    **b. Stage II:** 80% to 85%

    **c. Stage III:** 70% to 75%

    **d. Stage IV:** 60% to 65%

    **e. Stage V:** 50%

**C. Congenital mesoblastic nephroma** is a distinct renal tumor of infancy related to Wilms' tumor.

**1.** To date about 70 cases have been reported.

**2.** The tumor usually presents soon after birth as an abdominal mass.

**3.** Nephrectomy alone is the current therapy and is curative.

**D. Neuroblastoma** is a neoplasm of adrenal and neural crest origin.

**1.** It occurs in 1 of every 10,000 live births and is the most common extracranial solid tumor of childhood.

**2.** It occurs in the early age-group, with 50% to 60% presenting by age 2 years.

**3.** There are several **major variants** of neuroblastoma.

    **a. Classic neuroblastoma** is a highly undifferentiated, immature malignant tumor that is unencapsulated and diffusely infiltrates the surrounding tissue.

    **b. Ganglioneuroma** is a benign, well-encapsulated tumor containing fully differentiated mature ganglia cells.

    **c. Ganglioneuroblastoma** is an intermediate or transitional form consisting of both primitive undifferentiated neuroblasts and mature differentiated ganglia cells. It can occur with or without encapsulation.

**4.** While they may occur anywhere along the sympathetic chain, the majority (65%) of these tumors arise from adrenal or nonadrenal retroperitoneal sites.

    **a.** Therefore, most patients **present** with a complaint of an abdominal mass.

    **b.** Neurologic symptoms may occur, resulting from compression of nerve trunks or from extension of the tumor into the extradural space (**"dumb-bell" tumor**).

    **c.** Horner's syndrome has been reported.

    **d.** Other symptoms include acute cerebellar ataxia and **opsoclonus** (sustained, irregular, multidirectional spontaneous conjugate eye movements).

**5. Metastatic spread** can involve the liver, lungs, skin, bone marrow, and bone.

    **a.** Skin lesions are firm, nontender, and bluish; biopsy will provide the diagnosis.

    **b.** The orbit is a common site of bony metastasis, with consequent periorbital ecchymosis and proptosis.

**6. Diagnosis** of the tumor may be obtained by various laboratory means.
    **a.** Bone marrow aspiration may reveal typical neuroblastoma cells.
    **b.** The tumor may synthesize various catecholamines.
        **(1)** The excretion products include vanillylmandelic acid (VMA) and homovanillic acid.
        **(2)** These can be checked in both spot urine samples and in 24-hour urine collections.
    **c. Radiologic studies**
        **(1)** Skeletal surveys or bone scans may show metastatic lesions.
        **(2)** Chest x-rays will confirm or rule out pulmonary metastasis.
        **(3)** The mainstay of radiologic testing for adrenal neuroblastoma is **intravenous pyelography**. This will show a suprarenal mass compressing the kidney and causing the collecting system to take on a "drooping lily" appearance.
        **(4)** Calcifications are seen much more often on abdominal x-rays in neuroblastoma than in Wilms' tumor.
        **(5)** Sonography may be of aid in identifying the mass.
        **(6)** A CT scan may not only aid in localizing the primary tumor but also may be a sensitive test for identifying hepatic metastasis.
    **d.** Liver function is documented and routine blood studies are done. Anemia will be present in about 40% to 60% of the patients at the time of diagnosis.

**7. Staging** for neuroblastoma is as follows.
    **a. Stage I:** The tumor is confined to the organ or structure of origin and is completely excised.
    **b. Stage II:** The tumor extends beyond the organ or structure of origin, but does not cross the midline.
    **c. Stage III:** The tumor extends across the midline.
    **d. Stage IV:** Remote disease is present and involves the skeleton, organs, soft tissue, or a distant lymph node group.
    **e. Stage IV-S:** The tumor is stage I or II; remote disease is present but is confined to one or more of the following sites: liver, skin, or bone marrow.

**8.** A rational approach to the **treatment** of neuroblastoma requires a **combined approach** employing the surgeon, radiation oncologist, chemotherapist, and pediatrician.
    **a.** While complete **surgical removal** is desirable, the majority (60%) of patients will present with metastatic disease. Neuroblastoma is unlike Wilms' tumor, in which aggressive surgery in the face of advanced disease is associated with good results. Such is not the case with neuroblastoma.
    **b. Radiation** is used as an adjuvant for resected or partially resected primary tumors and as palliative therapy for symptomatic metastases.
    **c.** Current **chemotherapy** includes the use of cyclophosphamide, vincristine, adriamycin, and dacarbazine (DTIC). The exact therapeutic protocol has not been developed, and other agents are currently under investigation.

**9. Prognosis.** Neuroblastoma remains as one of the few childhood tumors that has not responded dramatically to modern antitumor therapy. A child diagnosed today has the same dismal prognosis as a child diagnosed over 20 years ago.
    **a. Factors that influence survival** include:
        **(1) Age.** The younger the child at diagnosis, the better the outlook; this is independent of staging.
        **(2) Stage.** The more advanced the disease, the worse the prognosis; however, stage IV-S has a relatively good prognosis (60% survival).
        **(3) Location.** Abdominal neuroblastoma has a worse outlook than extra-abdominal neuroblastoma.
        **(4) Site of metastasis.** Patients presenting with bony lesions have a mortality rate near 100%.
        **(5) Presentation.** Patients presenting with opsoclonus have a higher survival rate than those presenting without it.
    **b. Overall survival rates** are as follows:
        **(1) Stage I:** 64%
        **(2) Stage II:** 54%
        **(3) Stage III:** 28%
        **(4) Stage IV:** 5%
        **(5) Stage IV-S:** 61%

# Part IX
# Study Questions

## QUESTIONS

**Directions:** Each question below contains five suggested answers. Choose the **one best** response to each question.

1. The most common causative factor in tendon ruptures is

(A) overuse
(B) severe trauma
(C) a stab wound
(D) a fall from a height
(E) a congenital defect

2. The diagnosis of Parinaud's syndrome could be based on all of the following findings EXCEPT

(A) papilledema
(B) hydrocephalus, visible on computed tomography (CT) scan
(C) a mass lesion involving the right cerebral hemisphere
(D) a mass lesion in the posterior part of the third ventricle
(E) upward gaze palsy

3. A traumatic hip dislocation commonly occurs with all of the following injuries EXCEPT

(A) fractured femur
(B) fractured lumbar spine
(C) fractured calcaneus
(D) fractured patella
(E) fractured tibia

4. All of the following statements concerning malrotation of the gut are true EXCEPT

(A) two potential problems are intestinal obstruction at the duodenum, and midgut volvulus that produces obstruction and ischemia of the small intestine
(B) malrotation is a diagnosis of exclusion and is considered only after other causes of obstruction are ruled out
(C) bilious vomiting is a common presenting symptom
(D) the "double-bubble" sign is often seen on plain films of the abdomen
(E) the long-term outlook is very good in patients treated for simple malrotation without volvulus

5. A 24-year-old man sustains a crush injury to his right shoulder. On examination, a 3-inch laceration is found, extending into the axilla and with no apparent involvement of the underlying muscles. Neurologic examination of the right upper extremity shows deltoids to be $2^+$ and triceps to be $2^+$. No other muscle contractions are seen. The proper management of this patient should include all of the following measures EXCEPT

(A) evaluation of the vascular supply to the limb
(B) immediate exploration of the brachial plexus
(C) thorough debridement of the wound and primary closure
(D) tetanus prophylaxis
(E) periodic neurologic examinations of the limb

6. What is the weak link of the musculoskeletal system in children?

(A) The growth plate of long bone
(B) The metaphyseal portion of long bone
(C) Ligamentous tissue
(D) Muscle fiber
(E) Tendinous tissue

7. Which of the following statements concerning breast reconstruction is true?

(A) The percentage of women who request reconstruction diminishes over time following mastectomy
(B) Reconstruction should never be performed at the time of mastectomy
(C) Silastic implants are placed beneath the skin to reconstruct breast fullness
(D) Although breast fullness can be accomplished, the nipple-areolar complex can never be reconstructed
(E) Reduction mammoplasty is seldom necessary for the opposite breast to achieve symmetry

8. A small boy who is brought to the emergency room by his parents is found to have a spiral fracture of the femur with a variety of ecchymoses. What is the most likely cause of the injuries?

(A) An automobile hit-and-run accident
(B) A fall from a tree
(C) Child abuse
(D) A fall from a bicycle
(E) A hockey-stick injury

9. Which of the following statements best describes basal cell carcinoma?

(A) It is an uncommon skin tumor
(B) It grows rapidly
(C) It frequently involves lymph nodes
(D) It has a poor prognosis
(E) It is frequently associated with prolonged exposure to sunlight

10. All of the following techniques are part of the management of chronic osteomyelitis EXCEPT

(A) use of antibiotics
(B) debridement
(C) bone graft (Papineau)
(D) plaster cast immobilization
(E) use of muscle flaps

**Directions:** Each question below contains four suggested answers of which **one or more** is correct. Choose the answer

    **A**  if **1, 2, and 3** are correct
    **B**  if **1 and 3** are correct
    **C**  if **2 and 4** are correct
    **D**  if **4** is correct
    **E**  if **1, 2, 3, and 4** are correct

11. Staging evaluation of a patient with a testicular tumor should include

(1) chest tomography
(2) determination of serum acid phosphatase levels
(3) determination of serum $\alpha$-fetoprotein levels
(4) excretory urography

12. Wilms' tumor has been associated with which of the following conditions?

(1) Aniridia
(2) Hemihypertrophy
(3) Hypertension
(4) Beckwith's syndrome

13. A 4-week-old white male whose mother has been breast-feeding him is noted to be jaundiced. The history reveals an increasing intolerance to feeding, nonbilious vomiting, and weight loss. There is no relevant family history, as this is the first-born child. What can be said about the management of this case?

(1) The vomiting and jaundice call for an immediate workup to identify or exclude biliary atresia
(2) Palpation of the abdomen in this patient would reveal a mass
(3) The infant needs to be changed to a formula, since feeding intolerance accompanied by jaundice has been related to breast milk
(4) Both physical examination and serum electrolytes in this infant would reveal findings of pyloric stenosis

14. Full- and split-thickness skin grafts have which of the following characteristics?

(1) Split-thickness skin grafts contain only the epidermis
(2) Full-thickness skin grafts contain the epidermis and the full thickness of dermis without subcutaneous fat
(3) Full-thickness skin grafts are useful for covering large surface areas
(4) Split-thickness skin grafts are cosmetically inferior to full-thickness skin grafts

15. A 50-year-old man presents with a complaint of gross painless hematuria. Workup of this patient should include

(1) screening for urinary nitrate reduction
(2) culture of urine
(3) evaluation of clotting parameters initially
(4) evaluation for a urinary tract neoplasm

16. The survival of a skin graft requires

(1) an adequate vascular bed for the graft
(2) good contact of the skin graft with the recipient bed
(3) absence of infection in the recipient bed
(4) the careful removal of periosteum from bone prior to grafting

17. Which of the following statements can be made about a neonatal tracheoesophageal fistula?

(1) Associated congenital defects are common, with the heart the most commonly involved organ
(2) Failure to pass a nasogastric tube into the stomach is very suggestive of a tracheoesophageal fistula
(3) The length between the blind pouch and the fistula is important in determining the time of surgery
(4) Gastroesophageal reflux is uncommon and has no bearing on the development of esophageal stricture

18. Common warts (verrucae vulgaris) have which of the following characteristics?

(1) They occur most frequently in the third decade of life
(2) They are caused by papovaviruses
(3) Most will not resolve spontaneously and require treatment such as desiccation
(4) The fingers are the most common location

19. Evaluation of a patient with erectile failure should include determination of

(1) urinary esterase
(2) serum testosterone levels
(3) serum chorionic gonadotropin levels
(4) penile blood pressure

20. In children with neuroblastoma, several factors are used to predict prognosis. These include the

(1) patient's age
(2) location of the tumor
(3) site of metastasis
(4) presence of calcifications on x-ray

21. Indications for excision of a pigmented nevus include

(1) a sudden change in color, size, or shape
(2) development of pain in the lesion
(3) the appearance of satellite lesions in the area of a previously existing nevus
(4) unexplained regional adenopathy

22. Indications for surgery in a newborn infant with either active or resolved necrotizing enterocolitis include which of the following?

(1) Free intraperitoneal air
(2) Portal vein gas
(3) Ileal stricture documented on barium studies
(4) A serum sodium level of 128 mEq/L and a platelet count of 80,000 at the time of diagnosis

23. Factors indicating the extent of tumor and the prognosis in a patient with a papillary transitional cell carcinoma of the bladder include

(1) cytologic grade of the tumor
(2) abnormal urinary cytology
(3) depth of invasion of the muscularis of the bladder
(4) presence of hematuria

24. True statements about diaphragmatic hernias include which of the following?

(1) They occur in approximately 1 in 4000 births
(2) They occur consistently on the right side
(3) They cause respiratory distress, a scaphoid abdomen, and a gas-bubble pattern in the affected hemithorax on chest x-ray
(4) They require complete stabilization with ventilatory support before surgical reduction

## ANSWERS AND EXPLANATIONS

**1. The answer is A.** (*Chapter 32 III F 1*) Disruptions of the musculotendinous unit are most commonly associated with overuse. The typical patient is middle-aged or older, and often gives a history of unusual, strenuous exertion. Torn or ruptured tendons require surgical repair.

**2. The answer is C.** (*Chapter 31 IV B 5; IX B 2*) Parinaud's syndrome consists of upward gaze paralysis, usually resulting from pressure in the pretectal area. A pineal tumor could cause obstructive hydrocephalus, leading to Parinaud's syndrome, and would be seen on the computed tomography (CT) scan as a lesion in the posterior part of the third ventricle. A tumor involving a cerebral hemisphere would be unlikely to produce Parinaud's syndrome.

**3. The answer is E.** (*Chapter 32 III A 2 a, E 2*) High-velocity injuries, especially those caused by automobile accidents, often include hip dislocation. Falling from a height is another common cause. Associated injuries in automobile accidents include ipsilateral fractures of the femur and patella and contralateral hip fractures. Associated injuries in falling accidents include fractures of the calcaneus or the thoracolumbar spine.

**4. The answer is B.** (*Chapter 33 V*) Simple duodenal obstruction is the more common of the two potential problems of malrotation, but volvulus with ischemia of the midgut is the more critical since delay in treatment may cause complete loss of the midgut. If a diagnosis of malrotation is entertained, the infant must quickly be evaluated, and if malrotation cannot be excluded rapidly, then an immediate surgical exploration is carried out. Bilious vomiting is an early and common symptom and dictates a surgical evaluation. Simple malrotation, once treated, has no long-term sequelae associated with it, and the outlook is excellent.

**5. The answer is B.** (*Chapter 31 VIII; Chapter 32 III B 3 b*) The patient obviously has a brachial plexus injury. In this case, the peripheral pulses should be evaluated, and if they are present, exploration of the brachial plexus would not be done. If there is any vascular injury that requires operative repair, it would be reasonable to inspect the brachial plexus at the time that the repair is made. In general, crush injuries of peripheral nerves do not require acute intervention.

**6. The answer is A.** (*Chapter 32 III A 1 a*) The weak link in the musculoskeletal system varies with age. In the skeletally immature child, the weak link is the growth plate in the ends of long bones. In young but skeletally mature persons, the weak link is the ligamentous tissue supporting the joints. In the elderly, the weak link is the metaphyseal portion of the long bones. Therefore, the consequence of trauma depends to some extent on the age of the patient.

**7. The answer is A.** (*Chapter 30 I F 4*) The percentage of women requesting reconstruction diminishes as the time since mastectomy increases. Reconstruction may be performed at the time of mastectomy if plastic surgeons skilled in this technique are available. The Silastic implants are placed beneath the pectoralis muscle and not beneath the skin. The nipple-areolar complex can be reconstructed, usually with tissue taken from the opposite breast or from the labia. It is frequently necessary to do a reduction mammoplasty on the opposite breast to achieve symmetry. Women can now be offered satisfactory breast reconstruction following mastectomy, and postmastectomy reconstrution represents one of the major areas of advancement in plastic surgery in recent times.

**8. The answer is C.** (*Chapter 32 III C 1 d*) The spiral fracture of a long bone, combined with the variety of bruises, should lead one to suspect a case of child abuse. Other suspicious lesions include unusual oblique fractures, fractures of various ages in different extremities, and burns or scrapes in various locations and of various ages. Inconsistencies between the type of lesion seen and the history of how it occurred can also be a clue. Abuse of a child is now reportable by law in all states.

**9. The answer is E.** (*Chapter 30 II F 1*) Basal cell carcinoma is the most common malignant skin tumor. It is usually localized and slow-growing and rarely metastasizes to lymph nodes. It is strongly linked with excessive exposure to sunlight. In general, it has a very favorable prognosis.

**10. The answer is D.** (*Chapter 32 II B 3*) Chronic osteomyelitis can be difficult to cure. Therapeutic principles include removal of all foreign material, thorough debridement of infected, devascularized bone, correction of bone defects with a bone graft, good local wound care, and prolonged use of intravenous antibiotics. Muscle flaps and split-thickness skin grafts are employed after the infection is controlled. The affected region is not immobilized in a plaster cast; this would reduce blood circulation to a site that is already poorly vascularized and therefore would hinder, not promote, control of the infection.

**11. The answer is B (1, 3).** (*Chapter 29 VII E 4 a, b*) Staging evaluation of a patient with a testicular tumor should include chest tomography and determination of serum levels of α-fetoprotein. Pulmonary metastases are often the first to be detected by radiologic studies. Sensitivity can be increased by examining lung tomograms or computed tomography (CT) scans of the chest. Chest x-rays should also be employed routinely in the follow-up of patients treated for testicular tumors. Elevated serum levels of both α-fetoprotein and human chorionic gonadotropin are accurate markers of testicular tumors, indicating the presence of microscopic metastases and giving early evidence of recurrence. False-negatives occur since not all testicular tumors produce these markers. Serum acid phosphatase determinations and excretory urography are used in the staging of prostatic, not testicular, tumors.

**12. The answer is E (all).** (*Chapter 33 X B*) Wilms' tumor has been associated with a number of congenital anomalies, including aniridia, hemihypertrophy, Beckwith's syndrome, sexual ambiguity, cryptorchidism, and other genitourinary defects. Hypertension is seen in about 10% of the patients with this common childhood tumor of the kidney. Wilms' tumor, which has an estimated incidence of 500 new cases per year, represents an outstanding example of successful management among the tumors of childhood.

**13. The answer is C (2, 4).** (*Chapter 33 IX A*) This infant has a typical history of pyloric stenosis. Jaundice occurs in about 10% of these infants, and it resolves after pyloromyotomy. The diagnosis is usually made by palpation of a mobile midepigastric mass. Correction of dehydration as well as correction of serum potassium and serum carbon dioxide deficits is necessary before surgery.

**14. The answer is C (2, 4).** (*Chapter 30 I D 1*) Split-thickness skin grafts contain the epidermis and a portion of the dermis. Advantages of split-thickness skin grafts are: they are useful in covering large defects, they are easy to harvest, and they can be stored for later use. The disadvantages of split-thickness grafts are: they are cosmetically inferior to full-thickness grafts, they are not as durable, and they are more prone to hyperpigmentation. Full-thickness grafts contain the epidermis and the full thickness of the dermis without subcutaneous fat. They yield a good color match and are especially useful for repairing defects on the face and hands.

**15. The answer is D (4).** (*Chapter 29 VII B 3 a, C 4 a, D 3 a*) The patient with gross painless hematuria must be evaluated for a urinary tract neoplasm. The majority of patients with urothelial neoplasms or renal parenchymal tumors experience hematuria in the course of the neoplasm. However, the absence of hematuria cannot be considered to rule out a urologic tumor.

**16. The answer is A (1, 2, 3).** (*Chapter 30 I D 3*) A well-vascularized recipient bed is essential to provide nourishment for the transplanted graft. The graft is initially supported by plasma imbibition and within several days will become vascularized through a process of vascular budding. Contact between the graft and the vascular bed is essential, and any infected wound will not support a skin graft. Bone denuded of periosteum will not support a skin graft, nor will cartilage denuded of perichondrium.

**17. The answer is A (1, 2, 3).** (*Chapter 33 IV*) In tracheoesophageal fistula there is a high incidence of associated defects. Affected organs include the heart (most commonly involved), the kidneys, and bone. Other gastrointestinal anomalies are also common. The hallmark of tracheoesophageal fistula is a blind proximal pouch that will not allow passage of a nasogastric tube. A gap of greater than 2 cm (2½ vertebral bodies) may require delayed repair. Gastroesophageal reflux is now felt to be the primary reason for postoperative stricture formation in the patient with tracheoesophageal fistula.

**18. The answer is C (2, 4).** (*Chapter 30 II B 1*) Common warts occur most frequently in the second decade of life and may be transmitted by direct or indirect contact. They are caused by a member of the papovavirus family. The fingers are the most common location, and the lesions have a characteristic rough, elevated surface and can become tender. Many of these warts will resolve spontaneously, and only problematic lesions should be treated. This is usually accomplished by electrodesiccation or by chemotherapy with caustic topical agents.

**19. The answer is C (2, 4).** (*Chapter 29 X B 5*) The evaluation of the patient with erectile failure should include serum testosterone and penile blood pressure determinations. Measuring serum levels of testosterone, follicle-stimulating and luteinizing hormones, and prolactin may indicate hormonal abnormalities which can be treated appropriately. Penile blood pressure determinations may indicate inadequate penile blood flow. When this is related to obstruction of major pelvic vessels, revascularization procedures can be used. Because revascularization of small vessels has not been particularly successful, treatment by implantation of a prosthesis may be indicated.

**20. The answer is A (1, 2, 3).** (*Chapter 33 X D 9*) The presence of calcifications is more common in neuroblastoma than in Wilms' tumor, but the finding carries no known prognostic significance. By contrast, the patient's age, the location of the tumor, and the site of metastasis all have significant prognostic implications.

**21. The answer is E (all).** (*Chapter 30 II D 4*) Malignant melanoma can arise from preexisting nevi, particularly those that have a junctional component. Sudden changes in color, size, and shape as well as pain, satellite lesions, and unexplained regional adenopathy all warrant immediate excision and pathologic examination of the nevus.

**22. The answer is B (1, 3).** (*Chapter 33 IX C 7*) The absolute indications for surgery in an infant with necrotizing enterocolitis include intestinal perforation, as demonstrated by free intraperitoneal air, and a stricture requiring resection to relieve the bowel obstruction. Perforation occurs in active necrotizing enterocolitis and may require formal laparotomy or placement of an intraperitoneal drain. Strictures usually develop approximately 6 weeks after resolution of necrotizing enterocolitis. Portal vein gas and the low serum sodium level and platelet count are findings associated with the disease; by themselves they have no surgical implications.

**23. The answer is B (1, 3).** (*Chapter 29 VII D 4*) The cytologic appearance of a transitional cell carcinoma, or the grade, can be correlated with the malignant behavior of the lesion. The higher the grade, the greater the chance of invasion and of metastasis. The depth of invasion of a transitional cell carcinoma is related to the probability of metastasis. Treatment is based partially on the depth of invasion.

**24. The answer is B (1, 3).** (*Chapter 33 II B*) The majority of diaphragmatic hernias are through the foramen of Bochdalek and are left-sided. The incidence is approximately 1 in 4000 live births. The usual early presentation is respiratory distress. Because the abdominal contents are located in the hemithorax, the abdomen is scaphoid and the chest x-ray will show an abnormal gas-bubble pattern as more air enters the gastrointestinal tract. The most important factor in the initial improvement of respiratory function is the rapid surgical reduction of the gastrointestinal tract out of the hemithorax and into the abdomen.

# Post-test

## QUESTIONS

**Directions:** Each question below contains five suggested answers. Choose the **one best** response to each question.

1. A patient has had a persistent area of pneumonitis in the right lung for 2 months. What is the next step in the workup?

(A) Continuous observation with monthly chest roentgenograms
(B) Workup with multiple fungal skin tests and begin antifungal therapy
(C) Bronchoscopy with biopsy brushings and washings
(D) Addition of broad-spectrum antibiotics
(E) Repetition of sputum cultures and accordant treatment

2. An average-sized (70-kg), 60-year-old man with normal renal function underwent a vagotomy and hemigastrectomy for an obstructing duodenal ulcer. Intraoperative fluid losses were appropriately replaced, and he was considered normovolemic. On the first postoperative day, his nasogastric tube drained 5000 ml of bile-stained fluid. What volume of parenteral fluids should be ordered for this patient over the next 24 hours?

(A) 2500 ml
(B) 5000 ml
(C) 7500 ml
(D) 10,000 ml
(E) 12,000 ml

3. All of the following disorders are pre- or intrasinusoidal causes of portal hypertension EXCEPT

(A) alcoholic cirrhosis
(B) acute alcoholic hepatitis
(C) schistosomiasis
(D) Budd-Chiari syndrome
(E) postnecrotic cirrhosis

4. Which of the following statements is true concerning soft tissue injuries in the trauma patient?

(A) Palpable pulses rule out arterial injury
(B) Fasciotomies are frequently required in conjunction with vascular repair
(C) Stab wounds or missile tracts near major vessels can be closed if there is no sign of major arterial or venous hemorrhage
(D) Exposed nerves can be left open, as granulation tissue will readily cover them
(E) Attached bones should be removed in order to speed healing

5. Which of the following conditions in a potential cadaver donor would make the kidneys unacceptable for transplantation?

(A) Deep coma
(B) Colon cancer 3 years previously
(C) Serum creatinine level of 1.5 mg/dl (the normal level is up to 1.4 mg/dl)
(D) A gunshot wound to the head
(E) Endotracheal intubation

6. Wound contraction is caused by which of the following mechanisms?

(A) Collagen formation
(B) Myofibroblasts
(C) Elastic fibers
(D) Ground substance
(E) Granulation tissue

7. Massive bleeding from the lower gastrointestinal tract is occurring in a 55-year-old, otherwise healthy man. Initial management, after continued bleeding equivalent to 1 unit of blood, would be

(A) emergency laparotomy and total colectomy with ileoproctostomy
(B) emergency laparotomy and colostomy with operative endoscopy
(C) arteriography for identification of the bleeding site after anoscopy and sigmoidoscopy have ruled out a distal site
(D) infusion of vitamin K and fresh frozen plasma
(E) colonic irrigation with iced saline solution

8. Which of the following statements concerning the treatment of pulmonary embolism with anticoagulation therapy is true?

(A) Thrombolytic therapy with streptokinase may be used with patients who have life-threatening pulmonary embolism complicated by intracranial hemorrhage
(B) Heparin is most effective when administered intermittently, especially to elderly patients
(C) Pulmonary embolism recurs despite anticoagulation therapy in 30% of cases
(D) Warfarin is most useful for long-term anticoagulation therapy, as associated drug interactions are minimal
(E) None of the above statements is true

9. All of the following complications of renal transplantation are likely to threaten the patient's life EXCEPT

(A) active peptic ulcer disease
(B) acute diverticulitis
(C) pulmonary aspergillosis
(D) glomerulonephritis
(E) angina pectoris

10. A woman has undergone a cholecystectomy and common duct exploration. Two stones were removed and a T tube was placed in the common duct. On the seventh postoperative day her serum bilirubin level remains elevated and she has an episode of crampy pain that radiates to her back. What is the next step in the management of this patient?

(A) Begin therapy with drugs to "dissolve" gallstones
(B) Remove the T tube
(C) Clamp off the T tube
(D) Return the patient to the operating room
(E) Perform T tube cholangiography

11. Patients requiring surgery should be treated by blood transfusions to maintain a hemoglobin level (Hb) of 10 g/dl in all of the following situations EXCEPT

(A) Hb of 8 g/dl in a patient with coronary artery disease
(B) Hb of 8 g/dl in a patient with a ruptured spleen
(C) Hb of 7 g/dl in a patient on parenteral nutrition for a small bowel fistula
(D) Hb of 7 g/dl in a patient with chronic renal failure
(E) Hb of 8 g/dl in a patient with a history of congestive heart failure

12. A 21-year-old man who was involved in an automobile accident is brought to the emergency room. On admission, his blood pressure is 80/60, respirations are purely diaphragmatic, and he has a right-sided Horner's syndrome. Cervical spine x-rays show a $C_4$ on $C_5$ fracture dislocation but $C_7$ is not visualized. Which of the following statements about management of this patient is correct?

(A) Repeat cervical spine films are not necessary as there is very little likelihood of fracture at another level
(B) Vasopressor agents have to be administered immediately to raise the blood pressure
(C) Attention must be given to maintaining an adequate airway
(D) Administration of mannitol is unnecessary
(E) The nature of the cervical injury is a contraindication to the use of traction as part of therapy

13. Which of the following studies of pulmonary function is most reliable in predicting whether a 70-year-old man will tolerate the hemodynamic effects following pneumonectomy?

(A) History and physical examination
(B) Arterial blood gases
(C) Tidal volume
(D) Balloon catheter occlusion of the pulmonary artery of the affected lung
(E) Chest roentgenography

14. Hoarseness following radiation therapy for a left superior sulcus lung carcinoma is usually secondary to

(A) vocal cord paralysis due to radiation injury
(B) radiation scarring of the larynx
(C) tumor involvement of the left recurrent laryngeal nerve
(D) continued cigarette smoking
(E) central nervous system metastasis

15. The treatment for benign mixed tumors of the parotid gland is

(A) primary irradiation
(B) excision of the gross tumor
(C) radical excision of the parotid gland including the facial membrane
(D) local excision of the tumor followed by radiation
(E) excision of the tumor with a margin of normal tissue and preservation of the facial nerve

16. A patient who has been admitted to the hospital for an elective surgical procedure has a recent history of heavy aspirin use. The safest course of action in this case is to

(A) proceed with the surgery, paying particular attention to meticulous hemostasis
(B) proceed with the surgery, after ensuring that properly crossmatched platelets are available should excess bleeding occur
(C) proceed with the surgery, after transfusion of 1 unit of platelets immediately prior to the incision
(D) delay the surgery for 7 days, instructing the patient to avoid all aspirin and aspirin-containing products
(E) delay the surgery if it involves additional anticoagulation, such as open heart surgery

17. During a pre-employment physical examination, a 50-year-old man is found to have an asymptomatic thyroid nodule. The nodule is well circumscribed and freely moveable. There is no associated cervical lymphadenopathy, and no family history of thyroid malignancy. Which of the following studies will best determine the nature of the thyroid enlargement?

(A) Technetium-99m ($^{99m}$Tc) thyroid scan
(B) Iodine-131 ($^{131}$I) thyroid scan
(C) Thyroid ultrasonography
(D) Fine-needle aspiration of the thyroid
(E) Serum thyrocalcitonin assay

18. In a patient with hemorrhage from a suspected diverticulum in the colon, what is the minimal rate of hemorrhage that can usually be visualized by selective mesenteric angiography?

(A) 0.1 ml per minute
(B) 0.5 ml per minute
(C) 5 ml per minute
(D) 15 ml per minute
(E) 50 ml per minute

19. A hollow viscus forms part of the wall of the hernia sac in a

(A) pantaloon hernia
(B) sliding hernia
(C) direct inguinal hernia
(D) Richter's hernia
(E) Littre's hernia

20. After a thorough diagnostic workup, a patient is found to have Zollinger-Ellison syndrome. Which of the following statements can be made about this syndrome?

(A) It is a postoperative complication of ulcer surgery leading to postprandial vomiting
(B) It is also known as "cast syndrome" and is due to duodenal obstruction by the superior mesenteric artery
(C) It is an obstruction of the gastric outlet caused by a pyloric ulcer
(D) It is a form of severe duodenal ulcer disease caused by a gastrin-secreting pancreatic tumor
(E) It is seen in psychotic persons who repeatedly ingest foreign objects

21. Upon abdominal exploration, a patient is found to have a nonobstructing carcinoma of the transverse colon and apparent liver metastases. The best treatment is to

(A) biopsy the liver nodules, then close the abdomen
(B) close the abdomen
(C) resect the colon lesion only
(D) resect the colon lesion and biopsy the liver lesion
(E) perform a colostomy

22. In a patient who presents with Cushing's syndrome, with elevated plasma cortisol levels and low plasma adrenocorticotropic hormone (ACTH) levels, the most likely cause of the syndome is

(A) a basophilic adenoma of the pituitary gland
(B) an oat cell carcinoma of the lung
(C) bilateral adrenal cortical hyperplasia
(D) an adrenal cortical adenoma
(E) a malignant non-beta islet cell tumor of the pancreas

23. Aortoiliac vascular reconstruction is indicated by all of the following clinical presentations EXCEPT

(A) impotence related to bilateral internal iliac artery occlusion
(B) rest pain in the foot
(C) complete occlusion of the external iliac artery
(D) gangrene of the toes
(E) emboli in the leg originating from the distal aorta

24. A patient was referred by his family physician because of a mass in his leg. All of the following radiologic studies are part of the initial workup of this patient EXCEPT

(A) plain radiography
(B) computed tomography (CT) of the mass and area
(C) CT of the chest
(D) a scan of the liver and spleen
(E) a bone scan

25. Which of the following is the most acceptable surgical procedure for a carcinoma of the splenic flexure of the colon?

(A) Wedge resection of the lesion
(B) Left hemicolectomy
(C) Total colectomy
(D) Abdominoperineal resection
(E) Anterior resection

26. A patient who has had a previous appendectomy presents in the emergency room with a history of abdominal pain, cramps, vomiting, and anorexia. A mechanical small bowel obstruction is seen on the abdominal roentgenogram. He has no fever, his white blood count is normal, and he has no acidosis or hypotension, although his serum potassium level is 2.8 mEq/L. Which of the following is the best treatment?

(A) Immediate surgery for lysis of adhesions
(B) Correction of hypokalemia over 3 to 6 hours, followed by surgery
(C) Correction of hypokalemia over 24 hours, followed by surgery
(D) Observation for signs of complications due to intestinal obstruction
(E) Insertion of a gastrointestinal tube into the small bowel

27. Curability of carcinoma of the pancreas is principally determined by the

(A) type of procedure performed (Whipple versus total pancreatectomy)
(B) type of chemotherapy used
(C) use of radioactive seed implants
(D) biologic activity of the tumor
(E) degree of serum bilirubin present

28. A biliary tract tumor such as a Klatskin tumor occurring at the hepatic duct confluence is most accurately diagnosed with which of the following tests?

(A) An upper GI series
(B) Intravenous cholangiography
(C) Percutaneous transhepatic cholangiography
(D) Hepatic scintiscanning
(E) Liver biopsy

**Directions:** Each question below contains four suggested answers of which **one or more** is correct. Choose the answer

A  if **1, 2, and 3** are correct
B  if **1 and 3** are correct
C  if **2 and 4** are correct
D  if **4** is correct
E  if **1, 2, 3, and 4** are correct

29. A patient who has undergone surgical repair of a stress ulcer has developed an enterocutaneous fistula that is draining 300 ml of fluid daily. Management of this patient would include

(1) contrast radiography of the gut
(2) prompt operative repair of the fistula
(3) control of external drainage
(4) increase in the oral fluid and nutrient intake

30. Joint arthroplasty, or total joint replacement, is a recent addition to the operative management of joint diseases. True statements about this useful new procedure include which of the following?

(1) It is limited to rheumatoid arthritis
(2) It is a permanent repair
(3) It is indicated for young, active patients
(4) It is used to relieve pain

31. If a patient receives a penetrating injury to the arm, what is the correct management protocol?

(1) If active immunization occurred more than 5 years previously, a toxoid booster is recommended
(2) If the wound is clean and the patient has never been immunized, it is safe to give tetanus toxoid in three separate doses
(3) If the wound is dirty and the patient has never been immunized, passive immunization with human tetanus immune globulin is recommended
(4) Adequate debridement of devitalized tissue is essential

32. True statements concerning transplant rejection include

(1) acute rejection involves lymphocytic infiltration of the kidney
(2) hyperacute rejection involves preformed antibodies against the new kidney
(3) chronic rejection involves vascular intimal thickening and scarring
(4) accelerated acute rejection usually involves a second-set, or anamnestic, response

33. An association has been found between hepatocellular carcinoma and a number of prior diseases and environmental factors. Which of the following would belong in that category?

(1) Chronic alcohol abuse
(2) Hepatitis B surface antigen
(3) Aflatoxins
(4) Oral contraceptives

34. A patient develops fever, chills, and a red streak over a saphenous vein, beginning at the site of an intravenous catheter. Pus can be expressed from both the vein and the venous cutdown. Proper management of this patient's infection includes

(1) removal of the intravenous catheter
(2) excision of the involved segment of the saphenous vein
(3) intravenous administration of antibiotics after culturing and Gram-staining the pus
(4) intravenous administration of heparin to prevent venous thrombosis

35. True statements regarding relapsing pancreatitis include which of the following?

(1) A positive Nardi provocative test is likely
(2) It usually is associated with alcohol abuse
(3) Sphincteroplasty of the pancreaticobiliary septum may be helpful
(4) It is the most common cause of pancreatic ascites

36. After hospitalization for a knife wound in the chest, a young man is being monitored for cardiac tamponade. Which of the following findings should be watched for?

(1) Distended neck veins
(2) Hypotension
(3) Pulsus paradoxus
(4) Increased heart sounds

37. Factors that may increase the risk of developing cancer of the breast include

(1) chronic cystic mastitis
(2) previous contralateral breast cancer
(3) breast cancer in a maternal grandmother
(4) breast cancer in a paternal grandmother

38. Causes of an inguinal hernia include

(1) vesical outlet obstruction
(2) ascites
(3) chronic obstructive lung disease
(4) gastric ulcer disease

39. A patient who had a gastrectomy has developed problems. His surgeon tells the patient that he has dumping syndrome. Which of the following statements might the surgeon make about this syndrome?

(1) It can cause epigastric pain due to small bowel distention
(2) It causes the patient's symptoms of nausea, dizziness, and palpitations
(3) It occurs because rapid emptying of the stomach causes jejunal distention from fluid accumulation
(4) It can be controlled by dietary modifications

SUMMARY OF DIRECTIONS

| A | B | C | D | E |
|---|---|---|---|---|
| 1, 2, 3 only | 1, 3 only | 2, 4 only | 4 only | All are correct |

40. A 4-year-old girl presents with a smooth in-tranasal lesion. True statements about this lesion include

(1) if unilateral, it should be biopsied
(2) if bilateral, smooth, and glistening, a sweat chloride test should be obtained
(3) if reddish in color, excision should be undertaken immediately
(4) signs of expansion of the lesion should be sought during straining, crying, or a Valsalva maneuver

41. Absolute indications for splenectomy include

(1) primary splenic tumors
(2) splenic abscess
(3) hereditary spherocytosis
(4) autoimmune hemolytic anemia

42. Which of the following nutrients must be replaced parenterally after resection of the terminal ileum in a patient with Crohn's disease?

(1) Vitamin E
(2) Iron
(3) Bile salts
(4) Vitamin $B_{12}$

43. Which of the following characteristics would favor the diagnosis of a benign lesion in a patient with a solitary pulmonary nodule?

(1) A diameter greater than 5 cm
(2) Cavitation
(3) A peripheral location
(4) Calcification within the lesion

44. True statements concerning Hodgkin's disease include

(1) the prognosis for affected individuals remains poor
(2) stage II classification indicates involvement of the nodal regions on both sides of the diaphragm
(3) the spleen should not be removed during staging laparotomy
(4) staging laparotomy reveals unsuspected abdominal disease in 25% of stage I or II patients

45. Important procedures in treating perforated diverticulitis with abscess formation include

(1) administration of systemic antibiotics
(2) drainage of the abscess
(3) avoidance of a primary anastomosis
(4) mechanical bowel preparation

46. A child who got into a playground scuffle decided not to report it. Some time later her teacher noticed the child protecting her elbow. Examination showed an abrasion with a red streak extending towards the armpit. The school nurse diagnosed lymphangitis. It is important for the nurse to tell the child's parents that

(1) septicemia may occur if the process is not arrested by the lymph nodes
(2) *Escherichia coli* is the most commonly isolated organism
(3) any source of infection such as a paronychia or other collections should be drained
(4) exercising the affected limb to promote lymphatic drainage is mandatory

47. Surgical complications following elective or emergency aortic surgery include which of the following?

(1) Renal failure
(2) Leg ischemia
(3) Spinal cord ischemia
(4) Impotence in men

**Directions:** The groups of questions below consist of lettered choices followed by several numbered items. For each numbered item select the **one** lettered choice with which it is **most** closely associated. Each lettered choice may be used once, more than once, or not at all.

**Questions 48–52**

For each sentence describing a soft tissue sarcoma match the appropriate neoplasm.

(A) Liposarcoma
(B) Fibrosarcoma
(C) Pleomorphic rhabdomyosarcoma
(D) Kaposi's sarcoma
(E) Lymphangiosarcoma

48. This lesion is of vascular origin and has been found in association with acquired immune deficiency syndrome (AIDS)

49. There is no effective treatment for this tumor, and the prognosis for patients is dismal

50. When well differentiated, this tumor is associated with a 70% 5-year survival rate

51. This tumor is the second most common soft tissue sarcoma and usually presents as a hard, round mass in an extremity

52. This tumor is associated with a 30% 5-year survival rate

**Questions 53–55**

Match each phrase describing the incidence of congenital heart defects with the correct disease.

(A) Patent ductus arteriosus
(B) Coarctation of the aorta
(C) Atrial septal defect
(D) Ventricular septal defect
(E) Tetralogy of Fallot

53. The most common congenital heart defect

54. Occurs twice as often in females as in males

55. Occurs twice as often in males as in females

**Questions 56–60**

For each urologic neoplasm listed below, select the diagnostic study that is appropriate for that neoplasm.

(A) Acid phosphatase
(B) Arteriography
(C) Human chorionic gonadotropin
(D) Cystoscopy
(E) Retrograde ureteropyelography

56. Testicular tumor

57. Prostatic carcinoma

58. Renal cell carcinoma

59. Transitional cell carcinoma of the renal pelvis

60. Carcinoma of the bladder

## ANSWERS AND EXPLANATIONS

**1. The answer is C.** [*Chapter 27 I B 2 b (1)*] Persistent pneumonitis should be aggressively investigated as an indicator of an occult carcinoma impinging upon a bronchial segment. Bronchoscopy and further workup should be performed. If the question remains unresolved, then lung biopsy or resection should be carried out.

**2. The answer is C.** [*Chapter 1 I F 3–4, G 1 b (1), 2*] In a patient who is normovolemic, the first priority of fluid therapy is volume-for-volume replacement. Since the patient described in the question lost 5000 ml of fluid through nasogastric drainage, then 5000 ml of water and electrolyte therapy is necessary to replace this loss. The second priority is maintenance therapy—that is, administration of the fluid and electrolytes necessary to satisfy normal requirements; normal daily requirements are calculated according to weight. In this case, the patient will require 2500 ml of fluids for maintenance. Thus, the total fluid requirement for a 24-hour period is 7500 ml.

**3. The answer is D.** (*Chapter 9 I E 3*) The Budd-Chiari syndrome is a postsinusoidal cause of portal hypertension, not a pre- or intrasinusoidal cause. It is a syndrome characterized by hepatic venous thrombosis, resulting in marked hepatic congestion and hepatomegaly. The most common etiologic factors in this disorder are oral contraceptives, tumors, trauma, and hematologic disorders associated with increased thrombogenicity. The Budd-Chiari syndrome is a rare cause of portal hypertension. By far the most common cause is cirrhosis of the liver: It is the etiology in 85% of portal hypertension cases in the United States.

**4. The answer is B.** (*Chapter 2 I C 6 e*) Palpable pulses do not rule out arterial injury, as intimal tears can be present with intact pulses distally. Fasciotomies will almost always be required for vascular injuries, particularly if any length of time has passed before repair. The reason is that postoperative swelling will be extensive and will lead to necrosis of muscle in closed fascial spaces. Stab wounds or missile tracts near major vascular structures require arteriography to rule out injury to the structures. This should be done whether or not obvious bleeding is seen. Exposed nerves must be covered with normal muscle or fat following repair. Attached bones should generally be left in situ to speed healing.

**5. The answer is B.** (*Chapter 16 I C 2*) A history of cancer in a potential donor is an absolute contraindication to organ donation. The only exception to this would be a preexisting primary central nervous system tumor restricted to the cranial vault. The minimally elevated creatinine level is not a contraindication to organ donation.

**6. The answer is B.** (*Chapter 1 IV A 3*) Contraction occurs in the tissues of a wound, helping the wound to close by decreasing its surface area. The myofibroblasts exert a contractile force within the wound and are responsible for wound contraction. Collagen formation, granulation tissue, elastic fibers, and ground substance are all important in wound repair but are not responsible for wound contraction.

**7. The answer is C.** (*Chapter 4 IV B, C*) Arteriography is most often used as the initial evaluation step for continued bleeding after anorectal bleeding sources have been eliminated by endoscopy. Arteriography allows identification of diverticular bleeding as well as an angiodysplastic lesion of the right colon. Barium enema may also be used in the initial management. Surgery is generally not indicated until 4 to 6 units of blood have been shed. Coagulation products are of no use unless the patient has abnormal clotting studies. Saline lavage of the colon is not a routine procedure.

**8. The answer is E.** (*Chapter 14 II F 1–4, G 1, 2*) Thrombolytic therapy with streptokinase or urokinase may be used in patients with acute life-threatening pulmonary embolism; however, it is contraindicated in patients with recent intracranial hemorrhage, recent surgery, or other bleeding disorders. Heparin as an anticoagulant should be administered as an initial bolus of 10,000 to 20,000 units and continued as an intravenous drip at approximately 1000 units per hour for a minimum of 7 days. The risk of hemorrhage is greatest if heparin is administered intermittently or is given to elderly or severely hypertensive patients. Although warfarin can be used for long-term anticoagulation therapy, its effectiveness can be severely altered by its interactions with other drugs. Despite anticoagulation therapy, pulmonary embolism recurs in 1% to 8% of patients.

**9. The answer is D.** (*Chapter 16 II B, E, G 3, 4; VI C, D 1*) Although the recurrent development of glomerulonephritis may destroy the transplanted kidney, it is not directly life-threatening. An acute or chronic infection, whether bacterial, viral, or fungal, and myocardial infarction are the most common causes of death in transplant recipients.

**10. The answer is E.** (*Chapter 9 II H 1 e*) The patient probably has a biliary blockage, secondary to either a retained common duct stone or to some mechanical problem related to the surgery or the T tube. It is most important to maintain adequate drainage; thus, the T tube should not be clamped or removed. A cholangiogram should be obtained. Decisions about further management will be based on the findings.

**11. The answer is D.** (*Chapter 3 I C 3; III B 3 a*) Most physicians accept a hemoglobin level of 10 g/dl of blood prior to major surgery. Thus, preoperative blood replacement is recommended when excessive blood loss is anticipated, when the patient has significant coronary artery disease or a history of congestive heart failure, after a preoperative hemorrhage, in hypoxia, and in the presence of sepsis or malnutrition. However, the patient with chronic renal failure and no other complications tolerates a hemoglobin level of 7 to 8 g/dl well for most surgical procedures.

**12. The answer is C.** (*Chapter 31 VII A–E*) In cases of suspected cervical spine trauma, the importance of visualizing all cervical vertebrae cannot be overemphasized. When there is difficulty in visualizing the $C_7$ vertebra, using special views (e.g., Swimmer's) or simply pulling the arms down and taking a lateral film may be beneficial. High cervical cord injuries result in a sympathectomy and thus may give rise to a Horner's syndrome and systemic hypotension as a result of peripheral vasodilatation. In these cases adequate blood pressure is restored by volume replacement rather than by the use of vasopressor agents. Hematomas can develop in front of the vertebral bodies, jeopardizing the airways. Therefore, attention must be given to maintaining adequate airways. It has been postulated that cord edema develops following the initial injury, which further embarrasses the microcirculation and aggravates the injury. Thus, osmotic agents such as mannitol are administered to decrease the cord edema and reduce the extent of injury. Fracture dislocations of the cervical spine are treated by traction, applied by means of skull tongs and weights.

**13. The answer is D.** (*Chapter 3 II C 3 a*) Patients undergoing resection must be evaluated to determine if they will tolerate removal of part or all of a lung. In addition to measuring forced expiratory volume, vital capacity, maximal inspiratory and expiratory flows, pulmonary vascular measurement should be made. Pulmonary artery pressure should be measured with a Swan-Ganz catheter. If the pulmonary artery pressure rises significantly when the pulmonary artery of the affected lung is occluded with a balloon catheter, it reliably predicts an inability to tolerate pneumonectomy. A detailed history, a physical examination, arterial blood gases, tidal volume, and chest x-ray can suggest but not predict the intraoperative effect of pneumonectomy.

**14. The answer is C.** (*Chapter 27 I B 2 a*) Tumor involvement of the left recurrent laryngeal nerve within the thorax is the usual cause of hoarseness in superior sulcus lung carcinoma. Therefore, when hoarseness develops after radiation therapy, it indicates failure of therapy to control the tumor.

**15. The answer is E.** (*Chapter 26 II C*) The benign mixed tumor of the parotid gland often seems to "shell out" at surgery. This means that it easily separates from the surrounding normal tissue of the glands. In fact, a resection of normal tissue around the tumor is necessary to prevent recurrence, since nests of tumor cells will be left behind by a lesser procedure. The facial nerve should be spared, if possible, during surgery for benign parotid neoplasms.

**16. The answer is D.** [*Chapter 1 V A 2 d, B 1 c, C 1 a (1), b (1) (d) (i), (2)*] In a truly elective situation, patients should stop aspirin use at least 1 week prior to surgery. The platelet deficit caused by aspirin lasts for the full life of the platelets—that is, about 7 days. After this time, if aspirin is avoided, the platelets will be normal. Although disorders of platelet function are treated by transfusions of normal platelets preoperatively if the surgery is urgent, the cost and the potential complications from their use are not justified in an elective case.

**17. The answer is D.** (*Chapter 18 VI D 1–6*) Technetium-99m ($^{99m}$Tc) and iodine-131 ($^{131}$I) scans of the thyroid will help to distinguish functioning from nonfunctioning thyroid nodules, but although most thyroid malignancies are nonfunctioning, radionuclide scans do not distinguish benign from malignant nonfunctioning thyroid nodules. Thyroid ultrasonography is helpful in distinguishing solid from cystic lesions, but it does not distinguish malignant from benign solid lesions. In the absence of a family history of thyroid malignancy, it is unlikely that a thyrocalcitonin assay will be positive. Fine-needle aspiration of the thyroid nodule will provide cytopathologic material to help in the diagnosis of the thyroid nodule and in deciding on its management. If the cytopathologic findings are those of a benign colloid nodule or adenomatous hyperplasia, then careful clinical observation would be indicated.

**18. The answer is B.** [*Chapter 4 IV C 2 b (1)*] Most angiograms are sensitive down to a level of 0.5 ml per minute. The technetium-99m ($^{99m}$Tc) radionuclide scan is much more sensitive, detecting to a level of 0.05 ml per minute, but it is much less specific in determining the site of bleeding. If bleeding is proceeding at a rate of 50 ml per minute, immediate surgery is indicated.

**19. The answer is B.** (*Chapter 1 X A 3 g–i, B 3, 4*) Hernias may be described according to physical or operative findings. In a sliding hernia, the wall of the hernia sac, rather than being formed completely by peritoneum, is formed by the wall of another intra-abdominal structure, such as the colon or the bladder. In a Richter's hernia, one side of the bowel wall is trapped in the hernia rather than the entire loop of bowel. In Littre's hernia, a Meckel's diverticulum is incarcerated in the hernia. A direct inguinal hernia is a direct protrusion of abdominal structures into the floor of the canal posterior to the spermatic cord. A pantaloon hernia is a combination of a direct and indirect hernia in which the hernia sac passes around the inferior epigastric vessels both medially and laterally.

**20. The answer is D.** (*Chapter 5 III B 3 d; Chapter 22 II C*) The Zollinger-Ellison syndrome causes a virulent form of duodenal ulcer disease. The syndrome is due to the oversecretion of gastrin by a gastrinoma, a tumor of the non-beta islet cells of the pancreas. Because the cells of origin are part of the amine precursor uptake and decarboxylation (APUD) system, gastrinomas and other types of tumors arising from cells of this system are known as apudomas. In the Zollinger-Ellison syndrome, the excess gastrin production causes an overproduction of gastric acid, which leads to the severe ulcer symptoms.

**21. The answer is D.** (*Chapter 7 XII F 1 c, e*) The colonic lesion should always be resected because surgery is still capable of controlling local disease and preventing local recurrence. Thus, resection should be done because otherwise eventual colonic obstruction is inevitable. The liver lesion should be biopsied to document metastasis.

**22. The answer is D.** (*Chapter 19 VII B, E*) Each of the conditions listed in the question can cause Cushing's syndrome. However, each of the conditions except an adrenal cortical adenoma causes Cushing's syndrome by the production of increased levels of adrenocorticotropic hormone (ACTH). Basophilic adenomas of the pituitary cause bilateral adrenal cortical hyperplasia as a result of increased ACTH production. Adrenal cortical hyperplasia does not occur de novo but results from excessive stimulation of the adrenals by ACTH from an extra-adrenal source, whether it be pituitary or nonpituitary in origin. Both oat cell carcinoma of the lung and malignant islet cell tumors of the pancreas are sources of ectopic ACTH production and result in increased plasma levels of ACTH. Adrenal cortical adenomas autonomously produce increased amounts of cortisol without being dependent on ACTH production, and they actually suppress endogenous ACTH production.

**23. The answer is C.** (*Chapter 13 III B 1–4*) Indications for surgery in aortoiliac occlusive disease are limited to only a few situations, including severe claudication or rest pain, tissue necrosis of the lower extremities or toes, formation of distal arterial emboli, and impotence secondary to bilateral internal iliac occlusion. Aortoiliac vascular reconstruction is an inadequate procedure for complete occlusion of the external iliac artery because it will not restore sufficient blood flow to the affected limb. Also, there is a high risk of thrombosis of the graft limb that feeds the affected side because of inadequate outflow.

**24. The answer is D.** (*Chapter 32 IV B 2*) A mass in the extremity is a common presentation of a bone tumor, and bone tumors warrant thorough, logical workups. A plain film of the involved area will suggest whether the tumor is benign or malignant. Other appropriate studies include computed tomography (CT) of the involved are a to delineate the anatomic relationships of the mass, a bone scan to identify the extent of the tumor within the bone, and CT of the chest to determine possible metastatic disease.

**25. The answer is B.** (*Chapter 7 XII F*) A left hemicolectomy is usually necessary to remove a splenic flexure lesion. A wedge resection has inadequate margins, and there is a risk of local recurrence. Total colectomy, abdominoperineal resection, and anterior resection are not appropriate.

**26. The answer is B.** (*Chapter 4 I H 6*) As long as the patient has no evidence of a strangulating process, which usually causes acidosis, leukocytosis, and hypotension, it is safe to postpone exploration for several hours while fluids and electrolytes are corrected. It is potentially dangerous to begin general anesthesia in the presence of hypokalemia, and it is certainly unwarranted to observe the patient for complications because the most common complications of intestinal obstruction would be perforation of the bowel followed by sepsis. Most surgeons do not initially treat small bowel obstruction with a long intestinal tube.

**27. The answer is D.** (*Chapter 10 III A 5*) Most pancreatic tumors are incurable under present conditions. This incurability is principally determined by the high malignant biologic activity of the tumor and the fact that it has usually spread before the time of diagnosis, even when it appears to be cured at the time of surgery.

**28. The answer is C.** (*Chapter 9 II J 3 b*) Of the choices listed in the question, percutaneous transhepatic cholangiography is the most precise method of visualizing the area of the bile duct at the hepatic duct confluence. The procedure is usually successful when biliary obstruction is present. At the time of the study, a biopsy using a brush or forceps can be performed, establishing the diagnosis. The other invasive procedure that can be helpful is endoscopic retrograde cholangiography.

**29. The answer is B (1, 3).** (*Chapter 8 IV; V*) Radiography, with contrast medium given either by mouth, rectum, or fistula, is important in defining the location and dimensions of the fistula. The use of suction catheters or various bags as collection devices to control the drainage from fistulas is important to prevent skin excoriation and further morbidity. Prompt operative intervention to repair the fistula is usually not indicated, although early surgery to drain an abscess may be necessary. With the availability of means for long-term parenteral nutrition, the intravenous route is usually preferred for fluid and nutritional maintenance in patients with high-output fistulas.

**30. The answer is D (4).** (*Chapter 32 IV C*) Joint arthroplasty, which is indicated for the relief of pain, can be used to repair a joint destroyed by any of the arthritides except, perhaps, postinfectious arthritis. It is used predominantly in patients over the age of 65, in part at least, because the repair is not permanent. The "life expectancy" of an arthroplasty implant is about 10 to 12 years at present. By contrast, the results of arthrodesis are long-lasting. In this procedure, the joint surfaces are fused so that the joint heals in a fixed position. Because the results are more durable, arthrodesis rather than arthroplasty is the preferred procedure for young, active patients.

**31. The answer is E (all).** (*Chapter 1 VII A 4*) Any person with a penetrating injury must receive tetanus prophylaxis if previous immunization was not recent or cannot be documented. A previously immunized person should be given a booster dose if none has been given within the past 5 years. A patient with a clean injury who has never been immunized may be give tetanus toxoid in three separate doses. A patient with a dirty wound who has never been immunized should be given passive immunization with homologous tetanus immune globulin. Adequate debridement of devitalized tissue and removal of all foreign matter is also essential. The efficacy of antibiotics for prophylaxis of tetanus-prone wounds is unproven.

**32. The answer is E (all).** (*Chapter 16 VI A 2*) There are four types of renal transplant rejection, classified according to the time of rejection in relation to the operation and the type of immune response involved. Hyperacute rejection results from preformed antibody and complement deposition on vascular endothelium followed by activation of the coagulation system; it occurs in the operating room. Accelerated acute rejection occurs within 1 week following transplantation and probably is a second-set, or anamnestic, response involving both cellular and humoral elements. Acute rejection usually occurs within 3 months following the operation and is characterized by T-lymphocyte–mediated infiltration of vascular and interstitial renal elements. Chronic rejection occurs over a period of months to years and involves both cellular and humoral destructive events. Chronic rejection is associated with vascular intimal thickening and tubular atrophy.

**33. The answer is A (1, 2, 3).** [*Chapter 9 I B 2 a (2)*] Chronic alcohol abuse, hepatitis B surface antigen, and aflatoxins are clearly associated with the development of hepatocellular carcinoma. Oral contraceptives, by contrast, have shown an association with focal nodular hyperplasia and hepatocellular adenoma but not carcinoma.

**34. The answer is A (1, 2, 3).** (*Chapter 1 VII C 1–4*) The patient described in the question has the classic signs and symptoms of cellulitis (i.e., red tender streaks, fever, and leukocytosis), an inflammation of the dermal and subcutaneous tissues as a result of a puncture wound or any other type of skin infection. Proper management of this infection includes removal of the foreign body (catheter), excision and drainage of the infected vein site, and administration of appropriate antibiotics.

**35. The answer is B (1, 3).** (*Chapter 10 II D*) Relapsing pancreatitis is generally associated with biliary tract disease and not with alcohol abuse. It is best diagnosed from the history, and the diagnosis may be confirmed by the Nardi test (narcotic-induced spasm of the sphincter of Oddi with subsequent amylase elevation and abdominal pain). If the test is positive, a sphincteroplasty may improve or resolve the symptoms. Pancreatic ascites is most commonly associated with a leaking pancreatic pseudocyst with resultant spillage of pancreatic duct contents into the peritoneal cavity.

**36. The answer is A (1, 2, 3).** (*Chapter 17 I G 1 b*) Injury to the heart may result in bleeding into the pericardial sac, which may result in tamponade. This is a true emergency that must be diagnosed and treated promptly. The classic findings are distended neck veins, hypotension, and pulsus paradoxus. The heart sounds are characteristically decreased. If tamponade is suspected, the pericardial sac should be aspirated, which will usually result in a rapid improvement in the patient's blood pressure. Definitive treatment of the underlying cause of tamponade can then be undertaken.

**37. The answer is A (1, 2, 3).** (*Chapter 23 III A 3*) Family history and antecedent contralateral breast cancer are the most significant risk factors for developing breast cancer. As far as is known presently, however, only maternal family history is significant; paternal family history of female breast cancer does not carry an increased risk of developing the disease. A patient with chronic cystic mastitis has only a slightly increased risk.

**38. The answer is A (1, 2, 3).** (*Chapter 1 X A 2*) Hernias can occur as a result of a variety of factors. Congenital defects in the abdominal wall are common. Loss of tissue strength and elasticity, especially due to aging, can also result in herniation. Trauma, especially operative trauma in which normal tissue strength is destroyed surgically can lead to the development of a hernia. Any condition that increases intra-abdominal pressure can result in a hernia, such as coughing, chronic obstructive lung disease, asthma, vesical outlet obstruction (e.g., benign prostatic hypertrophy), constipation, pregnancy, ascites, and obesity.

**39. The answer is E (all).** (*Chapter 5 X C*) Dumping syndrome is a complication of gastrectomy. It is characterized by epigastric fullness or pain, nausea, tachyarrhythmia, and diarrhea. These occur because premature gastric emptying ("dumping") releases hypertonic chyme into the small bowel, with consequent jejunal distention from the rapid accumulation of fluid. Dumping syndrome affects most postgastrectomy patients to a mild degree and can usually be managed by dietary control.

**40. The answer is C (2, 4).** (*Chapter 24 III D 4, G; IV C, F*) The lesion in question may be an encephalocele, nasal dermoid, vestibular papilloma, or nasal polyps. In children the presence of an encephalocele must be ruled out prior to the biopsy of such a lesion. Finding bilateral polyps in a child this young raises the question of cystic fibrosis.

**41. The answer is A (1, 2, 3).** (*Chapter 11 IV A–C; V C*) Primary splenic tumors, splenic abscess, and hereditary spherocytosis are absolute indications for splenectomy. Idiopathic autoimmune hemolytic anemia occurs most often in women over 50 years of age. Antibodies against red blood cells are found, and the direct Coombs' test is positive. The disease may be self-limiting and mild. If it persists, it should be treated with steroids; splenectomy is considered if steroids are ineffective or contraindicated.

**42. The answer is D (4).** (*Chapter 6 IV A; VII D 6*) Vitamin $B_{12}$ is the only nutrient absorbed exclusively in the terminal ileum; therefore, parenteral replacement is necessary after resection of this area. Although bile salts are also absorbed primarily in the terminal ileum, they usually do not require replacement either enterally or parenterally.

**43. The answer is D (4).** (*Chapter 27 VI B 6*) Calcification within a so-called coin lesion, especially if it is in a concentric or popcorn-like pattern, favors a benign diagnosis. No growth shown on chest x-rays taken over 1 or 2 years also suggests a benign lesion. A diameter greater than 1 or 2 cm suggests a malignant lesion. All coin lesions are peripheral, and so this location would not help to distinguish a benign from a malignant lesion. Cavitation occurs with both carcinoma and infection.

**44. The answer is D (4).** (*Chapter 11 V I*) Hodgkin's disease is now treatable, and patients have a good chance of cure or long-term survival. Proper staging is essential. A classification of stage II Hodgkin's disease indicates two or more involved nodal areas on the same side of the diaphragm. The spleen should be removed during laparotomy; if it is not, it may need to be radiated, a procedure that may damage the left kidney and left lung, which are both in the field of radiation. Histologic examination may reveal involvement of the spleen and change the staging of the disease.

**45. The answer is A (1, 2, 3).** (*Chapter 7 XVII E 2 d*) The infection must be treated by drainage and use of systemic antibiotics. In the presence of infection, a primary anastomosis of the colon is very prone to break down and leak, and it therefore should be avoided. Although mechanical preparation of the bowel is useful in elective surgery for diverticulitis, the presence of a perforated colon with an abscess usually does not allow the time required for an adequate bowel preparation.

**46. The answer is B (1, 3).** (*Chapter 12 III*) Lymphangitis is an acute inflammation of the lymphatic channels. Staphylococci and $\beta$-hemolytic streptococci are the usual causative pathogens. Septicemia can occur if the lymph nodes do not arrest the infection. Any source of infection must be adequately drained. The extremity should be at rest, and exercise is contraindicated since it will propel the bacteria through the lymph channels, which is likely to exacerbate the situation.

**47. The answer is E (all).** (*Chapter 13 IX C 1–6*) Surgical complications unfortunately are not infrequent following aortic surgery. Postoperative renal failure occurs in 21% of cases of ruptured aneurysms and in 2.5% of aneurysms treated surgically, with mortality rates of up to 90%. Acute leg ischemia accompanied by muscular compartment syndrome occurs postoperatively in 7% of cases but can be treated successfully by fasciotomy if it is recognized early. Spinal cord ischemia, a rare complication, is most common in cases of ruptured aneurysm (0.25% of cases). It results from injury to the artery of Adamkiewicz and can lead to paraplegia. Impotence in men can result if pudendal nerve branches that mediate erection and ejaculation are divided accidentally during surgery.

**48–52. The answers are: 48-D, 49-E, 50-A, 51-B, 52-C.** [*Chapter 30 II G 2 a (4), b (1), c (2) (c), d, e*] Sarcomas of the soft tissue constitute only 1% of malignant tumors. They can occur anywhere in the body and often present as an enlarging, but painless, mass. The diagnosis usually is made from an excisional biopsy, if the tumor is small, and from a wedge biopsy, if the tumor is large. Soft tissue sarcomas frequently have a pseudocapsule, which can lead the unwary surgeon to assume falsely that the tumor can be removed easily. In reality, these tumors must be removed by wide excision well away from what appear to be the margins of the tumor. Local recurrence is common, and when metastasis occurs, it usually is by the hematogenous route.

Liposarcoma is the most common of the soft tissue sarcomas. Only 1% arise from preexisting benign lipomas. Liposarcomas are treated by wide excision and, when well differentiated, are associated with a 70% 5-year survival rate.

Fibrosarcoma, the second most common soft tissue sarcoma, usually is found as a hard, round mass in an extremity. These tumors are more common among men than among women and, when adequately treated (wide excision), are associated with a 77% 5-year survival rate.

Rhabdomyosarcoma arises from skeletal muscle and occurs in two forms—juvenile and adult. Pleomorphic rhabdomyosarcoma, the type occurring in adults, is associated with a 30% 5-year survival rate. Patients with embryonal rhabdomyosarcoma—the juvenile form—have recently enjoyed an increase in 5-year survival to a rate of 70% due to treatment that combines surgery, radiotherapy, and multidrug chemotherapy.

Kaposi's sarcoma is a malignant lesion of vascular origin, which, until recently, was seen in the lower extremities of older men. Currently, this lesion often is seen in connection with acquired immune deficiency syndrome (AIDS).

Lymphangiosarcoma develops in areas of chronic lymphedema. There is no effective treatment for this peculiar tumor, and the patient prognosis is dismal.

**53–55. The answers are: 53-D, 54-C, 55-B.** (*Chapter 17 II C 1, 3 c, D 1, 4, E 1, 5 b*) Ventricular septal defect is the most common type of congenital heart defect. Small ventricular septal defects rarely cause significant symptoms in infancy or early childhood and may close spontaneously before they are recognized. Cardiac catheterization is essential for locating the defect precisely. Surgical closure should be carried out in an infant with significant cardiac failure or increased pulmonary vascular resistance. Children who are asymptomatic should have the defect corrected surgically if it has not closed by the age of 2 years. The operative mortality risk is generally less than 5% and is related to the degree of preoperative pulmonary vascular disease.

Atrial septal defects occur twice as often in females as in males. The ostium secundum defect, which is found in the midportion of the atrial septum, accounts for the majority of atrial septal defects. The diagnosis is made by cardiac catheterization, which measures the step-up in oxygen saturation in the right atrium. From this oxygen difference, the left-to-right shunt can be calculated. Surgical closure of the defect is indicated if the pulmonary blood flow is one and one-half to two times greater than the systemic blood flow.

Coarctation of the aorta is found twice as often in males as in females. It may be fatal in the first few months of life if it is left untreated. Cardiac catheterization is required to define the location of the coarctation and any associated cardiac defects. Surgical correction is indicated for all patients, but is delayed until age 5 or 6 years if the patient is asymptomatic.

**56–60. The answers are: 56-C, 57-A, 58-B, 59-E, 60-D.** (*Chapter 29 VII B 3 d, C 4 d, D 3 c, E 3 c, F 5 d*) Some testicular tumors have been shown to produce human chorionic gonadotropin and α-fetoprotein. These markers have accurately indicated the presence of microscopic metastases and recurrences. In prostatic carcinoma, serum prostatic acid phosphatase is an early and reliable tumor marker. It has accurately indicated extracapsular extensions, metastases, and recurrences. Renal cell carcinoma can be diagnosed and partially staged by renal arteriography. The tumor is usually indicated by neovascularity with contrast pooling and a vascular blush.

Transitional cell carcinoma of the renal pelvis can be demonstrated by retrograde pyelography. A filling defect seen on excretory urography can be outlined more clearly by the retrograde technique, which can differentiate an obstructing calculus or a neoplasm filling the pelvis of a nonfunctioning kidney. In carcinoma of the bladder, cystoscopy is essential. Bladder endoscopy should be performed in the evaluation of all patients with gross painless hematuria and in the follow-up after treatment of a urothelial neoplasm of the bladder, ureter, or renal pelvis. The mucosal surface of the bladder can be inspected directly and much greater accuracy in diagnosis can be obtained than with radiologic studies.

# Index